# ANESTHESIA and ANALGESIA

## for Veterinary Technicians

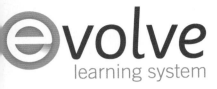
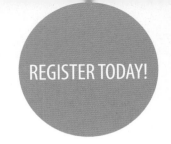

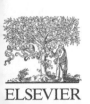

# ANESTHESIA and ANALGESIA

## for Veterinary Technicians

### Fourth Edition

**John A. Thomas, DVM**
Assistant Professor, Veterinary Technology
Cuyahoga Community College
Cleveland, Ohio

**Phillip Lerche, BVSc, PhD, Dipl ACVA**
Assistant Professor
Department of Veterinary Clinical Sciences
The Ohio State University
Columbus, Ohio

*With 300 illustrations*

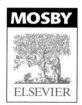

MOSBY

ELSEVIER

3251 Riverport Lane
St. Louis, Missouri 63043

---

**Notice**

Knowledge and best practice in this field are constantly changing. As new research and experience broaden
our understanding, changes in research methods, professional practices, or medical treatment may become
necessary.
Practitioners and researchers must always rely on their own experience and knowledge in evaluating and
using any information, methods, compounds, or experiments described herein. In using such information
or methods they should be mindful of their own safety and the safety of others, including parties for whom
they have a professional responsibility.
With respect to any drug or pharmaceutical products identified, readers are advised to check the most
current information provided (i) on procedures featured or (ii) by the manufacturer of each product to be
administered, to verify the recommended dose or formula, the method and duration of administration,
and contraindications. It is the responsibility of practitioners, relying on their own experience and knowledge
of their patients, to make diagnoses, to determine dosages and the best treatment for each individual patient,
and to take all appropriate safety precautions.
To the fullest extent of the law, neither the Publisher nor the authors, contributors, or editors, assume any
liability for any injury and/or damage to persons or property as a matter of products liability, negligence
or otherwise, or from any use or operation of any methods, products, instructions, or ideas contained in the
material herein.

---

**Library of Congress Cataloging-in-Publication Data**

Thomas, John A. (John Alfred), 1956-
  Anesthesia and analgesia for veterinary technicians / John A. Thomas, Phillip Lerche. — 4th ed.
     p. ; cm.
  Rev. ed. of: Veterinary anesthesia and analgesia / Diane McKelvey, K. Wayne Hollingshead. 3rd ed. ©2003.
  Includes bibliographical references and index.
  ISBN 978-0-323-05504-8 (pbk. : alk. paper)  1. Dogs—Surgery. 2. Cats—Surgery. 3. Veterinary anesthesia.
4. Analgesia. I. Lerche, Phillip. II. McKelvey, Diane. Veterinary anesthesia and analgesia. III. Title.
  [DNLM: 1. Surgery, Veterinary. 2. Analgesia—veterinary. 3. Anesthesia—veterinary.  SF 914 T458a 2010]
  SF911.M39 2010
  636.089'796—dc22                                                              2010007601

*Vice President and Publisher:* Linda Duncan
*Publisher:* Penny Rudolph
*Acquisitions Editor:* Teri Merchant
*Publishing Services Manager:* Patricia Tannian
*Senior Project Manager:* Sarah Wunderly
*Design Direction:* Amy Buxton

Printed in the United States of America

Last digit is the print number:  9  8  7  6  5  4

# Dedication

To my family, Lisa, Tim, and Liz, for their support and understanding during the many days, evenings, and weekends spent working on this book.
To Dr. Joanna Bassert and Teri Merchant, to whom I will always be grateful for believing in me and opening the doors that led to my authorship of this volume.

**J.T.**

To my family and friends for their constant support.
To John, who invited me along for the ride. Without his vision, patience, and attention to detail, this book would not have been possible.

**P.L.**

# Contributors

**Paul Flecknell, MA, VetMB, PhD, DLAS, DECVA, DECLAM, (Hon) DACLAM, (Hon) FRCVS**
Professor of Laboratory Animal Science
Comparative Biology Centre
Newcastle University
Newcastle, Tyne and Wear, UK

**K. Wayne Hollingshead, MSc, DVM**
Cats at Home Veterinary Clinic
Surrey, British Columbia, Canada

**Diane McKelvey, BSc, DVM, Dipl ABVP (Feline)**
Kamloops Veterinary Clinic
Kamloops, British Columbia

For many years, the text *Veterinary Anesthesia and Analgesia* by Diane McKelvey and K. Wayne Hollingshead has been highly respected and heavily used by veterinary technician educators. Under new authorship, the fourth edition, entitled *Anesthesia and Analgesia for Veterinary Technicians,* has not only a new name that reflects its intended audience, but also many changes designed to enhance accessibility, content, and practical application for instructors, students, and practicing anesthetists. While attention has been given to preservation of the many valuable features of previous editions, this volume represents a significant departure in several ways.

## New to This Edition

Readers familiar with previous editions will note that this text is organized somewhat differently. Following a brief introduction (Chapter 1) covering history, terms and definitions, and the veterinary technician's role as veterinary anesthetist, Chapters 2 through 6 cover the fundamentals of veterinary anesthesia.

- Chapter 2—Patient Preparation
- Chapter 3—Anesthetic Agents and Adjuncts
- Chapter 4—Anesthetic Equipment
- Chapter 5—Anesthetic Monitoring
- Chapter 6—Special Techniques
  Local anesthesia, assisted and controlled ventilation, and neuromuscular blocking agents are included in this chapter
- Chapter 7—Analgesia

The next four chapters cover application of these fundamentals to specific species or species groups.

- Chapter 8—Canine and Feline Anesthesia
- Chapter 9—Equine Anesthesia
- Chapter 10—Ruminant and Swine Anesthesia
- Chapter 11—Rodent and Rabbit Anesthesia

The final chapters cover practical application of the following topics in all practice settings.

- Chapter 12—Anesthetic Problems and Emergencies
- Chapter 13—Workplace Safety

The content of the fourth edition has been substantially updated to reflect the many changes that have occurred in the practice of anesthesia since publication of the previous edition, including new drugs, equipment, and techniques. Rather than being a small animal anesthesia text with large animals addressed separately, this edition is a true multispecies text in which each of the common domestic species (dogs, cats, horses, swine, and cattle) is given balanced treatment throughout. Readers will find the following features in this edition that were present in the previous edition:

- Learning objectives at the beginning of each chapter
- Key points at the end of each chapter
- Suggested readings
- Review questions and answers

Readers will also find many new enhancements designed to provide rapid access to information required for effective learning and successful practice of anesthesia:

- Key terms and a chapter outline at the beginning of each chapter
- 240 new full-color photos and 60 full-color line illustrations
- Technician notes that emphasize important points and practical tips gleaned from the narrative
- More than 60 reference tables and boxes designed to facilitate rapid access to key information such as fluid administration rates, properties of anesthetic drugs, oxygen flow rates, anesthetic protocols, and normal and abnormal monitoring parameters. Also added to this edition are 20 anesthetic protocols and 5 case studies
- 49 step-by-step descriptions of common procedures used during each phase of an anesthetic event, including patient preparation, IV catheter placement, anesthetic induction techniques, endotracheal intubation, anesthetic maintenance techniques, and anesthetic recovery
- A complete glossary with definitions of all key terms
- All new appendices with supplemental and reference information

## Evolve Resources

In addition to these features, readers will also have access to the following online resources through Evolve, Elsevier's online portal for instructors and students.

### Instructor Resources
- Image collection from the text that can be included in classroom presentations
- PowerPoint lecture outlines

### Student Resources
- Anesthesia machine tutorial that demonstrates care and maintenance of anesthesia machines
- Drug dosage calculators
- Image collection from the text, which can be used for review and study

With these updates, changes, and enhancements, this established and respected text provides veterinary technician educators, students, and anesthetists with the tools necessary to maximize learning in the classroom and beyond. It is our earnest hope that readers will find this book to be an accessible, useful, and highly valued resource and will realize as much personal and professional growth from reading it as we have realized in writing it.

## Acknowledgments

The authors would like to thank the following individuals for their contributions to the production of this volume.

Steven Ahern, AA, AAB, and William Fogarty, M Ed, for their help in producing many of the illustrations in Chapters 2, 3, 4, 5, and 8.

The Cuyahoga Community College Veterinary Technology Program students, (class of 2009), and Linda DeHoff, RVT, for their help with new photographs in chapters 2, 3, 4, 5, and 8. Special thanks to veterinary technology student Stephanie Maskovyak, and to Audrey Kukwa, RVT, who graciously volunteered to assist with the acquisition of numerous photographs.

Heather Cruea, RVT, Christina Duffey, RVT, Amanda English, RVT, Theresa Hand, RVT, Suzanne Huck, RVT, Gladys Karpa, RVT, Carl O'Brien, RVT, Zachary Schell, RVT, Kim Morrison, RVT, Liz Santschi, DVM, Michael Rings, DVM, MS, Turi Aarnes, DVM, MS, Lisa Sams, DVM, Rebecca Krimins, DVM, and students of the class of 2010 of The Ohio State University College of Veterinary Medicine, for their help with photographs in several chapters.

Diane McKelvey and K. Wayne Hollingshead, authors of the first three editions, for setting a high standard for veterinary technician educators, and for laying the foundation on which this edition rests.

Contributing authors, Paul Flecknell, K. Wayne Hollingshead, and Diane McKelvey for sharing their knowledge, expertise, and experience.

To Teri Merchant, acquisitions editor at Elsevier, for her guidance and support during the many months spent planning, writing, and producing this text.

John A. Thomas
Phillip Lerche

# Contents

1. Introduction to Anesthesia *1*

2. Patient Preparation *5*

3. Anesthetic Agents and Adjuncts *50*

4. Anesthetic Equipment *96*

5. Anesthetic Monitoring *138*

6. Special Techniques *183*

7. Analgesia *206*

8. Canine and Feline Anesthesia *233*

9. Equine Anesthesia *265*

10. Ruminant and Swine Anesthesia *283*

11. Rodent and Rabbit Anesthesia *298*
    *Paul Flecknell*

12. Anesthetic Problems and Emergencies *319*
    *K. Wayne Hollingshead*

13. Workplace Safety *351*
    *Diane McKelvey*

Answer Key *365*

Glossary *381*

Index *389*

## Appendixes

A American College of Veterinary Anesthesiologists Monitoring Guidelines Update, 2009 *367*

B Nitrous Oxide *370*

C Use of Nonprecision Vaporizers *373*

D Procedure for Operation of a Closed Rebreathing System *375*

E Standard Volumes, Weights, Measures, and Equivalents *376*

F Equipment and Drugs for Use in an Emergency Crash Kit *379*

# ANESTHESIA and ANALGESIA

for Veterinary Technicians

# Introduction to Anesthesia

1

## KEY TERMS

Analgesia
Anesthesia
Balanced anesthesia
Epidural anesthesia
General anesthesia
Hypnosis
Local anesthesia
Narcosis
Noxious
Regional anesthesia
Sedation
Surgical anesthesia
Therapeutic index
Topical anesthesia
Tranquilization

## OUTLINE

History and Terminology of Anesthesia, 1
The Veterinary Technician's Role in the
   Practice of Anesthesia, 3

## LEARNING OBJECTIVES

*When you have completed this chapter, you will be able to:*
- Define anesthesia, and differentiate topical, local, regional, general, and surgical anesthesia.
- Differentiate sedation, tranquilization, hypnosis, and narcosis.
- Explain the concept of balanced anesthesia and the advantages of this approach.
- List common indications for anesthesia.
- Describe fundamental challenges and risks associated with anesthesia.
- List the qualities and abilities of a successful veterinary anesthetist.

## HISTORY AND TERMINOLOGY OF ANESTHESIA

On October 16, 1846, at Massachusetts General Hospital, Boston dentist William T. G. Morton gave the first successful demonstration of the pain-relieving properties of diethyl ether in the presence of a group of physicians and medical students. On receiving the ether, the patient, who was undergoing a tumor removal, entered a state of insensibility during which the surgical pain was alleviated. During the next several months, additional experiments conducted by Morton and others confirmed the value of ether as an effective pain-relieving agent in surgery patients.

Although ether had been used experimentally as early as 1842, Dr. Morton's demonstration is particularly significant because it attracted the attention of the prominent physician Oliver Wendell Holmes Sr., who, in a letter to Dr. Morton dated November 21, 1846, suggested that the state of insensibility to pain produced by this agent be called *anesthesia.* The name was adopted by the medical community, and over the next few years the practice of anesthesia spread widely throughout North America and Europe. The veterinary community, however, did not embrace the use of anesthetics as rapidly. Although reports began to appear in the veterinary literature regarding the use of inhalation anesthetics such as ether and chloroform within the following decade, inhalation anesthesia was not an accepted practice until early in the twentieth century. Only after the development of injectable barbiturates in the 1930s did the use of anesthetics in veterinary patients become commonplace.

The term **anesthesia** (derived from the Greek word *anaisthesia* which means "without feeling" or "insensibility") may be defined as "a loss of sensation." By providing a loss of sensation, or more specifically the loss of sensitivity to pain, the development and use of anesthetics during the mid-nineteenth century solved one of the primary problems associated with surgery. Since then, the practice of anesthesia has gradually evolved from an experimental technique to a highly sophisticated science. Now, over 160 years after its introduction, anesthesia is used daily in most veterinary practices to provide sedation, tranquilization, immobility, muscle relaxation, unconsciousness, and pain control for a diverse range of indications including surgery, dentistry, grooming, diagnostic imaging, wound care, and capture and transport of wild animals, just to name a few. So although the literal definition of the term *anesthesia* accurately describes one of its fundamental effects, when viewed from the perspective of current practice the word falls far short of capturing the many facets of this complex discipline.

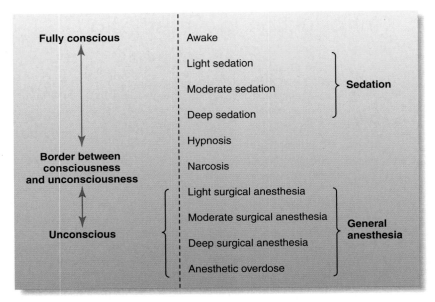

Notes:
- In addition to CNS depression, most anesthetics cause a variety of other effects such as analgesia and muscle relaxation.
- Although most anesthetics cause CNS depression as noted above, some agents such as dissociatives may also stimulate the CNS (see Chapter 3 for a discussion of these agents).
- Transient excitement may also occur during some stages of anesthesia (see Chapter 5 for a discussion of the stages and planes of general anesthesia).

**FIGURE 1-1**    The continuum of levels of central nervous system depression induced by anesthetic agents.

---

TECHNICIAN NOTE    Anesthesia is used daily in most veterinary practices to provide sedation, tranquilization, immobility, muscle relaxation, unconsciousness, and pain control for a diverse range of indications.

Most people associate the word *anesthesia* with general anesthesia, which is only one extreme in a continuum of levels of central nervous system (CNS) depression that can be induced by administration of anesthetic agents (Figure 1-1). **General anesthesia** may be defined as a reversible state of unconsciousness, immobility, muscle relaxation, and loss of sensation throughout the entire body produced by administration of one or more anesthetic agents. While under general anesthesia, a patient cannot be aroused even with painful stimulation. For this reason, general anesthesia is commonly used to prepare patients for surgery or other acutely painful procedures. **Surgical anesthesia** is a specific stage of general anesthesia in which there is a sufficient degree of **analgesia** (a loss of sensitivity to pain) and muscle relaxation to allow surgery to be performed without patient pain or movement.

Other states within the continuum of CNS depression include *sedation* and *tranquilization*. **Sedation** refers to drug-induced CNS depression and drowsiness that vary in intensity from light to deep. A sedated patient generally is minimally aware or unaware of its surroundings but can be aroused by **noxious** stimulation. Sedation is often used to prepare patients for diagnostic imaging,

grooming, wound treatment, and other minor procedures. **Tranquilization** is a drug-induced state of calm in which the patient is reluctant to move and is aware of but unconcerned about its surroundings. Although the terms *tranquilization* and *sedation* are not exactly the same in meaning, they are often used interchangeably.

The terms *hypnosis* and *narcosis* are also used to describe anesthetic-induced states. **Hypnosis** is a drug-induced sleeplike state that impairs the ability of the patient to respond appropriately to stimuli. This meaning of this term is somewhat imprecise, as it is used to describe various degrees of CNS depression. In this text, hypnosis will be used to mean a sleeplike state from which the patient can be aroused with sufficient stimulation. The term **narcosis** refers to a drug-induced sleep from which the patient is not easily aroused and that is most often associated with the administration of narcotics.

The effect of anesthetic agents may be selectively directed to affect specific areas or regions of the body. Smaller areas can be targeted by use of local or topical anesthesia. **Local anesthesia** refers to loss of sensation in a small area of the body produced by administration of a local anesthetic agent in proximity to the area of interest. Infiltration of local anesthetic into the tissues surrounding a small tumor to facilitate removal is an example of local anesthesia. **Topical anesthesia** is the loss of sensation of a localized area produced by administration of a local anesthetic directly to a body surface or to a surgical or traumatic wound. Use of ophthalmic local anesthetic drops in the eye before an ophthalmic examination or application of local anesthetic to an open declaw incision for the purpose of pain control are examples of topical anesthesia.

Larger areas can be targeted by use of **regional anesthesia,** which refers to a loss of sensation in a limited area of the body produced by administration of a local anesthetic or other agent in proximity to sensory nerves. Regional anesthesia can be produced with a variety of techniques including nerve blocks and epidural anesthesia. For example, a brachial plexus block can be used to anesthetize the forelimb distal to and including the elbow; a maxillary nerve block can be used to anesthetize the upper dental arcade; and **epidural anesthesia** can be used to provide pain control of the rear quarters and pelvic region.

When anesthetics are administered, it is common practice to administer multiple drugs concurrently in smaller quantities than would be required if each were given alone. This technique, termed **balanced anesthesia,** maximizes the benefits of each drug, minimizes adverse effects, and gives the anesthetist the ability to produce anesthesia with the degree of CNS depression, muscle relaxation, analgesia, and immobilization appropriate for the patient and the procedure. Premedication with acepromazine, anesthetic induction with a combination of ketamine and diazepam, maintenance with isoflurane, and administration of a morphine and lidocaine infusion for analgesia is one example of balanced anesthesia.

> *TECHNICIAN NOTE* Balanced anesthesia maximizes benefits, minimizes adverse effects, and gives the anesthetist the ability to produce anesthesia with the degree of CNS depression, muscle relaxation, analgesia, and immobilization appropriate for the patient and the procedure.

## THE VETERINARY TECHNICIAN'S ROLE IN THE PRACTICE OF ANESTHESIA

Preparation, operation and maintenance of anesthetic equipment, administration of anesthetic agents, endotracheal intubation, and patient monitoring are considered part of the credentialed veterinary technician's scope of practice and are a required part of any accredited veterinary technology program's curriculum. Competency in each of these areas of responsibility requires an advanced knowledge and skill level that can be achieved only with a substantial commitment of time and effort on the part of the student. Before embarking on a study of anesthesia, the student must be aware of the following fundamental challenges and inherent risks she will face when acting as anesthetist.

- Most anesthetic agents have a very narrow **therapeutic index,** so the consequences of a calculation or administration error may be serious. Therefore care and attention to detail are critical when dosages are calculated and rates of administration are adjusted.

- Most anesthetic agents cause significant changes in cardiovascular and pulmonary function (e.g., decreased cardiac output, respiratory rate, tidal volume, and blood pressure), which can be dangerous or lethal if not carefully assessed and managed. These changes often occur quickly and without much warning. Vital signs and indicators of anesthetic depth must therefore be closely monitored.

- The anesthetist must accurately interpret a wide spectrum of visual, tactile, and auditory information from the patient, anesthetic equipment, and monitoring devices. To do this successfully, she must be able to rapidly assess multiple pieces of information and distinguish those that require action from those that do not.

- The anesthetist must have a comprehensive understanding of the significance of physical parameters and machine-generated data. The anesthetist must also be able to use her knowledge to make rapid and decisive judgments regarding patient management and to carry out corrective actions quickly and effectively.

- The potential for patient harm during administration of anesthetics is relatively high when compared with many other procedures. When serious anesthetic accidents occur, they are often devastating not only for the patient but also for the client and the anesthetist. In addition, after an accident, clients may choose to pursue legal action or file a complaint with the state veterinary medical board if they feel negligence was involved. These factors underscore the importance of maintaining a high standard to maximize the likelihood of a favorable outcome. This standard includes not only sound practices but also maintenance of detailed and accurate medical records, which are the cornerstone of a solid legal defense should a complaint arise. (See Chapter 5 for more information about anesthetic records.)

In view of each of these risks and challenges, the anesthetist must approach any anesthetic procedure with a genuine willingness to take personal responsibility for the well-being of the patient. Acceptance of this responsibility by the anesthetist is dependent on development of competence and confidence. Ultimately, competence and confidence are acquired only with much study, practice, persistence, an attitude of caring, and a dedication to excellence. Only then can the accomplished anesthetist use her skills and knowledge to protect and improve the life of each and every patient under her care in a way that is infinitely gratifying and singular to this complex and challenging discipline.

> *TECHNICIAN NOTE* The anesthetist must approach each and every anesthetic procedure with a genuine willingness to take personal responsibility for the well-being of the patient.

## KEY POINTS

1. General anesthesia is a reversible state of unconsciousness, immobility, muscle relaxation, and generalized loss of sensation, produced by administration of anesthetic agents. It is only one extreme in a continuum of levels of CNS depression produced by anesthetic agents, which also include sedation, hypnosis, and narcosis.

2. Many techniques including sedation, tranquilization, and topical, local, regional, and general anesthesia are used to produce specific effects appropriate to each patient.

3. Balanced anesthesia (the administration of multiple drugs in the same patient during one anesthetic event) is commonplace in the practice of anesthesia and produces many benefits not possible with administration of a single anesthetic.

4. Anesthesia involves a number of unique risks and dangers, of which the anesthetist must be conscious and aware.

5. The successful practice of anesthesia requires a high level of knowledge, competency, commitment, and acceptance of responsibility on the part of the anesthetist.

## REVIEW QUESTIONS

1. A drug-induced state of calm in which the patient is reluctant to move and is aware of but unconcerned about its surroundings.
   a. Sedation
   b. Hypnosis
   c. Narcosis
   d. Tranquilization

2. The term *regional anesthesia* refers to:
   a. Loss of sensation in a limited area of the body produced by administration of a local anesthetic or other agent in proximity to sensory nerves
   b. Loss of sensation in a small area of the body produced by administration of a local anesthetic agent in proximity to the area of interest
   c. Loss of sensation of a localized area produced by administration of a local anesthetic directly to a body surface or to a surgical or traumatic wound
   d. A drug-induced sleeplike state that impairs the ability of the patient to respond appropriately to stimuli

3. A sleeplike state from which the patient can be aroused with sufficient stimulation.
   a. Narcosis
   b. Sedation
   c. Hypnosis
   d. Tranquilization

4. The term *balanced anesthesia* refers to:
   a. The administration of two or more agents in equal volume
   b. Administration of multiple drugs concurrently in smaller quantities than would be required if each were given alone
   c. General anesthesia in which the patient's physiologic status remains stable
   d. The administration of a local and general anesthetic concurrently

For the following questions, more than one answer may be correct.
5. With sufficient stimulation, a patient can be aroused from:
   a. Sedation
   b. Narcosis
   c. General anesthesia
   d. Hypnosis

6. Which of the following statements about anesthesia is/are false?
   a. Anesthetic agents have wide therapeutic indices.
   b. There is always a risk to patient safety when anesthetics are administered.
   c. Most anesthetics cause significant changes in cardiopulmonary function.
   d. Administration of anesthetics is routine and thus requires no specialized skills.

## SELECTED READINGS

Muir WW, Hubbell JA, Bednarski RM: *Handbook of veterinary anesthesia*, ed 4, St Louis, 2006, Elsevier, pp 1-10.

Smithcors JF: The Early Use of Anesthesia in Veterinary Practice, *The British Veterinary Journal* 113:284-291, 1957.

Smithcors JF: *The veterinarian in America 1625-1975*. Santa Barbara, 1975, American Veterinary Publications.

Stevenson DE: The evolution of veterinary anesthesia, *The British Veterinary Journal* 119:477-483, 1963.

Thurmon JC, Short CE: History and overview of veterinary anesthesia. In Tranquilli WJ, Thurmon JC, Grimm KA, editors: *Lumb & Jones' veterinary anesthesia and analgesia*, ed 4, Ames, Iowa, 2007, Blackwell, pp 3-6.

Auscultation
Body condition score
Borborygmus
Cachexia
Cardiac output
Colloids
Comatose
Consent form
Constant rate infusion
Crystalloids
Cyanosis
Dead space
Debilitated
Drip rate
Dyspneic
Ecchymoses
Extra-label drug use
Gastric dilatation-
   volvulus
Homeostasis
Hypercarbia
Hypotension
Hypothermia
Hypoxemia
Hypoxia
Ileus
Infusion rate
Inotropy
Intact
Lethargic
Level of consciousness
Macrodrip
Microdrip
Minimum patient
   database
Miosis
Moribund
Obtunded
Oncotic pressure
Osmolarity
Osmotic pressure
Petechiae
Physical status
   classification
Purpura
Regurgitation
Reproductive status
Solutes
Signalment
Sloughing
Stridor
Stuporous
Syncope
Thrombocytopenia
Vasodilation
Vesicants
Veterinarian-in-charge
   (VIC)

# Patient Preparation

2

## OUTLINE

Communication—A Key to Success, 6
The Minimum Patient Database, 7
   *Patient History, 8*
   *Physical Examination and Physical*
      *Assessment, 13*
   *Preanesthetic Diagnostic Workup, 22*
Determination of the Physical Status
   Classification, 24
Selection of the Anesthetic Protocol, 24
   *Factors That Influence Selection, 25*
Preinduction Patient Care, 26
   *Withholding Food before*
      *Anesthesia, 26*
   *Patient Stabilization, 27*

Intravenous Catheterization, 27
   *Reasons for Intravenous Catheterization, 27*
   *Choosing and Placing an Intravenous*
      *Catheter, 27*
Fluid Administration, 28
   *Composition of Body Fluids, 28*
   *Fluid Homeostasis, 29*
   *Fluid Needs during Anesthesia, 30*
   *Classification of Intravenous Fluids, 30*
   *Intravenous Fluid Selection and*
      *Administration Rates, 33*
   *Adverse Effects of Fluid Administration, 35*
   *Calculating Fluid Administration Rates, 35*
Other Preanesthetic Care, 39

## LEARNING OBJECTIVES

*After you have completed this chapter, you will be able to:*
- Explain the importance of effective communication and the role of the veterinary technician in communication.
- List the reasons for preoperative patient evaluation.
- List the parts of a minimum patient database.
- Take a complete history, and identify findings that affect anesthetic event planning.
- Identify ways in which patient signalment influences the anesthetic procedure and patient management.
- Discuss the rationale for obtaining the owner's consent for anesthesia.
- Perform a preanesthetic physical assessment.
- Relate the patient signalment, body weight, and patient condition to the selection and use of anesthetic agents and adjuncts.
- Assign a patient to one of the five physical status classifications as specified by the American Society of Anesthesiologists.
- Describe the components of preanesthetic preparation, including diagnostic testing, choice of protocol, withholding of food, and correction of preexisting problems.
- List the reasons why an intravenous (IV) catheter is advisable for anesthetized patients.
- Describe the types of IV fluids that are used during anesthesia and why each might be chosen.
- Calculate IV fluid infusion rates.

All successful anesthetic procedures begin with careful patient preparation. Completion of this mundane but important aspect of anesthesia requires attention to several diverse tasks. First, the anesthetist must assist the **veterinarian-in-charge (VIC)** in developing a **minimum patient database**—a compilation of pertinent information gleaned from the patient history, physical examination, and diagnostic tests—which the VIC will use to determine the patient's physical status and anesthetic risk and to select an appropriate anesthetic protocol. Next, the anesthetist must ensure that the patient has been appropriately fasted. She must also provide preinduction care of the patient, including medication administration, intravenous (IV) catheterization, fluid administration, stabilization, and any other care ordered by the VIC. She must confirm that the necessary equipment and supplies are available and

| BOX 2-1 | **Patient Preparation "To-Do" List** |
|---|---|

**Patient History**
- Confirm the procedure to be performed ❑
- Gather historical information ❑
- Confirm compliance with fasting instructions ❑
- Confirm vaccines and other preventive care are current ❑
- Inquire about drug allergies or reactions ❑
- Determine the patient's condition the day of surgery ❑
- Note pertinent medical problems and communicate these to the VIC ❑

**Client Communication**
- Present the standard consent form and obtain the client's signature ❑
- Present a fee estimate and obtain the client's signature ❑
- Complete any financial transactions (deposits, payments, insurance) ❑
- Answer the client's questions ❑
- Inform the client of the nature of the procedure, the expected outcome, and the expected time of completion ❑
- Communicate the date and time of discharge if known ❑
- Determine an emergency communication protocol including client phone number, availability, and schedule ❑

**Physical Examination**
- Double-check the patient identity ❑
- Weigh the patient ❑
- Confirm the patient's sex and reproductive status ❑
- Determine the patient's hydration status ❑
- Determine the vital signs ❑
- Perform a physical assessment focusing on the cardiovascular and pulmonary systems ❑
- Determine the patient's pain score and physical status class ❑
- Communicate to the VIC any pertinent physical abnormalities ❑
- Note any concurrent conditions that may be best treated while patient is under anesthesia ❑

**Direct Patient Preparation**
- If patient is hospitalized, make arrangements for preanesthetic fasting ❑
- Perform diagnostic tests, convey results to the VIC, and highlight abnormal data ❑
- Determine and have VIC approve the anesthetic protocol ❑
- Give medications ordered by the VIC ❑
- Place IV catheter and administer fluids if indicated ❑
- Administer preanesthetic medications ❑
- Make any necessary preparations for postoperative care ❑

**Equipment Preparation**
- Gather all necessary equipment ❑
- Prepare the anesthetic machine ❑
- Check that all equipment is in good working order ❑

*IV*, Intravenous; *VIC*, veterinarian-in-charge.

in good working order (further described in Chapter 4). Finally, she must administer preanesthetic medications ordered by the veterinarian and monitor the patient until the time of induction. Box 2-1 lists "to-do" items during the preanesthetic period. Like the pieces of a puzzle, each step is necessary to create a finished whole, and if any step is missed, the likelihood of a positive outcome decreases.

## COMMUNICATION—A KEY TO SUCCESS

A key element of successful preparation is effective communication. Veterinarians depend on accurate information at all stages of the procedure to make effective patient care decisions. Clients need clear instructions and answers to questions before the procedure, as well as progress reports and home care instructions after the procedure. In addition, the technician often acts as a liaison between the doctor and client, conveying necessary information between these two parties.

The bond between most clients and pets is very strong. Surveys of pet owners over the past several decades consistently show that a vast majority of dog and cat owners consider their pets to be members of the family. Consequently, most clients are very protective of, and concerned about, the well-being of their animals and are very attuned to real or perceived risks to their safety. The risks inherent in the practice of anesthesia often produce or heighten feelings of anxiety.

## CASE 2-1 CASE PRESENTATION

Pixie, a 9-year-old Yorkshire terrier, was presented for a dental cleaning. A minimum patient database was acquired, and the patient was prepared in a routine manner. The client was educated regarding the condition of the oral cavity, the nature of the procedure including the probable need for extractions, and follow-up care. The consent form was signed, and a phone number with which the client could be reached during the procedure was obtained.

The dental cleaning was performed, and during the process of assessing the oral cavity, the patient was determined to have grade IV periodontal disease, 10 teeth with advanced mobility, and several more with end-stage, irreversible damage to the periodontal tissues. A total of 17 teeth were extracted with minimal effort. The client was not called because the possibility of extractions was discussed at the preoperative interview.

It was routine in this clinic to have the veterinary technician meet with the owner at discharge to review what was done and to provide instructions for home care. During the exit interview the owner became agitated and very angry and demanded to see the doctor immediately. He expressed anger over the large number of extractions, and grave concerns that the patient would be unable to eat normally. He refused to listen to any explanation of the importance of removal of these teeth or the dangers associated with leaving them in. The owner left the clinic in a state of extreme agitation, vowing never to come back to the clinic. Although the doctor followed up by phone 1 week later to check on the patient's progress, the client's anger had not abated.

This case illustrates how easily seemingly small omissions in communication can lead to misunderstandings, dissatisfaction, anger, and even the loss of a client. The client's perception of the quality of care is most often closely related to whether or not his or her expectations have been met, so if there is an unexpected outcome, the client may react strongly. In this situation, even though the owner was informed that extractions would be necessary, he assumed perhaps two or three at the most, and he had no previous experience to prepare him for the large number that was needed in this case. Consequently, the gap between his expectation and the outcome was wide.

With experience, veterinary professionals learn to anticipate circumstances that have the potential to lead to misunderstandings and to circumvent unmet expectations with good communication. Options in this case would have been to write an estimated number of extractions on the release form and call the client if the actual number was going to exceed this figure, or to call the client in any case when it was clear that the number of extractions was going to be high. If the clients had been warned and had not been surprised with this information during the exit interview, it is likely that he would have left happy, satisfied, and confident that everything possible had been done to protect the health of his pet.

---

These feelings can be minimized, however, when the relationship between health care providers and the client is strong. A strong relationship is based not only on confidence in the competency of the veterinarian and staff, but also on assurance that they truly care about the welfare of the patient. The saying, "Clients don't care how much you know until they know how much you care," has become an oft-repeated adage in the veterinary community. Although not originally used in reference to the veterinary profession, anyone with even a little practice experience can tell you that it accurately reflects the way most clients feel.

Exceptional communication is probably the best way to convey the caring that clients desire and expect. They feel more confident and less anxious about the procedure when informed. When unanticipated complications occur, clients are thus more able to come to terms with the outcome. A few extra minutes spent answering questions and explaining the risks and benefits before a procedure is well worth the time in terms of increased client satisfaction and lessening of the sadness, anger, and disappointment that occur when events do not go as hoped and that, if not adequately addressed, can result in ill will, the loss of a client, or even legal action.

In fact, there is no better predictor of success than the technician's communication skills, and for this important reason communication will remain a centerpiece of this text. (See Case Presentation 2-1 for an example of the importance of good communication.)

## THE MINIMUM PATIENT DATABASE

Technicians soon become accustomed to wide variety in size, age, temperament, conformation, and condition among the patients they see. Veterinary patients can range in size from 20 g to over 1000 kg and may be neonatal, pediatric, mature, or geriatric. They may be docile, spirited, fearful, agitated, or aggressive. They may be emaciated, lean, obese, brachiocephalic, deep-chested, or pregnant. Some are healthy, and others have varying degrees of illness ranging from mild to critical. Some are brought in for minor procedures; others will undergo complicated and lengthy operations. Given this diversity, it is unrealistic to assume that the same anesthetic techniques will work for all patients. Furthermore, it is dangerous to expect all patients to react to a given anesthetic agent in the same way.

Therefore the veterinarian and technician must gather as much information as possible to uncover any factors that might lead to anesthetic complications. The information, collectively referred to as a *minimum patient database,* is used to make patient care decisions. If the information obtained about a given animal reveals a potential problem, the veterinarian may choose to alter, postpone, or even cancel the anesthetic procedure.

The minimum patient database consists of the following:
1. Patient history including the patient signalment
2. Complete physical examination findings
3. Results of a preanesthetic diagnostic workup

Many veterinary clinics routinely recommend that animals scheduled for elective surgery be brought into the clinic for an appointment before the day of surgery so that this information can be gathered. During the visit, the veterinarian may also administer necessary vaccinations, give information about preanesthetic fasting of the animal, obtain signed consent forms, and present a fee estimate. If such an appointment is scheduled several days before the planned procedure, unforeseen problems can be discovered and addressed well in advance of surgery.

> **TECHNICIAN NOTE** An appointment should be scheduled several days before the planned procedure to acquire the minimum patient database, so that unforeseen problems can be discovered and addressed well in advance of surgery.

Before embarking on a study of anesthesia, the student should be familiar with the process required to obtain a patient history as well as the procedures required to perform a complete physical examination and diagnostic workup. Consequently the sections that follow will focus specifically on how the anesthetist can best obtain information needed to make effective and safe anesthetic management decisions. Emphasis will be placed on specific historical questions to ask, physical findings to focus on, and diagnostic test results that are most pertinent to anesthetic procedures, as well as the ways in which common abnormal findings from each of these sources of information affect outcomes.

## Patient History

A patient history is information about the patient's health acquired by asking the client questions. A thorough patient history is an essential part of a minimum patient database and, in fact, is often considerably more important for making effective patient care decisions than results of diagnostic testing.

Obtaining a thorough patient history requires skill and care, and, like all arts, it must be continually practiced and refined. The technician must know the most important questions to ask as well as the most effective way to frame those questions. Otherwise the patient history will be incomplete or misleading.

> **TECHNICIAN NOTE** When taking a patient history, emphasize open-ended questions. Avoid leading questions or questions that can be answered "yes" or "no."

A common error is to ask a question that can be answered "yes" or "no." For instance, the question "Does your dog drink a normal amount of water?" will yield a "yes" or "no" answer that reflects that owner's assumption regarding what is normal, as opposed to facts that can be accurately evaluated. In contrast, the question "About how much water does your dog drink per day?" prompts the owner to quantify the amount of water consumed but not to judge whether he or she believes the amount to be normal. If the client replies, "About 1 quart (or liter)," the VIC will then be able to determine whether or not this volume is excessive, despite the owner's opinion regarding its significance.

Another common error is to ask leading questions. In the previous example, the question "Your dog doesn't drink much water, does she?" might bias the owner toward a particular response such as "No, I guess not," resulting in misleading information.

In a busy practice it is often difficult to set aside adequate time to obtain a good history. Under these circumstances, the technician may be tempted to take shortcuts or omit questions altogether—an inadvisable practice that will lead to unpleasant surprises. For instance, an owner may not realize that coughing and exercise intolerance may be associated with a heart problem. If an adequate history is not taken, the preexisting heart disease may not be detected, and the technician may become aware of the problem only when the anesthetized animal is in danger.

When inquiring about signs of illness, the technician not only should note information the client freely offers but should always strive to get as much detail as possible. For instance, if a client indicates that the patient is vomiting, the doctor will want to know other details in order to interpret its significance. No matter what the sign (for example vomiting, coughing, diarrhea, polyuria, seizures, or weakness), it is always helpful to know the following four points,* which give the doctor specific information necessary to arrive at a diagnosis:
1. The duration (how long has it been going on?)
2. The volume or severity (how much or how severe?)
3. The frequency (how often?)
4. The character or appearance (what does it look like?)

---

*Note that although not all of these points may apply to every sign, they apply to most.

---

> **TECHNICIAN NOTE** When gathering historical information about signs of illness (e.g., vomiting or coughing), always ask about the following:
> 1. The duration (how long has it been going on?)
> 2. The volume or severity (how much or how severe?)
> 3. The frequency (how often?)
> 4. The character or appearance (what does it look like?)

## Confirmation of the Scheduled Procedure

Because miscommunications occur and clerical errors may be made on medical charts, in appointment books, and on surgery schedules, the technician must verbally confirm the procedure to be performed. Periodically stories appear in the news about devastating consequences of a miscommunication in the human medical field such as amputation of the wrong limb or administration of chemotherapy to the wrong patient. Similar errors may occur in veterinary patients and frequently result in ill will, patient harm, or legal proceedings.

Attention to this simple but important element of effective communication will prevent these and other embarrassing, dangerous, or potentially devastating errors such as a missed diagnosis from failing to submit a biopsy sample, anesthetizing the wrong patient, neglecting to perform a necessary procedure, or performing a procedure the patient does not need. When confirming the procedure, check the following specifics:

- When performing surgery on a limb, confirm the affected limb (left or right; fore or hind).
- When a tumor is being removed, be sure that the exact location of the tumor is known. Skin tumors can be obscured by the hair coat, and if small can be extremely difficult to locate unless pointed out by the client. Once the tumor has been located, mark the location by clipping the hair or using a surgical marker.
- If removing tumors or other mass lesions, confirm the owner's wishes regarding histopathology (biopsy) or cytology.
- Determine if the client wishes the doctor to use his or her judgment regarding decisions that must be made during the procedure (such as the number of teeth that need to be extracted during a dental cleaning) or if the client would like a telephone call before proceeding.

After confirming this information with the client, be sure it is accurately transferred to the medical record and communicated to the VIC.

> **TECHNICIAN NOTE** Always reconfirm the nature of the scheduled procedure when the patient is admitted, including the exact location of tumors or lesions, the affected limb (for procedures involving a limb), and the owner's wishes regarding testing (such as histopathology).

## Obtaining a Patient History

When a complete patient history is being obtained, the following specific questions should be asked.

### What Are the Species, Breed, Age, Sex, and Reproductive Status of the Patient?

The species, breed, age, sex, and reproductive status are collectively known as the **signalment**. The signalment is important in planning the anesthetic procedure, as each data point influences the anesthetic plan, drug doses, and many other actions related to patient management as noted in the following sections.

**Species.** Each species has unique responses to anesthetic agents and adjuncts as well as unique needs associated with anesthesia. Following are examples of notable species differences that must be considered:

- Horses and cats are more sensitive to opioids than dogs and ruminants. Therefore some of these agents must be used with caution, at lower doses or not at all in these species.
- Each species has unique dosing requirements (e.g., cats require a lower dose of lidocaine but are more resistant to the effects of phenothiazine tranquilizers than dogs).
- Horses tend to have rougher recoveries from inhalant anesthetics than other species.
- The use of anticholinergics should be avoided in ruminants, as it can make their saliva thick and ropy, which can lead to airway occlusion. Ruminants may also regurgitate at any point during anesthesia, and the anesthetist should take steps to avoid aspiration.
- Ruminants are more sensitive to xylazine, requiring about one tenth the dose of horses.
- Cats can tolerate administration of dissociative agents alone, whereas dogs may experience seizure-like activity unless the dissociative is combined with another agent.
- Large animals are prone to respiratory depression and dependent atelectasis and thus often require ventilatory support.
- Large animals experience pressure necrosis of tissues lying over pressure points such as the shoulder and hip and thus require measures to pad dependent areas when in lateral recumbency.
- Horses may fracture limbs during anesthetic recovery and thus require special attention during the recovery period.
- Cats, small dogs, and small animal pediatric patients are prone to hypoxemia and **hypercarbia** caused by increased mechanical **dead space**.
- Cats and ruminants are prone to airway blockage because of development of excess airway secretions.
- Ruminants are prone to bloat.

- Exotic animals such as birds and reptiles must be managed very differently than common domestic species. The technician should consult appropriate references and the veterinarian before administering anesthetics to these animals.

**Breed.** Differences in anatomy and physiology among the various breeds also may affect the animal's response to anesthetic agents and procedures.

- Sighthounds such as greyhounds and salukis are sensitive to barbiturates (e.g., thiopental sodium) because of their relative lack of body fat and slow metabolism of these agents compared with other breeds. Consequently these drugs must be used cautiously or not at all in these patients.
- Boxers and giant breeds are more sensitive to acepromazine than other breeds, whereas terriers are resistant.
- Brachycephalic animals are difficult to intubate and must be watched closely to ensure a patent airway before, during, and after any anesthetic procedure. Also, members of these breeds often require use of smaller endotracheal tubes than most other breeds.
- Many exotic or rare breed animals are perceived to be sensitive to anesthetics by their owners, although many of these idiosyncrasies are not proven.
- Draft horses are typically sensitive to sedatives in the same way that giant breed dogs are. They are also more likely to experience complications during recovery because of their large body mass compared with average-sized horses.

**Age.** The age of the patient can be an important consideration when deciding what drugs to use. Neonates (up to 2 weeks of age) or pediatric patients (2 to 8 weeks of age) are much less capable of metabolizing injectable drugs than are adult animals because the necessary liver metabolic pathways are not fully developed. Geriatric patients may be unable to tolerate normal doses of some drugs because of poor hepatic or renal function. The result in either case may be a slow recovery from anesthesia, particularly if doses of injectable drugs are not adjusted accordingly. In addition, young patients are more difficult to intubate and to catheterize, are more subject to dosing errors, are more prone to **hypothermia** and **hypoxia,** and have a weaker respiratory drive. As patients age, they become less able to tolerate the demands that anesthesia places on their major organ systems. These factors put neonatal, pediatric, and geriatric patients at higher risk for complications.

> *TECHNICIAN NOTE*  Patients that are very large, very small, very young (<8 weeks old), or very old (>75% of the normal lifespan) respond to anesthetic procedures differently than other animals and have special needs of which the anesthetist must be aware.

**Sex and Reproductive Status.** Always confirm the patient's sex by physical examination. Owners often are not aware of their pet's sex or may misidentify it. If not corrected, misidentification of the patient's sex can lead to an undesirable outcome. For instance, attempting to spay a male cat (because the patient's sex was misidentified by the client and not confirmed by the technician) is unnecessary for the patient and very embarrassing and difficult to explain to the client.

**Reproductive status** refers to whether or not the patient has been spayed or castrated and, if the patient is **intact,** whether or not the patient is being used for breeding. For intact female patients, it also includes the current estrous cycle status and pregnancy status. These points are of particular importance in terms of the anesthetic plan as well as patient management as indicated in the following examples:

- When an intact female animal is in heat, the uterus is enlarged and has a more extensive blood supply. These patients also may bleed excessively because of the effects of estrogen on the clotting cascade. For an ovariohysterectomy, these factors increase the length, difficulty, risk, and often the cost of the surgery.
- During pregnancy, the gravid uterus and its blood supply gradually enlarge, reaching a size many times larger than a nongravid uterus. As is the case with estrus, these changes substantially increase the length, difficulty, and risk of an ovariohysterectomy. The prospect of spaying a pregnant animal also creates an ethical dilemma that must be discussed with the client before proceeding.
- Acepromazine is considered to be contraindicated by many clinicians in stallions because it may cause penile prolapse, which can lead to permanent injury.
- Xylazine has been shown to cause uterine contractions in the third trimester of pregnancy in sheep and cattle.

> *TECHNICIAN NOTE*  When obtaining the history, determine each of the following:
> - The signalment
> - Current and past illnesses
> - Medications currently being administered
> - Allergies or drug reactions
> - The status of preventive care

### Is the Patient Receiving or Has It Recently Received Treatment with Any Drugs, Neutraceuticals, or Pesticides?

Many medications, including anticonvulsants, behavior-modifying drugs, drugs that affect the autonomic nervous system, and antibiotics may influence the effect of anesthetics.

- Sympathomimetics such as epinephrine increase the incidence of cardiac arrhythmias when given with cyclohexamines, xylazine, barbiturates, and halothane.

- Tricyclic antidepressants such as amitriptyline and clomipramine may predispose patients to cardiac arrhythmias and excessive responses to anticholinergics and central nervous system (CNS) depressants.
- The antibiotic chloramphenicol may decrease biotransformation of barbiturate anesthetics, leading to significantly prolonged recovery, and may prolong the action of propofol and ketamine.
- When given within 14 days of one another, some monoamine oxidase inhibitors such as amitraz and selegiline may increase the effects of morphine and other opioids.
- Some antihistamines can increase CNS and respiratory depression when given with opioids and other anesthetic agents that depress these body systems.

### Is There Any History of Allergies or Drug Reactions?

Past adverse reactions to drugs must be documented in the medical record and conveyed to the VIC. Severe allergic reactions such as anaphylaxis preclude the use of the offending drug in the future. A past history of prolonged recovery, personality changes, organ dysfunction, or other postanesthetic adverse reactions may influence a decision to use these agents and must be brought to the veterinarian's attention. For example, some cats will have prolonged recoveries from ketamine and other dissociatives that can last several days. Some dogs can experience behavioral changes after sedation with acepromazine that can result in bites. It may be best to choose another agent in the future for a patient experiencing these and other adverse reactions.

### Is the Patient up to Date on Routine Preventive Care?

Check the date and type of vaccines administered and the results of fecal analysis and routine testing for contagious diseases such as heartworm disease in dogs and cats and feline leukemia and feline immunodeficiency virus in cats. The last date of tetanus antitoxoid administration to an equine patient should be known. Many veterinary clinics require current vaccinations before hospitalization to prevent the spread of contagious diseases.

### Has the Patient Ever Had or Does It Currently Have Any Illness or Medical Problems, and, If So, What Was the Medical or Surgical Treatment?

Information about current and past medical problems is obtained from the patient's medical record or verbally from the client. Animals with preexisting disease may be at increased risk for anesthetic complications. Sick animals may also introduce pathogens into the hospital,

posing a risk to other patients unless they are placed in an isolation ward.

Asking if the patient has any of the signs listed in the following paragraphs helps the VIC make a diagnosis, determine risk, and guide patient management decisions. These common signs of disease often indicate a variety of problems, which must be explored and acted on through physical examination, diagnostic testing, patient treatment and stabilization, or even postponement of the procedure. Remember to determine the details regarding duration, volume or severity, frequency, and appearance or character.

**Anorexia, Vomiting, Diarrhea, Coughing, Sneezing, Polyuria, Polydipsia, Tenesmus, or Dysuria.** Anorexia, vomiting, diarrhea, coughing, sneezing, polyuria, polydipsia, tenesmus, or dysuria may indicate one of many disorders, which may need to be stabilized before anesthesia. Parvovirus in dogs, upper respiratory infections in cats, inflammatory bowel disease, urinary blockage, endocrine disease, and organ dysfunction are examples of problems associated with these signs.

**A Change in Behavior.** Changes in behavior may be a sign of CNS disease, pain, systemic illness, and many other conditions.

**Exercise Intolerance.** Exercise intolerance may indicate a variety of problems including heart disease, anemia, and musculoskeletal pain.

**Weakness.** Weakness is a nonspecific sign caused by many disorders and always warrants investigation to determine a cause.

**Fainting or Seizures.** Both fainting episodes and seizures vary widely in appearance and sometimes may be difficult to tell apart. In many cases these disorders can be differentiated by careful observation, but other cases require careful analysis of information derived from the patient history, physical examination, and diagnostic tests. Despite any similarities in appearance, these disorders have completely different causes. Fainting (also called **syncope**) often indicates hypoxemia, low blood pressure, or cardiac disease, whereas seizures are often associated with CNS disease, toxin ingestion, or metabolic disorders such as hypoglycemia.

**Bleeding.** Any unexplained bleeding including bruising, blood in the urine or stool, or prolonged bleeding after venipuncture or surgery may be a sign of a coagulation disorder, which, if unidentified, will increase a patient's risk for intraoperative and postoperative hemorrhage.

### Other Considerations

Before the procedure, it is advisable to give the owner a written estimate of the expected charges. It is also customary to obtain a signed **consent form** authorizing anesthesia and surgery. It is illegal in most jurisdictions to undertake surgery or anesthesia on an animal without the owner's written or oral consent, and in any case is unadvisable. Such consent must be informed, meaning that the owner is warned beforehand of risks associated with the procedure. Standard consent forms (available from practice management consultants and from state and provincial veterinary associations) often state that anesthesia and surgery are never without risk (Figure 2-1).

*TECHNICIAN NOTE*    Before any anesthetic procedure, *always* give the owner a written estimate of the expected charges and obtain a signed consent form authorizing anesthesia and surgery.

VETERINARY HOSPITAL OF THE
UNIVERSITY OF PENNSYLVANIA

**CONSENT FOR TREATMENT AND/OR
ADMISSION**

CLIENT PLATE

I, the undersigned owner, or owner's agent, of the pet identified above, certify that **I am/I am not** (circle one) over **eighteen** years of age, and hereby consent to the examination of my pet by staff veterinarians at VHUP. I also agree that after consultation with me, VHUP's doctors may prescribe medication for, treat, hospitalize, anesthetize, sedate, and/or perform surgery on my animal. I understand that some risks always exist with anesthesia, surgery, and/or certain diagnostic procedures and treatments and that I am encouraged to discuss any concerns I have about those risks with my attending veterinarian before the procedure is initiated. Should some unexpected life-saving emergency care be required and my attending veterinarian be unable to reach me, VHUP's staff has my permission to provide such treatment, and I agree to pay for such care.

I understand that an estimate of the costs of veterinary services will be provided to me and that I am encouraged to discuss all fees attendant to such care before services are rendered and during my pet's ongoing medical treatment. If my pet is hospitalized, I agree to pay a deposit of one half of the estimated fees and assume financial responsibility for the balance of all services rendered on a cash, credit card or check basis at the time my pet is discharged from the hospital. In the event my pet is hospitalized for more than 48 hours and my attending doctor is unable to reach me, I understand it is my responsibility to call the hospital at least every 48 hours to inquire as to the medical status of my pet and the fees incurred for medical services up to that day. In the event of an open balance, I agree to pay a monthly billing fee equal to 1.5% of the unpaid balance.

I understand that VHUP faculty and staff have teaching and research functions in addition to their clinical duties. In fulfilling their mission, they may generate photographs, x-rays or other images of patients and/or make use of blood or tissue samples in performing their studies. I consent to the taking of photographs and other images and the use of such images and blood or tissue samples for teaching and research purposes provided that 1) they are obtained as part of the normal diagnostic and therapeutic work-ups and 2) neither my animal nor I are identified in any publications, reports or presentations without permission. I understand that staff members will not obtain additional samples nor perform additional procedures beyond those necessary for the clinical care of my pet without additional oral or written consent.

I further agree that I, or an authorized agent of mine, will pick up my pet and pay for all accrued charges within 5 days after receiving written or oral notification that my pet is ready to be discharged from the hospital. Such notice will be given at the address maintained on the hospital's patient/client record or the address listed below. I agree that if I fail to comply with this policy, VHUP may handle the abandonment of my pet in the best interests of the animal and the hospital.

**HAVE YOU TALKED WITH YOUR VETERINARIAN
ABOUT THE FOLLOWING?**

- The reasonable medical and/or surgical treatment options for your pet?
- Sufficient details of the procedures for you to understand what will be performed?
- How fully your pet might respond or recover and how long it could take?
- The most common complications and how serious they might be?
- The length and type of follow-up care and restraint required?
- How much all of the care is expected to cost?

_____    _____
Signature of Owner or Agent          Date

_____    _____
Signature of Parent or Legal Guardian    Date
if owner/agent less than 18 years of age

**FIGURE 2-1**    Standard consent for treatment and/or authorization for admission to the hospital.

Many consent forms also include a statement giving the veterinarian permission to perform cardiopulmonary-cerebrovascular resuscitation (CPCR) if the patient's condition requires it. Owners should be asked to provide a telephone number at which they may be reached during the day, in case an emergency or unforeseen complication should arise. Consent forms may also state that some anesthetic drugs may be used that have not received approval from the Food and Drug Administration for this purpose. This is termed **extra-label drug use** and is common in veterinary anesthesia.

It is ironic that although cell phones have become ubiquitous, clients are often difficult to reach because they rely on voice mail and don't always feel compelled to answer their phones promptly. An inability to contact a client presents a problem, particularly with procedures such as exploratory surgery, in which the diagnosis is not known. In these situations decisions that require the client's input (such as whether to biopsy or remove a tumor or whether to proceed with a difficult, high-risk, or expensive procedure) must sometimes be made quickly. Therefore it is imperative that the client knows to be present and available by phone at the time of surgery, so that he or she can be contacted immediately should the need arise.

Obviously a great deal of information must be exchanged before anesthesia is initiated. Although it may be appropriate for a trained receptionist to assist in gathering this information, particularly when a young, healthy animal is scheduled for an elective operation such as castration or ovariohysterectomy, the veterinarian or technician should handle more complex cases. The hospital employee who admits a patient and speaks to the owner must not just obtain this information but must also relay that information to the anesthetist by means of a written record or oral report.

In some cases it may be difficult to obtain the history in person. Some clinics prefer to have the owner fill out a prepared history form, particularly if the clinic has a high volume of patients. In any practice, difficulties may arise when an animal's owner is in a hurry and reluctant to stop and answer questions. However, it is usually possible to obtain a telephone number and call for more information at a prearranged time. Occasionally the person bringing the animal into the clinic is not the owner and is unfamiliar with the pet. In this case, every effort should be made to contact the owner by telephone to obtain the required information.

## Physical Examination and Physical Assessment

A physical examination is a complete evaluation of a patient's physical condition using the hands, eyes, ears, and nose. Although the basic technique used to perform a physical examination is the same whether the examination is performed by a veterinarian or veterinary technician, there is a qualitative difference in the way the results of the examination are used by these two parties. A veterinarian uses the physical findings to arrive at a diagnosis and plan treatment. In contrast, a veterinary technician uses physical findings to provide effective patient care, respond to patient needs, and alert the veterinarian to changes in patient condition that influence patient management. Coordinated application of these two very different but complementary approaches enables the veterinary team to provide high-quality care at a level that would not otherwise be possible.

In order to differentiate this contrast in purpose, in this text the term *physical examination* (PE) will be used to indicate evaluation by a veterinarian for the purpose of diagnosis and treatment planning, and the term *physical assessment* (PA) will be used to indicate evaluation by a technician for the purpose of maximizing quality of care and influencing patient management through communication with the VIC. No value judgment is implied in either term, as both physical examinations and assessments as defined herein are interdependent techniques—equally necessary and of equal importance in delivery of high-quality patient care. With this in mind, discussion of this vital part of the minimum patient database follows.

A complete physical examination should be conducted on every animal scheduled for anesthesia. Although a veterinarian usually does this before scheduling a procedure, the technician should, in addition, always perform a brief physical assessment immediately before the procedure. Following are common examples of findings revealed during physical examination or physical assessment that will influence patient anesthetic management.

- *Dehydration* increases the risk for anesthetic complications including **hypotension,** poor tissue perfusion, and kidney damage.
- *Anemia* decreases the oxygen-carrying capacity of the blood and predisposes the patient to **hypoxemia.**
- *Bruising lesions* on the skin or mucous membranes, in the absence of trauma, often indicate a clotting disorder, which will increase the risk of potentially life-threatening intraoperative and postoperative bleeding.
- *Respiratory or cardiovascular disease* increases the risk of anesthetic complications and death.
- *Abnormalities of abdominal organs* such as an enlarged liver or abnormally small kidneys may be associated with abnormal organ function and a reduced ability to metabolize or excrete anesthetic agents.
- *General conditions that require veterinary attention* such as ear mite or flea infestations, otitis externa, dental disease, overgrown nails, and anal sac impaction. These conditions are often most easily treated during the anesthetic procedure. Owners are often not aware these conditions are present and, once informed, will frequently authorize treatment.

- *Physical abnormalities that may influence the procedure.* One example of this is an abdominally retained testicle in a patient presented for castration. This condition increases the complexity and cost of surgery, so the owner must be informed before the veterinarian proceeds.

In most jurisdictions, veterinary technicians must perform a physical assessment under the supervision of a licensed veterinarian. The veterinary medical licensing board practice act should be consulted to determine the laws regulating technician duties in your state or province.

> **TECHNICIAN NOTE**    The technician should *always* perform a brief physical assessment immediately before the procedure, to uncover hidden problems that may increase risk or alter patient management.

There are many different ways to approach a physical examination or physical assessment. Any technique is valid as long as the patient is examined entirely and in a systematic manner (e.g., from head to tail or by organ system). Include each element listed in the following sections, with emphasis on the nervous, cardiovascular, and pulmonary systems, as these systems are generally most affected by anesthetic agents and most directly influence outcome. When possible, it is helpful to have the owner present during the physical examination or physical assessment to give pertinent history about any physical abnormalities that are found. Any unusual findings must be brought to the attention of the veterinarian, because ultimately it is the veterinarian's responsibility to make a diagnosis, formulate an appropriate treatment plan, and advise the owner and hospital staff accordingly.

### Patient Identification

In practice, inattention to seemingly simple considerations, such as proper patient identification, may result in undesirable outcomes, because they are easily overlooked. Examination of the news will occasionally reveal stories of accidents at human hospitals related to patient identification such as a surgery performed on the wrong patient. Needless to say, serious errors such as these can and do occur in veterinary medicine.

In a busy animal hospital, patients may easily be confused if not positively identified with cage tags and patient identification collars, as well as documentation of external characteristics such as species, breed, size, hair coat length, color, and other visual identifying characteristics. This is because most individuals within a particular breed look very similar. Patients may be placed in the wrong cage, or one may simply be mistaken for another. Therefore, careful attention must always be given to patient identification.

Tags on the front of each cage should identify the patient so that those passing the cage can quickly identify the patient before opening the cage. Identification collars

confirm patient identification in case a patient is inadvertently placed in the wrong cage.

> **TECHNICIAN NOTE**    Identification collars must be placed on *all* patients on admission to the hospital. Before anesthetizing a patient, do whatever you need to do to make sure the animal in your hands is the correct one!

Before performing any procedure, make positive patient identification by matching the cage tag, the ID collar, and the patient's external characteristics with the information contained in the medical record. In other words, do whatever needs to be done to make sure the animal in your hands is the correct one!

### Body Weight

Anesthetic agents as a rule have very narrow therapeutic indexes. Therefore accurate dosing is critical to a successful outcome. With the exception of inhalant anesthetics, most drug dosages and IV fluid administration rates are calculated according to body weight. All animals should therefore be accurately weighed immediately before any anesthetic procedure. Animals under 5 kg should be weighed on a pediatric scale, and those under 1 kg should be weighed on a gram scale. It is not appropriate to estimate a body weight for purposes of anesthetic administration unless working with a large animal that cannot be weighed because of temperament or lack of a large animal scale. In this case, techniques will be used to estimate weight based on experience, or measurement of girth and length in horses, but must also take into account the patient's body condition score. The basic formula for determining the body weight in horses is as follows:

$$\text{Body weight}\,(\text{kg}) = \frac{\text{Heart girth}\,(\text{cm})^2 \times \text{Length}\,(\text{cm})}{11880}$$

where heart girth equals the circumference of the chest behind the point of the elbow, and length equals the distance from the point of the shoulder to the point of the pelvis.

The current weight should be compared with previous weights (found in the patient's medical record) to determine whether weight gain or loss has occurred. Changes in weight may reflect changes in the patient's food intake, hydration, activity level, or overall state of health.

> **TECHNICIAN NOTE**    All animals should be accurately weighed *immediately* before any anesthetic procedure. Animals under 5 kg should be weighed on a pediatric scale, and those under 1 kg should be weighed on a gram scale.

## Body Condition Score

A **body condition score** is a numeric assessment of the patient's weight compared with the ideal body weight. Some professionals use a five-level system, and others use a nine-level system. In the nine-level system, the number 5 in cats and 4 or 5 in dogs represents ideal body weight. Lower numbers and higher numbers represent a body weight less than or greater than the ideal weight respectively, with a score of 1 representing extreme **cachexia** and 9 representing overt obesity (Figure 2-2). Although it has fewer gradations, the five-level system is similar to

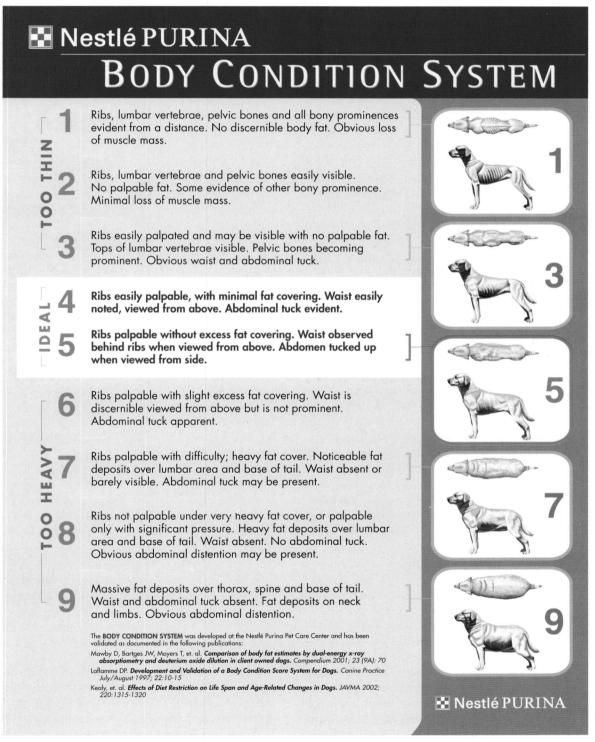

A

**FIGURE 2-2**   Nine-level body condition scoring for dogs and cats. **A,** Body condition scoring system for dogs.

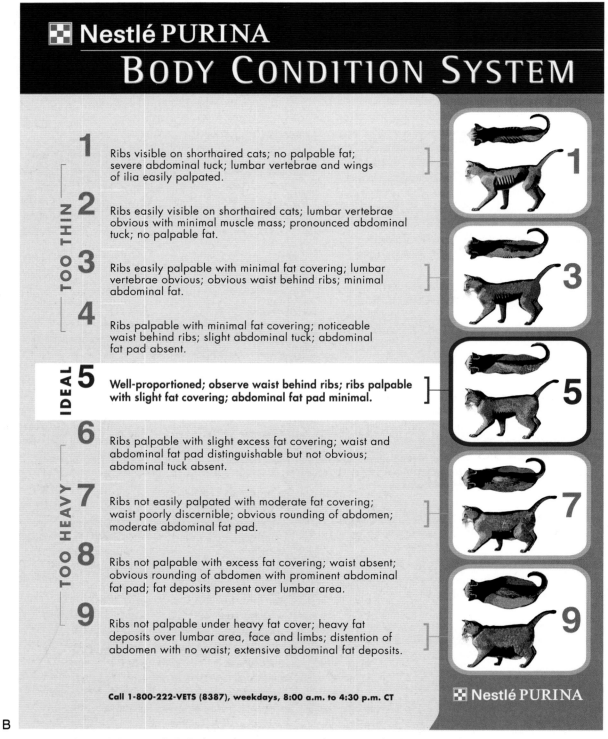

## Nestlé PURINA

# BODY CONDITION SYSTEM

**TOO THIN**

**1** Ribs visible on shorthaired cats; no palpable fat; severe abdominal tuck; lumbar vertebrae and wings of ilia easily palpated.

**2** Ribs easily visible on shorthaired cats; lumbar vertebrae obvious with minimal muscle mass; pronounced abdominal tuck; no palpable fat.

**3** Ribs easily palpable with minimal fat covering; lumbar vertebrae obvious; obvious waist behind ribs; minimal abdominal fat.

**4** Ribs palpable with minimal fat covering; noticeable waist behind ribs; slight abdominal tuck; abdominal fat pad absent.

**IDEAL**

**5** **Well-proportioned; observe waist behind ribs; ribs palpable with slight fat covering; abdominal fat pad minimal.**

**TOO HEAVY**

**6** Ribs palpable with slight excess fat covering; waist and abdominal fat pad distinguishable but not obvious; abdominal tuck absent.

**7** Ribs not easily palpated with moderate fat covering; waist poorly discernible; obvious rounding of abdomen; moderate abdominal fat pad.

**8** Ribs not palpable with excess fat covering; waist absent; obvious rounding of abdomen with prominent abdominal fat pad; fat deposits present over lumbar area.

**9** Ribs not palpable under heavy fat cover; heavy fat deposits over lumbar area, face and limbs; distention of abdomen with no waist; extensive abdominal fat deposits.

Call 1-800-222-VETS (8387), weekdays, 8:00 a.m. to 4:30 p.m. CT

## Nestlé PURINA

B

**FIGURE 2-2, cont'd**   B, Body condition scoring system for cats. (Used with permission from Nestle-Purina.)

the nine-level system, except that a score of 3 represents normal weight and 5 represents overt obesity.

The body condition score is important because changes in body weight influence patient management. Excessive thinness may indicate the presence of an underlying disorder such as hyperthyroidism or chronic parasitism, which may increase patient risk. Animals with little body fat are more sensitive to the effects of some anesthetics such as the ultra–short-acting barbiturates and also are more prone to hypothermia than patients of normal body weight.

Obesity also poses difficulties for the anesthetist. Obese animals may have compromised cardiovascular function

| TABLE 2-1 | Physical Signs Associated with Dehydration |
|---|---|

| Percent Dehydration | Physical Signs |
|---|---|
| <5 | Not detectable |
| 5-6 | Mild loss of skin elasticity |
| 6-8 | Definite loss of skin elasticity<br>May have dry mucous membranes<br>May have depressed globes within orbits |
| 8-10 | Persistent skin tent with slow return because of loss of skin elasticity |
| 10-12 | Persistent skin tent because of loss of skin elasticity<br>Depressed globes within orbits<br>Dry mucous membranes<br>Signs of perfusion deficits (CRT >2 sec, tachycardia) |
| 12-15 | Signs of shock<br>Death |

From DiBartola S: *Fluid, electrolyte, and acid-base disorders,* ed 3, St Louis, 2006, Elsevier.
*CRT,* Capillary refill time.

and decreased functional lung volume. In addition, venipuncture and auscultation are more difficult in obese patients. When patients are significantly overweight, anesthetics should be dosed according to lean body weight (excluding body fat) instead of the total body weight. This is because body fat increases the total body weight, but not the volume or weight of the nervous tissue on which anesthetics exert their effect. Administration of a dose calculated using total body weight results in an anesthetic overdose. Therefore the anesthetist must use the body condition score along with the actual patient weight to estimate lean body weight.

## Assessment of Hydration

Hydration status is assessed using physical parameters that enable the anesthetist to estimate percent dehydration. Table 2-1 outlines these parameters including skin turgor, position of the eye in the orbit, mucous membrane color, refill and moisture level, heart rate, and pulse strength. As these parameters are affected by body fat content, age, and other factors, assessment of hydration is a somewhat subjective procedure at best and is naturally subject to many inaccuracies. For instance, young and obese patients appear more hydrated than they really are, whereas old and cachectic patients appear less hydrated. Panting may dry mucous membranes, causing the patient to appear less hydrated. Therefore these physical parameters can be expected to give the anesthetist only a general idea of hydration and must be used with other clinical data such as careful serial monitoring of body weight. This is an excellent indicator of hydration, with a sudden loss of 1 kg corresponding to 1 L of fluid loss.

Some clinical chemistry and hematology tests such as the plasma protein and hematocrit also reflect hydration status and will be discussed in the following section on diagnostic testing.

In any case, if the animal appears significantly dehydrated, this should be corrected before anesthesia, because dehydration will impair tissue perfusion and predispose the patient to hypotension. Fluid therapy is further discussed on p. 28.

> **TECHNICIAN NOTE** Serial monitoring of body weight is an excellent indicator of hydration, with a sudden loss of 1 kg corresponding to 1 L of fluid loss.

## Level of Consciousness

**Level of consciousness** (LOC) refers to the patient's responsiveness to stimuli or how easily it can be aroused, and is used to assess brain function. A decreased LOC indicates abnormal brain function and is caused by a variety of factors including hypoxia, drugs, dehydration, and neurologic disease.

Consciousness of healthy patients is often described as alert and responsive or alert and oriented. Patients can further be classified as "bright" if noticeably engaged and interested in the environment, or "quiet" or "subdued" if this is not the case. Therefore "B/A/R" is an abbreviation that may be used to describe patients that are bright, alert, and responsive, and "Q/A/R" may be used for patients that are quiet, alert, and responsive.

Patients with a mildly decreased LOC that can be aroused with minimal difficulty are said to be **lethargic.** The word *lethargy* is a noun describing this state. Patients that are more depressed and that cannot be fully aroused are referred to as **obtunded** (noun form *obtundity*). A **stuporous** patient (noun form *stupor*) is in a sleeplike state and can be aroused only with a painful stimulus. A **comatose** patient (noun form *coma*) cannot be aroused and is unresponsive to all stimuli including pain.

A system commonly used in human patients is referred to as the *AVPU scale.* Each letter represents one of four levels of consciousness: *A* for alert (which includes the classifications B/A/R, Q/A/R, and lethargic); *V* for a patient that responds to a verbal stimulus (equivalent to obtunded); *P* for a patient that responds to only a painful stimulus (equivalent to stuporous); and *U* for an unresponsive patient (equivalent to comatose). Although this system is not currently in common use in veterinary medicine, it can easily be applied to veterinary patients. Table 2-2 summarizes the methods used to assess LOC.

## Pain Score

Assessment of the patient's level of pain should be included as a routine part of the patient assessment. The pain score will help guide selection of preanesthetic and anesthetic agents. Refer to Chapter 7 for a discussion of methods used to determine the pain score.

| TABLE 2-2 | Assessment of Level of Consciousness (LOC) | | |
|---|---|---|---|
| Signs | | LOC (Traditional) | AVPU Scale |
| Fully conscious, alert, engaged and interested in the environment. | | Bright, alert, responsive (B/A/R) | A (Alert) |
| Fully conscious and alert but not engaged, owing to fear, pain, illness, or any other cause. Subdued or quiet. | | Quiet, alert, responsive (Q/A/R) | A (Alert) |
| Mildly depressed. Is aware of surroundings. Can be aroused with minimal difficulty (verbal or tactile stimulus). | | Lethargic | A (Alert) |
| Very depressed. Uninterested in surroundings. Responds to but cannot be fully aroused by a verbal or tactile stimulus. | | Obtunded | V (Responds to a verbal stimulus) |
| A sleeplike state. Nonresponsive to a verbal stimulus. Can be aroused only by a painful stimulus. | | Stuporous | P (Responds only to a painful stimulus) |
| Sleeplike state. Cannot be aroused by any means. | | Comatose | U (Unresponsive) |

| TABLE 2-3 | Normal Vital Signs in Nonanesthetized Patients | | | |
|---|---|---|---|---|
| Species | Body Temperature | Heart Rate | Heart Rhythm | Respiratory Rate and Character |
| Dog | 100°-102.5° F (37.8°-39.2° C) | 60-180* | NSR or SA | 10-30 (panting is normal) |
| Cat | 100°-102.5° F (37.8°-39.2° C) | 120-240 | NSR only | 15-30 |
| Horse | 99°-100.5° F (37.2°-38° C) | 30-45 | NSR, SA, or first- or second-degree AV block | 8-20 |
| Cow | 100°-102.5° F (37.8°-39.2° C) | 60-80 | NSR or SA | 8-20 |
| Sheep/goat | 102°-104° F (38.9°-40° C) | 60-90 | NSR or SA | 16-24 |
| All species | | | | Normal effort and $V_T$ |

*AV, Atrioventricular; NSR, normal sinus rhythm; SA, sinus arrhythmia; $V_T$, tidal volume.*
*Owing to the extreme variability of size, large dogs tend to have lower rates, whereas small dogs and puppies have higher rates.

## Body Temperature

Body temperature is best determined using a rectal thermometer. Table 2-3 shows normal body temperatures in nonanesthetized animals. A high body temperature most commonly indicates an inflammatory condition, which must be identified and may require pretreatment with antibiotics, antiinflammatories, or other medication. A significantly low body temperature may be associated with one of a number of serious systemic disorders.

## General Condition

The patient's general condition refers to findings that are revealed by visually examining the patient at a distance including gait, temperament, and activity level.

### Gait

*Gait* refers to the manner in which the patient moves. A patient with a normal gait places approximately equal weight on all limbs as it walks. A lame patient places unequal weight on the limbs, limps or carries a limb, and may have sensitive or painful areas. Any of these signs may indicate a musculoskeletal disorder that may require treatment during the procedure or, in some cases, may indicate a nervous or systemic disorder that would increase anesthetic risk.

### Temperament and Activity Level

The animal's temperament and activity level will affect the selection of anesthetic agents. For instance, an animal that is anxious or excited may override the effects of a phenothiazine tranquilizer. In this case, combining a phenothiazine tranquilizer with an opioid or giving a more potent agent such as an alpha$_2$-agonist may be preferable. An ill patient may be excessively sedated with a standard dose of acepromazine, and the veterinarian may choose to reduce the dose of acepromazine, give a milder agent, or omit sedation entirely. Special handling techniques such as anesthetic chamber inductions, oral administration of ketamine, or the use of intramuscular (IM) alpha$_2$-agonists or Telazol (tiletamine-zolazepam) may be necessary to restrain feral or extremely aggressive patients without endangering hospital staff.

Exercise intolerance or weakness can indicate a variety of disorders that may affect anesthetic outcome including anemia, heart disease, or electrolyte disturbances. When observed from a distance, a weak patient will be reluctant to rise, may not stand for long, or may appear unsteady on its feet. An exercise-intolerant patient will tire quickly. These patients may require alternative anesthetic protocols or treatment before the anesthetic procedure.

## Examination of Exterior Surfaces

Examination of exterior surfaces consists of examination of the hair coat, the skin, lymph nodes, mammary glands, and body openings.

### Coat Condition

The hair coat should be shiny, full, and smooth. A rough hair coat, alopecia, and external parasites should be noted and reported. Although external infestations with ear mites, lice, fleas, ticks, or other parasites may not directly affect the anesthetic management, affected animals may require treatment during or after the anesthetic procedure.

### Skin

Part the hair and examine the skin over the entire body including ventral surfaces. Run your hands over the entire body surface, as many masses may be hidden in the fur or on a part of the body difficult to see such as the axilla or groin. Redness, inflammation, masses, or wounds should be noted and reported. **Ecchymoses, purpura,** or **petechiae** on the skin or mucous membranes, in the absence of trauma, indicate a clotting disorder, which will increase the risk of potentially life-threatening intraoperative and postoperative bleeding.

### Lymph Nodes and Mammary Glands

Examine the superficial lymph nodes and mammary glands for masses or swellings. This is best done with a combination of visual examination and palpation. Lymph nodes, if normal, should be very small or nonpalpable in small animal patients. Enlarged lymph nodes in any patient may indicate the presence of infection, inflammation, or neoplasia.

### Body Openings

Examine all body openings for odors and discharges. In intact females, examine the patient for signs of estrus or milk production. Common causes of putrid (foul smelling) odors include dental disease, external ear infections, abscesses, urogenital infections, diarrhea, and skin infections. Patients with severe kidney failure may have azotemic (urine-like) breath, and patients with ketonemia from complicated diabetes mellitus may have a characteristic odor to the breath. Some of the conditions that cause odors or discharges, such as kidney failure and diabetes, may necessitate treatment before anesthesia. Some, such as pyometra, may necessitate a change in the anesthetic protocol, and many others including dental disease, abscesses, and ear infections may require treatment while the patient is anesthetized.

## Examination of the Eyes, Ears, Nose, and Oral Cavity

The eyes, ears, nose, and oral cavity are often referred to as the "eyes, ears, nose, and throat" or EENT. Normal patients should not have discharges, inflammation, or swelling involving the oral cavity, ears, or nose. The eyes should be central, corneas should be clear, and eye discharge or redness should not be present.

Air should move freely and quietly through the nares during breathing. **Stridor** may indicate an upper airway infection or obstruction. Any disorder that could impede endotracheal intubation, such as the presence of redundant tissue in the oropharynx, tumors, or jaw fractures, should be noted, because it may be necessary to intubate a patient so affected through a tracheotomy incision. The gingivae and mucous membranes should be pink and should not be inflamed, bleed, or show bruising.

Note the amount of dental tartar. Because dental cleanings must be performed using chemical restraint, it is commonplace to clean the teeth during the same anesthetic event used to perform another surgery or procedure as long as there is no anticipated detrimental effect of performing both procedures together. Combining two procedures minimizes the number of anesthetic events, decreases the number of visits to the clinic, and in most cases also costs less. Therefore identification of dental disease before anesthesia increases safety, value, convenience, and client satisfaction.

> **TECHNICIAN NOTE** Dental cleanings are commonly performed during the same anesthetic event used to perform another surgery or procedure. Combining two procedures minimizes the number of anesthetic events, decreases the number of visits to the clinic, and in most cases also costs less.

### Assessment of the Pupillary Light Reflex

To check the pupillary light reflex (PLR), first observe and compare the size of both pupils, which should be of equal diameter. The size depends on the amount of ambient light entering the eye, the patient's level of excitement, patient health, and the effect of medications. Next direct a bright light (usually from a penlight or other portable light source) into the right eye with the beam directed toward the medial aspect of the retina, as this region is more sensitive to light. Note the size of the right pupil (direct reflex). Pupil constriction (**miosis**) is normal, whereas failure to constrict in the presence of light is abnormal. While still directing the light in the right eye, observe the pupil size in the left eye (consensual reflex); in a normal patient the left pupil should constrict the same amount as the right pupil (Figure 2-3). Finally repeat the process on the left eye, looking for both a direct and consensual response. Note that the PLR may be diminished in excited animals or after the administration of some anesthetic agents and adjuncts including anticholinergics and opioids.

## Cardiovascular System Examination

### Determination of the Heart Rate and Rhythm

The heart rate and rhythm are generally most easily evaluated by **auscultation** of the heart over the left chest wall at the point of maximal intensity. With experience, the heart rate in beats per minute (bpm) can be accurately determined in small animals by counting the number of beats in 10 seconds and multiplying the number by 6. Large animal patients have slower heart rates; therefore

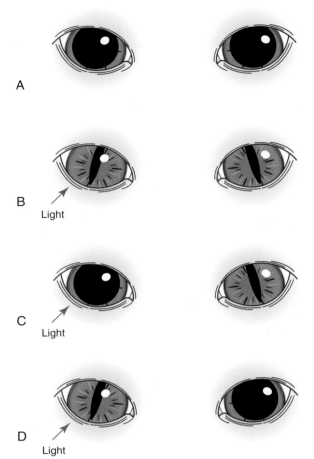

**FIGURE 2-3** Pupillary light reflex. **A,** Normal pupils. **B,** Direct and consensual light reflex (normal). **C,** Consensual but no direct light reflex (abnormal). **D,** Direct but no consensual light reflex (abnormal).

counting for a period of 30 seconds and multiplying by 2 is more accurate. The heart may be difficult to assess, however, in obese patients, panting dogs, and purring cats, so the anesthetist must be familiar with techniques to deal with these situations. In obese patients (especially cats) the audible intensity of the heartbeat is often decreased. Sometimes palpation for the apical pulse is helpful to locate the optimal area for placement of the diaphragm of the stethoscope. When the apical pulse is not palpable, the anesthetist must carefully search in the region of the left axilla for a spot where the heart is most audible. This requires systematic, small measured changes in the position of the stethoscope head until the optimal area is located. A decreased heart sound intensity in a nonobese patient may indicate pericardial or pleural effusion. Suspicion of either of these conditions should be communicated to the VIC.

> **TECHNICIAN NOTE** The heart rate in beats/minute (bpm) can be accurately determined in small animals by counting the number of beats in 10 seconds and multiplying the number by 6 or in large animals by counting the number in 30 seconds and multiplying by 2.

When panting prevents determination of a dog's heart rate, the muzzle can be gently held closed for a brief time to stop the pant, although this will cause some patients to struggle. In these patients, blow gently in the nose or distract the patient. One of these actions may stop the panting long enough to determine the rate. Do not attempt these techniques in aggressive patients if you are concerned for your safety.

Purring in cats can sometimes be stopped by distracting the patient or by turning on the tap in a sink and allowing the patient to see a gentle stream of running water from a distance. If this does not work, gradually bring the patient closer to the stream or increase the flow until the purring stops. Use caution as some cats are more fearful of water than others and may scratch or bite if brought too close to the water.

Normal heart rates (see Table 2-3) are generally inversely proportional to body size (faster in smaller species and breeds and slower in larger species and breeds). In all species, pediatric patients tend to have higher rates than adults. Exercise or the stress of handling may cause the heart rate to increase. The heart rate should be measured when the patient is calm, not after stressful events such as inserting a rectal thermometer or collecting a blood sample.

Normal heart rhythms vary according to the species (see Table 2-3). Normal dogs may have either a normal sinus rhythm (NSR) or a sinus arrhythmia (SA). Cats and most other exotic mammals such as rabbits, ferrets, and rodents should always have an NSR, as an SA is not normal in these species. Horses and ruminants usually have an NSR or SA. Horses may also exhibit first- or second-degree block when at rest but will have an NSR after exercise. The sound of these rhythms is summarized below in the following paragraphs.

**Normal Sinus Rhythm.** Normal sinus rhythm is a completely regular rhythm with no irregularities or pauses between beats, although the rate may change in response to excitement level.

**Sinus Arrhythmia.** Sinus arrhythmia is a rhythm in which the heart rate cyclically increases during inspiration and decreases during expiration. This rhythm may be pronounced in young, healthy dogs and can sound to the inexperienced anesthetist as if there are skipped or premature beats. Abnormal rhythms can be differentiated from sinus arrhythmia by observing the respirations while listening to the heart. Abnormal rhythms are not associated with the breathing.

**First-Degree Atrioventricular Heart Block.** First-degree atrioventricular (AV) heart block is caused by a conduction delay through the AV node and is recognized by a prolonged PR interval on an electrocardiographic tracing. This rhythm causes no noticeable change in the heart sounds and therefore can be detected only by electrocardiography.

**Second-Degree Atrioventricular Heart Block.** Second-degree AV heart block is caused by a periodic block of electrical conduction through the AV node and is recognized by missing QRS complexes. On auscultation, periodic pauses representing skipped beats are audible. Note that it is not normal for more than one beat to be skipped in a row.

Any abnormal rhythms must be reported to the VIC, as they may be exacerbated or become life-threatening during anesthesia. (More detail regarding these rhythms may be found in Chapter 5.)

> **TECHNICIAN NOTE**  Sinus arrhythmia is a rhythm in which the heart rate cyclically increases during inspiration and decreases during expiration. This rhythm may be pronounced in young, healthy dogs and can sound to the inexperienced anesthetist as if there are skipped or premature beats. Abnormal rhythms can be differentiated from sinus arrhythmia by observing the respirations while listening to the heart.

## Examination for Murmurs

During auscultation, also check for heart murmurs. Listen over each valve and place the stethoscope diaphragm into the cranial-most aspect of the left axilla, as some murmurs including those associated with patent ductus arteriosus are often audible only in this location. Murmurs are caused by turbulence associated with abnormal flow of blood and often indicate a variety of conditions such as a leaking valve, a stenotic valve or vessel, or an abnormal communication between heart chambers, any of which may increase anesthetic risk.

## Palpation of the Pulse and Comparison with the Heart Rate

In the conscious dog and cat the pulse is most easily palpated at the femoral artery, on the medial side of the rear leg. The patient should be standing quietly, and the femoral artery should be located by cupping the hand around the medial aspect of the thigh with the pad of the first or second finger in the groin just over the femur (see Figure 5-17, *B*). Other sites that may be palpable on medium to large dogs include the metatarsal and metacarpal arteries. In large animals the pulse may be palpated at the facial artery, digital artery, ventral tail, and auricular artery.

A strong, regular pulse should closely follow each audible heartbeat. If there are more heartbeats than pulses, a pulse deficit exists, which may indicate the presence of cardiovascular disease.

Palpation of the pulse also may give a crude estimate of blood pressure. A weak or nonpalpable pulse suggests hypotension, whereas an exaggerated pulse suggests hypertension. Realize that this is not always reliable because many other factors including body conformation, drugs, patient temperament, and excitement may affect either the strength of the pulse or the ability of the anesthetist to feel it.

## Assessment of Mucous Membrane Color and Capillary Refill Time

The standard site for assessment is the gingiva at the base of a tooth. Normal mucous membrane color is sometimes described as "bubblegum pink." Capillary refill time is assessed by applying digital pressure on the gingiva until blanching occurs, releasing pressure, and then observing the amount of time it takes for the return of normal color (see Figure 5-16). Normal refill time is less than 2 seconds. Pale mucous membranes or prolonged capillary refill time is indicative of decreased perfusion from shock, vasoconstriction, hypotension, or a variety of other conditions. Pale mucous membranes can also be associated with anemia. Cyanotic mucous membranes indicate reduced oxygen saturation, which is a medical emergency. Any of these conditions will increase anesthetic risk and must be treated before the procedure. If the gingivae are pigmented, mucous membrane color and capillary refill time may be observed at other sites, such as the conjunctiva of the lower eyelid, the entrance to the vulva, or the tip of the prepuce.

> **TECHNICIAN NOTE**  Pale mucous membranes or prolonged capillary refill time are indicative of decreased perfusion from shock, vasoconstriction, hypotension, or a variety of other issues. Pale mucous membranes can also be associated with anemia. Cyanotic mucous membranes indicate reduced oxygen saturation, which is a medical emergency.

## Respiratory System Examination

### Determination of Respiratory Rate and Character

The respiratory rate in breaths per minute and respiratory character are best evaluated by visually observing chest excursions. In most cases the respiratory rate can be accurately determined in small and large animals by counting the breaths in 30 seconds and multiplying the result by 2. Auscultation is not a particularly useful tool for assessing respirations. As with the heart rate, the respiratory rate is generally inversely proportional to body size and age and will be affected by exercise or stress. Normal dogs may pant during examination. In this situation, as long as respiratory effort is normal, the rate may be entered in the medical record as "pant" instead of attempting to count the rate. (See Table 2-3 for normal respiratory rates in nonanesthetized animals.)

*Respiratory character* refers to other aspects of respirations including effort, relative length of inhalation and exhalation, and regularity. Patients with a normal respiratory cycle should inhale, immediately exhale, and then briefly rest before the next inhalation. Exhalation should be about twice as long as inhalation. Normal respirations should be even, smooth, and minimally visible when the patient is at rest.

Dyspneic patients may exhibit mouth breathing, flared nostrils, excessive panting, exaggerated chest or abdominal movements on inspiration, wheezing, and reluctance to lie down. In extreme cases a dyspneic animal may exhibit **cyanosis. Dyspnea** and cyanosis are both medical emergencies and should be brought to the veterinarian's attention immediately. Avoid stressing dyspneic or cyanotic patients, as they are very intolerant of handling and can die during examination.

> **TECHNICIAN NOTE**  Dyspnea and cyanosis are both medical emergencies and should be brought to the veterinarian's attention immediately. Avoid stressing dyspneic or cyanotic patients, as they are very intolerant of handling and can die during examination.

### Auscultation of the Lungs

Assess the lungs by auscultating each of the four quadrants of the thorax (the right and left anteroventral lung fields and the right and left dorsal lung fields). In normal, calm patients the lung sounds should be very quiet. The presence of discontinuous lung sounds (crackles, rales, or rhonchi) or continuous sounds (wheezes) may indicate either pulmonary conditions (including pneumonia, bronchial disease, or asthma) or heart failure.

### Abdominal Palpation and Auscultation

The normal abdomen should be soft to the touch and not painful. In small animals, most normal organs are difficult to feel except for a full urinary bladder, full colon, and, in cats, kidneys. Any firm or painful structure or any organ that feels larger than normal should be reported. Abdominal distention may indicate ascites, pregnancy, organ enlargement, or the presence of tumors. In large animals abdominal auscultation is used to detect normal **borborygmus** (gut sounds). Borborygmus should be present in all four abdominal quadrants in horses. In ruminants, normal contraction of the rumen is audible in the left paralumbar fossa.

### Preanesthetic Diagnostic Workup

After the history and physical examination are completed, the veterinarian will decide which diagnostic tests (if any) are recommended for a given patient. The technician will then obtain appropriate samples (blood, urine, feces, or other samples) and will either perform the tests or forward the samples to a diagnostic laboratory for testing.

There are no universal guidelines for preanesthetic diagnostic tests, but each facility has standard policies. Some tests may be routinely recommended for every animal scheduled for anesthesia; different test groupings may be recommended for different patient groups such as geriatric patients, patients undergoing elective surgeries, and sick patients; or recommended tests may be based on

| TABLE 2-4 | Preanesthetic Diagnostic Test Recommendations | | |
|---|---|---|---|
| Species | ASA Physical Status Classification | Age | Recommended Tests |
| Dogs*/ cats† | P1 and P2 | <5 Years | PCV and PP |
| | P1 and P2 | >5 Years | CBC/chemistry profile |
| | P3-P5 | Any age | As ordered by the VIC |
| Ruminants | P1 and P2 | Any age | PCV and PP |
| | P3-P5 | Any age | As ordered by the VIC |
| Horses | P1 and P2 | Any age | CBC and PP |
| | P3-P5 | Any age | As ordered by the VIC |

*ASA*, American Society of Anesthesiologists; *CBC*, complete blood count; *PCV*, packed cell volume; *PP*, plasma protein.
*Heartworm testing is recommended for all dogs. Some clinics may extend this requirement to feline patients as well.
†All cats should be screened for feline leukemia virus (FeLV) and feline immunodeficiency virus (FIV) before anesthesia.

the physical status class. The veterinarian may customize tests on the basis of the patient's age, the history, and the results of the physical examination. Financial and other considerations may affect the number and type of tests the client chooses to approve. If the client declines one or more tests, a waiver should be signed indicating that the client understands the risk of proceeding without the information that would be provided by the declined tests. Table 2-4 lists sample preanesthetic diagnostic testing recommendations.

Common preanesthetic diagnostic tests and procedures include the complete blood count (CBC), blood chemistries, parasite screens, complete urinalysis, serologic tests, coagulation screen, electrocardiogram (ECG), and thoracic radiographs. Other tests may be ordered based on other conditions or illnesses that may be present. All test results must be recorded in the medical record and reviewed by the VIC before commencement of the procedure.

### Complete Blood Cell Count

The CBC is a comprehensive evaluation of blood cell numbers and morphology that includes packed cell volume (PCV), plasma protein (PP), hemoglobin, and total red blood cell (RBC), white blood cell (WBC), platelet, and absolute leukocyte counts. Normal values for these parameters are given in Table 2-5.

The PCV is a measurement of the percent of the total blood volume that is made up of whole RBCs. The total RBC count (erythrocyte count) is a direct measurement of the total number of RBCs in a fixed volume of blood.

| TABLE 2-5 | Normal Hematologic Values | | | |
|---|---|---|---|---|
| | Dog | Cat | Horse | Cow |
| Plasma protein (g/dL) | 5.7-7.2 | 5.6-7.4 | 6.5-7.8 | 7-9 |
| PCV (%) | 36-54 | 25-46 | 27-44 | 23-35 |
| Hb (g/dL) | 11.9-18.4 | 8.0-14.9 | 9.7-15.6 | 8.3-12.3 |
| RBC ($10^{12}$/L) | 4.9-8.2 | 5.3-10.2 | 5.1-10.0 | 5-7.5 |
| Total leukocytes ($\times 10^9$/L) | 4.1-15.2 | 4.0-14.5 | 4.7-10.6 | 3.0-13.5 |
| Neutrophil— segmented ($\times 10^9$/L) | 3-10.4 | 3-9.2 | 2.4-6.4 | 0.7-5.1 |
| Neutrophil— band ($\times 10^9$/L) | 0-0.1 | 0-0.1 | 0-0.1 | 0-0.1 |
| Lymphocytes ($\times 10^9$/L) | 1-4.6 | 0.9-3.9 | 1-4.9 | 1.1-8.2 |
| Monocytes ($\times 10^9$/L) | 0-1.2 | 0-0.5 | 0-0.5 | 0-0.6 |
| Eosinophils ($\times 10^9$/L) | 0-1.3 | 0-1.2 | 0-0.3 | 0-1.5 |
| Basophils ($\times 10^9$/L) | 0 | 0-0.2 | 0-0.1 | 0-0.1 |
| Platelets ($\times 10^9$/L) | 106-424 | 150-600 | 125-310 | 192-746 |

Modified from Muir WW, Hubbell JA, Bednarski RM: *Handbook of veterinary anesthesia*, ed 4, St Louis, 2006, Mosby.
*Hb*, Hemoglobin; *PCV*, packed cell volume; *RBC*, red blood cells.

Both tests are indicators of the oxygen-carrying capacity of the blood.

An elevated PCV or RBC count is most often caused by dehydration and is of concern to the anesthetist because of the associated decrease in blood volume, which may adversely affect cardiac output, blood pressure, and tissue perfusion.

In contrast, a decreased PCV or RBC count indicates anemia caused by decreased production, loss, or destruction of RBCs. Anemia results in a decreased capacity to supply oxygen to the tissues. Because the effects of anesthesia often increase the risk of tissue hypoxia, anemia must not be ignored. When a significant anemia is present, the veterinarian may recommend that anesthesia be postponed until it is corrected. A PCV less than 25% in a dog or less than 20% in a cat, horse, or cow should be reported immediately.

The PP is a measurement of blood protein including albumin, globulins, and fibrinogen. As with an elevated PCV, hyperproteinemia may be associated with dehydration and the same potential adverse consequences mentioned previously.

Hypoproteinemia usually results from decreased protein production by the liver or increased loss from the gastrointestinal tract or kidneys or from blood loss. Many anesthetics circulate in the blood partially bound to plasma proteins and partially free. Only the portion of the drug that is free and unbound can exert an effect. In patients with hypoproteinemia, the unbound portion proportionately increases, increasing drug potency. Hypoproteinemic patients also have difficulty maintaining adequate blood volume and may develop tissue edema because of the decreased oncotic pressure in the vascular system. For these reasons, a PP less than 4.0 in a patient of any species should be reported immediately.

The total WBC and absolute leukocyte counts (calculated from the total WBC and the differential WBC counts) measure the total number of leukocytes and the numbers of each type of leukocyte (neutrophils, lymphocytes, monocytes, eosinophils, and basophils). Changes in these counts may be associated with infection, parasitism, leukemias, and many other conditions that may be exacerbated by anesthesia and surgery or may increase anesthetic risk. The blood smear evaluation reveals changes in blood cell morphology, inclusions, parasites, and other conditions that may influence preanesthetic patient management. Interpretation of these tests is complex and beyond the scope of this chapter.

The platelet count is necessary to evaluate the mechanical component of blood coagulation. Patients with **thrombocytopenia** are at higher risk for abnormal intraoperative and postoperative bleeding, and their condition must be stabilized before surgery. Any decrease in platelet numbers should be reported to the VIC immediately.

*TECHNICIAN NOTE* The following findings should be reported to the VIC immediately:
- A PCV <25% in a dog or <20% in a cat, horse, or cow
- A PP <4.0 in any species
- Any decrease in the platelet count
- Any coagulation test result outside the normal range

## Urinalysis

The complete urinalysis provides information about both the urinary and nonurinary systems.

The kidney function is of particular interest to the anesthetist, as it plays an important role in regulating electrolyte and water balance, blood pressure, and elimination of many anesthetics. If there is protein in the urine or if the urine specific gravity is less than 1.030 in a canine sample, 1.035 in a feline sample, or 1.025 in a large animal sample, the veterinarian should be notified because further tests may be needed to accurately assess kidney function.

Abnormalities in the macroscopic examination findings (color, clarity, and odor), biochemical analysis, and microscopic examination findings also may reveal evidence of diabetes mellitus, liver or kidney disease, or other systemic disorders that may affect patient anesthetic management. Abnormalities in any of these parts of the urinalysis should be reported and investigated.

## Blood Chemistry Tests

A wide variety of blood chemistry tests are available that assess circulating enzymes, electrolytes, proteins, and metabolites. These tests give information about organ health and function, help the veterinarian formulate the anesthetic plan, screen for conditions that increase patient risk, influence patient perianesthetic management, and allow preparation for potential complications. Chemistry tests are often grouped in preanesthetic profiles that may assess one body organ such as the kidney, the liver, or the pancreas or may provide a comprehensive evaluation of all organ systems. The interpretation of these tests is complex, so any abnormalities should be reported to the veterinarian.

## Blood Coagulation Screens

Blood coagulation screens evaluate the chemical, and sometimes mechanical components of blood coagulation. This is particularly important before nonelective surgeries because various disorders may adversely affect blood coagulation and put surgery patients at high risk for intraoperative and postoperative hemorrhage. A coagulation panel, including a prothrombin time (PT) and activated partial thromboplastin time (APTT), should be performed on any patient that may have a preexisting coagulation disorder (such as those with end-stage liver disease) or animals of breeds known to be commonly affected by hereditary coagulation disorders, such as Doberman pinschers, Rottweilers, and Scottish terriers. Coagulation panels may be performed at reference laboratories or in house. Any abnormal coagulation test result should be reported to the VIC immediately. The buccal mucosal bleeding time is an in-house screening test that can be used in patients, including those with normal platelet counts and coagulation panels, to determine the likelihood of perioperative bleeding (Procedure 2-1, p. 42).

> *TECHNICIAN NOTE* The buccal mucosal bleeding time is a simple in-house screening test that is an excellent indicator of the likelihood of perioperative bleeding.

## Electrocardiogram

The ECG records the electrical activity of the heart, allowing the veterinarian to assess heart rhythm. Although not routine, an ECG is recommended for those patients with known or suspected heart disease, chest trauma, **gastric dilatation-volvulus,** splenic disease, or electrolyte disturbances or that are on medications that affect heart rhythm. The ECG also can be used to screen for cardiac disease in geriatric or other high-risk patients. Because most anesthetic agents alter heart rate, cardiac output, and oxygen consumption to some degree, patients with heart disease are at much greater risk for anesthetic complications. (ECGs are further discussed in Chapter 5.)

## Radiography

Although not routine, thoracic radiography is warranted in animals that show signs of cardiac or pulmonary disease.

Thoracic and abdominal radiographs are indicated for animals with major trauma (such as having been hit by a car) to rule out conditions that could increase patient risk or require modification of the protocol such as diaphragmatic hernia, pneumothorax, pleural effusion, pulmonary contusions, bladder rupture, or intraabdominal bleeding.

## Miscellaneous Tests

Depending on patient need, existing illness, the geographic location of the practice, and other factors, other diagnostic tests may be routinely performed before anesthesia. For example, most veterinary practices in areas where heartworm disease is endemic require a heartworm test for all dogs and in some cases cats before any anesthetic procedure.

## DETERMINATION OF THE PHYSICAL STATUS CLASSIFICATION

Before selecting the anesthetic protocol, the VIC should evaluate the minimum patient database and assign a **physical status classification.** The most widely accepted classification system is the one adopted by the American Society of Anesthesiologists (ASA), which is summarized in Table 2-6. This system rates patient risk from minimal (class P1) to extreme (class P5) based on the patient's health.

In general, class P1 and class P2 patients can be safely anesthetized with standard anesthetic protocols. Class P3 to P5 patients often require special protocols, and their condition should be stabilized before surgery if possible. Patients undergoing emergency anesthesia may also be assigned an additional letter E regardless of class (e.g., P2E or P5E).

Classification of risk is somewhat subjective and may change over time. Two anesthetists might disagree, for example, on whether a patient with a moderate anemia should be assigned to class P2 (low risk) or class P3 (moderate risk). A patient in shock might be downgraded to a lower risk classification after receiving appropriate IV fluid therapy. Nevertheless, this system gives the anesthetist some basis for making patient management decisions that will minimize risk. The physical status class should be recorded in the animal's medical record and in the anesthetic logbook.

> *TECHNICIAN NOTE* In general, class P1 and class P2 patients can be safely anesthetized with standard anesthetic protocols. Class P3 to P5 patients often require special protocols, and their condition should be stabilized before surgery if possible.

## SELECTION OF THE ANESTHETIC PROTOCOL

As mentioned in the previous sections, the technician acting as anesthetist should not hesitate to discuss abnormal findings from the minimum database with

**TABLE 2-6 American Society of Anesthesiologists Physical Status Classifications**

| Classification | Risk | Criteria | Representative Conditions |
|---|---|---|---|
| P1 | Minimal | Normal, healthy patient | Patients undergoing elective procedures (ovariohysterectomy, castration, or declaw) |
| P2 | Low | Patient with mild systemic disease | Neonatal, geriatric, or obese patients Mild dehydration Skin tumor removal |
| P3 | Moderate | Patient with severe systemic disease | Anemia Moderate dehydration Compensated major organ disease |
| P4 | High | Patient with severe systemic disease that is a constant threat to life | Ruptured bladder Internal hemorrhage Pneumothorax Pyometra |
| P5 | Extreme | Moribund patient that is not expected to survive without the operation | Severe head trauma Pulmonary embolus Gastric dilatation-volvulus End-stage major organ failure |

From Bassert JM, McCurnin DM: *McCurnin's clinical textbook for veterinary technicians,* ed 7, St Louis, 2010, Elsevier.

the veterinarian because such information may lead to changes in the planned anesthetic protocol. The presence of severe disease does not necessarily require that the procedure be postponed or canceled, although this may be the wisest course in some situations. It does often require selection of agents with which the anesthetist may be less familiar but that are less likely to produce adverse effects. For example the VIC may choose to use etomidate instead of propofol in a geriatric dog with heart failure because etomidate is much less likely to adversely affect cardiovascular function.

If the patient is very ill, the veterinarian may decide that the animal's condition must be stabilized before an anesthetic is administered. Patients that are severely dehydrated, are profoundly anemic, or have a serious systemic disease or electrolyte imbalance are poor anesthetic risks.

Every attempt should be made to correct these conditions before anesthesia, if time allows. If the planned procedure is not immediately necessary to save the patient's life, it is possible that anesthesia may safely be postponed.

## Factors That Influence Selection

In all jurisdictions in the United States and Canada, the veterinarian is the only health care provider legally allowed to choose (that is, prescribe) anesthetic drugs for animals. In most hospitals however, the veterinarian establishes one or two standard anesthetic protocols for physical status class P1 and P2 patients, with which the technician will quickly become familiar. However, each patient must be evaluated individually based on the minimum patient database, and changes must be made to the standard protocol when necessary. Although a technician with a strong knowledge base can help the veterinarian make an appropriate choice by communicating observations and suggestions regarding the patient, ultimately the VIC bears responsibility for the patient and must make the final decision regarding the anesthetic protocol.

When choosing the anesthetic protocol, the following factors must be considered.

### Facilities and Equipment

Some anesthetic protocols require the use of specialized equipment. For example, isoflurane and sevoflurane require the use of a precision vaporizer and an oxygen supply. In some circumstances such as equine field anesthesia, use of a machine is impractical or impossible.

### Familiarity with the Agent

Although for most patients any one of several anesthetic protocols is likely to result in a successful outcome, practitioners frequently choose the protocol with which they are most familiar. It is seldom advisable to anesthetize a high-risk patient with a new combination of drugs that the anesthetist may have heard or read about but has never tried before.

### Nature of the Procedure

Procedures vary in their duration and complexity. They also require different degrees of analgesia, immobilization, muscle relaxation, and CNS depression. For example, local anesthesia may be suitable for short procedures such as a skin biopsy in which the patient requires only anesthesia of the biopsy site and physical restraint but no CNS depression. On the other hand, general anesthesia is required for thoracic or abdominal surgery, which necessitates unconsciousness, immobility, generalized visceral and somatic analgesia, and muscle relaxation.

### Circumstances Specific to the Procedure

Anesthetics that may be appropriate for animals undergoing a routine operation (such as ovariohysterectomy or orchiectomy) may not be appropriate for a nonelective surgical procedure. For example, a cesarean section will require a protocol that minimizes respiratory depression in the neonates. In contrast, excellent muscle relaxation may be important for a fracture repair.

## Cost

In a situation in which two agents are comparable in terms of patient safety, it is reasonable to choose the less expensive option. In other situations such as the presence of cardiac disease, it may be important to choose a cardiac-sparing drug such as etomidate even though it is considerably more expensive than thiobarbiturates or propofol.

## Degree of Urgency

Critically injured animals may require rapid induction of anesthesia to initiate emergency therapy. For example, a patient that is in danger of shock because of ongoing uncontrolled hemorrhage cannot wait 15 to 20 minutes for a premedication given subcutaneously or intramuscularly to take effect. Selection of agents that allow for preservation of adequate blood pressure and rapid induction is desirable in this case.

## PREINDUCTION PATIENT CARE

During the preinduction period the technician should ensure that the patient is fasted and receives appropriate nursing care, fluid therapy, medication administration, and any other care ordered by the veterinarian. All treatments should be recorded in the medical record. A checklist of procedures may be helpful, particularly if more than one person is responsible for preanesthetic care.

## Withholding Food before Anesthesia

Animals that are anesthetized without prior fasting are prone to a variety of mild to serious complications that result from reflux of stomach contents into the distal esophagus, aspiration of stomach contents into the pulmonary tree, and bloating in ruminants (see Chapter 10).

Esophageal reflux commonly occurs during the anesthetic period as a result of decreased lower esophageal sphincter tone and flow of stomach acid into the esophagus that occurs when a patient is in a prone position. Esophageal reflux may cause irritation, inflammation, or, in extreme cases, severe tissue damage of the distal esophagus, resulting in stricture, and is recognized as a common cause of postoperative nausea, dysphagia, vomiting, and anorexia.

Vomiting is an active expulsion of stomach contents, preceded by retching, that occurs only in conscious patients. In contrast, **regurgitation** is a passive process that may occur in an unconscious or conscious patient, is not preceded by retching, and results in flow of stomach contents into the esophagus and mouth. Pulmonary aspiration occurs if the patient vomits or regurgitates during

| TABLE 2-7 | Fasting Recommendations | |
| --- | --- | --- |
| Species | Food Withholding Time (Hours) | Water Withholding Time (Hours) |
| Dogs and cats | 8-12* | 2-4 |
| Horses | 8-12 | 0-2 |
| Cattle | 24-48 | 8-12 |
| Small ruminants | 12-18 | 8-12 |
| Neonatal and pediatric patients (<8 weeks old) | None | None |

*Note that patients under 2 kg should be fasted for shorter lengths of time.

a time when the swallowing reflex is decreased or absent. Pulmonary aspiration is always serious and may lead to pneumonia that is difficult to treat, permanent disability, and in some cases even immediate respiratory arrest and death.

To prevent vomiting and minimize reflux during the anesthetic period, food should be withheld from most patients except for neonatal, pediatric, and some exotic patients. Table 2-7 lists fasting recommendations. The technician must ensure that fluids are administered as prescribed, because fasted patients are at higher risk for dehydration, especially if ill.

If a patient is known to have eaten within 12 hours of the proposed surgery and the surgery cannot be postponed, the veterinarian may choose to administer a preanesthetic with antiemetic properties (such as acepromazine), administer an agent that is likely to induce vomiting (such as xylazine in small animals) in order to empty the stomach, or proceed with heightened monitoring for regurgitation or vomiting.

> *TECHNICIAN NOTE* Pulmonary aspiration is always serious and may lead to pneumonia that is difficult to treat, permanent disability, and in some cases even immediate respiratory arrest and death of the patient. Unless told otherwise by the VIC, food should be withheld from all patients except for neonatal, pediatric, and some exotic patients.

Even if fasting recommendations are observed, vomiting may occur during the anesthetic or recovery period. Fasted patients sometimes vomit foam, bile, or mucus. At other times food may be vomited if a disorder exists that prevents the stomach from emptying, such as a foreign body, **ileus,** or a stricture. If vomiting occurs in the anesthetized patient, there is some protection against aspiration if a cuffed endotracheal tube is in place. This is the reason that the endotracheal tube must be left in place during recovery until the animal regains the swallowing reflex. (Methods for preventing and managing vomiting during anesthesia are discussed further in Chapter 12.)

Animals undergoing gastrointestinal procedures such as enterotomy, colonoscopy, or intestinal biopsy may require longer withholding times, enemas, or cathartics to minimize the amount of ingesta within the gastrointestinal tract at the time of surgery.

The anesthetist should be aware that although preanesthetic fasting is recommended, prolonged fasting is detrimental. Many seriously ill animals are anorexic and may refuse to eat. For example, a dog with severe trauma that requires prolonged hospitalization may be too uncomfortable, frightened, or weak to eat, and by the time it is released it may have gone without eating for several days. This lack of adequate intake impedes the healing process and prolongs recovery. For these reasons, efforts should be made to reestablish caloric intake by hand-feeding palatable foods, feeding by syringe bolus, or using feeding tubes or total parenteral nutrition.

## Patient Stabilization

Seriously ill patients may require significant nursing care before surgery for stabilization. For example, a patient with a pneumothorax and femoral fracture will need to have the pneumothorax stabilized before the fracture repair is performed. This care can be labor- and time-intensive but is a very important part of minimizing patient risk. Veterinary technicians are usually intimately involved in this process of stabilization. At times (for example, with a patient with a gastric torsion or uncontrolled internal bleeding) the veterinarian may decide that the risk of delaying surgery outweighs the increased anesthetic risk and will elect to proceed. These patients often pose the greatest test of the technician's skills and knowledge.

## INTRAVENOUS CATHETERIZATION

### Reasons for Intravenous Catheterization

Not all animals are catheterized before anesthesia; however, the presence of an IV catheter is of benefit to both the patient and the anesthetist for the following reasons:

1. Fluid administration helps to maintain blood volume and support blood pressure. Although not mandatory for routine operations in healthy patients, fluid administration is highly recommended under the following circumstances:
   - Patients undergoing any procedure that may result in significant blood loss (such as a cesarean section or removal of a splenic tumor).
   - **Debilitated** or dehydrated patients.
   - Patients with organ dysfunction or failure.
   - Patients with electrolyte abnormalities (for example, hyperkalemia).
   - Prolonged anesthesia (more than 1 hour).
   - Patients at risk for hypotension or shock. Even mild hypotension is a potential problem in anesthetized animals because it leads to decreased blood flow to the kidneys and other vital organs.
2. IV access allows rapid administration of emergency drugs such as epinephrine.
3. An IV catheter can be used for **constant rate infusion** (CRI) of anesthetics, analgesics, electrolytes, or other drugs such as insulin. CRI is slow, continuous administration of a drug at a rate sufficient to achieve the desired effect. For example, propofol is administered by CRI to maintain general anesthesia or to control seizures in patients with status epilepticus. Drugs given by CRI are either administered through an IV catheter with a syringe pump or added to an IV fluid bag and administered via an administration set and IV catheter.

   The use of an IV catheter is necessary for safe CRI of drugs because it is difficult to keep a needle seated in a vein for more than a few minutes, especially if the patient is moved from one location to another. Therefore attempting to administer CRIs via a needle and syringe is likely to result in perivascular drug injection.
4. **Vesicants** (anesthetic agents that damage tissues if injected perivascularly, such as thiopental) can be administered safely. Some vesicants are so irritating to tissues that injection of even an extremely small amount can cause tissue irritation and **sloughing.** Perivascular injection is much more likely when a syringe and needle are used.
5. Incompatible drugs can be administered more easily via an IV catheter. For example diazepam and hydromorphone will precipitate when mixed because hydromorphone is water-soluble and diazepam is not. When administering this drug combination intravenously, each drug must be injected separately with saline flush in between to prevent mixing. Sequential injections are very cumbersome to administer by venipuncture with a needle and syringe without the risk of inadvertent perivascular injection or without breaking aseptic technique.

### Choosing and Placing an Intravenous Catheter

Two main types of IV catheters are in common use for fluid and drug administration in veterinary patients: through-the-needle catheters and over-the-needle catheters. Although commonly used in critical care patients, through-the-needle catheters are not frequently used for anesthesia because they are more complex, expensive, and time-consuming to place, especially if the technician is not experienced with their use.

Over-the-needle catheters are more commonly used in general practice for patients receiving anesthesia and in most cases serve this purpose well because they are inexpensive, readily available, and relatively easy to place. Procedure 2-2, p. 44, shows the sequence of events used to place a catheter in a small animal patient. Typically, 16- to 24-gauge, ¾- to 2-inch catheters are used in small animal anesthesia, and 12- to 16-gauge, 5¼-inch catheters are used in cattle and horses.

---

*TECHNICIAN NOTE*    When placing and maintaining an IV catheter for use during surgery:

- Choose a catheter of sufficient length to minimize the risk of dislodgement.
- Choose a catheter of large diameter.
- Choose a location that will not interfere with the procedure.
- Use an administration set with an injection port.
- After positioning the patient, check that fluids are flowing freely.
- Avoid excessive catheter and patient movement during transfer.
- Administer IV drugs slowly.
- Use saline flush following IV injection of a drug.

---

When used for anesthetic management, the basic principles of catheter placement and maintenance are no different than when used for any other purpose. However, there are several special considerations that apply specifically to catheter maintenance and fluid administration during anesthesia:

- It is important to choose a catheter of sufficient length and to secure it carefully to prevent it from being dislodged during patient transfer (such as from surgical preparation to the operating room to recovery).
- When possible, choose a large-diameter catheter in case rapid fluid administration is necessary, as would be the case with excessive blood loss or hypotension.
- The catheter must be placed in a location that will not interfere with the procedure. For instance, if an orthopedic procedure is to be performed on the left front limb, the catheter must be placed in the right front limb, a rear limb, or some other site.
- Be sure to use an administration set with an injection port, so that IV medications can be administered when necessary. Procedure 2-3, p. 46, shows the sequence of events used to administer medications through an IV administration set port.
- Because surgery patients are placed in various positions most conducive to exposure of the surgery site, limb ties or the limb position itself may impede flow of fluids. This must be kept in mind when positioning and securing the patient to ensure that fluids are flowing freely.
- Movement of the catheter and patient during patient transfer may result in the introduction of air into the vein (known as an *air embolism*) through the administration line. This must be avoided, because a large air embolus is life-threatening.
- Drugs administered via a catheter must be given slowly. Most drugs should be given over a period of 15 to 60 seconds, although some, such as sodium bicarbonate and potassium chloride, must be given much more slowly.
- When administering drugs IV, be sure to flush the entire dose of drug into the vein after each bolus. This will prevent dosage errors.

## FLUID ADMINISTRATION

All animals have a fundamental physiologic need for a constant source of oxygen delivered to all body tissues in quantities necessary to perform basic metabolic functions. An absence of adequate oxygen will rapidly damage any tissues so deprived and will result in cell death in high-demand tissues such as the brain and heart muscle within minutes.

One of the primary functions of the cardiovascular and respiratory systems is to supply this need by extracting oxygen from the air and conveying it directly to every cell in the body. For this reason, agents that adversely affect cardiopulmonary function have the potential for decreasing oxygen delivery. As nearly all anesthetic agents adversely affect these systems, constant attention to cardiopulmonary support is one of the cornerstones of the successful practice of anesthesia.

There are several specific ways in which anesthetic agents affect cardiopulmonary function. Almost all anesthetic agents decrease the force of heart muscle contraction (referred to as **inotropy**) and cause bradycardia. These factors in turn decrease the flow of blood from the heart (**cardiac output**). Almost all agents also relax the muscle tone of blood vessels, which in turn causes an increase in the intravascular volume (vasodilatation). Together the decreased cardiac output and vasodilatation cause hypotension and decrease the perfusion of tissues with blood.

Administration of intravenous fluids is one of the primary tools available to the anesthetist to support oxygen delivery. Fluids increase circulating blood volume and cardiac output—two physiologic changes that support blood pressure and tissue perfusion.

### Composition of Body Fluids

Water is the most prevalent substance in the body. In adult animals, about 60% of the body weight is water. Because of variation associated with age and body fat content, young and lean patients have a somewhat higher percentage, whereas old and obese patients have a somewhat lower percentage. Body water is separated by cell membranes into intracellular (within the cells) and extracellular (outside of the cells) fluid compartments.

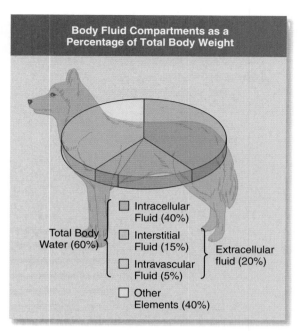

**Body Fluid Compartments as a Percentage of Total Body Weight**

- ☐ Intracellular Fluid (40%)
- ☐ Interstitial Fluid (15%)
- ☐ Intravascular Fluid (5%)
- ☐ Other Elements (40%)

Total Body Water (60%)

Extracellular fluid (20%)

**FIGURE 2-4** Body fluid compartments.

The extracellular fluid compartment is subdivided by the vascular endothelium into the interstitial fluid compartment (fluid in the tissues outside of the cells) and the intravascular compartment (fluid within the vascular system).

Of the 60% of the body weight that consists of water, about two thirds (or 40% of the body weight) is intracellular fluid (ICF). Although estimates of extracellular fluid (ECF) vary widely (about 15% to 30% of body weight for small animals), most clinicians use the figure 20% for the purpose of calculating fluid needs. About three fourths of the ECF (15% of the body weight) is interstitial fluid (fluid between the cells), and one fourth (5% of the total body weight) is intravascular fluid (plasma) (Figure 2-4). When blood cells are added, blood volume is considered to be 8% to 9% of body weight in dogs and large animals and 6% to 7% of body weight in cats. For this reason the figures 90 mL/kg for dogs and large animals and 60 mL/kg for cats are commonly used for the purpose of calculating blood volume.

Body fluids consist of water and **solutes.** Body fluid solutes are either atoms or molecules dissolved in body water. The solutes most important in fluid therapy are small–molecular-weight electrically charged particles called *ions,* large–molecular-weight plasma proteins called **colloids,** and small nonionic particles such as glucose and small proteins.

Electrolytes are substances that when dissolved separate into positively charged ions, called *cations* (so called because they migrate toward the cathode during electrolysis), and negatively charged ions, called *anions* (so called because they migrate toward the anode). Sodium chloride (NaCl or table salt) is an example of an electrolyte; when dissolved, it separates into the cation sodium and the anion chloride. Important cations in body fluids include sodium ($Na^+$), potassium ($K^+$), magnesium ($Mg^{2+}$) and calcium ($Ca^{2+}$). Important anions include chloride ($Cl^-$), bicarbonate ($HCO_3^-$), phosphates ($HPO_4^{2-}$, $H_2PO_4^-$), and proteins.

Solutes serve diverse purposes. Electrolytes provide osmotic pressure and are essential for many fundamental physiologic processes such as blood clotting, heart function, and neuromuscular function. Proteins participate in a wide variety of processes including drug transport, regulation of blood pressure by providing oncotic pressure, and blood clotting. Glucose provides energy to the cells.

## Fluid Homeostasis

**Homeostasis** refers to a constant state within the body created and maintained by normal physiologic processes. Maintenance of fluid homeostasis is a highly delicate and dynamic process. In health, water and solutes constantly move through cell membranes between fluid compartments as needed to maintain solute concentrations within a narrow and specific range. Many solutes move freely between body compartments by passive diffusion along gradients from areas of high concentration to those of low concentration. Others are confined to or concentrated in a particular space. For instance, owing to its extremely large size, albumin does not travel freely through the normal vascular endothelium but tends to concentrate within the intravascular space. Another example is potassium, which, because of active transport through the cell membranes, is concentrated within the cells (98% of $K^+$ is located within the cells). In contrast, sodium is largely excluded from the cells and thus is found in high concentrations in the extracellular space.

Consequently, the concentration of each of the major solutes often differs widely among the fluid compartments. For instance, ICF is very rich in potassium, magnesium, protein, and phosphate when compared with ECF. In contrast, ECF has much higher concentrations of sodium, chloride, and bicarbonate (Figure 2-5).

The balance of water and solutes in body fluids is governed by a number of principles, which, if known, help the anesthetist administer fluids in a way that is most beneficial to the patient. Some of these principles are as follows:

- At any given time, the number of negatively and positively charged particles in any given fluid compartment must be equal. Thus if the number of positively charged particles in a compartment increases, the number of negatively charged particles must increase by the same amount. This state of electrical balance in any fluid compartment is called *electroneutrality.*
- In health, a solute concentration or **osmolarity** of approximately 300 mOsm/L is maintained in all body fluids. Conditions including dehydration,

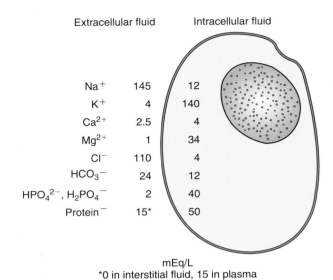

| Extracellular fluid | | Intracellular fluid |
| --- | --- | --- |
| $Na^+$ | 145 | 12 |
| $K^+$ | 4 | 140 |
| $Ca^{2+}$ | 2.5 | 4 |
| $Mg^{2+}$ | 1 | 34 |
| $Cl^-$ | 110 | 4 |
| $HCO_3^-$ | 24 | 12 |
| $HPO_4^{2-}, H_2PO_4^-$ | 2 | 40 |
| Protein$^-$ | 15* | 50 |

mEq/L
*0 in interstitial fluid, 15 in plasma

**FIGURE 2-5** Comparison of the average electrolyte concentrations in the extracellular and intracellular fluid compartments. (Modified from DiBartola S: *Fluid, electrolyte, and acid-base disorders,* ed 3, St Louis, 2006, Elsevier.)

exercise, heat stroke, and some cases of vomiting and diarrhea that involve primarily water loss will increase the osmolarity, and others such as chronic congestive heart failure, in which large quantities of solutes are lost, will decrease it.

- The solutes in each fluid compartment provide **osmotic pressure,** which draws water into that compartment in proportion to the number of particles present. For example, if the osmolarity in the vascular space increases or decreases, water will follow, increasing or decreasing the blood volume respectively.
- Small particle solutes such as ions diffuse freely through vascular endothelium, taking water with them. Thus they equilibrate relatively quickly between the intravascular and interstitial fluid spaces. The interstitial fluid compartment is at least twice the size of the intravascular compartment. Therefore at most only about one third of fluid administered intravenously remains in the vascular space after equilibration.
- Colloids including albumin do not diffuse freely through vascular endothelium. Their presence in the vascular space provides colloid osmotic pressure (also called **oncotic pressure**) that tends to draw water into the blood vessels and is thus important for maintenance of blood volume and pressure.
- The plasma concentration of certain solutes such as potassium and calcium must be kept in a very narrow range in order to maintain normal muscle and heart function. Relatively small deviations in levels of these cations can cause significant clinical signs and can endanger the patient.

> *TECHNICIAN NOTE*   The plasma concentration of certain solutes such as potassium and calcium must be kept in a very narrow range in order to maintain normal muscle and heart function. Relatively small deviations in levels of these cations can cause significant clinical signs and can endanger the patient.

## Fluid Needs during Anesthesia

During anesthesia, many factors including disease conditions, surgery, and effects of drugs often disrupt fluid homeostasis and require the anesthetist to intervene. Appropriate fluid therapy requires knowledge of the nature of fluid losses associated with disease conditions. Following are some common associations with general anesthesia:

- Fluid losses that occur from dehydration and many general disease conditions initially deplete the ECF space. For this reason, when replacing recent fluid losses in patients with disease, dehydration, or anorexia, fluids should be chosen with solute profiles similar to ECF.
- Perioperative hemorrhage involves fluid loss from the intravascular space, part of the ECF space. Thus, as in the previous example, fluids should be chosen with solute profiles similar to ECF, unless hemorrhage is profound.
- Profound perioperative hemorrhage involves significant loss of albumin, blood cells, and other constituents of blood in addition to electrolytes and water. To support patients experiencing severe perioperative hemorrhage, administration of blood products may be necessary to provide RBCs or hemoglobin to support oxygen-carrying capacity, and in some cases clotting factors and platelets to support normal coagulation.
- Patients with perioperative hemorrhage may also benefit from hypertonic saline or colloid solutions, both of which draw water into the vascular space and raise blood pressure.
- Patients with low albumin may require colloids or blood plasma (fluids containing large solutes), which provide oncotically active particles that remain in the vascular space for longer periods and help maintain blood volume and pressure.

## Classification of Intravenous Fluids

All IV fluids are solutions consisting of one or more solutes dissolved in water. Most IV fluids contain one or more electrolytes. Dextrose, a naturally occurring form of glucose, is another ingredient present in some fluids. Some fluids also contain the buffers lactate, gluconate, or acetate, which are converted to $HCO_3^-$ by the liver and help regulate pH. Others contain colloids (large–molecular-weight solutes).

There are many intravenous solutions, each with different solute profiles. These fluids are most commonly classified as either **crystalloids** or colloids based in the molecular weight of the primary solutes they contain.

## TABLE 2-8  Solute Composition of Selected Commercially Available Crystalloid Fluids

| Fluid | Dextrose (g/L) | Na+ (mEq/L) | Cl− (mEq/L) | K+ (mEq/L) | Ca2+ (mEq/L) | Mg2+ (mEq/L) | Buffer* (mEq/L) | Osmolarity (mOsm/L) | pH kCal/L | Fluid Type† |
|---|---|---|---|---|---|---|---|---|---|---|
| 0.9% NaCl | 0 | 154 | 154 | 0 | 0 | 0 | 0 | 310 | pH 5.0 0 kCal/L | R/U/I |
| Lactated Ringer's solution | 0 | 130 | 109 | 4 | 4 | 0 | 28 (L) | 272 | pH 6.5 9 kCal/L | R/B/I |
| Plasma-Lyte R | 0 | 140 | 103 | 10 | 5 | 3 | 8 (L) 47 (A) | 312 | pH 5.5 17 kCal/L | R/B/I |
| Normosol-R and Plasma-Lyte A pH 7.4 | 0 | 140 | 98 | 5 | 0 | 3 | 27 (A) 23 (G) | 294 | pH 7.4 18 kCal/L | R/B/I |
| Isolyte S pH 7.4 | 0 | 141 | 98 | 5 | 0 | 3 | 29 (A) 23 (G) | 295 | pH 7.4 | R/B/I |
| Normosol-M w/5% Dextrose Plasma-Lyte 56 w/5% dextrose | 50 | 40 | 40 | 13 | 0 | 3 | 16 (A) | 368 (111 w/o D) | pH 5.5 170 kCal/L | M/I or H‡ |
| 5% Dextrose | 50 | 0 | 0 | 0 | 0 | 0 | 0 | 253 | pH 4.0 170 kCal/L | D/I or H‡ |
| 3% NaCl | 0 | 513 | 513 | 0 | 0 | 0 | 0 | 1030 | pH 5.0 0 kCal/L | HTS |
| 5% NaCl | 0 | 855 | 855 | 0 | 0 | 0 | 0 | 1710 | pH 5.0 0 kCal/L | HTS |

Modified from Plumb D: *Plumb's veterinary drug handbook*, ed 6, Ames, 2008, Blackwell.
*Buffers used: A = acetate; G = gluconate; L = lactate.
†Fluid types: B = balanced; D = dextrose solution; H = hypotonic; HTS = hypertonic saline; I = isotonic; M = maintenance; R = replacement; U = unbalanced.
‡Note that because of the rapid metabolism of dextrose, these solutions may be classified as hypotonic.

Either crystalloids or colloids may also be classified according to the mix and quantity of solutes as replacement or maintenance; balanced or unbalanced; and isotonic, hypotonic, or hypertonic. Replacement fluids have high concentrations of Na+ and Cl− (as ECF does) and are designed to replace fluid losses. Maintenance fluids have lower concentrations of Na+ and Cl− but somewhat more K+ (as total body water does) and are designed to maintain fluid balance over a longer period. Balanced fluids contain a solute profile similar to that of ECF, whereas unbalanced fluids do not. Isotonic fluids have an osmolarity near that of blood plasma (300 mOsm/L). Hypotonic and hypertonic fluids have an osmolarity significantly lower or higher than plasma, respectively.

TECHNICIAN NOTE  Replacement fluids have high concentrations of Na+ and Cl− (as ECF does) and are designed to replace fluid losses. Maintenance fluids have lower concentrations of Na+ and Cl− but somewhat more K+ and are designed to maintain fluid balance over a longer period.

## Crystalloid Solutions

Crystalloid solutions (also referred to as *crystalloids*) contain water and small–molecular-weight solutes such as electrolytes that pass freely through vascular endothelium.

In addition to electrolytes, some crystalloids contain dextrose and alkalinizing agents (buffers). Table 2-8 shows the composition of selected commercially available crystalloid fluids. Other constituents are sometimes added to commercially available crystalloids, including 50% dextrose, potassium, and B-complex vitamins. Crystalloids are routinely used in most anesthetized patients, except those that have low blood protein, low RBC mass, or a low platelet count. These solutions are generally appropriate, provided the PCV is 20% or greater and the plasma protein is 3.5 g/dL or greater. There are five basic types of crystalloid solutions.

### Isotonic, Polyionic Replacement Solutions

As the name implies, isotonic, polyionic replacement solutions are balanced solutions that contain several ions (most often sodium, potassium, and chloride and in some cases magnesium and/or calcium) in concentrations that reflect the solute composition of ECF. Lactated Ringer's solution (LR), Normosol-R (NR), Plasma-Lyte A and R (PA and PR), and Isolyte S (IS) are examples of some commonly used solutions in this class. They all have somewhat similar solute profiles with the following exceptions. Each contains one or two buffers (lactate, gluconate, and/or acetate), but the concentration of buffer differs among these five solutions. PA, PR, NR, and IS contain magnesium, whereas LR does not. LR and PR

Patients with excessive bleeding or hypotension will need significantly higher rates of administration. Healthy young dogs tolerate an IV infusion rate of 40 mL/kg/hr for a maximum of 1 hour, with half of this given over the first 15 minutes. Cats are more susceptible to overhydration than dogs, and for this reason the infusion rate should

kg slowly over a 5-minute period, followed by administration of isotonic crystalloids. If hypertonic solutions are given too quickly, serious side effects can occur, including hypotension, bradycardia, rapid, shallow breathing, and bronchoconstriction. Therefore the rate of administration must be monitored carefully.

contain calcium, whereas NR, PA, and IS do not. Because calcium may cause transfused blood to clot, LR and PR may not be administered with blood products.

### Isotonic, Polyionic Maintenance Solutions

polyionic solutions containing 2.5% or 5% dextrose are available or may be mixed in house. Once infused, the dextrose in these solutions is rapidly metabolized to $CO_2$ and water, and then most of the remaining plain water diffuses into the interstitial compartment. For this reason,

| TABLE 2-9 | | Quick Reference Chart for Standard Fluid Administration Rates during Surgery | | | | | | | | |
|---|---|---|---|---|---|---|---|---|---|---|
| Body Weight | | Infusion Rate | Drip Rate Macrodrip (10 gtt/mL) | | | Drip Rate Macrodrip (15 gtt/mL) | | | Drip Rate Microdrip (60 gtt/mL) | | |
| lb | kg | mL/hr | gtt/min | gtt/sec | sec between drops | gtt/min | gtt/sec | sec between drops | gtt/min | gtt/sec | sec between drops |
| 1 | 0.5 | 5 | — | — | — | — | — | — | 5 | 0.1 | 13.2 |
| 2 | 0.9 | 9 | — | — | — | — | — | — | 9 | 0.2 | 6.6 |
| 3 | 1.4 | 14 | — | — | — | — | — | — | 14 | 0.2 | 4.4 |
| 4 | 1.8 | 18 | — | — | — | — | — | — | 18 | 0.3 | 3.3 |
| 5 | 2.3 | 23 | — | — | — | — | — | — | 23 | 0.4 | 2.6 |
| 6 | 2.7 | 27 | — | — | — | — | — | — | 27 | 0.5 | 2.2 |
| 7 | 3.2 | 32 | — | — | — | — | — | — | 32 | 0.5 | 1.9 |
| 8 | 3.6 | 36 | — | — | — | — | — | — | 36 | 0.6 | 1.7 |
| 9 | 4.1 | 41 | — | — | — | — | — | — | 41 | 0.7 | 1.5 |
| 10 | 4.5 | 45 | — | — | — | — | — | — | 45 | 0.8 | 1.3 |
| 12 | 5.5 | 55 | — | — | — | 14 | 0.2 | 4.4 | 55 | 0.9 | 1.1 |
| 14 | 6.4 | 64 | — | — | — | 16 | 0.3 | 3.8 | 64 | 1.1 | 0.9 |
| 16 | 7.3 | 73 | — | — | — | 18 | 0.3 | 3.3 | 73 | 1.2 | — |
| 18 | 8.2 | 82 | — | — | — | 20 | 0.3 | 2.9 | 82 | 1.4 | — |
| 20 | 9.1 | 91 | 15 | 0.3 | 4.0 | 23 | 0.4 | 2.6 | 91 | 1.5 | — |
| 25 | 11.4 | 114 | 19 | 0.3 | 3.2 | 28 | 0.5 | 2.1 | 114 | 1.9 | — |
| 30 | 13.6 | 136 | 23 | 0.4 | 2.6 | 34 | 0.6 | 1.8 | 136 | 2.3 | — |
| 35 | 15.9 | 159 | 27 | 0.4 | 2.3 | 40 | 0.7 | 1.5 | 159 | 2.7 | — |
| 40 | 18.2 | 182 | 30 | 0.5 | 2.0 | 45 | 0.8 | 1.3 | 182 | 3.0 | — |
| 45 | 20.5 | 205 | 34 | 0.6 | 1.8 | 51 | 0.9 | 1.2 | — | — | — |
| 50 | 22.7 | 227 | 38 | 0.6 | 1.6 | 57 | 0.9 | 1.1 | — | — | — |
| 60 | 27.3 | 273 | 45 | 0.8 | 1.3 | 68 | 1.1 | 0.9 | — | — | — |
| 70 | 31.8 | 318 | 53 | 0.9 | 1.1 | 80 | 1.3 | — | — | — | — |
| 80 | 36.4 | 364 | 61 | 1.0 | 1.0 | 91 | 1.5 | — | — | — | — |
| 90 | 40.9 | 409 | 68 | 1.1 | 0.9 | 102 | 1.7 | — | — | — | — |
| 100 | 45.5 | 455 | 76 | 1.3 | — | 114 | 1.9 | — | — | — | — |
| 120 | 54.5 | 545 | 91 | 1.5 | — | 136 | 2.3 | — | — | — | — |
| 140 | 63.6 | 636 | 106 | 1.8 | — | 159 | 2.7 | — | — | — | — |
| 160 | 72.7 | 727 | 121 | 2.0 | — | 182 | 3.0 | — | — | — | — |
| 180 | 81.8 | 818 | 136 | 2.3 | — | 205 | 3.4 | — | — | — | — |
| 200 | 90.9 | 909 | 152 | 2.5 | — | 227 | 3.8 | — | — | — | — |
| 250 | 113.6 | 1136 | 189 | 3.2 | — | 284 | 4.7 | — | — | — | — |
| 300 | 136.4 | 1364 | 227 | 3.8 | — | 341 | 5.7 | — | — | — | — |
| 350 | 159.1 | 1591 | 265 | 4.4 | — | 398 | 6.6 | — | — | — | — |
| 400 | 181.8 | 1818 | 303 | 5.1 | — | 455 | 7.6 | — | — | — | — |
| 450 | 204.5 | 2045 | 341 | 5.7 | — | 511 | 8.5 | — | — | — | — |
| 500 | 227.3 | 2273 | 379 | 6.3 | — | 568 | 9.5 | — | — | — | — |
| 600 | 272.7 | 2727 | 455 | 7.6 | — | — | — | — | — | — | — |

*Continued*

| TABLE 2-9 | Quick Reference Chart for Standard Fluid Administration Rates during Surgery—cont'd | | | | | | | | | | | | | |
|---|---|---|---|---|---|---|---|---|---|---|---|---|---|---|

| Body Weight | | Infusion Rate | Drip Rate Macrodrip (10 gtt/mL) | | | Drip Rate Macrodrip (15 gtt/mL) | | | Drip Rate Microdrip (60 gtt/mL) | | |
|---|---|---|---|---|---|---|---|---|---|---|---|
| lb | kg | mL/hr | gtt/min | gtt/sec | sec between drops | gtt/min | gtt/sec | sec between drops | gtt/min | gtt/sec | sec between drops |
| 800 | 363.6 | 3636 | 606 | 10.1 | — | — | — | — | — | — | — |
| 1000 | 454.5 | 4545 | 758 | 12.6 | — | — | — | — | — | — | — |

## USING THIS CHART

- The third column shows the calculated infusion rate (mL/hr) based on a standard prescribed rate of 10 mL/kg/hr for the first hour. Use half this rate for each additional hour.
- The remaining three groups of three columns show the drip rate for administration sets with drip ratings of 10 gtt/mL, 15 gtt/mL, and 60 gtt/mL.
- In each group, the left, middle, and right columns express the drip rate in gtt/min, gtt/sec, and seconds between drops, respectively.
- When the calculated drip rate is significantly under 1 drop per second, the flow can be very difficult to set accurately. In these cases it is often easier to use the alternative figure "seconds between drops," which is in the third column of each group. A setting of 3 seconds between drops means that one drop should fall every 3 seconds.

> **TECHNICIAN NOTE** For blood volume expansion in large and small animals, administer 7% hypertonic saline IV at a rate of 3 to 4 mL/kg slowly over a 5-minute period, followed by administration of isotonic crystalloids.

## Colloids

Synthetic colloids are administered IV in moderate volumes (10 to 20 mL/kg/day for dogs and for large animals and 5 to 10 mL/kg/day for cats). Because colloids expand blood volume, the infusion rate and total volume of colloids administered must be watched closely to prevent volume overload. These agents can also infrequently cause coagulation disorders and rarely allergic reactions. If given too rapidly, hetastarch can induce nausea and vomiting. Therefore colloids are usually administered to dogs and large animals as a slow bolus over 15 to 60 minutes and to cats as a slow bolus over 30 to 60 minutes. These solutions may also be administered as a CRI of 1 to 2 mL/kg/hr.

> **TECHNICIAN NOTE** Synthetic colloids are administered IV at a rate of 10 to 20 mL/kg/day for dogs and for large animals as a slow bolus over 15 to 60 minutes, and 5 to 10 mL/kg/day for cats as a slow bolus over 30 to 60 minutes.

## Adverse Effects of Fluid Administration

If fluid administration is too rapid, the volume may overwhelm the circulation and cause problems such as pulmonary or cerebral edema. This condition is known as *volume overload.* Animals weighing less than 5 kg and those with cardiac or renal disease are at greatest risk. For these patients, a slower infusion rate of 3 to 5 mL/kg/hr of crystalloid fluids during surgery may be more appropriate. When monitoring any anesthetized patient that is receiving IV fluids, the anesthetist should be alert for signs of overhydration. These include ocular and nasal discharge, chemosis (edema and swelling of the conjunctiva), subcutaneous edema, increased lung sounds, increased respiratory rate, and dyspnea. When the patient is awake, coughing and restlessness may be seen. Although not commonly done, measurement of central venous pressure (see Chapter 5) allows early detection of overhydration and is recommended for patients receiving more than this amount.

Another potential adverse effect of excessive fluid administration is dilution of the RBCs and plasma proteins, a condition known as *hemodilution.* Anemic patients, hypoproteinemic patients, and patients that lose a lot of blood from tissue oozing during surgery are particularly at risk. In these patients, fluid therapy should therefore be based on careful monitoring of the packed cell volume (PCV), plasma protein (PP), and physical parameters.

> **TECHNICIAN NOTE** Signs of overhydration include ocular and nasal discharge, chemosis (edema and swelling of the conjunctiva), subcutaneous edema, increased lung sounds, increased respiratory rate, and dyspnea. When the patient is awake, coughing and restlessness may be seen.

To avoid overhydration, fluids should either be administered using a fluid pump or monitored carefully. In either case, the fluid bag should be labeled with a scale indicating the starting fluid level and anticipated fluid levels by the hour so that the volume of fluid administered can be closely monitored. The use of a burette is advisable in small patients because it allows accurate measurement and administration of small volumes of fluids rather than direct administration from a bag or bottle. See Figure 2-6 for an illustration of an infusion pump, a scale, and a burette.

## Calculating Fluid Administration Rates

When fluids are administered, the prescribed rates (in volume/body weight/unit time) listed in the previous section must be converted into a form that will allow

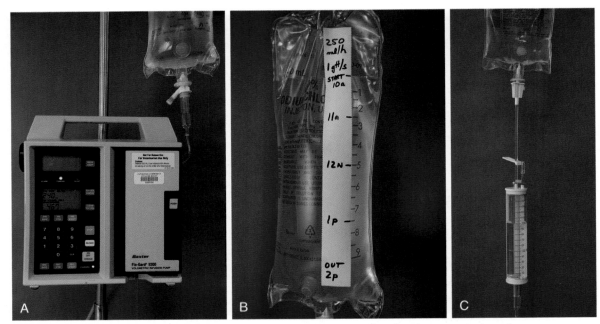

**FIGURE 2-6**    Infusion pump, tape scale, and burette. **A,** Infusion pump. Place the administration set line in the pump as indicated on the owner's manual. Most pumps require an infusion rate in milliliters per hour, and a total volume to be infused (VTBI) in milliliters. Note that this pump is programmed to deliver 240 mL/hr, and the VTBI is 467 mL. Most pumps will stop and sound an alarm if an occlusion or air bubble is detected in the line. Consequently, infusion pumps must be monitored frequently to ensure proper operation. **B,** Tape scale used to monitor the fluid administration rate. The tape should be labeled with the infusion rate (250 mL/hr in this case) and the drip rate (1 gtt/sec in this case) and should have lines drawn indicating the expected fluid level each hour. This way, any staff member can determine if the patient has received the proper volume of fluids. **C,** Burette. Used to administer small volumes of fluids to small, pediatric, or exotic patients. The burette is filled with the total volume of fluids to be infused by opening the clamp between the burette and the fluid bag. When it is filled to the desired level (in this case 100 mL), the upper clamp is closed. The lower clamp is then opened to allow the fluids to flow into the patient at the desired rate.

## BOX 2-2    Terms Related to Fluid Administration Rate Calculations

### Prescribed Rate
- The fluid administration rate ordered by the doctor.
- Expressed in **milliliters per unit body weight per unit time.** Most often **mL/kg/hr.**

### Infusion Rate
- The rate at which fluids should be administered expressed in **milliliters per unit time.** Most often **mL/hr.** (Determined by multiplying the following: **Patient body weight × Prescribed rate.** May also require a conversion factor to change pounds to kilograms.)

### Delivery Rate
- The number of drops of fluid that must fall inside the drip chamber of an administration set to deliver 1 mL of fluid expressed in drops per milliliter **(gtt/mL).** (Determined by looking on the packaging of the administration set [see Figure 2-7].)

### Drip Rate
- The rate at which fluids should be administered expressed in **drops per unit time.** Most often **gtt/min.** (Determined by multiplying the following: **Infusion rate × Conversion factor for hours to minutes × Delivery rate.**)
- If necessary to make it easier to set the rate, this figure may be reduced to **drops per 10 or 15 seconds** (usually calculated using a proportion) or **drops per second** (usually calculated by multiplying the drip rate [drops per minute] by the conversion factor for minutes to seconds).

### Infusion Time
- The total time over which the fluids will be administered expressed in **hours.**

### Infusion Volume
- The total volume of fluids to be administered expressed in **milliliters** or **liters.** (Determined by multiplying the following three values: **Patient body weight × Prescribed rate × Infusion time.**)

Note: Before fluid infusion rates are calculated, units must be converted so that they are the same (e.g., if working in milliliters per kilogram per hour, then all values involving body weight must be in kilograms).

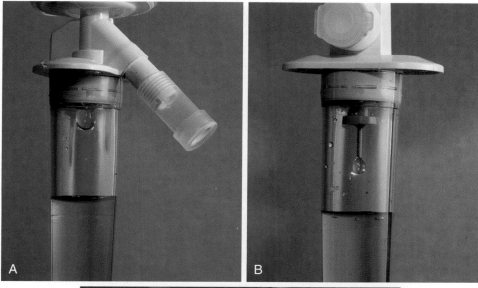

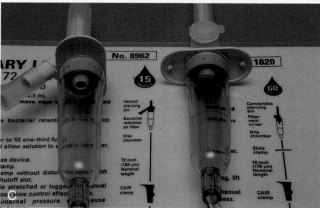

**FIGURE 2-7**   Fluid administration set chambers, comparing the size of the drops delivered. **A,** Macrodrip set chamber (15 gtt/mL). Used for infusion rates ≥100 mL/hr. Compare the size of this drop with **B,** Microdrip set chamber (60 gtt/mL). Used for infusion rates of <100 mL/hr. **C,** Macrodrip (15 gtt/mL) and microdrip (60 gtt/mL) fluid administration sets on the left and right, respectively. Note that the delivery rate in gtt/mL is listed on the package.

the anesthetist to program an infusion pump or set the roller clamp on an infusion set. Conversion requires use of mathematic formulas. Any discussion of fluid rate calculations can be confusing, however, because the terminology of fluid administration is not standard throughout the literature. So to avoid confusion, the discussion that follows will begin with a list of terms and definitions related to fluid administration rate calculations (Box 2-2).

The **infusion rate** (mL/hr) is the value used to program an IV infusion pump, and the **drip rate** (gtt/min or gtt/sec) is the value used to adjust the administration set. In order to perform the necessary calculations, the anesthetist must be familiar with the formulas used to determine these rates as well as the delivery rates of available administration sets.

There are two general types of administration sets. **Macrodrip** sets deliver fluids at a rate of 10 or 15 drops per milliliter and are used to deliver fluids at infusion rates equal to or greater than 100 mL/hr. **Microdrip**

sets deliver fluids at a rate of 60 drops per milliliter and are used for infusion rates less than 100 mL/hr (Figure 2-7).

As an alternative, the appropriate set can be chosen based on patient body weight. Macrodrip sets are appropriate for patients that weigh 10 kg or more, and microdrip sets are appropriate for patients that weigh less than 10 kg. This guideline works well unless delivering fluids at very high rates as for shock therapy, in which case the guideline based on the infusion rate will work better. If the appropriate set is not used, the anesthetist will find it difficult to adjust the drip rate accurately.

Calculation of fluid administration rates may be divided into two basic steps. (1) Use the patient body weight and the prescribed rate to calculate the infusion rate in milliliters per hour. (2) Using the infusion rate, the delivery rate, and conversion factors, calculate the drip rate in drops per minute or some other unit. Box 2-3 and Figure 2-8 summarize the steps required to

## BOX 2-3   Calculating Fluid Administration Rates

**Step 1: Calculate the Infusion Rate**
a. Determine the patient body weight (lb or kg).
b. Determine the prescribed rate (mL/kg/hr).
c. Calculate the infusion rate (mL/hr).

*Example 1*
The doctor orders IV fluids for a **35-lb dog** at a rate of **10 mL/kg/hr** for a 1-hour surgery. What is the infusion rate in mL/hr?
   Set up the problem this way:

$$\boxed{\text{Patient wt (lb)}} \times \boxed{\text{lb to kg conversion factor}} \times \boxed{\text{Prescribed rate (mL/kg/hr)}} = \boxed{\text{Infusion rate (mL/hr)}}$$

$$\text{weight (lb)} \times \frac{1\ (kg)}{2.2\ (lb)} \times \frac{(mL)}{(kg/hr)} = \text{Answer} \frac{(mLs)}{(hr)}$$

$$35\ \cancel{lb} \times \frac{1\ \cancel{kg}}{2.2\ \cancel{lb}} \times \frac{10\ mL}{1\ \cancel{kg}/hr} = 159\ \frac{mL}{hr}$$

*Example 2*
The doctor orders IV fluids for treatment of shock in a **12-lb** cat at a rate of **25 mL/lb (55 mL/kg) as rapidly as possible**. What is the infusion rate in milliliters?
   Set up the problem this way:

$$\boxed{\text{Patient wt (lb)}} \times \boxed{\text{Prescribed rate (mL/lb)}} = \boxed{\text{Infusion rate (mL)}}$$

$$\text{Weight (lb)} \times \frac{(mL)}{(lb)} = \text{Answer (mL) as rapidly as possible}$$

$$12\ \cancel{lb} \times \frac{25\ mL}{1\ \cancel{lb}} = 300\ mL \text{ as rapidly as possible}$$

Because this cat is being treated for shock, the calculated dose of fluids will be given as rapidly as possible instead of at a constant rate.

**Step 2: Calculate the Drip Rate**
a. Choose the appropriate administration set, and note the delivery rate (in drops per milliliter) by looking at the package.
   • Choose a *microdrip* set if the rate is <100 mL/hr (all microdrip sets deliver **60 gtt/mL**).
   • Choose a *macrodrip* set if the rate is ≥100 mL/hr (the delivery rate will be **10 or 15 gtt/mL** depending on the set chosen).
b. Calculate the drip rate (gtt/min).

*Example 1 (Continued)*
The **35-lb dog** in step 1, Example 1 requires an infusion rate of **159 mL/hr**. What administration set should you use, and what is the drip rate?
   Set up the problem this way:

$$\boxed{\text{Infusion rate (mL/hr)}} \times \boxed{\text{Conversion (1 hr/60 min)}} \times \boxed{\text{Delivery rate (gtt/mL)}} = \boxed{\text{Drip rate (gtt/min)}}$$

$$\frac{mL}{hr} \times \frac{1\ hr}{60\ min} \times \frac{gtt}{mL} = \text{Answer} \frac{gtt}{min}$$

You should choose a macro administration set, because the infusion rate is >100 mL/hr

$$159\ \frac{\cancel{mL}}{\cancel{hr}} \times \frac{1\ \cancel{hr}}{60\ min} \times \frac{15\ gtt}{\cancel{mL}} = \frac{40\ gtt}{min}$$

| BOX 2-3 | Calculating Fluid Administration Rates—cont'd |
|---|---|

*Example 1 (Continued)*

c. If desired, convert the drip rate to gtt/sec, gtt/10 sec, or gtt/15 sec.

It is often easier to set the drip rate if you convert it to a smaller unit of time (number of drops in 10 or 15 seconds or drops/sec). Conversion to drops per second:

$$\frac{40 \text{ gtt}}{\cancel{\text{min}}} \times \frac{1 \cancel{\text{min}}}{60 \text{ sec}} = 0.67 \frac{\text{gtt}}{\text{sec}}$$

Conversion to drops in 15 seconds: cross-multiply and solve for the unknown.

$$\frac{40 \text{ gtt}}{60 \text{ sec}} = \frac{\text{gtt}}{15 \text{ sec}}$$

$$40 \text{ gtt} \times 15 \text{ sec} = \text{gtt} \times 60 \text{ sec}$$

$$\text{gtt} = \frac{40 \text{ gtt} \times 15 \text{ sec}}{60 \text{ sec}}$$

Answer = 10 gtt in 15 seconds or 2 gtt in 3 seconds

---

calculate infusion rates and drip rates during the perioperative period for routine administration during surgery and for treatment of blood loss, hypotension, and shock.

> **TECHNICIAN NOTE** Use macrodrip sets (10 or 15 gtt/mL) for infusion rates equal to or greater than 100 mL/hr or for patients weighing 10 kg or more. Use microdrip sets (60 drops/mL) for infusion rates less than 100 mL/hr or for patients weighing less than 10 kg.

## OTHER PREANESTHETIC CARE

In addition to the care summarized on the previous pages, the veterinarian may direct the technician or another staff member to provide additional preoperative nursing care including administration of medications.

Antibiotics are often ordered for animals that have infections or that are scheduled for procedures involving a contaminated area (such as gastrointestinal or dental procedures). Administration of pain medication before painful procedures, a practice known as *preemptive analgesia* (discussed further in Chapter 7), is proven to be considerably more effective than waiting until the pain is manifest and significantly improves patient recovery.

Some patients may require a variety of other medications such as insulin, anticonvulsants, or antiemetic or antiinflammatory drugs. The technician should actively seek specific instructions from the veterinarian regarding care required, as the well-being of the patient and the outcome of the procedure are significantly influenced by the attention that is given to this final but important facet of patient preparation.

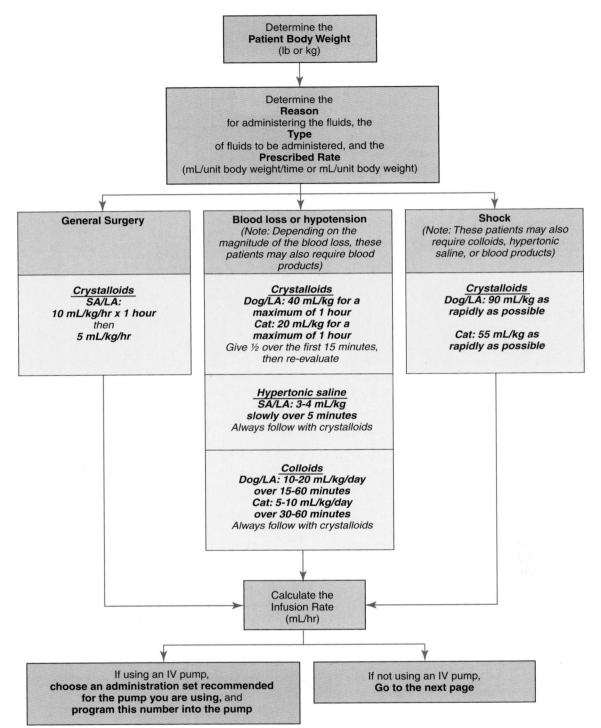

**FIGURE 2-8**    Flow chart for fluid rate calculations.

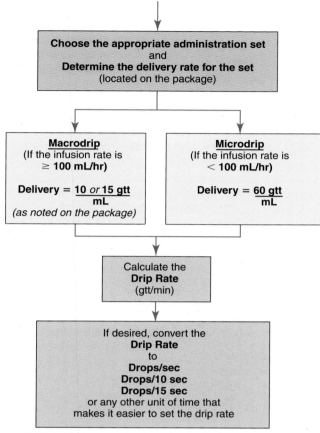

**FIGURE 2-8, cont'd** Flow chart for fluid rate calculations.

## KEY POINTS

1. Effective communication is key to the ability of the veterinary health care team to provide high-quality patient care. The veterinary technician often acts as a liaison between the veterinarian-in-charge (VIC), the client, and other members of the health care team.

2. During the preanesthetic period, the technician has many duties. He or she must help the VIC develop a minimum patient database, ensure that fasting instructions were followed, place an intravenous (IV) catheter, administer fluids, stabilize the patient, prepare equipment, and administer medications.

3. An accurate and complete patient history is at least as important, if not more important, than results of diagnostic tests in shaping patient management. Acquisition of a patient history requires skill in choosing and framing questions.

4. There are many ways in which patient signalment influences response to anesthesia. The anesthetist must consider these factors when managing patients.

5. Dehydration, anemia, abnormal bleeding, respiratory or cardiovascular system disease, kidney or liver dysfunction, and conditions that require treatment while the patient is under anesthesia are physical findings that may influence anesthetic management.

6. Immediately before any procedure, definitively identify and weigh the patient; assess body condition, hydration, level of consciousness, vital signs, and general condition; and determine a pain score.

7. Before any procedure, always present a consent form and fee estimate and acquire signatures.

8. No single anesthetic protocol is ideal for all patients. Rather, the anesthetic techniques and agents used are tailored to the needs of the individual patient. Factors such as previous or concurrent illness, nature of the procedure, urgency, and preference of the veterinarian are all considered in selecting a protocol.

9. Diagnostic tests such as the complete blood cell count (CBC), chemistries, urinalysis, radiography, and electrocardiography may provide valuable information regarding the patient's ability to tolerate anesthesia.

10. The risk of anesthesia to the patient should be assessed before initiating any procedure. The patient should be assigned to a class on the basis of physical condition, as outlined by the American Society of Anesthesiologists.

11. The patient should be in stable condition, when possible, before being anesthetized. Preexisting problems such as dehydration or shock should be corrected.

12. IV catheter placement in surgery patients gives the anesthetist the ability to safely administer IV anesthetics, provide fluid support, maintain anesthesia via constant rate infusion (CRI), and administer emergency drugs if needed.

13. Knowledge of fluid homeostasis and composition of body fluids enables the anesthetist to administer fluids safely and effectively.

14. Crystalloids may be classified according to the mix and quantity of solutes as replacement or maintenance; balanced or unbalanced; and isotonic, hypotonic, or hypertonic.

15. Crystalloids are routinely used in most anesthetized patients, except those with a plasma protein level less than 3.5 g/dL, a packed cell volume (PCV) less than 20%, or a low platelet count.

16. Colloids and/or blood products are used to support expansion of blood volume, blood pressure, oxygen-carrying capacity, and/or blood coagulation in patients with low plasma protein, PCV, and/or platelet count.

17. Although IV catheterization and fluid administration increase patient safety, the procedure is associated with the risk of accidental overhydration. A fluid infusion rate of 10 mL/kg/hr for the first hour followed by 5 mL/kg/hr for each additional hour is considered safe for most patients.

## PROCEDURE 2-1 Mucosal Bleeding Time

The *buccal mucosal bleeding time* is an in-house coagulation screen that gives an estimation of platelet function. It can be easily performed on any anesthetized animal but may also be performed on conscious patients.

This test primarily evaluates platelet function, but findings may be abnormal in patients with other problems such as thrombocytopenia and von Willebrand's disease. In contrast, results may be normal in patients with other coagulation disorders.

### Equipment
- Spring-loaded lancet that makes two side-by-side cuts of a standard length and depth, such as the Simplate II (0.5 mm deep × 2.5 mm long for cats and small dogs or 1 mm deep × 5 mm long for larger dogs)
- Stopwatch
- Filter paper
- Roll gauze

### Procedure
1. Place the patient in lateral recumbency.
2. Fold the lip back and tie with gauze so the mucosa of the lip cranial to the tie is slightly engorged (Figure 1).

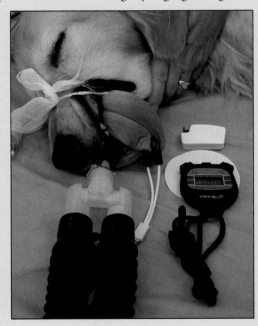

**FIGURE 1**

## PROCEDURE 2-1 Mucosal Bleeding Time—cont'd

3. Activate the lancet on the lip cranial to the tie, but away from major blood vessels.
4. Start the stopwatch (Figure 2).

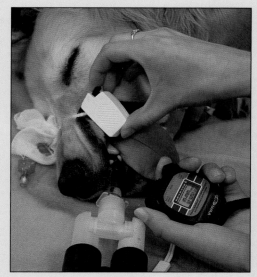

**FIGURE 2**

5. Wick blood from the area with the filter paper (without touching the incisions) at 5-second intervals until blood no longer appears from the incisions (Figure 3).

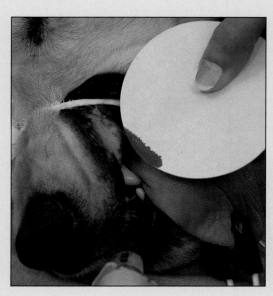

**FIGURE 3**

6. Stop the stopwatch when the bleeding stops.
7. Release the gauze.
8. Report the time from when the incision was made to blood clotting (Figure 4).

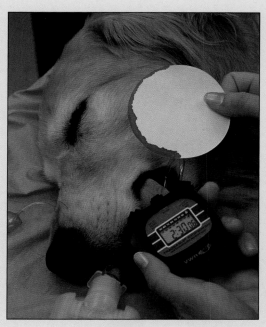

**FIGURE 4**

9. If clotting takes longer than 15 minutes, stop the test, release the gauze, apply pressure to the cuts, and report as ">15 minutes."

*Note.* Normal values: Dog, approximately 2-4 minutes; cat, approximately 1-3 minutes.

## PROCEDURE 2-2  Placing an IV Catheter in a Small Animal Patient

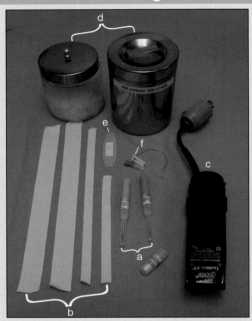

Equipment (letters in list correspond to those in figure)

- a, Catheter (20 to 24 gauge, ¾ to 1 ½ inches long for cats; 16 to 22 gauge, 1 to 2 inches long for dogs)
- b, Two approximately 6-inch-long strips of 1-inch porous adhesive tape, one approximately 6-inch-long and one approximately 3-inch-long strip of ½-inch tape
- c, Clipper with #40 blade
- d, 1:1 Chlorhexidine surgical scrub/water-soaked cotton balls and alcohol-soaked cotton balls
- e, ½-inch plastic strip with antiseptic ointment
- f, T-port, cap, or administration set (both the catheter and T-port should be flushed with saline before catheterization)

*Procedure*

1. Clip a generous area over the vein from the medial to lateral aspect of the limb. Prepare the area using standard aseptic technique with three chlorhexidine/water-soaked cotton balls, followed by three alcohol-soaked cotton balls. Place a 6-inch strip of ½-inch tape over the catheter hub. Have assistant hold off the vein. Locate the vein, apply tension in a ventral direction to tense skin, and position the catheter with the needle fully inserted and with the bevel up (Figure 1).

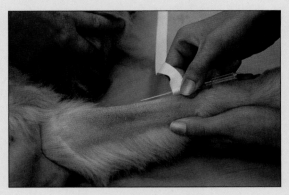

**FIGURE 1**

2. Advance the catheter and needle assembly as a unit through the skin, and the near wall of the vein. Blood will flash back into the needle hub when the vein is entered. Advance the unit a few more millimeters until the end of the catheter is firmly seated in the vein (Figure 2).

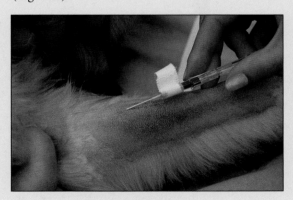

**FIGURE 2**

**PROCEDURE 2-2 Placing an IV Catheter in a Small Animal Patient—cont'd**

3. Holding the needle stationary, advance the catheter over the end of the needle until inserted to the hub. Remove the needle. Have the assistant apply pressure at the insertion site to prevent bleeding (Figure 3).

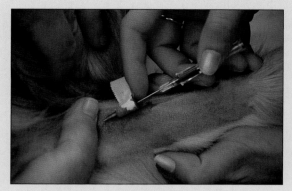

FIGURE 3

4. Quickly attach a T-port, cap, or administration set line to the catheter hub. Apply the first piece of tape to secure the catheter (Figure 4).

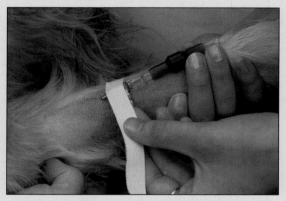

FIGURE 4

5. Flush the catheter with several milliliters of normal saline through the injection port. Twist the 3-inch-long strip of ½-inch tape into a "bow-tie" configuration (Figure 5).

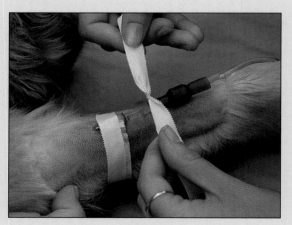

FIGURE 5

6. Apply the tape under and then around the catheter hub in a crisscross fashion (Figure 6).

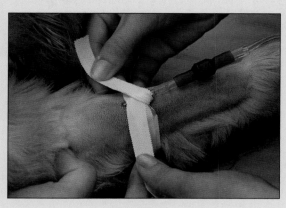

FIGURE 6

7. Apply a small amount of chlorhexidine ointment to the plastic strip (Figure 7).

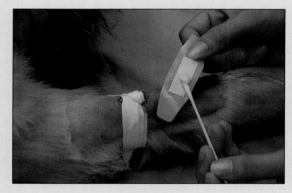

FIGURE 7

8. Apply the plastic strip over the insertion site (Figure 8).

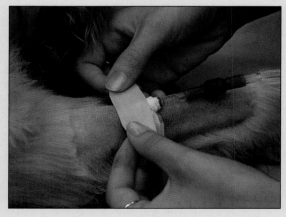

FIGURE 8

*Continued*

## PROCEDURE 2-2  Placing an IV Catheter in a Small Animal Patient—cont'd

9. Tear a ½-inch V in a 6-inch length of 1-inch tape about 1 inch from the end. Slip it under the catheter, with the torn area directly under the catheter hub (Figure 9).

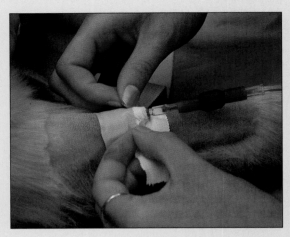

FIGURE 9

10. Apply the remainder of this length of tape over the plastic strip to secure (Figure 10).

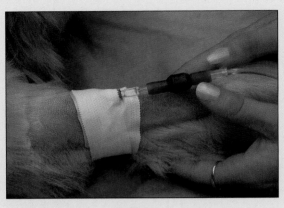

FIGURE 10

11. Apply the remaining 6-inch long strip of 1-inch tape around the administration set line or T-port to create a tension loop (see Procedure 2-3, Figure 1).

## PROCEDURE 2-3  Giving an IV Injection through an IV Administration Set Port

*Procedure*

1. Prepare the medication or induction agent. Cleanse the injection port with alcohol. IV fluids should be flowing at the standard infusion rate (Figure 1).

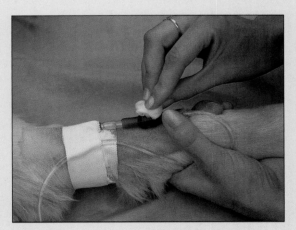

FIGURE 1

2. Insert the needle in the injection port. Pinch off the administration set line between the injection port and the fluid bag to prevent backflow of agent into the fluid bag during injection. (Figure 2)

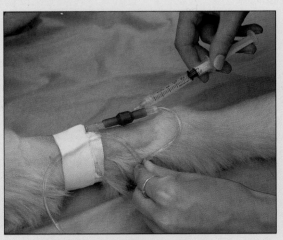

FIGURE 2

## PROCEDURE 2-3  Giving an IV Injection through an IV Administration Set Port—cont'd

3. Give the medication at an appropriate rate as dictated by the VIC. For most medications, a slow IV bolus is appropriate. When inducing general anesthesia, inject an appropriate initial volume following the guidelines in Chapters 8, 9, and 10 (Figure 3).

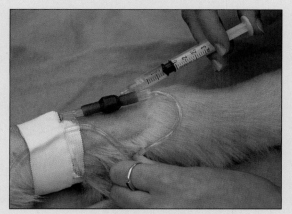

**FIGURE 3**

4. After injection, release the administration set line, so that the entire dose of medication is flushed into the patient. This is necessary because typically as much as 0.5 to 2 mL of agent will remain in the fluid line and catheter until flushed out (Figure 4).

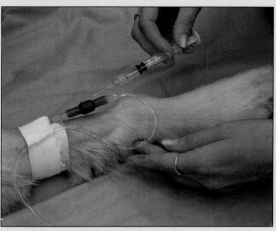

**FIGURE 4**

When administering an induction agent, administer additional doses to effect by following steps 2, 3, and 4. As soon as the patient is at an adequate anesthetic depth to permit intubation, remove the needle and syringe to prevent accidental overdose.

## REVIEW QUESTIONS

1. In gathering a patient history, which of the following would be the best way to frame a question about a patient's exercise level?
   a. "Your dog does not exercise much, does he, Mrs. Jones?"
   b. "Does your dog exercise, Mrs. Jones?"
   c. "How many times a week does your pet go for a walk or exercise, Mrs. Jones?"
   d. "You don't give your dog as much exercise as you should, do you, Mrs. Jones?"

2. Which of the following examples of species associations is not correct?
   a. Horses and cats are more sensitive to opioids than dogs and ruminants.
   b. The use of anticholinergics is recommended in ruminants to avoid airway occlusion.
   c. Horses may fracture limbs during anesthetic recovery and thus require special attention during the recovery period.
   d. Large animals are prone to respiratory depression and dependent atelectasis and thus often require ventilatory support.

3. Which of the following statements regarding physical examination findings is incorrect?
   a. Dehydration increases the risk for hypotension.
   b. Anemia predisposes the patient to hypoxemia.
   c. Patients with bruising may be at higher risk for potentially life-threatening intraoperative and postoperative bleeding.
   d. A dog with a body condition score of 8/9 will require more anesthetic per unit body weight than a dog of the same breed with a body condition score of 5/9.

4. You are evaluating a patient's LOC and find the patient in a sleeplike state, nonresponsive to a verbal stimulus but arousable by a painful stimulus. This patient is:
   a. Lethargic
   b. Obtunded
   c. Stuporous
   d. Comatose

5. You are evaluating a patient's hydration. The skin elasticity is somewhat slowed, the patient's mucous membranes are tacky, the CRT is 1.5 seconds, but the eyes are in a normal position in the orbit. Your patient is:
   a. Approximately 5% to 6% dehydrated
   b. Approximately 6% to 8% dehydrated
   c. Approximately 8% to 10% dehydrated
   d. Approximately 12% to 15% dehydrated

6. Which of the following fasting times is least advisable?
   a. Dog: 8 to 12 hours
   b. Horse: 2 to 4 hours
   c. Cow: 24 to 48 hours
   d. Small ruminant: 12 to 18 hours

7. Which of the following is not a crystalloid solution?
   a. Lactated Ringer's solution
   b. Normal saline solution
   c. Dextran
   d. 5% dextrose

8. Using the ASA Physical Status Classification system, a patient that is moderately anemic or moderately dehydrated would be classified as:
   a. Class P1
   b. Class P2
   c. Class P3
   d. Class P4
   e. Class P5

9. Which of the following signs of disease in a calm canine patient would be most significant in terms of the potential to increase the risk of anesthesia?
   a. Increased respiratory effort
   b. Lethargy
   c. A body temperature of 103.4° F
   d. A sinus arrhythmia

10. Which of the following species or breeds must be watched especially closely during any anesthetic procedure to ensure a patent airway?
    a. Brachiocephalic breeds
    b. Exotic breeds
    c. Cats and horses
    d. Sighthounds

11. Using the standard fluid infusion rate of 10 mL/kg/hr for the first hour, and a macrodrip administration set with a delivery rate of 15 gtt/mL, a 53-lb patient would require which of the following infusion and drip rates?
    a. 530 mL/hr; 2.2 gtt/sec
    b. 240 mL/hr; 2 gtt/sec
    c. 240 mL/hr; 1 gtt/2 seconds
    d. 240 mL/hr; 1 gtt/sec

12. Which of the following statements regarding IV catheter placement and use in surgery patients is incorrect?
    a. Choose an administration set with an injection port.
    b. Give all IV drugs slowly unless told otherwise.
    c. Always follow IV injections through a catheter with sterile saline flush.
    d. Choose a catheter that is small in diameter to minimize the risk of bleeding.

13. Which of the following general guidelines about body fluids in a normal adult animal is incorrect?
    a. About 40% of the body weight is water.
    b. About two thirds of the total body water is inside the cells.
    c. Blood plasma makes up about 5% of the total body weight.
    d. Dogs have a larger total blood volume than cats.

14. The fluid type most appropriate to replace moderate losses from dehydration would be:
    a. Colloids
    b. Hypertonic saline
    c. Isotonic crystalloids
    d. 50% Dextrose

15. Which of the following figures represents a fluid "infusion rate" as defined in this chapter?
    a. 10 mL/kg/hr
    b. 100 mL/hr
    c. 1 gtt/sec
    d. 500 mL total

16. The delivery rate of a microdrip administration set is:
    a. 10 gtt/mL only
    b. 10 or 15 gtt/mL
    c. 20 or 60 gtt/mL
    d. 60 gtt/mL

17. Which of the following statements regarding electrolyte composition of fluids is incorrect?
    a. Extracellular fluid contains more sodium than intracellular fluid.
    b. Intracellular fluid contains more potassium than intravascular fluid.
    c. The osmolarity of intracellular fluid is similar to that of extracellular fluid.
    d. Intravascular fluid has more negatively charged particles than positively charged particles.

18. Regarding fluid infusion rates:
    a. Standard shock doses of fluids are about the same as doses used during routine surgery.
    b. Surgery patients with blood loss may require colloids instead of crystalloids.
    c. Crystalloids are generally given at lower administration rates than colloids.
    d. Hypertonic saline is administered in large volumes to patients in shock.

19. Which of the following is *not* a sign of fluid overload?
    a. Ocular and nasal discharge
    b. Hypotension
    c. Increased lung sounds and respiratory rate
    d. Dyspnea

20. Which of the following heart rhythms is not normal in a resting horse?
    a. NSR
    b. SA
    c. Second-degree AV block
    d. Third-degree AV block

## SELECTED READINGS

Arnell K: Postanesthesia regurgitation in a dog, *Clinician's Brief* 6(11): 47-50, 2008.

Battaglia AM: Patient's lifeline: intravenous catheter. In Battaglia AM, editor: *Small animal emergency and critical care for veterinary technicians*, ed 2, St. Louis, 2007, Saunders, pp 33-47.

Davis H: Management of the patient in shock. In Battaglia AM, editor: *Small animal emergency and critical care for veterinary technicians*, ed 2, St Louis, 2007, Saunders, pp 180-187.

DiBartola S, Bateman S: Introduction to fluid therapy. In DiBartola S, editor: *Fluid, electrolyte, and acid-base disorders*, ed 3, St Louis, 2006, Saunders, pp 325-344.

Hansen BD: Technical aspects of fluid therapy. In DiBartola S, editor: *Fluid, electrolyte, and acid-base disorders*, ed 3, St Louis, 2006, Saunders, pp 376-391.

Haskins SC: Fluid, electrolyte, and acid-base balance: maintenance in the perioperative period. In Paddleford RR, editor: *Manual of small animal anesthesia*, ed 2, Philadelphia, 1999, Saunders, pp 247-265.

Jenkins-Perez J: Dispelling common myths about anesthesia, *Veterinary Technician* 28(12):752-760, 2007.

Lake T, Green N: *Essential calculations for veterinary nurses and technicians*, ed 2, Edinburgh, 2009, Elsevier.

Looney AL: Evaluation preoperative, protocols anesthetic. In Morgan RV, editor: *Handbook of small animal practice*, ed 5, St Louis, 2007, Saunders, pp 1-10.

Lucero R: Anesthesia: minimizing risks in senior pets, *Veterinary Technician* 30(4):24-28, 2009.

Macintire D, Drobatz K, Haskins S, Saxon W: *Manual of small animal emergency and critical care medicine*, Philadelphia, 2005, Lippincott Williams and Wilkins, pp 55-70.

Mathews KA: Monitoring fluid therapy and complications of fluid therapy. In DiBartola S, editor: *Fluid, electrolyte, and acid-base disorders*, ed 3, St Louis, 2006, Saunders, pp 377-391.

Mosley C: Fluid, electrolytes and acid-base. In Doherty T, Valverde A, editors: *Manual of equine anesthesia and analgesia*, Ames, 2006, Blackwell, pp 1-10, 86-104.

Muir WW: Considerations for general anesthesia. In Tranquilli WJ, Thurmon JC, Grimm KA, editors: *Lumb & Jones' veterinary anesthesia and analgesia*, ed 4, Ames, Iowa, 2007, Blackwell, pp 7-30, pp 3-6.

Muir WW, Hubbell JA, Bednarski RM: *Handbook of veterinary anesthesia*, ed 4, St Louis, 2006, Mosby, pp 1-22, 485-536.

Paddleford RR: *Manual of small animal anesthesia*, ed 2, Philadelphia, 1999, Saunders, pp 1-11.

Pascoe PJ: Perioperative management of fluid therapy. In DiBartola S, editor: *Fluid, electrolyte, and acid-base disorders*, ed 3, St Louis, 2006, Saunders, pp 391-419.

Plumb DC: *Plumb's veterinary drug handbook*, ed 6, Ames, 2008, Blackwell Publishing Professional, pp 1053-1054.

Ritchie AM: Fluid therapy. In Battaglia AM, editor: *Small animal emergency and critical care for veterinary technicians*, ed 2, St Louis, 2007, Saunders, pp 48-67.

Seeler DC: Fluid, electrolyte, and blood component therapy. In Tranquilli WJ, Thurmon JC, Grimm KA, editors: *Lumb & Jones' veterinary anesthesia and analgesia*, ed 4, Ames, Iowa, 2007, Blackwell, pp 183-201.

Thurmon JC, Tranquilli WJ, Benson GJ: *Essentials of small animal anesthesia and analgesia.*, Baltimore, 1999, Lippincott Williams & Wilkins, pp 326-366.

Wellman ML, DiBartola SP, Kohn CW: Applied physiology of body fluids in dogs and cats. In DiBartola S, editor: *Fluid, electrolyte, and acid-base disorders*, ed 3, St Louis, 2006, Saunders, pp 3-26.

# 3

# Anesthetic Agents and Adjuncts

## OUTLINE

Introduction to Anesthetic Agents and
    Adjuncts, 50
    *Agonists, Partial Agonists, Mixed Agonist-*
        *Antagonists, and Antagonists, 51*
    *Analgesic Effects of Anesthetics and*
        *Adjuncts, 51*
    *Using Drugs in Combination, 52*
    *Regulatory Considerations for Controlled*
        *Substances, 53*
Preanesthetic Medications, 54
    *Reasons for the Use of Preanesthetic*
        *Medications, 54*
    *Anticholinergics, 56*
    *Tranquilizers and Sedatives, 59*
    *Opioids, 66*

Injectable Anesthetics, 70
    *Barbiturates, 70*
    *Propofol, 76*
    *Dissociative Anesthetics, 78*
    *Etomidate, 82*
    *Guaifenesin, 83*
Inhalation Anesthetics, 84
    *Diethyl Ether, 84*
    *Halogenated Organic Compounds, 84*
    *Nitrous Oxide, 91*
Central Nervous System and Respiratory
    Stimulants, 92
    *Doxapram, 92*

## LEARNING OBJECTIVES

*After completion of this chapter, the reader will be able to:*

- Classify anesthetic agents and adjuncts based on route of administration, time of administration, principal effect, or chemistry.
- Differentiate agonists, partial agonists, agonist-antagonists, and antagonists based on their action and effect. List anesthetics and adjuncts that can be reversed.
- Apply principles of safe administration of anesthetic agents and adjuncts.
- List anesthetic agents and adjuncts commonly used as preanesthetic medications, and describe their indications, mode of action, effects, adverse effects, and use.
- List injectable anesthetic drugs in common use, and describe their indications, mode of action, effects, adverse effects, and use.
- Describe the effect of ionization, protein binding, lipid solubility, and redistribution on barbiturate pharmacokinetics and pharmacodynamics.
- Define dissociative anesthesia; describe the actions and effects of dissociative anesthetics, and explain ways in which these drugs differ from other injectable anesthetics.
- List the inhalation anesthetic agents in common use, and describe their indications, mode of action, effects, adverse effects, and use.
- Define vapor pressure, partition coefficient, minimum alveolar concentration (MAC), and rubber solubility; and explain the ways in which these properties affect the action and use of inhalant anesthetic agents.
- Describe the uptake, distribution, and elimination of the commonly used inhalation anesthetic agents.

## KEY TERMS

Adjunct
Agonist-antagonists
Agonists
Analeptic agent
Anesthetic agent
Antagonists
Anticholinergics
Apnea
Apneustic respiration
Ataxia
Bagging
Cataleptoid state
Colic
Cortisol
Dead space
Dysphoria
Enantiomers
Fasciculations
Hypoventilation
Mydriasis
Neuroleptanalgesia
Neuromuscular
  blockers
Nystagmus
Parasympatholytics
Partial agonists
Pharmacodynamics
Pharmacokinetics
Preanesthetic
  medications
Reversal agents
Somatic analgesia
Status epilepticus
Tachycardia
Tidal volume
Visceral analgesia

## INTRODUCTION TO ANESTHETIC AGENTS AND ADJUNCTS

An **anesthetic agent** may be defined as any drug used to induce a loss of sensation with or without unconsciousness. The term **adjunct** is used to describe a drug that is not a true anesthetic but that is used during anesthesia to produce other desired effects such as sedation, muscle relaxation, analgesia, reversal, neuromuscular blockade, or parasympathetic blockade. Because adjuncts are used as a part of balanced anesthesia, they are traditionally included in the study of anesthetic agents. Anesthetic agents and adjuncts may be classified a number of ways.

First, they may be classified based on the route of administration. Inhalant agents are administered from an anesthetic machine into the lower respiratory tree via an endotracheal tube or mask. Injectable agents are injected intravenously, intramuscularly, subcutaneously, intraperitoneally, intralesionally, or into a number of other locations. Oral agents are given by mouth, and topical agents are applied to a body surface such as the skin or mucous membranes.

Another way these agents may be classified is based on the time period at which they are given during the course of an anesthetic procedure. Drugs given before general anesthesia are referred to as **preanesthetic medications.** Drugs used to induce general anesthesia are referred to as *induction agents,* and those used to maintain general anesthesia are referred to as *maintenance agents.*

A third way anesthetic agents and adjuncts may be classified is according to the principal effect. Local anesthetics induce a loss of sensation in a localized area of the body. In contrast, general anesthetics induce a loss of sensation over the entire body, accompanied by unconsciousness. Sedatives and tranquilizers are agents that cause sedation and tranquilization, respectively. Analgesics prevent and control pain. Muscle relaxants decrease muscle tone. **Neuromuscular blockers,** although infrequently used in general practice, are used to relax or paralyze skeletal muscles during ophthalmic, orthopedic, or other surgeries. Anticholinergic agents are used to decrease effects of parasympathetic nervous system (PNS) stimulation such as bradycardia and excessive salivation. Finally, **reversal agents** lessen or abolish the effects of other anesthetic agents and are therefore used to "wake" the patient after sedation or anesthesia.

Many of the agents used in anesthesia cause two or more of these effects, depending on the dose and the circumstances under which they are used. For instance, morphine causes sedation and is an excellent analgesic. The injectable drug dexmedetomidine causes moderate to profound sedation, analgesia, and good muscle relaxation when given alone but can be used in combination with other agents to induce general anesthesia. The intravenous (IV) anesthetic propofol induces general anesthesia at higher doses but can be used as a sedative when given as a low-dose constant rate infusion (CRI). As a consequence, classification of these agents based on the principal effect is somewhat arbitrary.

The final way anesthetic agents and adjuncts may be classified is based on their chemistry. For the student, this is perhaps the most useful method of classification because the agents within a given class tend to have similar properties and effects. For this reason, the anesthetic agents and adjuncts discussed herein will be presented this way. Tables 3-1 to 3-4 summarize the principal effects and adverse effects of the anesthetic agents and adjuncts.

## Agonists, Partial Agonists, Mixed Agonist-Antagonists, and Antagonists

Before embarking on a study of anesthetic agents and adjuncts, a general knowledge of **pharmacokinetics** (the effect the body has on a drug) and **pharmacodynamics** (the effects a drug has on the body) is necessary. After administration, most drugs are distributed throughout the body by the blood. Each drug binds to specific receptors in one or more "target tissues." After binding to specific receptors, the drug stimulates the receptor, causing one or more specific effects. In the case of anesthetic agents and adjuncts, the primary target tissue is most often the central nervous system (CNS), and the most common effect is depression and/or stimulation of one or more parts of the CNS.

Anesthetic agents and adjuncts differ according to the degree to which they stimulate target tissue receptors. **Agonists** bind to and stimulate tissue receptors. Most anesthetics and adjuncts are classified as agonists.

Some drug classes such as the alpha$_2$-adrenergics and opioids include drugs that are classified as antagonists. **Antagonists** bind to but do not stimulate receptors. These drugs are given after an agonist of the same class to "wake" the patient after anesthesia or sedation. They are therefore called *reversal agents* because they reverse the effects of the corresponding agonist. Specifically, most antagonists competitively bind to receptors and displace the corresponding agonist, blocking further action.

The opioid class also includes some partial agonists and agonist-antagonists. **Partial agonists** bind to and partially stimulate receptors. **Agonist-antagonists** bind to more than one receptor type and simultaneously stimulate at least one and block at least one. Both partial agonists and agonist-antagonists are sometimes used to partially block the effects of pure agonists.

> *TECHNICIAN NOTE*  Many commonly used general anesthetics are not analgesics but indirectly provide pain control during the anesthetic period by producing a state of unconsciousness. Therefore when these agents are used, analgesia in the preoperative and postoperative periods must be provided by the use of true analgesics such as the opioids.

## Analgesic Effects of Anesthetics and Adjuncts

When an anesthetic protocol is being chosen for animals that are experiencing pain or that are undergoing a painful procedure, it must be kept in mind that analgesia must be provided before, during, and after the anesthetic event. Many commonly used general anesthetics, including halogenated inhalant agents, propofol, and etomidate, produce unconsciousness but little to no pain control and so are not true analgesics.

| TABLE 3-1 | **Principal Central Nervous System Effects of Anesthetic Agents and Adjuncts** | | | | |
|---|---|---|---|---|---|
| Agent Class | CNS Activity* | Intracranial Pressure | Analgesia | Body Temperature | Other CNS Effects |
| Anticholinergics | - (atropine) 0 (glycopyrrolate) | | 0 | 0 | |
| Acepromazine | - - (Ca, Eq, Bo) - (Fe) | | 0 | Decreased | Excitement; aggression; decreased seizure threshold |
| Benzodiazepines | - (old, ill) + (young, healthy) | 0 to - | 0 | | Disorientation; aggression; ataxia; anticonvulsant activity |
| Alpha$_2$-agonists | - - - (especially SA, small Ru, foals) | + (because of vomiting) | ++ (short duration, somatic, and visceral) | Decreased | Aggression; ataxia; cattle lie down; muscle tremors (Eq) |
| Opioids | - to - - - (Ca) - to +++ (Fe, Eq, Ru) | 0 (+ only if hypoventilating) | +++ (agonists) ++ (agonist-antagonists) (somatic and visceral) | Decreased (Ca) Increased (Fe, possibly Eq, Ru) | Disorientation (Ca, if not in pain); excitement, dysphoria (Fe, Eq, Ru) |
| Barbiturates | - to - - - (+ at low doses) | - (0 if normal respirations) | 0 | Decreased | Excitement during recovery and induction, especially if given too slowly |
| Propofol | - to - - - | - | 0 | Decreased | Muscular activity that resembles seizures |
| Dissociatives | Both + and - (dissociative anesthesia) | + | ++ (somatic) 0 to + (visceral) | Decreased | Seizure-like activity; intact reflexes |
| Etomidate | - to - - - | 0 | 0 to + | | Anticonvulsant activity; decreased $O_2$ consumption |
| Guaifenesin | - | | 0 | | |
| Halogenated inhalants | - to - - - | + | 0 | Decreased | Halothane: malignant hyperthermia in susceptible patients |

*Bo*, Bovine; *Ca*, canine; *CNS*, central nervous system; *Eq*, equine; *Fe*, feline; *Ru*, ruminants; *SA*, small animals.
*- = depression; + = stimulation.
Notes on use of this table:
- 0 indicates minimal to no effect.
- - indicates a decrease in the parameter indicated (where - is mild; - - is moderate; - - - is marked).
- + indicates an increase in the parameter indicated (where + is mild; ++ is moderate; +++ is marked).
- Effects of drugs depend on many factors, including species, differences among specific agents within a class, dose, and drug interactions. Therefore quantifications of the principal effects (mild, moderate, marked) are approximations.
- The information regarding opioids includes those of agonists, partial agonists, and agonist-antagonists. When reading this, note that effects of agonists are generally more pronounced than those of agonist-antagonists or partial agonists).

As animals do not feel pain while unconscious, general anesthetics indirectly provide analgesia by producing a state of unconsciousness. In other words, when these agents are used, pain is not perceived while the patient is "asleep" but recurs with the return of consciousness. Therefore these agents do not provide adequate pain control at subhypnotic or subanesthetic doses, and their use must be preceded and followed by administration of true analgesics if preoperative or postoperative pain control is necessary.

In contrast, true analgesics such as the opioid agonists produce analgesia regardless of the patient's level of consciousness. In other words, these agents work whether the patient is "asleep" (unconscious) or "awake" (conscious) and are used to provide analgesia during the pre-, intra-, and post-operative periods.

## Using Drugs in Combination

Two or more anesthetic agents and/or adjuncts are often used in combination. Some drugs can be safely mixed in the same syringe, whereas others cannot. Incompatible mixtures can produce a variety of harmful or even fatal adverse effects because of loss of

**TABLE 3-2  Principal Cardiovascular Effects of Anesthetic Agents and Adjuncts**

| Preanesthetic Agent Class | Heart Rate | Cardiac Output | Blood Pressure | Cardiac Arrhythmias | Other Cardiovascular Effects |
|---|---|---|---|---|---|
| Anticholinergics | ++/+++ | 0/+ | 0/+ | ++ (atropine) + (glycopyrrolate) | Atropine, low doses: temporary bradycardia |
| Acepromazine | - or + secondary to hypotension | - | - -/- - - | - (protects against arrhythmias) | Vasodilatation; high doses may cause low HR (Ca) |
| Benzodiazepines | 0 (- if given rapidly IV) | 0 | 0 (- if given rapidly IV) | 0 | |
| Alpha$_2$-agonists | - - - | - -/- - - | - -/- - - | ++ (especially early) | Initial hypertension resulting from vasoconstriction; pale mucous membranes |
| Opioids | - to - - - | 0 | 0 | 0 | Morphine: hypotension secondary to histamine release |
| Barbiturates | - or + | - to - - - (dose-dependent) | - to - - - (dose-dependent) | +++ (especially bigeminy) | |
| Propofol | - | - | - (transient); - - in some patients | 0 (alone) + (with epinephrine) | |
| Dissociatives | + | + | + | + | Increased O$_2$ consumption; decreased inotropy |
| Etomidate | 0 | 0 | Transient -/then 0 | 0 | |
| Guaifenesin | Mild + (transient) | 0 | - (transient) | 0 | |
| Halogenated inhalants | Variable | -/- - (dose-dependent) | -/- - | 0 (except halothane: ++) | Vasodilatation |

*Ca, canine; HR, heart rate; IV, intravenously.*
- = depression; + = stimulation.
Notes on use of this table:
- 0 indicates minimal to no effect.
- - indicates a decrease in the parameter indicated (where - is mild; - - is moderate; - - - is marked).
- + indicates an increase in the parameter indicated (where + is mild; ++ is moderate; +++ is marked).
- Effects of drugs depend on many factors, including species, differences among specific agents within a class, dose, and drug interactions. Therefore quantifications of the principal effects (mild, moderate, marked) are approximations.
- The information regarding opioids includes those of agonists, partial agonists, and agonist-antagonists. When reading this, note that effects of agonists are generally more pronounced than those of agonist-antagonists or partial agonists).

potency, change in chemistry, precipitation of one or more of the drugs, or other untoward interactions. For this reason, the anesthetist must observe some general guidelines when faced with a decision to mix two or more drugs.

With the exception of diazepam (a benzodiazepine tranquilizer), most anesthetic agents and adjuncts are water-soluble. In general, two or more water-soluble drugs can be safely mixed, but a water-soluble drug and a non–water-soluble drug cannot. The sole exception to the rule is the combination of the water-soluble drug ketamine and diazepam, which can be safely mixed and administered unless visible precipitation occurs. Regardless of these guidelines, *do not mix two or more drugs unless you have reliable evidence that it is safe to do so.* Usually this information can be found in professional publications such as anesthesia textbooks and peer-reviewed journals as well as from experienced anesthetists.

*TECHNICIAN NOTE*  With the exception of diazepam, most anesthetic agents and adjuncts are water-soluble. In general, two or more water-soluble drugs can be safely mixed, but a water-soluble drug and a non–water-soluble drug cannot. For this reason, when using two or more drugs in the same patient, *do not mix them unless you are sure that it is safe to do so.*

## Regulatory Considerations for Controlled Substances

Some of the agents covered in this chapter are subject to government (Drug Enforcement Administration [DEA]) regulation regarding purchase, handling, and dispensing. The benzodiazepines, dissociatives, barbiturates, and most opioids fall into this category. Any use of these "controlled substances" necessitates compliance with detailed

| TABLE 3-3 | **Principal Respiratory and Gastrointestinal System Effects of Anesthetic Agents and Adjuncts** | | | | |

| Preanesthetic Agent Class | Respiratory Rate | Tidal Volume | Salivary, Respiratory, GI Secretions | GI Motility | Other Respiratory and GI Effects |
|---|---|---|---|---|---|
| Anticholinergics | 0 | 0 | - (atropine) -- (glycopyrrolate) (except for Ru) | --/--- Colic (Eq); bloat (Ru) | Bronchodilatation; thickening of secretions (Fe, Ru) |
| Acepromazine | 0 (- with other agents) | 0 (- with other agents) | 0 | - | Antiemetic |
| Benzodiazepines | 0 (apnea if given rapidly IV) | 0 | 0 | | Appetite stimulation (Fe, Ru) |
| Alpha$_2$-agonists | - /-- (especially Ru) | -/-- (especially Ru) | 0 | - | ++ vomiting (Fe > Ca); gastric distension (Ca); bloat, regurgitation (Bo); bloat, ileus (Eq) |
| Opioids | - (minimal except at high doses) | - (minimal except at high doses) | +/++ (SA) | Stimulation (+), then ileus (-) | ++ vomiting (SA) diarrhea, then constipation |
| Barbiturates | --/--- (including apnea) | --/--- | ++/+++ | - then + | Sneezing and coughing |
| Propofol | --/--- (including apnea) | --/--- | 0 | | Antiemetic |
| Dissociatives | 0 | 0 | ++/+++ | | Apneustic respiration at high doses |
| Etomidate | 0 (temporary apnea), then may + | 0 | 0 | 0 | Nausea and vomiting (induction, recovery) |
| Guaifenesin | 0 | 0 | 0 | + | Apneustic respiration at high doses |
| Halogenated inhalants | - to --- | - to --- | 0 | - | Isoflurane: may vomit Desflurane: coughing |

*Bo*, Bovine; *Ca*, canine; *Eq*, equine; *Fe*, feline; *GI*, gastrointestinal; *IV*, intravenously; *Ru*, ruminants; *SA*, small animals.
- = depression; + = stimulation.
Notes on use of this table:
- 0 indicates minimal to no effect.
- - indicates a decrease in the parameter indicated (where - is mild; -- is moderate; --- is marked).
- + indicates an increase in the parameter indicated (where + is mild; ++ is moderate; +++ is marked).
- Effects of drugs depend on many factors, including species, differences among specific agents within a class, dose, and drug interactions. Therefore quantifications of the principal effects (mild, moderate, marked) are approximations.
- The information regarding opioids includes those of agonists, partial agonists, and agonist-antagonists. When reading this, note that effects of agonists are generally more pronounced than those of agonist-antagonists or partial agonists).

record-keeping requirements owing to the potential for abuse or theft. In the United States, the Controlled Substances Act assigns each drug to one of five drug schedules according to its potential for abuse. In a similar way, Canadian legislation has classified each opiate as a narcotic, controlled, or prescription drug. Agents classified as narcotics in Canada or as Schedule II substances in the United States cannot be dispensed or drawn into a syringe except under the direct supervision of a licensed veterinarian.

All controlled substances must be kept in a double-locked cabinet, safe, or other secure storage place and must not be left on countertops or in other public areas. After a dose is withdrawn from a bottle containing a controlled substance, the bottle should be immediately returned to locked storage. Usage must be accurately recorded in a drug logbook, and inventory must be periodically checked to ensure that no drug is unaccounted for.

## PREANESTHETIC MEDICATIONS

The following agent classes are traditionally classified as preanesthetic medications because they are most commonly administered during the preanesthetic period. These agents are often given alone or in combination as a part of balanced anesthesia.
- Anticholinergics
- Tranquilizers and sedatives
  - Phenothiazines
  - Benzodiazepines
  - Alpha$_2$-adrenoceptor agonists (alpha$_2$-agonists)
- Opioids

### Reasons for the Use of Preanesthetic Medications

The principal reasons for giving commonly used preanesthetic medications follow. Table 3-5 summarizes these benefits.

| TABLE 3-4 | **Other Principal Effects of Anesthetic Agents and Adjuncts** | | | | |
|---|---|---|---|---|---|
| Preanesthetic Agent Class | Ocular Effects | Muscle Tone | Urogenital System Effects | Cross Placental Barrier | Other Effects |
| Anticholinergics | +/++ Mydriasis (Fe > Ca) | 0 | | Yes (atropine); minimally (glycopyrrolate) | PLR may be depressed; decreased lacrimal secretions |
| Acepromazine | Third eyelid prolapse; decreased IOP | 0 | Penile prolapse (Eq, Bo) | Yes—slowly | antihistamine effect; decreased PCV |
| Benzodiazepines | Decreased IOP | - - - | | Yes | Muscular fasciculations (Eq); IM injection painful |
| Alpha$_2$- agonists | Increased IOP because of vomiting | - - - | Premature parturition (Bo); increased urine production | Yes | Transient hyperglycemia; reaction to loud noises; sweating, muscle tremors (Eq) |
| Opioids | Miosis (Ca); mydriasis (Fe, LA); increased IOP | 0 | Urine retention; decreased urine production | Yes—slowly | Reactions to loud noises; sweating (Eq); increased motor activity (Eq) |
| Barbiturates | Decreased IOP | 0/- | | Yes | Tissue irritation if not injected IV |
| Propofol | Decreased IOP | - -/- - - | | Yes | Muscle twitching during induction (Ca) |
| Dissociatives | Open, central, dilated; 0/+ nystagmus; increased IOP | 0 to +++ (muscle twitching) | | Yes | Increased sensitivity to sensory stimuli; behavior changes during recovery |
| Etomidate | 0/increased IOP | - - | | Yes | Excitement and muscle activity during induction, recovery; intravenous injection painful |
| Guaifenesin | | - - | | Yes | Excitement during induction if used alone; tissue irritation if not injected IV |
| Halogenated inhalants | -/- - (isoflurane) | | | Yes | Sevoflurane: excitement, muscle fasciculations during recovery |

*Bo,* Bovine; *Ca,* canine; *Eq,* equine; *Fe,* feline; *IM,* intramuscular; *IOP,* intraocular pressure; *IV,* intravenously; *LA,* large animals; *PCV,* packed cell volume; *PLR,* pupillary light reflex; *Ru,* ruminants; *SA,* small animals.

- = depression; + = stimulation.

Notes on use of this table:

- 0 indicates minimal to no effect.
- - indicates a decrease in the parameter indicated (where - is mild; - - is moderate; - - - is marked).
- + indicates an increase in the parameter indicated (where + is mild; ++ is moderate; +++ is marked).
- Effects of drugs depend on many factors, including species, differences among specific agents within a class, dose, and drug interactions. Therefore quantifications of the principal effects (mild, moderate, marked) are approximations.
- The information regarding opioids includes those of agonists, partial agonists, and agonist-antagonists. When reading this, note that effects of agonists are generally more pronounced than those of agonist-antagonists or partial agonists).

1. To calm or sedate an excited, frightened, or vicious animal. Sedation not only enhances patient comfort and reduces anxiety, but also simplifies patient restraint.
2. To minimize adverse effects of concurrently administered drugs. All anesthetic agents and adjuncts cause undesirable adverse effects in addition to their desired action. For example, ketamine causes excessive salivation in some patients, and alpha$_2$-agonists may cause profound bradycardia or heart block. Anticholinergics are sometimes given to decrease these exaggerated parasympathetic effects.
3. To reduce the required dose of concurrently administered agents. For example, administration of a sedative during the preanesthetic period will often decrease the amount of general anesthetic required to produce surgical anesthesia.
4. To produce smoother anesthetic inductions and recoveries. During induction and recovery, patients pass through a period of involuntary excitement. While passing through this stage, they can be dangerous to themselves and to personnel, inflicting bites or experiencing bone fractures or other serious injuries in extreme situations.

| TABLE 3-5 | **Principal Reasons for Giving Preanesthetic Agents** | | | | | |
|---|---|---|---|---|---|---|
| Preanesthetic Agent Class | Provide Tranquilization and/or Sedation | Ease Induction and Recovery | Decrease Adverse Effects and Amount of General Anesthetic Required | Provide Muscle Relaxation | Minimize Bradycardia and Salivation | Provide Analgesia |
| Anticholinergics | 0 | 0 | 0 | 0 | +++ | 0 |
| Acepromazine | ++ | ++ | + | 0 | 0 | 0 |
| Benzodiazepines | +/0 | ++ | + | ++ | 0 | 0 |
| Alpha$_2$-agonists | +++ | +++ | +++ | ++ | 0 | ++ |
| Opioid agonists; partial agonists; agonist-antagonists | +/++ | ++ | ++ | 0 | 0 | +++ |

0 = does not have the effect listed

+, ++ or +++ = produces the effect to a slight, moderate or great degree respectively.

5. To decrease pain and discomfort before, during, and after surgery. As noted above, most general anesthetic agents have limited or no analgesic effect, so in many cases adjuncts must be given to provide the necessary level of pain control.

6. To produce muscle relaxation. Muscle relaxation is particularly important during some procedures including orthopedic and ocular surgery. Preanesthetic medications such as benzodiazepines and alpha$_2$-agonists are often given concurrently with general anesthetics to produce the desired amount of muscle relaxation.

Preanesthetic medications also have other uses. For example, tranquilizers are used to calm patients for transport, physical examination, radiographic procedures, and wound treatment. They are helpful in preventing animals from chewing wounds and bandages. The benzodiazepine diazepam stimulates the appetite in cats and ruminants, phenothiazines have antiemetic properties, and many opioids are effective cough suppressants.

The veterinarian will decide which preanesthetic medications to give based on the nature of the procedure, patient need, personal preference, and other factors, as well as the route and time of administration.

Preanesthetic medications are usually given via the IV, intramuscular (IM), or subcutaneous (SC) route, but the onset of action, duration of action, and dose vary with each of these routes. Of these three routes, SC administration is associated with the slowest onset of action and longest duration. IM administration results in a somewhat faster onset (15 to 20 minutes in most cases) and a somewhat shorter duration than SC administration. Patients given sedatives by the IM or SC route should be left undisturbed until peak action is reached because excitement or stimulation can sometimes cause the patient to override the effects of these agents when either of these routes is used. Drugs given intravenously generally act within seconds to a few minutes and have a shorter duration than if given either intramuscularly or subcutaneously but should be administered slowly and cautiously because potency and the potential for adverse effects are increased when drugs are given by this route. In general, IV doses are typically about one half IM or SC doses.

Although some agents such as ketamine can be given by mouth, effects of orally administered drugs are unpredictable. For this reason, this route of administration is usually reserved for patients too aggressive to be handled or for other situations in which it is impossible to inject the drug.

> **TECHNICIAN NOTE** Patients given sedatives by the IM or SC route should be left undisturbed until peak action is reached because excitement or stimulation can sometimes cause the patient to override the effects. Drugs given intravenously should be administered slowly and cautiously because potency and the potential for adverse effects are increased when drugs are given by this route.

## Anticholinergics

Also known as **parasympatholytics, anticholinergics** are most commonly used to prevent and treat bradycardia and to decrease salivary secretions arising from parasympathetic stimulation. The two anticholinergic agents commonly used in veterinary medicine are atropine and glycopyrrolate. Atropine is a relatively old drug, derived from the deadly nightshade plant, that was used for many years to decrease excessive respiratory secretions and laryngospasm caused by the irritating effects of ether, and the excess secretions caused by the barbiturates. Glycopyrrolate is a newer synthetic quaternary ammonium compound. Both drugs may be given by the IV, IM, SC, or intratracheal (IT) route. When these drugs are used as preanesthetics, the IM and IV routes are most commonly employed. The IT and IV routes are used in emergency situations in which rapid action is essential. Atropine is approved for use in several domestic species, and glycopyrrolate is approved for use in dogs and cats.

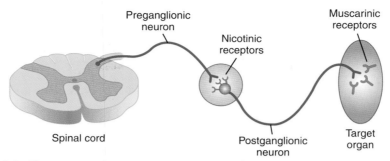

**FIGURE 3-1**   The parasympathetic nervous system. Preganglionic neuron releases acetylcholine at the nicotinic receptors. Postganglionic neuron releases acetylcholine at the muscarinic receptors of the target organ. Anticholinergics affect only the muscarinic receptors.

## Mode of Action and Pharmacology

Acetylcholine is the primary neurotransmitter in the PNS responsible for parasympathetic effects (also referred to as *cholinergic effects*). The PNS has two types of receptors for acetylcholine. The nicotinic receptors are located on the postganglionic neurons at the junction with the preganglionic neurons, and the muscarinic receptors are located on the target organs (Figure 3-1). Anticholinergics competitively block binding of the neurotransmitter acetylcholine at the muscarinic receptors.

The vagus nerve (tenth cranial nerve) provides parasympathetic innervation to numerous target organs including the heart, lungs, gastrointestinal (GI) tract, some secretory glands, and the iris of the eye. During surgery the vagus nerve may be stimulated by endotracheal intubation, traction on visceral organs during abdominal surgery (known as the *viscerovagal reflex*), and manipulation of the eye during ocular surgery (known as the *oculovagal reflex*) and by some drugs including the alpha$_2$-agonists, opioids, and common general anesthetics. Increased binding of acetylcholine to the muscarinic receptors caused by vagal stimulation results in observable parasympathetic effects at the target organs, such as bradycardia, bronchoconstriction, excess tear and saliva production, excess production of respiratory system secretions, increased GI motility, and miosis. By blocking the muscarinic receptors, anticholinergics help to reverse and prevent these parasympathetic effects (thus the alternative name, *parasympatholytics*).

After IM injection, atropine begins to act in about 5 minutes, reaches peak effect in about 10 to 20 minutes, and has a duration of action of 60 to 90 minutes. Glycopyrrolate has a similar onset of action, reaches peak effect in about 30 to 45 minutes, and has a duration of action of 2 to 3 hours, although salivary secretions can be suppressed for up to 7 hours. In order to allow time for peak effect, either agent should be administered intramuscularly at least 20 to 30 minutes before anesthetic induction. When given intravenously, the onset of action of atropine is about 1 minute and peak effect is about 3 to 4 minutes after injection. This makes this drug ideal for treatment of bradycardia in emergency situations such as cardiopulmonary-cerebrovascular resuscitation (CPCR).

### Effects on Major Organ Systems

#### Central Nervous System

Anticholinergics are not sedatives and therefore have limited CNS effects, although atropine can cause mild sedation in some patients at therapeutic doses. Glycopyrrolate is less likely to cause CNS effects because it does not cross the blood-brain barrier.

#### Cardiovascular System

These agents prevent bradycardia, which is often associated with anesthesia and surgery, and routinely cause the heart rate to increase.

### Other Effects

- Reduction of respiratory tract, GI tract, and salivary secretions. Several anesthetic agents, particularly ketamine and thiobarbiturates, induce copious production of saliva. Endotracheal intubation often induces excess airway mucous production, especially in cats. Accumulation of these excessive secretions can lead to airway obstruction.
- **Mydriasis.** This effect is not commonly seen when dogs are given the usual preanesthetic doses but may be seen in cats. When monitoring patients, the anesthetist must remember that the pupillary light reflex (PLR) may be depressed and therefore unreliable in patients given anticholinergics.
- Reduction of lacrimal secretions. Corneal drying is a risk of general anesthesia because the patient's eyes remain open. Corneal drying, if severe or prolonged, will result in keratitis and corneal ulceration. For this reason, the corneas of animals receiving anticholinergics should be protected from drying by instilling a ¼- to ½-inch strip of ophthalmic lubricating ointment in each eye every hour.
- Bronchodilatation. Anticholinergics increase the diameter of bronchioles. This results in increased anatomic **dead space,** which may put the patient at risk for hypoxemia (low blood oxygen).

## Adverse Effects

### Cardiovascular System

- Arrhythmias. After IV injection, anticholinergics may induce temporary first- or second-degree atrioventricular (AV) block, followed by sinus **tachycardia.** Although glycopyrrolate is less arrhythmogenic than atropine, either drug may also induce other cardiac arrhythmias including ventricular arrhythmias. For these reasons, these drugs should be avoided in animals with preexisting rapid heart rates (more than 140 beats per minute [bpm] in dogs, 180 bpm in cats, 60 bpm in horses, and 100 bpm in ruminants) or heart disease (such as congestive heart failure or hyperthyroid-associated cardiomyopathy in cats).
- When given at low doses, atropine may induce a temporary bradycardia. This is because atropine blocks a second type of muscarinic receptor located on presynaptic nerve terminals that normally inhibits acetylcholine release. The atropine-induced blockade of these receptors releases acetylcholine, resulting in bradycardia until the postsynaptic receptors are also blocked.

### Respiratory System

- Thickening of respiratory and salivary secretions. The use of anticholinergics in cats is associated with the production of thick mucous secretions within the airways. So even though these drugs decrease the volume of the secretions, the increased viscosity may predispose the patient to airway blockage. For this reason, some veterinarians do not use anticholinergics in this species. Anticholinergics are not recommended in ruminants at all except to treat intraoperative bradycardia or for CPCR. This is because these drugs do not decrease the amount of salivary secretions in these species but instead cause the saliva to become thick and ropy, which places these patients at risk for respiratory obstruction.

### Other Adverse Effects

- Anticholinergics inhibit intestinal peristalsis. This can cause gut stasis and **colic** in horses and bloat in ruminants even at clinical doses. Therefore use of these agents should be avoided in these species.

## Use of Anticholinergics

Atropine and glycopyrrolate are still commonly used by veterinary anesthetists, although less so now than in the past. Many modern anesthetic agents do not cause excessive secretions, and bradycardia is well tolerated by most patients. Because of the potential for significant adverse effects, particularly tachycardia, thickening of mucous secretions, decreased tear production, and mydriasis, many authorities question the routine use of these agents. However, anticholinergics are beneficial for some patients (e.g., those with severe bradycardia, heart block, or excessive salivary secretions).

Atropine or glycopyrrolate is often included in preanesthetic and sedative protocols such as the "BAG" and "SuperBAG" protocols (see Chapter 8). Either agent can also be used to prevent adverse effects associated with reversal of nondepolarizing neuromuscular blocking agents. (See Chapter 6 for more information about neuromuscular blocking agents.)

Although the agents are similar, there are subtle differences between atropine and glycopyrrolate. Glycopyrrolate is slightly less likely to induce cardiac arrhythmias, suppresses salivation more effectively than atropine, and only minimally crosses the placental barrier in pregnant animals. For these reasons many practitioners prefer this drug as a preanesthetic despite its greater expense. Atropine is still considered to be the better choice as an emergency treatment for bradycardias associated with cardiopulmonary arrest, however, because of its faster onset.

Veterinary-labeled atropine products are available in two strengths: 0.54 mg/mL (sometimes listed on the label as 1/120 grain/mL) and 15 mg/mL. After calculating a dose, remember to draw the drug of the correct strength into the syringe or an incorrect amount will be administered to the patient. For example, a volume of 0.5 mL of atropine drawn from a solution with a concentration of 15 mg/mL contains nearly 30 times the amount of drug as compared with a solution with a concentration of 0.54 mg/mL.

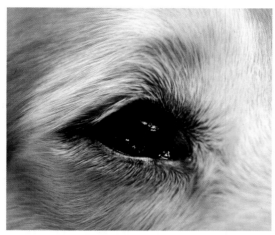

**FIGURE 3-2**  Prolapse of the third eyelid. Note that the cornea is partially covered.

## Tranquilizers and Sedatives

As mentioned in the introduction, a sedative and a tranquilizer are not exactly the same thing. A tranquilizer is a drug that reduces anxiety but does not necessarily decrease awareness and wakefulness. A sedative is a drug that causes reduced mental activity and sleepiness. Most veterinarians use the terms *sedative* and *tranquilizer* interchangeably, however. This is because the effects of these drugs often overlap, as most of these drugs produce both effects to some degree. For instance, tranquilizing effects predominate in the drug diazepam, whereas dexmedetomidine has primarily sedative effects.

Three classes of tranquilizers or sedatives are commonly used in veterinary medicine: phenothiazines, benzodiazepines, and alpha$_2$-adrenoceptor agonists (alpha$_2$-agonists). In addition to tranquilization and sedation, some also cause other effects including **ataxia** and prolapse of the nictitating membrane (also called the *third eyelid*) (Figure 3-2). Phenothiazines protect against cardiac arrhythmias and are antiemetics. In contrast, alpha$_2$-agonists are analgesics and can produce vomiting in some patients. Both alpha$_2$-agonists and benzodiazepines are good muscle relaxants.

There are some general risks to using these medications of which the technician must be aware. After receiving these drugs, patients should not be left unattended on a table or in a cage with an open door because they can easily fall and be injured. Sedatives relax the tissues in the pharynx, which may cause serious and life-threatening respiratory distress in brachycephalic dogs, especially those that exhibit significant respiratory stridor when awake. There are also risks to personnel and owners. Sedated animals may exhibit unusual behavior such as aggression or may suddenly become aroused and aggressive, particularly if stimulated suddenly (e.g., by pain).

## Phenothiazines

Phenothiazines are a group of noncontrolled, water-soluble drugs with somewhat diverse indications. Acepromazine maleate is used in a wide variety of large and small animal species as an anesthetic adjunct. Triflupromazine, a drug used only in humans, is an antipsychotic and antiemetic drug used to treat schizophrenia and vomiting. Chlorpromazine, a drug with similar indications to triflupromazine in human patients, is also used in veterinary patients as an antiemetic but not as an anesthetic adjunct.

Acepromazine maleate (also known as acepromazine or "ace") is used alone or in combination with other drugs as a preanesthetic in many species to provide sedation, to decrease the dose of general anesthetic required, and to ease induction and recovery. It is also used alone or in combination with opioids to provide a mild to moderate level of sedation and tranquilization for minor procedures including wound treatment, grooming, and noninvasive diagnostic tests such as radiography. It is approved for use in dogs, cats, and horses.

When used as a preanesthetic and sedative, acepromazine is usually administered by the IV or IM route. Although it is also available in oral tablet form for tranquilization and sedation of small animals, this route is seldom used in anesthesia. There is currently no available reversal agent.

### Mode of Action and Pharmacology

Acepromazine has a complex mechanism of action that is not fully understood. Major effects include depression of the reticular activating center of the brain and blockage of alpha-adrenergic, dopamine, and histamine receptors. It is metabolized by the liver and crosses the placental barrier slowly. Onset of action is about 15 minutes after IM injection in dogs or IV injection in horses, and peak effect occurs within 30 to 60 minutes. The duration of action is 4 to 8 hours in small animals but may be longer (up to 48 hours) if higher doses are used or if the drug is given to old, sick, or debilitated patients or patients with liver disease. The duration of action in horses is shorter (1 to 3 hours).

### Effects on Major Organ Systems

**Central Nervous System**

- Calming, sedation, reluctance to move, and decreased interest in the patient's surroundings. Sedation is less pronounced in cats than in dogs and horses and is less pronounced than that seen with alpha$_2$-agonists in all species.
- Acepromazine does not provide pain control but does decrease anxiety in patients in pain that are receiving analgesics concurrently.

**Cardiovascular System**

- Peripheral vasodilatation. This causes hypotension, a reflexive increase in heart rate, and increased heat loss, leading to hypothermia. Acepromazine also directly decreases cardiac output.
- Antiarrhythmic effect. Some anesthetics, such as barbiturates, have a potential to cause cardiac arrhythmias, which may decrease cardiac output. Phenothiazines protect against ventricular arrhythmias.

### Respiratory System

• Acepromazine does not cause significant respiratory depression but worsens depressive effects of other sedative and anesthetic agents.

### *Other Effects*

• Antiemetic effect. Even at very low doses, acepromazine helps prevent vomiting during the anesthetic period. It can also be used to prevent vomiting caused by motion sickness.
• Antihistamine effect. Histamine is a chemical released during an allergic response. Acepromazine prevents the release of histamine and therefore decreases allergic reactions. For this reason, acepromazine should not be used to sedate animals that are to undergo allergy testing.

 **TECHNICIAN NOTE** Major effects of phenothiazines are as follows:
• Calming, sedation
• Peripheral vasodilatation
• Antiarrhythmic effects
• Antiemetic effects

### *Adverse Effects*

#### Central Nervous System

• Reduction of the seizure threshold. Although it was reported to have antiseizure activity by some researchers, acepromazine is now generally believed to have the ability to induce seizures in patients with epilepsy or seizures from other causes.
• Occasionally acepromazine may induce excitement or aggression rather than sedation. This effect may persist into the postanesthetic period but usually resolves within 48 hours. Owners should be warned that behavioral changes sometimes occur, and care should be used when handling patients returning home within 48 hours of anesthesia.

#### Cardiovascular System

• Severe hypotension. Hypotension produced by acepromazine is dose-dependent and more pronounced in frightened or excited patients. In animals receiving isoflurane, a significant drop in blood pressure (as much as 20% to 30%) occurs. This contributes to intraoperative hypotension commonly seen in patients given this combination.

#### Other Adverse Effects

• Penile prolapse. Acepromazine has been reported to cause prolapse of the penis in horses and other large animals, which can lead to injury and subsequent permanent paralysis of the retractor penis muscle. For this reason, some veterinarians choose not to use acepromazine in breeding stallions.
• Decreased packed cell volume (PCV). In horses and dogs the PCV drops within 30 minutes, likely because of increased uptake of red blood cells (RBCs) by the spleen.

 **TECHNICIAN NOTE** Major adverse effects of phenothiazines are as follows:
• Reduction of the seizure threshold
• Hypotension
• Penile prolapse in horses and other large animals
• Decreased PCV

### *Use of Acepromazine*

Patients should be placed in a quiet location free from stimulation between administration and peak effect, because the sedative effects can be overridden if the patient is stimulated to a sufficient degree.

It has been suggested that the manufacturer's recommended dose for acepromazine is higher than that actually required for preanesthesia and that the dose should be reduced to minimize the danger of adverse effects. The commonly accepted doses are about 0.05 to 0.1 mg/kg in small animals with a maximum dose of 3 mg in dogs and 1 mg in cats, and 0.03 to 0.05 mg/kg in horses. Higher doses will increase hypotension but not sedation.

The anesthetist should be particularly aware that phenothiazines have increased potency or duration in geriatric animals, neonates, animals with liver or cardiac dysfunction, and generally debilitated patients. Responses to this drug are also species- and breed-dependent. Doses should be reduced 25% in collies and Australian shepherds to minimize the possibility of exaggerated or prolonged sedation. Giant breed dogs, greyhounds, and boxers can be very sensitive to this drug and may experience severe bradycardia and hypotension. Terriers and cats are more resistant to its effects. Severe hypotension and bradycardia are treated with IV fluid therapy and anticholinergics.

In horses, care must be taken to ensure that acepromazine is injected into a vein. Inadvertent injection into the carotid artery can cause severe CNS excitement or depression, seizures, and death. The location of the needle can be checked by the following maneuver. After venipuncture, remove the syringe from the needle. Release digital pressure on the vein. If the needle is in the jugular vein, blood flow from the hub will cease. If it is in an artery, blood flow will continue from the hub despite the release in digital pressure.

Although acepromazine has a relatively low toxicity, severe overdoses require treatment. Hypotension resulting from overdose is worsened by epinephrine and should instead be treated with phenylephrine or norepinephrine.

**TECHNICIAN NOTE** The commonly used dose of acepromazine (about 0.05 to 0.1 mg/kg in small animals with a maximum dose of 3 mg in dogs and 1 mg in cats; 0.03 to 0.05 mg/kg in horses) is significantly less than the labeled dose. Higher doses will increase hypotension but not sedation.

## Benzodiazepines

The benzodiazepines, also referred to as *minor tranquilizers,* are a group of controlled, reversible drugs most often used in combination with other agents for their muscle relaxant, anticonvulsant, and appetite-stimulating properties. These drugs produce unreliable sedative effects and in dogs, cats, and horses may instead produce **dysphoria,** excitement, and ataxia, especially when administered to young, healthy animals.

Diazepam, zolazepam (a component of Telazol), and midazolam are the most commonly used anesthetic adjuncts in this class. Although not used for anesthesia, lorazepam is used in dogs as an alternative to diazepam to treat status epilepticus. Of these agents, only zolazepam is licensed for use in animals in the United States and Canada.

Benzodiazepines are commonly administered intramuscularly or intravenously, although diazepam is irritating and poorly absorbed when administered intramuscularly.

### Mode of Action and Pharmacology

Benzodiazepines depress the CNS. Although the exact mechanism of action is not known, benzodiazepines exert their primary effects by increasing activity of endogenous gamma-aminobutyric acid (GABA), an inhibitory neurotransmitter in the brain.

The commercially prepared injectable diazepam is mixed with 40% propylene glycol as well as several other ingredients. It is not water-soluble and cannot be mixed with water-soluble drugs except ketamine. Midazolam and zolazepam are water-soluble and so can be used in combination with other water-soluble drugs. Most benzodiazepines have a relatively rapid onset of action (less than or equal to 15 minutes after IM injection for midazolam and zolazepam) and short duration (1 to 4 hours).

### Effects on Major Organ Systems

#### Central Nervous System

- Antianxiety and calming effect. Benzodiazepines, unlike phenothiazines, do not cause significant sedation in healthy young animals unless used in combination with other drugs such as ketamine or opioids. Although their effect as a sole sedative in healthy young animals is inadequate, benzodiazepines are much more effective in geriatric or debilitated animals. Diazepam also enhances the sedation and analgesia of other agents, and its relative safety makes it a popular drug for combination protocols.
- The anesthetist should be aware that benzodiazepines, like phenothiazines, have no analgesic effect and when used alone will not be effective in calming animals that are experiencing pain.
- Anticonvulsant activity. To take advantage of this effect, many anesthetists use benzodiazepines in combination with other agents that have a potential to cause seizures, including ketamine and local anesthetics. Benzodiazepines are also preanesthetics of choice for some animals with seizure disorders. Diazepam and lorazepam can be given intravenously or intrarectally, and midazolam can be given intravenously for treatment of seizures.

#### Cardiovascular and Respiratory Systems

- At therapeutic doses, benzodiazepines have few effects on the cardiovascular and respiratory systems and therefore have a high margin of safety. Heart rate, blood pressure, and cardiac output are minimally affected. This property makes them particularly useful for anesthesia of high-risk and geriatric animals.

### Other Effects

- Skeletal muscle relaxation. Benzodiazepines are excellent skeletal muscle relaxants and often are used to counteract the muscle rigidity seen with agents such as ketamine and etomidate.
- Potentiation of general anesthetics. Premedication with diazepam decreases the requirements of many general anesthetics including the inhalant agents.
- Appetite stimulation in cats and ruminants. Diazepam and midazolam are commonly used as appetite stimulants in cats, and may also be effective appetite stimulants in many other species.

> **TECHNICIAN NOTE**   Major effects of benzodiazepines are as follows:
> - Antianxiety and calming *only* in old or ill patients
> - Anticonvulsant activity
> - Skeletal muscle relaxation
> - Appetite stimulation in cats and ruminants

### Adverse Effects

#### Central Nervous System

- The primary adverse effects of these drugs involve the CNS. Animals, especially those that are young and healthy, receiving these drugs alone may actually become more difficult to control. Dogs may become disoriented and excited, and cats may become dysphoric or aggressive. Horses may have muscle **fasciculations,** and animals of any large species may become ataxic or recumbent.

#### Other Adverse Effects

- Effect on neonates: Benzodiazepines cross the placenta and may cause CNS depression in neonates delivered by cesarean section.
- Adverse effects specific to diazepam: Diazepam is painful and poorly absorbed when administered intramuscularly. Diazepam should be given by slow IV injection, because if given rapidly it can cause pain, bradycardia, hypotension, and apnea. Cats receiving oral diazepam have been reported to develop hepatic failure within 5 to 11 days of commencing therapy.

*TECHNICIAN NOTE* Major adverse effects of benzodiazepines are as follows:
- Disorientation and excitement in young, healthy dogs
- Dysphoria and aggression in cats
- Ataxia or recumbency in large animals
- Muscle fasciculations in horses
- Pain on IM injection of diazepam

## Use of Benzodiazepines

Diazepam is not water-soluble and is therefore not physically compatible with most other agents. It should not be mixed in a single syringe with atropine, acepromazine, barbiturates, or opioids because a precipitate may form. Although not recommended by the manufacturer, diazepam is often combined in the same syringe with ketamine. Although this seldom results in adverse events, this combination should not be used if a precipitate forms and should not be stored in syringes or other plastic containers because diazepam is very soluble in plastic and over time is absorbed by syringes, IV bags, and IV tubing.

Diazepam and midazolam are both commonly used in combination with other agents to induce anesthesia. Although it is not possible to induce anesthesia in a healthy animal through the use of these drugs alone, they are an effective supplement to other agents. In particular, the combination of ketamine and diazepam has gained wide acceptance as a safe and effective IV induction agent in small animals and horses. When this combination is used in small animals, midazolam may be substituted for diazepam. Diazepam may also be administered concurrently with opioids, propofol, or thiopental (provided separate syringes are used) to achieve safe, smooth induction of high-risk patients. If diazepam is given in combination with opioids, thiopental, or propofol, an IV catheter should be used and a saline flush given after each drug.

Diazepam and midazolam are light-sensitive and for this reason are often provided in brown glass vials. If in a clear glass container, these drugs should be stored away from light.

Benzodiazepines are classified as controlled drugs in Canada and the United States. Some potential for human abuse and theft exists, so these drugs must be stored in a locked cabinet, and appropriate records must be kept in compliance with DEA requirements.

Midazolam has some advantages over diazepam. It is water-soluble and therefore can be mixed with other preanesthetic and anesthetic agents. It is less irritating to tissues and is also more reliably absorbed after IM or SC injection. Like diazepam, midazolam causes unreliable sedation in dogs when used alone but is an excellent sedative in swine and some exotics including ferrets, rabbits, and birds.

In dogs, small mammals, and birds, midazolam is usually used in combination with ketamine and/or opioids for sedation and intubation. It can also be administered before induction of anesthesia with thiopental, propofol, or etomidate to increase muscle relaxation and reduce adverse effects.

Zolazepam is available only mixed with tiletamine in the combination product Telazol. This powdered product requires reconstitution with sterile water and is discussed more in the section covering dissociative anesthetics on p. 82.

The benzodiazepine antagonist flumazenil can be administered to reverse the effects of benzodiazepines, although at the present time this drug is not commonly used in practice because of high expense and the very low incidence of complications seen with these agents.

Benzodiazepine agents are used for a variety of purposes in veterinary medicine other than anesthesia and seizure control. For instance, oral diazepam is sometimes used to modify undesirable behavior such as inappropriate urination in cats.

*TECHNICIAN NOTE* Diazepam should not be mixed in a single syringe with atropine, acepromazine, barbiturates, or opioids because a precipitate may form. Diazepam should not be stored in syringes, IV bags, or other plastic containers because it is absorbed.

## Alpha₂-Adrenoceptor Agonists

Alpha₂-adrenoceptor agonists (also written as *alpha₂-agonists* or *α₂-agonists*) are a group of noncontrolled agents used alone and in combination with other anesthetics and adjuncts in both large and small animal patients for sedation, analgesia, and muscle relaxation. They are commonly given before minor procedures such as radiography, wound treatment, or bandaging and subsequently reversed with an alpha₂-adrenoceptor antagonist. This allows the patient to be sequentially sedated and "awakened" so that it can be sent home a short time after completion of the procedure. Xylazine (Rompun, AnaSed), dexmedetomidine (Dexdomitor), detomidine (Dormosedan), and romifidine (Sedivet) are members of this class of drugs. Medetomidine (Domitor), a predecessor to dexmedetomidine, was recently discontinued in the United States. These drugs are most often administered intramuscularly or intravenously. SC injection is less reliable and not recommended.

### Mode of Action and Pharmacology

Alpha₂-agonists act on alpha₂-adrenergic receptors (also called *alpha₂-adrenoceptors*) of the sympathetic nervous system (SNS) both within the CNS and peripherally, causing a decrease in the release of the neurotransmitter norepinephrine. When these drugs are combined with other tranquilizers or analgesic agents, the result tends to be additive or synergistic (supraadditive) in nature.

The SNS has several different types of receptors (alpha, beta, and dopaminergic). In general, stimulation of the

SNS is associated with the "fight-or-flight response." For this reason, the CNS depression induced by alpha$_2$-agonists does not at first glance seem logical. This paradoxic effect occurs, however, because stimulation of the alpha$_2$-receptors does not cause the fight-or-flight response but instead causes sedation, analgesia, bradycardia, hypotension, and hypothermia. These unique effects make these particular SNS stimulants useful sedatives and analgesics.

Alpha$_2$-agonists are metabolized in the liver, and the metabolites are excreted in the urine. Adequate hepatic and renal function are therefore important requirements for any animal receiving these drugs.

The onset and duration of action are similar with all currently available alpha$_2$-agonists. After injection, sedation occurs rapidly (within 5 to 15 minutes of IV injection or 15 to 30 minutes of IM injection) and lasts about 1 to 2 hours in most cases. Complete recovery takes about 2 to 4 hours if the drug is not reversed.

### Effects on Major Organ Systems

#### Central Nervous System

- Alpha$_2$-agonists are potent sedatives. Sedation is dose-dependent and can be profound in small animals, small ruminants, and foals. In horses, effects include a lowered head ("knees-to-nose" position), relaxed facial muscles, and a drooping lower lip. When the drugs are combined with other agents, sedation may be sufficient for minor or even major surgical procedures (referred to as "standing sedation").
- Unlike phenothiazines and benzodiazepines, alpha$_2$-agonists also provide analgesia. When combined with other analgesics and sedatives, they may provide sufficient analgesia to allow surgical procedures to be performed. Although the sedative effect of alpha$_2$-agonists may last for several hours, the analgesia may be short-lived (approximately 20 minutes for xylazine) and should be supplemented with another agent, typically an opioid, if a prolonged effect is required.

#### Cardiovascular System

- Alpha$_2$-agonists have a significant effect on the cardiovascular system. After injection, there is an early dose-dependent vasoconstriction that results in a brief period of hypertension and reflex bradycardia, during which the mucous membranes may look pale. Various cardiac arrhythmias including first- and second-degree AV block may also occur during this time (see p.147 for a discussion of these arrhythmias). These effects are more pronounced when the drug is given intravenously. This phase is followed by a decrease in cardiac output, hypotension, and a further drop in heart rate owing to decreased sympathetic tone.

#### Respiratory System

- Alpha$_2$-agonists depress the respiratory system. Although the effect is minimal at lower doses, high doses can significantly decrease **tidal volume** and respiratory rate. Respiratory depression is most notable in ruminants.

### Other Effects

- Muscle relaxation. These drugs are useful adjuncts to general anesthetics for procedures in which muscle relaxation is necessary.
- Increased effects of other anesthetics. When these agents are given as a preanesthetic, or concurrently with general anesthetics, the required doses of the anesthetics are substantially reduced (e.g., up to an 80% reduction of thiopental and a 50% reduction of propofol and inhalant agents).
- Vomiting. Many cats and some dogs vomit within a few minutes of receiving these agents. Because affected patients may have decreased swallowing reflexes, the airway must be protected to prevent aspiration of stomach contents by placing the head in a dependent position as soon as retching is noted. Dexmedetomidine is less likely to cause vomiting than xylazine.
- Hyperglycemia. Alpha$_2$-agonists reduce the secretion of insulin by the pancreas, causing transient hyperglycemia, which is not harmful to the animal but may confound the interpretation of blood samples collected during this period.
- Hypothermia. Alpha$_2$-agonists decrease thermoregulation and shivering, leading to hypothermia.

 *TECHNICIAN NOTE* Major effects of alpha$_2$-adrenoceptor agonists are as follows:
- Dose-dependent sedation that can be profound
- Analgesia
- Decreased cardiac output, heart rate, and blood pressure
- Decreased respiratory rate and tidal volume
- Muscle relaxation
- Vomiting in dogs and cats

### Adverse Effects

Alpha$_2$-agonists have considerable potential for adverse effects. These are reported most commonly when the drugs are given by the IV route and include the effects discussed in the following paragraphs.

#### Central Nervous System

- Temporary behavior changes. Patients that are excited before administration may become agitated and aggressive when touched, and any patient may move or startle in response to loud noises. Horses may experience muscle tremors and may kick in response to loud noises. Cattle frequently lie down. Excessive doses given intravenously may cause falling from ataxia and sedation.

#### Cardiovascular System

- Alpha$_2$-agonists cause profound cardiovascular depression. Dramatic decreases in heart rate (e.g., down to 30 to 50 bpm in dogs), blood pressure, and cardiac output with a resultant decrease in tissue perfusion can occur with these agents especially when given at high doses. Because of these serious effects, the use of alpha$_2$-agonists should be avoided in animals that are debilitated or that have cardiovascular disease.

**Respiratory System**

- Respiratory system depression varies from animal to animal and is more severe when alpha$_2$-agonists are given with other drugs. Some animals show respiratory depression of sufficient magnitude to negatively affect ventilation. Brachycephalic dogs and horses with upper respiratory obstruction may become dyspneic. As a general rule, alpha$_2$-agonists should not be administered to animals showing signs of respiratory disease.

**Other Adverse Effects**

- Increased urination. Alpha$_2$-agonists may increase urination because they interfere with the release of antidiuretic hormone.
- GI effects. Dogs may develop gaseous distension of the stomach that is visible on radiographs and may need to be relieved. Cattle may salivate, bloat, and regurgitate stomach contents. Rarely, horses may develop gas, colic, or intestinal bloat.
- Premature parturition. Xylazine causes increased intrauterine pressure in cattle and has the potential to cause abortion in the last trimester.
- Horses may sweat.
- Accidental intraarterial injection in horses can result in excitement, seizures, and collapse.
- Alpha$_2$-agonists can be absorbed through skin abrasions and mucous membranes, and as little as 0.1 mL of dexmedetomidine can cause hypotension and sedation in humans. Hospital employees handling these agents should ensure that any of the drugs spilled on human or animal skin is immediately washed off.

*TECHNICIAN NOTE*  Major adverse effects of alpha$_2$-adrenoceptor agonists are as follows:
- Agitation or aggression when touched
- Reaction to loud noises
- Ataxia and falling in cattle
- Severe bradycardia, hypotension, and decreased cardiac output
- Severe respiratory depression

## Use of Alpha$_2$-Agonists

Careful monitoring of vital signs is always essential for patients receiving these drugs, all of which should be used with caution. All members of this class can be given in standard doses to young, healthy patients but should be avoided in geriatric, diabetic, pregnant, pediatric, or sick patients.

To reduce the incidence of bradycardia, some veterinarians give atropine or glycopyrrolate as a premedication. However, this is not always effective and may in fact increase the workload of the heart and myocardial oxygen consumption. If used, anticholinergics must be administered 10 to 20 minutes before these agents are given, or bradycardia may worsen and other arrhythmias may develop.

Anticholinergics should also be avoided with alpha$_2$-agonist–ketamine combinations, because prolonged tachycardia can occur. If bradycardia occurs, the best treatment is administration of an appropriate reversal agent.

*TECHNICIAN NOTE*  Administration of anticholinergics to reduce the incidence of alpha$_2$-agonist–induced bradycardia is not always effective and may in fact increase the workload of the heart, worsen bradycardia, or cause tachyarrhythmias. If bradycardia develops, the best treatment is administration of an appropriate reversal agent.

**Xylazine.**  Xylazine has been available for several decades and is the first widely used alpha$_2$-agonist in both large and small animal species. It is supplied as a 2% solution (20 mg/mL) for small animal use and as a 10% solution (100 mg/mL) for equine use. Therefore to avoid a serious overdose, it is very important to look carefully at the label before drawing up a dose.

For several decades xylazine has been frequently used alone or in various combinations with ketamine, opioids, and other agents in dogs, cats, and other small animals. It has now been largely replaced by dexmedetomidine in these species. It is still used in large animals as a preanesthetic and sedative, in combination with butorphanol for minor procedures, and in combination with ketamine and guaifenesin (a combination known as "triple drip") to produce total IV anesthesia. Cattle have a much lower tolerance for xylazine, requiring only about one tenth the dose of horses.

**Dexmedetomidine.**  Dexmedetomidine (Dexdomitor) is currently the most commonly used alpha$_2$-agonist in dogs and cats. It is closely related to medetomidine, which was recently discontinued in the United States. Medetomidine is a mixture of two molecules that are mirror images of each other (**enantiomers**). The dextrorotatory enantiomer is a molecule that rotates the plane of polarized light to the right, and a levorotatory molecule rotates it to the left. Dexmedetomidine is the dextrorotatory enantiomer of medetomidine and produces the sedative and analgesic effects we associate with this drug, whereas levomedetomidine (the levorotatory enantiomer) has no sedative or analgesic activity. Dexmedetomidine does not contain the inactive enantiomer and so has approximately twice the potency of medetomidine. In 2008 a new product approved for use in both dogs and cats containing only dexmedetomidine (Dexdomitor) was introduced in the United States.

Because dexmedetomidine is relatively new, at the time of this writing, experience with the use of this drug is limited. However, because it is the active form of medetomidine, current evidence suggests that it can be used in much the same way. Its use is summarized in the following paragraphs.

Dexmedetomidine has greater potency and fewer adverse effects than xylazine. It is supplied as a 0.5-mg/mL solution for sedation and analgesia in dogs and cats and as a preanesthetic in dogs and is marketed along with a corresponding antagonist atipamezole (Antisedan). These two products are packaged such that equivalent volumes of the two drugs can be used to sequentially sedate and wake a patient for short or minor diagnostic, surgical, or therapeutic procedures. Dexmedetomidine is labeled for IM use in dogs and cats and IV use only in dogs.

The manufacturer recommends that dexmedetomidine dose be determined according to body surface area in dogs, so that smaller patients receive relatively more and larger patients receive relatively less. Charts based on this dosage scheme are supplied with the drug, with progressively increasing doses listed for patients of various body weights for "sedation/analgesia in dogs" and "preanesthesia in dogs." Low doses of dexmedetomidine given as a preanesthetic are generally more effective than acepromazine in reducing general anesthetic requirements and do not cause as profound a degree of hypotension when given with isoflurane.

Like xylazine, dexmedetomidine is also used in combination with other agents. For instance, one combination in widespread use is dexmedetomidine (10 mcg/kg) and butorphanol (0.2 mg/kg). The two drugs can be mixed in the same syringe and given intramuscularly. Dexmedetomidine can also be mixed with other opioids or with ketamine.

Animals should be left in a quiet environment for 10 to 15 minutes after injection to allow the drug to take maximum effect. If a short, minimally invasive procedure is planned (such as an ear flush, bandage change, or radiography), the sedation provided by dexmedetomidine-butorphanol and other combinations may be adequate without a general anesthetic. The sedation can be supplemented with a local block if minor surgery such as suturing a laceration or removal of a superficial skin tumor is planned. Although these patients are usually too awake for intubation, some veterinarians choose to provide supplemental oxygen by facemask. Caution should be exercised when dexmedetomidine combinations are used for minor operations, because sudden arousal has been reported even in heavily sedated patients.

If the sedated animal is to undergo more extensive surgery, an injectable or inhalant general anesthetic (e.g., thiopental, propofol, or isoflurane) can be given. The dose of general anesthetic required will be significantly less than that required for a nonsedated animal, and caution must be exercised to avoid overdosage.

Pain may be associated with IM injection of dexmedetomidine. Do not give anticholinergics with high doses of dexmedetomidine because paradoxic bradycardia may result.

The parent drug medetomidine has been used extensively in many other species, including cats, horses, and exotic animals.

**Detomidine.** Detomidine is used in horses to produce sedation, analgesia, and muscle relaxation. This drug is similar to xylazine, producing similar beneficial and adverse effects, but has approximately twice the duration of action. It is commonly given with butorphanol to produce standing sedation. It is also used to provide analgesia for colic pain.

**Romifidine.** Romifidine is similar to other drugs in this class but produces less ataxia than either detomidine or xylazine.

### Alpha$_2$-Antagonists

Yohimbine, tolazoline, and atipamezole are alpha$_2$-antagonists that can be used to reverse the effects of alpha$_2$-agonists. Because of the adverse cardiovascular effects and long duration of sedation that can occur after administration of alpha$_2$-agonists, use of an antagonist is often desirable. Yohimbine and tolazoline are used to reverse the effects of xylazine in dogs, cats, ruminants, horses and exotic species. Atipamezole is used to reverse the effects of dexmedetomidine in dogs, cats, and exotic species.

#### Mode of Action and Pharmacology

These agents work by displacing the agonist from the alpha$_2$-receptors. Alpha$_2$-antagonists preferentially bind to the receptors, thus reversing the effect of the corresponding agonist.

#### Effects

The major effect of alpha$_2$-antagonists is reversal of the sedative and cardiovascular effects of the corresponding agonist.

#### Adverse Effects

Alpha$_2$-antagonists have few adverse effects at clinical doses but can have significant adverse effects if too much is given. Doses should be based on the amount of the agonist that was given and the length of time since agonist administration and should be reduced if more than 30 minutes have elapsed. Adverse effects are neurologic, cardiovascular, and GI and include excitement, muscle tremors, hypotension, tachycardia, salivation, and diarrhea. Because of the potential for tachycardia, these agents should not be given when anticholinergics have also been given.

> *TECHNICIAN NOTE* Alpha$_2$-antagonists have few adverse effects at clinical doses but can have significant adverse effects if too much is given. Doses should be based on the amount of the agonist that was given and the length of time since agonist administration and should be reduced if more than 30 minutes have elapsed. When given intravenously, these agents should be given *slowly!*

### Use of Alpha₂-Antagonists

Alpha$_2$-antagonists will reverse all of the clinical effects of alpha$_2$-agonists, both detrimental (bradycardia) and beneficial (analgesia). To maintain analgesia it may be necessary to administer another analgesic agent just before the reversal. The anesthetist must also realize that alpha$_2$-antagonists do not reverse the effects of other drugs given concurrently (e.g., dissociatives, opioids, general anesthetics). Because the duration of these drugs is generally short, resedation may occur, in which case an additional dose may be necessary.

The dose of these drugs is expressed as a ratio of the agonist dose to the antagonist dose. In other words, an agonist-antagonist ratio of 10:1 means that if 0.1 mg/kg of the agonist was given, then the correct dose for the antagonist is 0.01 mg/kg (one tenth the agonist dose). An agonist-antagonist ratio of 2:1 means that 0.1 mg of the agonist per kilogram should be followed by 0.05 mg of the antagonist per kilogram (half the agonist dose). When given intravenously, alpha$_2$-antagonists should be given slowly.

**Tolazoline.** Tolazoline is a nonspecific alpha-antagonist (it binds to both alpha$_1$ and alpha$_2$ receptors) primarily used to reverse the sedative and cardiovascular effects of xylazine in ruminants. The dose is calculated using a 1:10 agonist-antagonist ratio (0.1 mg of xylazine per kilogram is reversed with 1 mg of tolazoline per kilogram).

**Yohimbine.** Yohimbine is primarily used to reverse sedative and cardiovascular effects of xylazine in dogs, cats, horses, and exotic species. The calculated dose is based on a 10:1 agonist-antagonist ratio in dogs and horses and a 2:1 ratio in cats. (In a dog, 1 mg of xylazine per kilogram is reversed with 0.1 mg of yohimbine per kilogram.)

**Atipamezole.** Atipamezole (Antisedan) is packaged as a specific antagonist for dexmedetomidine and medetomidine. Atipamezole is labeled for IM injection only and should be given by this route unless IV administration is necessary for emergency resuscitation. The dose of atipamezole is based on an agonist-antagonist ratio of about 1:10. As the formulation of atipamezole is 10 times more concentrated than dexmedetomidine (atipamezole 5 mg/mL, dexmedetomidine 0.5 mg/mL), equal volumes of the two drugs should be administered to dogs. Cats are more sensitive to the effects of atipamezole, so about half of this dose should be used in this species (an agonist-antagonist ratio of 1:5). Because of marked side effects such as hypersalivation and CNS excitement, atipamezole should not be given intravenously in cats. Reversal of effects typically occurs 5 to 10 minutes after IM injection.

## Opioids

Opioids are derivatives of opium, an extract of a species of poppy called *Papaverum somniferum*. Opioids include both naturally derived compounds called *opiates* and synthesized compounds.

This is a versatile class of drugs used for analgesia, sedation, and, when combined with other agents, anesthetic induction. Opioids are classified as agonists, partial agonists, agonist-antagonists, or antagonists, depending on their predominant effects.

Commonly used opioids include the agonists morphine, hydromorphone, oxymorphone, fentanyl, and meperidine; the partial agonist buprenorphine; the agonist-antagonists butorphanol and nalbuphine; and the antagonist naloxone; as well as etorphine and carfentanil, two agonists used for wild animal capture. With the exception of the antagonists and nalbuphine, opioids are controlled drugs and include several that are Class II (including morphine, hydromorphone, oxymorphone, and fentanyl). They may be administered by a wide variety of routes including IV, IM, SC, oral, rectal, and transdermal, as well as subarachnoid and epidural routes (two different types of "spinal injections"). They have a wide safety margin and can be used on both healthy and debilitated patients. Information on the use of opioids as induction agents is found in Chapters 8, 9, and 10, and detailed information on specific opioid agents and their use for analgesia is presented in Chapter 7.

### Mode of Action and Pharmacology

Opioids produce similar effects as natural chemicals present in the body called *endogenous opioid peptides,* which include β-endorphin, dynorphins and enkephalins. Although the mode of action of opioids is not completely understood, it has been the subject of a great deal of research over the past several decades that has yielded much information. Although opioid receptors are found on neurons throughout the body, the analgesic and sedative effects are chiefly the result of their action on receptors located in the brain and spinal cord.

Three major types of opioid receptors have been identified: mu (μ), kappa (κ), and delta (δ), each of which has two or more subtypes. This variety of receptors produces a wide spectrum of effects because each opioid agent differs in its action at each of these sites and therefore in its overall effects on the body.

Opioid agonists exert their effects primarily by binding to and stimulating the mu and kappa receptors and are the best drugs available for moderate and severe pain. Partial agonists only partially stimulate the opioid receptors. Agonist-antagonists do not stimulate the mu receptors, but instead stimulate the kappa receptors. Pure antagonists bind to but do not stimulate mu or kappa receptors. They are therefore called *reversal agents,* because they displace agonists from the receptors and block their effect. These antagonists have no clinical effect on their own but are used to reverse the effects of the pure agonists, partial agonists, and mixed agonist-antagonists.

With few exceptions, opioids have a relatively short duration of action (½ to 3 hours). Exceptions are buprenorphine, which has a significantly longer duration

(6 to 8 hours), and morphine, which has a duration of 6 to 8 hours in horses.

## Effects on Major Organ Systems

### Central Nervous System

- Opioid agents may cause CNS depression or excitement. The exact effect depends on the dose, route, agent used, species, patient temperament, and pain status.
- In dogs the predominant effect is sedation, which tends to be greater with agonists and milder with partial agonists and agonist-antagonists. Most dogs exhibit CNS depression within 60 seconds of IV administration and 15 minutes after IM administration. If high doses of opioid agonists are given (particularly to a sick animal), a sleeplike state called *narcosis* may be produced.
- In contrast, cats, horses, and ruminants exhibit CNS stimulation that is more pronounced with pure agonists. This may include bizarre behavior patterns, including excitement, increased motor activity, or dysphoria (a state characterized by anxiety or restlessness), particularly if the drug is given intravenously. For this reason, some opioids (e.g., morphine) must be used at low doses in these species and IV injection is avoided. Dogs that are not in pain may show a similar reaction (e.g., whining and barking) after opioid administration, particularly if given by rapid IV injection or if a tranquilizing agent is not used concurrently.
- Analgesia. Opioids have long been considered to be the most effective agents for the treatment of pain. The degree of analgesia varies among members of the class: pure agonists such as morphine and hydromorphone are more effective for treatment of severe pain than the partial agonists such as buprenorphine or the mixed agonist-antagonists such as butorphanol. Opioids are particularly useful when included in premedication for patients undergoing surgery for painful conditions (e.g., repair of fractures).
- Because most commonly used general anesthetics have limited analgesic properties (e.g., isoflurane, sevoflurane, propofol, and barbiturates), the analgesic effect of opioids remains one of the chief indications in veterinary patients.

### Cardiovascular System

- Opioids typically cause bradycardia, which may be pronounced, especially if the drugs are given with other agents that slow the heart rate (such as alpha$_2$-agonists).

### Respiratory System

- Although these drugs have the potential to decrease respiratory rate and tidal volume, this effect is often minimal in the absence of preexisting CNS depression. Some dogs pant after administration of opioid agonists. This is because of a direct effect on the thermoregulatory center of the brain, which mistakenly interprets normal body temperature as being elevated.

### Other Effects

- Changes in pupil size. Opioids cause miosis in dogs and mydriasis in cats, ruminants, and horses.
- Changes in body temperature. Dogs become hypothermic as a result of resetting of the thermoregulatory center in the hypothalamus and panting. Cats become hyperthermic for unknown reasons.
- Increased responsiveness to noise. Some patients will startle in reaction to loud noises, requiring caution to ensure that the patient does not fall off a table or out of an open cage.
- Sweating in horses.
- Decreased urine production and urine retention.

**TECHNICIAN NOTE**   Major effects of opioids are as follows:
- CNS depression in dogs or excitement in cats and large animals
- Excellent somatic and visceral analgesia
- Bradycardia
- Panting in dogs
- Miosis in dogs and mydriasis in cats and large animals
- Increased responsiveness to noise

## Adverse Effects

Many of the adverse effects manifest as an exaggeration of the effects discussed previously.

### Central Nervous System

- As mentioned earlier, opioids can cause a variety of CNS effects including anxiety, disorientation, excitement, dysphoria, and increased motor activity in some patients (particularly horses), which can be problematic if exaggerated.

### Cardiovascular System

- Pronounced bradycardia can occur, resulting from increased vagal tone (a dose-related effect that is less pronounced in animals pretreated with atropine).

### Respiratory System

- A serious potential side effect of opioids is their tendency to depress respiration, particularly when used with tranquilizing agents. Although this effect is not seen at low dose rates (such as those used for pain control), opioids given at high dose rates may cause a decrease in both respiratory rate and tidal volume, resulting in decreased blood oxygen levels (Pa$_{O_2}$) and increased carbon dioxide levels (Pa$_{CO_2}$). This effect is particularly noticeable if the opioid is given in combination with another drug that is a respiratory depressant, such as dexmedetomidine or isoflurane. Respiratory depression is dose-dependent for many opioid agents, meaning the effect is more pronounced at high doses. Other opioids (e.g., butorphanol) exhibit a "ceiling effect" in that high doses cause no more respiratory depression than do low doses.

### Gastrointestinal System

• Opioids can cause several adverse GI effects, including salivation and vomiting in small animal patients. Initially many agents also cause an increase in peristaltic movement, resulting in diarrhea, vomiting, and flatulence. Pretreatment with atropine or acepromazine usually moderates this effect. After the initial stimulation of peristalsis, a prolonged period of GI stasis may occur, resulting in constipation. GI stasis or ileus is of particular concern in horses, as it can predispose them to developing colic. Because of the emetic effect of some opioid agents (particularly morphine), these drugs should be avoided in animals in which vomiting would be detrimental (e.g., animals with GI obstruction).

### Other Adverse Effects

• Physical dependence (addiction). Prolonged use of some opioid agents can lead to physical dependence. Human patients given morphine develop a tolerance for its effects in approximately 2 to 3 weeks. Not all opioids are addictive: those with minimal or antagonistic activity at mu receptors (e.g., butorphanol) have less potential for causing physical dependence.
• Morphine and meperidine may cause facial swelling and hypotension after rapid IV administration because of histamine release.
• Opioids tend to increase intraocular and intracranial pressure because of their tendency to depress ventilation, which in turn increases $PaCO_2$, and therefore should be avoided or used cautiously in patients with head trauma and other CNS disorders.
• Drug interactions. Some opioids, particularly meperidine, may cause a potentially fatal reaction known as *serotonin syndrome* when given to animals receiving monoamine oxidase inhibitors such as selegiline or tricyclic antidepressants such as clomipramine. Although the incidence of this reaction in veterinary patients is unknown, these combinations should be avoided until future studies clarify the risk.

> **TECHNICIAN NOTE** Major adverse effects of opioids are as follows:
> • Anxiety, disorientation, excitement, dysphoria, and increased motor activity
> • Pronounced bradycardia
> • Decreased respiratory rate and tidal volume
> • Salivation and vomiting in small animals
> • Initial diarrhea and flatulence, then ileus

## Use of Opioids

Opioid agonists, partial agonists, and agonist-antagonists are used in many ways in veterinary anesthesia. They are a common component of preanesthetic protocols. For high-risk patients, some anesthetists prefer to use an opioid such as morphine or hydromorphone as the sole preanesthetic agent. More commonly, however, opioids are mixed with a tranquilizer (such as acepromazine, diazepam, or dexmedetomidine) and/or an anticholinergic (atropine or glycopyrrolate) and given during the preanesthetic period. Many combinations are used; see Protocols 8-1 and 8-2 in Chapter 8 for common combinations used in small animals.

Ideally, these combinations should be chosen on the basis of individual patient need and drawn up into a syringe immediately before use. Some practices prepare these mixtures in advance and administer a set dose by IM or SC injection according to patient weight. This is more convenient than individual preparation, but there is some risk of inappropriate treatment, particularly if the patient is geriatric or debilitated or has significant organ dysfunction (e.g., liver disease).

Opioids are also used to prevent and treat postoperative pain (see Chapter 7 for a complete discussion of analgesia) and are often used in combination with a tranquilizer to achieve a state of profound sedation and analgesia termed **neuroleptanalgesia.**

### Neuroleptanalgesia

Neuroleptanalgesia is a state of profound sedation and analgesia induced by the simultaneous administration of an opioid and a tranquilizer. Neuroleptanalgesia is commonly used for procedures that require significant CNS depression and analgesia but not general anesthesia.

Opioids commonly used for neuroleptanalgesia include morphine, buprenorphine, butorphanol, and hydromorphone. Tranquilizers that may be combined with opioids include acepromazine, diazepam, midazolam, xylazine, and dexmedetomidine. Virtually any combination of these drugs may be used according to the veterinarian's preference.

Animals given neuroleptanalgesics generally lie quietly in lateral or sternal recumbency (adult horses stand quietly) but can be aroused by sufficient noise or surgical stimulation. Neuroleptanalgesics are commonly used to induce sedation in patients undergoing minor procedures including wound treatment, porcupine quill removal, and diagnostic procedures such as endoscopy or radiography. They are also used for induction of general anesthesia in dogs. Although this type of induction is slow and may cause some respiratory depression and bradycardia, it is safe for most patients, especially if the patient is subsequently intubated and ventilation is assisted.

Neuroleptanalgesics are generally not suitable for routine induction of anesthesia in healthy young dogs, because the level of sedation is not sufficient to permit intubation in these patients unless supplemented with an inhalation agent such as isoflurane or sevoflurane given by mask. However, neuroleptanalgesics may have a profound effect in high-risk or debilitated dogs (including those with hepatic, renal, and CNS disorders) and are a useful and safe alternative to propofol, barbiturate, or ketamine induction in these animals. Neuroleptanalgesics are seldom used to induce anesthesia in cats because of unacceptable side effects (excitement, mania).

The two drugs are often mixed in the same syringe (as long as diazepam is not included), although they may be injected separately. They are given intramuscularly or by slow IV injection and may be administered after pretreatment with anticholinergics, although this is not required, provided the heart rate is carefully monitored. If bradycardia is excessive, the anticholinergic can be administered later.

Neuroleptanalgesics provide a wide margin of safety in most patients, but care must be taken to administer them slowly intravenously, because if they are rapidly injected, CNS stimulation may occur. The anesthetist must also be prepared to intubate and ventilate the patient if necessary because respiratory depression may be profound.

Several procedures have been described for induction of anesthesia with neuroleptanalgesics. These include the following:
- Administration of an anticholinergic and tranquilizer intramuscularly 15 minutes before slow IV injection of the opioid.
- Administration of an anticholinergic intramuscularly, followed 15 minutes later by slow IV administration of the tranquilizer-opioid mixture. If diazepam is selected as the tranquilizing agent, the opioid should be given first, followed 1 to 2 minutes later by diazepam, because if diazepam is given before the opioid agent has taken effect, excitement may be seen. In young dogs, acepromazine offers more reliable sedation than diazepam and can be given at the same time as the opioid.
- Alternating small doses of hydromorphone or fentanyl and diazepam by slow IV injection until the animal is adequately anesthetized. Two syringes are used because these drugs cannot be mixed together.
- IM administration of the tranquilizer-opioid mixture.

When the procedure is over, the opioid in neuroleptanalgesic combinations can be reversed with naloxone. However, the tranquilizer component may or may not be reversible, depending on whether or not a specific antagonist is available. A detailed discussion of opioid reversal follows.

> **TECHNICIAN NOTE**   Neuroleptanalgesics must be administered intravenously slowly, because if rapidly injected, CNS stimulation may occur. The anesthetist must also be prepared to intubate and ventilate the patient if necessary, as respiratory depression may be profound.

## Opioid Antagonists

One distinct advantage of using opioids is their reversibility, which allows undesirable effects to be antagonized in situations in which the patient is in danger, or allows the anesthetist to "wake" or partially wake the patient after sedation with these agents. The opioid antagonist naloxone hydrochloride is commonly used to reverse the CNS and respiratory depression caused by administration of opioid agonists, partial agonists, or agonist-antagonists. It is administered by IM or slow IV injection and can be used in dogs, cats, horses, and exotic mammals. Although not used in domestic animals, naltrexone is a longer-lasting antagonist that is used in wild animals to reverse the effects of potent opioids such as etorphine.

Agonist-antagonists such as butorphanol can be also be used to partially reverse the effects of pure agonists. Realize that opioid antagonists are effective in reversing opioid agents only and cannot be used to reverse the effects of phenothiazines, benzodiazepines, or other nonopioid agents.

### Mode of Action and Pharmacology

Although, as with many other anesthetics and adjuncts, the exact mechanism of action of naloxone is not known, it is believed to competitively bind to the mu, kappa, and sigma receptors. Naloxone acts within 2 minutes of IV administration and 5 minutes of IM administration and has a duration of action of 30 to 60 minutes, and in some cases may last longer.

### Effects and Adverse Effects

The primary effect of naloxone is reversal of both the desirable and undesirable effects of an agonist, partial agonist, or agonist-antagonist, including sedation, dysphoria, panting, respiratory depression, hypotension, bradycardia, GI effects, and analgesia. The action of opioid antagonists is often dramatic, causing the patient to appear nearly unaffected shortly after administration. The respiratory depression caused by buprenorphine may be unresponsive, however, because this agent tightly binds to the mu receptors and is not easily displaced.

Adverse effects are rare at clinical doses, although sudden loss of analgesic effects resulting from routine use may precipitate excitement, anxiety, and SNS stimulation, resulting in tachycardia and cardiac arrhythmias. Total reversal of analgesia can be avoided by using an agonist-antagonist such as butorphanol that has some analgesic effect.

> **TECHNICIAN NOTE**   Opioid antagonists should be administered by IM or slow IV injection. They reverse both the desirable and undesirable effects of an agonist, partial agonist, or agonist-antagonist, including sedation and analgesia. The action of opioid antagonists is often dramatic, causing the patient to appear nearly unaffected shortly after administration.

## Use of Opioid Antagonists

Reversal of opioid effects through the use of an antagonist is not necessary for routine anesthesia. However, the technique is extremely useful in emergencies, after an overdose, or to reverse opioid effects after neuroleptanalgesia for nonpainful procedures. Opioid antagonists are also helpful in reviving neonates delivered by a cesarean section if the dam was given opioids. One drop of naloxone placed under the tongue of each puppy or kitten is usually sufficient to reverse the respiratory depression caused by fentanyl, morphine, or other opioid agonists.

In cases where the duration of action of the drug being reversed is longer than the duration of naloxone, signs of CNS or respiratory depression recur (a phenomenon referred to a *renarcotization*). In these cases, additional doses may be needed.

## INJECTABLE ANESTHETICS

Injectable anesthetics are drugs characterized by their ability to produce unconsciousness when given alone. They do not provide all the effects of general anesthesia (such as analgesia and muscle relaxation), however. Consequently these drugs must be used with other agents to produce the complete spectrum of effects of general anesthesia.

Injectable anesthetic agents include propofol, barbiturates, and etomidate, each of which is used to induce anesthesia. Through use of repeat boluses, or a CRI, propofol is also used to maintain general anesthesia. Barbiturates are used in both small and large animals. Propofol and etomidate are used only in small animals, small ruminants, and neonates of any species, but not in adult large animals because of the high expense of these agents.

Although they do not produce unconsciousness when given alone, dissociative agents are included in this discussion of injectable anesthetics because they are frequently used in combination with tranquilizers and opioids to produce general anesthesia.

With few exceptions, these agents are administered by IV injection to effect, instead of giving the entire calculated dose at once. "To effect" means that the drug is given in small boluses until the desired level of anesthesia is reached. More about this technique can be found in Chapter 8.

## Barbiturates

The barbiturates are a large class of controlled drugs, developed during the 1930s through the 1950s, that were commonly used general anesthetics for many decades because of their low cost, ease of use, and relative safety for healthy animals. Although these drugs are still used for certain indications, in recent years their use has decreased with the development of newer injectable agents such as propofol, and inhalant agents such as isoflurane and sevoflurane. Despite this decrease in popularity, there is a large body of knowledge about these agents based on the experience of more than seven decades of widespread use. Therefore the anesthetist must have a general knowledge of barbiturates not only to use them safely, but also as a point of reference against which other injectable anesthetics can be compared. In fact, some references still classify all injectable anesthetics as either barbiturates or nonbarbiturates.

## Classes of Barbiturates

All barbiturates in clinical use are derivatives of barbituric acid. They are placed into subclasses based on their duration of action (ultra–short-acting, short-acting, intermediate-acting, and long-acting). Two subclasses of barbiturates are used to induce general anesthesia in veterinary patients. The ultra–short-acting barbiturates thiopental sodium and methohexital are used to induce anesthesia primarily in dogs, cats, and horses, and the short-acting barbiturate pentobarbital is used to induce and maintain general anesthesia in laboratory animals. Most intermediate- and long-acting barbiturates are no longer used as anesthetics, although the long-acting barbiturate phenobarbital is commonly used as a sedative and anticonvulsant.

Barbiturates are also classified based on their chemical structure as oxybarbiturates (which include phenobarbital, pentobarbital, and methohexital) and thiobarbiturates (which include the ultra–short-acting agents thiopental and thiamylal).

> *TECHNICIAN NOTE*   Uses for barbiturates are as follows:
> - The ultra–short-acting barbiturates thiopental sodium and methohexital are used to induce anesthesia primarily in dogs, cats, and horses.
> - The short-acting barbiturate pentobarbital is used to induce and maintain general anesthesia in laboratory animals and to treat status epilepticus in small animals.
> - The long-acting barbiturate phenobarbital is used as a sedative and anticonvulsant.

## Action and Pharmacodynamics of Barbiturates

Although the precise mechanism of action of these drugs is not fully known, all barbiturates act on the neurons in a similar manner to the inhibitory neurotransmitter GABA. This action depresses nerve impulses in the cerebral cortex, resulting in CNS depression and a loss of consciousness. This effect is terminated when the agent leaves the brain and is either metabolized, excreted, or redistributed elsewhere in the body. To understand the differences in the potency and onset and duration of action of specific barbiturates, it is necessary to have some knowledge of the pharmacodynamics of these drugs.

### Ionization

All barbiturates exist in both ionized (polar) and nonionized (nonpolar) forms. Only the nonionized molecules can pass through cell membranes. When the blood pH is normal (7.4), barbiturates penetrate to the expected extent and consequently have the expected effects. When the blood pH is lower (a condition called *acidosis*), more of the drug is nonionized, causing increased diffusion into the brain. A normal dose of barbiturates may produce an exaggerated response in these animals. Therefore the dose of barbiturates required to anesthetize acidotic animals may be significantly less than that required to anesthetize healthy animals.

### Protein Binding

Barbiturates travel in the blood bound to plasma proteins and freely circulating. Only the free (unbound) molecules of barbiturate are able to enter the brain to induce anesthesia because the molecules bound to proteins are unable to cross cell membranes. In hypoproteinemic animals (that is, those with total plasma protein less than 3 g/dL) there is less plasma protein to bind barbiturate molecules and more barbiturate in the active, unbound form. The potency of barbiturates within the body is therefore increased in animals with low plasma protein levels. Doses of barbiturates suitable for healthy animals may cause prolonged unconsciousness or death in these patients.

### Lipid Solubility

The tendency of a drug to dissolve in fats, oils, or lipids is referred to as *lipid solubility* (also called *partition coefficient*) and is related to the ability to penetrate the fatty layer of the cell membranes. Highly lipid-soluble drugs (ultra–short-acting agents) pass into the brain cells more quickly, causing a faster onset of action as compared with drugs with low lipid solubility.

Lipid solubility is also related to duration of action. Drugs with high lipid solubility are rapidly removed from the brain by a process known as *tissue redistribution*. Drugs with moderate lipid solubility (the short-acting agents) are largely metabolized by the liver, a process that takes longer than redistribution; and drugs with low lipid solubility (the long-acting agents) are primarily excreted by the kidneys, a process that takes even longer.

### Redistribution

As mentioned, highly lipid-soluble ultra–short-acting agents such as thiopental sodium and methohexital are removed from the brain by a process known as *redistribution*. This process occurs because of the way in which these drugs are distributed to various tissues based on blood flow. After IV administration, absorption is most rapid in tissues with very high blood flow, known as the *vessel-rich group* (the CNS, heart, liver, kidney, and endocrine tissues),

which make up only about 10% of total body weight but receive about 75% of the total blood flow. Absorption is less rapid in muscle, which makes up about 50% of the body weight but receives only 20% of the blood flow, and slowest in fat, which makes up about 20% of body weight but receives a meager 5% of the blood flow (Figure 3-3).

The process of redistribution can be illustrated by using the example of administration of the drug thiopental sodium, the most commonly used drug in this class. Within seconds of IV injection, thiopental is dispersed throughout the body via the bloodstream. Large amounts of the drug rapidly reach the brain because of the excellent blood supply this organ receives. Thiopental is highly lipid-soluble, and its entry into brain tissue is enhanced by the high lipid content of the brain. The rapid absorption of thiopental into the brain causes the animal to lose consciousness within 30 seconds of injection.

Once the thiopental concentration in the blood falls below that in the brain tissue, the drug begins to leave the brain and reenter the circulation, where it is redistributed to muscle, fat, and other body tissues. Thiopental leaves the brain because it, like all drugs, diffuses from areas of high concentration to areas of low concentration. The animal shows signs of recovery (often within 10 to 15 minutes) as the concentration in the brain decreases, although the drug is still present in other tissues.

Over the next several hours, thiopental is gradually released from the muscle and fat and is eliminated from the body by liver metabolism and excretion of the metabolites in urine.

Because thiopental persists in muscle and fat for up to several hours and then is slowly metabolized over time, repeat administration can saturate the tissues. When this happens, drug levels may persist in the brain because the muscle and fat are "full" and unable to accommodate additional drug. This effect causes prolonged recovery. Therefore it is inadvisable to administer these drugs on a continuous or repeated basis.

The other commonly used barbiturates have different pharmacodynamics. Like thiopental, the ultra–short-acting agent methohexital has a short duration because of redistribution, but this drug is metabolized much more rapidly than thiopental. Consequently, repeat doses of methohexital can be given with minimal concern about prolonged recovery.

The long-acting barbiturate phenobarbital has low lipid solubility and is consequently slow to act, but effects are sustained because a decrease in brain levels depends primarily on excretion by the kidneys, a relatively lengthy process.

The short-acting barbiturate pentobarbital has intermediate lipid solubility when compared with thiopental and phenobarbital. It takes several minutes to reach its full effect and has a duration of action that is shorter than that of phenobarbital but longer than that of thiopental, because brain levels decrease as the drug is metabolized by the liver—which occurs faster than kidney excretion but more slowly than redistribution.

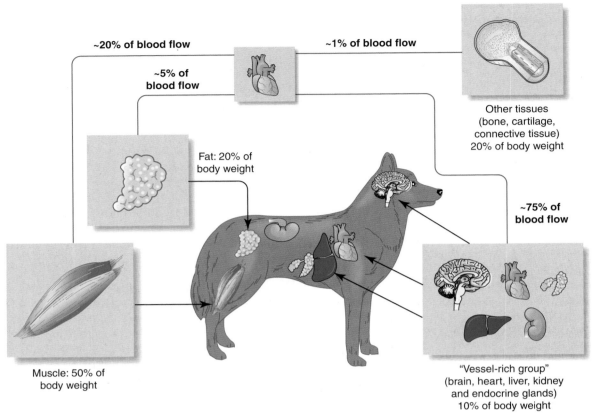

~20% of blood flow

~1% of blood flow

~5% of blood flow

Other tissues (bone, cartilage, connective tissue) 20% of body weight

Fat: 20% of body weight

~75% of blood flow

Muscle: 50% of body weight

"Vessel-rich group" (brain, heart, liver, kidney and endocrine glands) 10% of body weight

**FIGURE 3-3** A comparison of blood flow and tissue mass. Note that some tissues make up a small proportion of total body weight but receive a relatively large proportion of total blood flow (e.g., approximately 10% of total body weight and approximately 75% of total blood flow in the case of the vessel-rich group), whereas other tissues make up a relatively large proportion of total body weight but receive much less blood flow (e.g., approximately 20% of total body weight and approximately 5% of total blood flow in the case of fat).

## Use of Barbiturates

The convenience, relative safety, low cost, and rapid induction associated with the ultra–short-acting barbiturates led to their once common use in small and large animal anesthesia. Although their popularity has waned, thiopental and methohexital are both still used as induction agents to allow endotracheal intubation. After intubation, anesthesia is most often maintained with an inhalation anesthetic such as isoflurane or sevoflurane. Thiopental may also be used as the sole anesthetic agent for brief procedures, and methohexital can be used to maintain anesthesia for longer procedures with repeat boluses or a CRI. Regardless of the specific drug used, endotracheal intubation is strongly advised for all patients anesthetized with barbiturates, even for brief periods, to prevent aspiration of fluid or vomitus and to allow the anesthetist to support ventilation if necessary.

## Effects on Major Organ Systems
### Central Nervous System

- Barbiturates cause a full range of CNS depression, from mild sedation and hypnosis to complete unconsciousness. At low doses, they can also cause CNS excitement.

### Cardiovascular System

- Barbiturates cause cardiac depression, particularly shortly after IV injection. It has been shown in the dog that barbiturates cause a dose-dependent decrease in cardiac output and blood pressure that may be profound in patients that are already anesthetized.
- In addition, thiopental stimulates the PNS and the SNS, causing autonomic imbalances, and also increases the heart's sensitivity to the action of epinephrine, particularly in patients that are excited or stressed. This may lead to cardiac arrhythmias including ventricular premature complexes (VPC), tachycardia or bradycardia, and AV heart block.

### Respiratory System

- Barbiturates commonly depress the respiratory system, reducing respiratory rate and tidal volume and in some cases causing respiratory arrest. After IV administration of thiopental for anesthetic induction, a brief period of **apnea** is common, especially after rapid injection or administration of high doses. This occurs because of direct depression of the respiratory center in the medulla, the area of the brain that controls respiration. In the conscious animal the respiratory center responds to rising levels of carbon dioxide in arterial blood ($Pa_{CO_2}$) by sending impulses to the muscles that initiate inspiration. Barbiturates cause the respiratory center to become relatively insensitive to increased $Pa_{CO_2}$. Breathing resumes when the concentration of the drug in the plasma and brain decreases or when decreased blood oxygen stimulates breathing. Most healthy patients are not adversely affected by a brief period of apnea, but the other vital signs should be closely monitored to ensure that perfusion and oxygenation are maintained. Mucous membranes should remain pink, the heartbeat should be regular, the pulse should be strong, and oxygen saturation as measured by a pulse oximeter should be normal.

- During anesthesia induced with pentobarbital, the most common effect on respiration is a persistent reduction in tidal volume (that is, shallow breaths). The effect may be short-lived, or the patient's respirations may appear shallow throughout the anesthetic period. Patients with reduced tidal volume are predisposed to respiratory acidosis and poor tissue oxygenation, particularly if a barbiturate is used as the sole anesthetic agent and the patient does not receive oxygen supplementation.

### Other Effects

- Barbiturate induction is often accompanied by sneezing, laryngospasm, and coughing owing to increased salivation. Premedication with an anticholinergic minimizes these effects. Barbiturates also reduce GI motility at first, and then can increase it. Muscle relaxation with these drugs is not complete.

> **TECHNICIAN NOTE**  Major effects of barbiturates are as follows:
> - CNS depression from mild sedation to general anesthesia
> - Decreased cardiac output and blood pressure
> - Decreased respiratory rate and tidal volume
> - Increased salivation
> - Sneezing, laryngospasm, and coughing

### Adverse Effects

#### Cardiovascular System

- During the induction period, it is not uncommon for cardiac arrhythmias such as VPC to occur because of the combined effect of barbiturates, epinephrine, and hypoxia. A condition termed *bigeminy* in which each normal beat is followed by a single VPC is particularly common (Figure 3-4). These cardiac arrhythmias are not clinically significant in most patients; however, cardiac arrest has been reported, especially in animals that are stressed during induction. For these reasons, barbiturates should be used with caution in animals

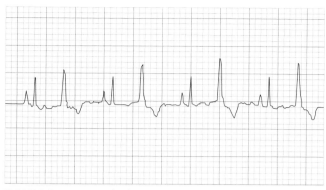

**FIGURE 3-4**  Ventricular bigeminy (cat). Note that normal complexes (the odd numbered complexes) alternate with ventricular premature complexes, which are early, are wider, and have a different shape than the normal complexes. 25 mm/sec; 1 cm/mV. (From Bonagura JD, Twedt DC: *Kirk's current veterinary therapy XIV*, St Louis, 2009, Elsevier.)

with known cardiac disease because a dose of barbiturate that is well tolerated by a healthy heart may severely stress a diseased heart.

- Adverse effects on the heart can be minimized by ensuring that barbiturates are given slowly and that dilute concentrations are used (e.g., 2% or 2.5%). Preoxygenating a patient for 3 to 5 minutes before inducing anesthesia with a barbiturate also helps to reduce the adverse cardiac effects of these drugs. If cardiac arrhythmias occur during induction, bagging the patient two or three times is often helpful to ensure adequate oxygenation.

#### Respiratory System

- Respiratory depression is related to dose and speed of administration and in some cases may be profound. If apnea persists for more than 1 to 2 minutes after administration, patients must be immediately intubated and bagged every 15 seconds to 1 minute until spontaneous breathing resumes.
- Respiratory depression of neonates is also a potential problem when barbiturates are used in cesarean deliveries. Barbiturates, like most anesthetic agents, readily cross the placenta and enter the fetal circulation and may interfere with the neonates' ability to breathe immediately after delivery. In fact, the newborn animal is more susceptible than the mother to the effect of barbiturates, and respiration may be completely inhibited by doses of barbiturates that are inadequate to anesthetize the dam.

#### Other Adverse Effects

- In addition to the cardiovascular and respiratory problems previously outlined, barbiturates may exhibit exaggerated and potentially dangerous potency in some animals. Classes of patients that are particularly sensitive to barbiturates include sighthounds, critically ill animals, and, as previously mentioned, hypoproteinemic and acidotic animals.

- *Effect on sighthounds.* Because of the redistribution of thiopental, prolonged recovery is common in very thin animals, including sighthounds (e.g., afghan hounds, whippets, salukis, borzoi, and greyhounds), especially if more than one dose is given. This is because the low fat stores in these patients quickly become saturated, preventing redistribution of the drug. Therefore drug levels in the brain remain high. Hepatic metabolism of barbiturates may also be slow in sighthounds, further delaying clearance from the body. For these reasons, thiopental is not recommended for use in sighthounds, although owing to rapid metabolism, methohexital is considered relatively safe in these breeds.

- *Effect on critically ill animals.* Animals with hepatic or renal disease and animals with hypothermia may exhibit prolonged recovery from thiopental and other barbiturates because metabolism and excretion are delayed. Barbiturates also show greater potency in animals that have hypotension or shock because blood flow to nonessential tissues (such as fat) is decreased, and blood flow to the brain and heart is increased. Thus the normal redistribution of these agents from the brain to body fat stores does not occur.

- *Tissue irritation and barbiturate sloughs.* Use of concentrations greater than 2.5% is toxic to capillary muscles and can cause thrombophlebitis. Barbiturate solutions are strongly alkaline (pH 10 to 11) and may cause significant tissue damage if injected perivascularly, particularly if the concentration of barbiturate exceeds 2.5%. Perivascular injection of concentrated barbiturate solutions may be followed within 48 hours by local swelling, pain, necrosis, and even tissue sloughing. The animal may chew at the area, thereby increasing tissue damage. Tissue sloughs are slow to heal and usually result in permanent scarring.

- A dilute solution of barbiturate should be used to avoid tissue irritation (in the case of thiopental 2% to 2.5%, although up to 10% is used in horses to decrease the volume that needs to be injected for induction of anesthesia). As an additional precaution, barbiturates are often administered through an IV catheter or winged infusion set. If perivascular injection occurs, the area should be immediately infiltrated with saline (in a volume at least equal to the volume of barbiturate injected) to dilute the barbiturate and reduce its irritating effect; 1 to 2 mL of 2% lidocaine without epinephrine may be added to the saline. The lidocaine causes vasodilatation, absorption of the barbiturate, and neutralization of the drug.

- Although uncommon, inadvertent intraarterial injections of thiopental must also be avoided, as they may cause vasoconstriction, pain, and tissue necrosis.

- *Excitement during induction or recovery.* Perivascular injection or excessively slow administration of some barbiturates may result in stage II excitement during induction. This occurs because the amount of barbiturate reaching the brain is insufficient to induce stage III

anesthesia. In this case additional drug must be administered immediately until the patient reaches surgical anesthesia. The use of barbiturates, particularly pentobarbital, is also associated with a high incidence of excitement during the recovery period. Paddling and vocalization are commonly seen but may be relieved by administration of IV diazepam. Use of preanesthetic medications is helpful in reducing the incidence and severity of excitement in the recovery period.

- *Interaction with other drugs.* Barbiturates enhance the neuromuscular blocking effect of muscle relaxants (see Chapter 6). Chronic administration of barbiturates (e.g., phenobarbital given daily to an epileptic dog or cat) increases the activity of some hepatic enzymes. This may lead to more rapid clearance and therefore shorter duration of effect of drugs that are metabolized in the liver such as diazepam and opioids. Concurrent administration of the antibiotic chloramphenicol may increase the effects of pentobarbital and phenobarbital.

 **TECHNICIAN NOTE** Major adverse effects of barbiturates are as follows:
- Cardiac arrhythmias, especially bigeminy
- Profound respiratory depression and apnea
- Prolonged recovery in sighthounds
- Increased potency in critically ill patients
- Tissue irritation and sloughing after perivascular injection
- Excitement during induction and recovery if patient is not premedicated

## Commonly Used Barbiturate Drugs
### Thiopental
Thiopental is an ultra–short-acting thiobarbiturate used for anesthetic induction of small animals and horses and can also be used as the sole anesthetic for brief procedures. Onset of action after injection is rapid (30 to 60 seconds), and duration of anesthesia is brief (10 to 15 minutes). Complete recovery usually occurs within 1 to 2 hours.

Thiopental is supplied as crystalline powder in multidose vials. Sterile water, normal saline, or 5% dextrose in water is added to the vial to make a 2% (20 mg/mL) or 2.5% (25 mg/mL) solution for small animals and a 5% (50 mg/mL) solution for large animals. All vials should be labeled with the percent concentration and date of reconstitution, because thiopental is unstable in solution and once reconstituted has a maximum shelf life of 1 week if refrigerated and 3 days at room temperature. Care should be taken to avoid injecting air into prepared solutions, because this may cause premature precipitation of the barbiturate. The solution should not be used if a precipitate is present.

The dose of thiopental used for induction varies depending on concurrent use of other agents and the depth of anesthesia required. Doses are commonly reduced by up to 80% in debilitated animals or in animals that have been heavily sedated.

Whether given alone or in combination with other drugs, thiopental is always given "to effect." Repeated administration is cumulative, and recovery can be greatly prolonged. For this reason it is not advisable to use this agent for anesthetic maintenance.

One method for IV induction with thiopental is described in Procedure 8-3. Another strategy is to give the antiarrhythmic drug lidocaine (2 mg/kg) intravenously, immediately followed by thiopental to reduce the incidence of arrhythmias. This technique is not suitable in cats because of their sensitivity to lidocaine. Thiopental can also be given at a dose of 8 mg/kg, after an IV injection of 0.2 mg/kg diazepam or midazolam (using separate syringes). Finally, thiopental can be mixed with propofol and given in the same syringe.

> TECHNICIAN NOTE Sterile water, normal saline, or 5% dextrose in water is added to thiopental powder to make a 2% (20 mg/mL) or 2.5% (25 mg/mL) solution for small animals and a 5% (50 mg/mL) solution for large animals. Thiopental is unstable in solution and once reconstituted has a maximum shelf life of 1 week if refrigerated and 3 days at room temperature.

### Methohexital

Methohexital is an ultra–short-acting methylated oxybarbiturate similar to thiopental in that the onset of action is rapid (15 to 60 seconds) and the duration of anesthesia is brief (5 to 10 minutes). In fact, animals induced with methohexital and subsequently connected to an anesthetic machine may show signs of recovery before the inhalation anesthetic has time to take effect. The rapid induction achieved with this agent is useful when anesthetizing a patient with a full stomach, because the anesthetist can intubate rapidly, decreasing the risk of aspiration of vomitus.

As with thiopental, methohexital is provided as a powder that must be reconstituted. A 1%-2.5% solution is commonly used in small animals. The reconstituted drug has a shelf life of at least 6 weeks when reconstituted with sterile water for injection, and does not require refrigeration. Methohexital is significantly more expensive than thiopental. The cost of thiopental required to anesthetize a 10-kg dog at the time of this writing is approximately $1 to $2, whereas the cost of methohexital is approximately $10 to $12.

Methohexital is administered in a manner similar to that of thiobarbiturates. In the premedicated patient, one third to one half of the calculated dose is given intravenously over 10 seconds. One injection is usually sufficient to allow intubation, but additional drug should be given in 30 seconds if an adequate plane of anesthesia is not reached. Further delay will result in a poor induction because of the rapid redistribution of the drug.

Methohexital may be used in sighthounds, because unlike thiopental it does not produce prolonged recoveries. Liver metabolism of methohexital is much faster than that of other barbiturates; therefore repeated administration is not cumulative.

Although methohexital is a useful drug for veterinary anesthesia, it should be used with caution. Methohexital can cause profound respiratory depression, and the lethal dose is only two to three times the anesthetic dose. Methohexital is also associated with excitement and seizures during induction (if given too slowly) or during recovery. Premedication with a tranquilizer helps to prevent seizures and is always recommended. Postoperative seizures may be controlled with IV diazepam. Animals with preexisting CNS disease, including epilepsy, should not receive methohexital.

### Pentobarbital

Pentobarbital is a short-acting barbiturate used in the treatment of **status epilepticus.** In recent years, propofol has become more widely used for this purpose owing to fewer adverse effects and smoother recoveries. Pentobarbital is also administered by intraperitoneal injection to produce general anesthesia in rodents (see Chapter 11); however, its potency and duration of effect are variable when given by this route. Before halogenated inhalant anesthetics were available, this drug was commonly used as the sole anesthetic agent for procedures such as ovariohysterectomy in the dog. Because of significant respiratory depression, difficulty controlling anesthetic depth, rough inductions and recoveries, and other adverse effects, the use of this agent for major surgical procedures is now rare in veterinary practice.

When treating status epilepticus, pentobarbital should be given at a rate of 3 to 15 mg/kg intravenously to effect, until the seizures stop and heavy sedation is achieved. It should be given very slowly in small doses, waiting several minutes before giving additional boluses. This agent must be used with caution because it has a narrow margin of safety; the euthanasia dose in healthy animals is only 60 mg/kg, which is approximately double the dose used for surgical anesthesia.

The onset of action is 30 to 60 seconds after IV injection, although the full effect may not be seen for several minutes. Animals anesthetized with pentobarbital will initially appear unable to raise the head. As more pentobarbital is given, the jaw and tongue become completely relaxed, but a pedal reflex is still present, indicating a light plane of anesthesia. As the animal achieves a moderate depth of anesthesia, the pedal reflex becomes sluggish. If the pedal reflex is lost, the animal likely requires intubation and respiratory support. Additional drug can be given to prolong anesthesia; however, repeated doses may be associated with excitement during the recovery period and with an extended recovery time. The anesthetic effect lasts 30 minutes to 2 hours, depending on dose and species. Pentobarbital is supplied as a 5% solution (50 mg/mL).

## Propofol

Propofol is an ultra–short-acting nonbarbiturate inject-able anesthetic with a wide margin of safety and is given intravenously for induction and short-term maintenance of general anesthesia in small animals, small ruminants, exotic animals, and neonates of any domestic species. Since its introduction to the veterinary market over a decade ago, its popularity has gradually increased, and now it is the most commonly used ultra–short-acting injectable agent in small animals for brief procedures or for anesthetic induction before intubation and mainte-nance with inhalant agents.

Propofol is also administered as an IV bolus followed by a CRI to treat status epilepticus in dogs and cats that do not respond to diazepam and phenobarbital.

### Mode of Action and Pharmacology

Propofol has a chemical structure unlike that of other anesthetic or preanesthetic agents. It is minimally water-soluble and is available in an egg lecithin, glycerin, and soybean oil aqueous emulsion at a concentration of 10 mg/mL. Although this agent has a milky appearance, it is the sole exception to the general rule that milky liquids should never be given intravenously.

Although the mode of action is not completely under-stood, propofol appears to affect GABA receptors in a simi-lar manner to barbiturates. Propofol has a rapid onset and short duration of action because it is highly fat-soluble. Propofol is rapidly taken up by vessel-rich tissues such as the brain, heart, liver, and kidneys but is very quickly redistributed to muscle and fat (see p. 71 for a discussion of redistribution) and is subsequently rapidly metabo-lized. This accounts for the rapid recovery and minimal residual sedative effects seen even after repeated injections.

The onset of action is about 30 to 60 seconds, and the duration of action is 5 to 10 minutes, with complete recovery in 20 minutes (dogs) and 30 minutes (cats).

### Effects on Major Organ Systems

#### Central Nervous System

- Propofol produces a dose-dependent CNS depression ranging from sedation to general anesthesia. Propofol is not an analgesic.

#### Cardiovascular System

- Propofol is a cardiac depressant, producing bradycar-dia, decreased cardiac output, decreased vascular resis-tance, and, as a result, transient hypotension.

#### Respiratory System

- Propofol is a potent respiratory depressant. High doses or rapid injection may cause significant respiratory depression, including apnea. To lessen the respiratory depression associated with the use of propofol, the anesthetist should give the initial bolus gradually over 1 to 2 minutes, carefully titrate the dose to effect, and monitor respiratory rate and depth carefully during the first few minutes after injection.

### Other Effects

- Some dogs may exhibit muscle twitching during induction. This reaction should not be interpreted as an indicator of inadequate anesthetic depth.
- Propofol results in good muscle relaxation.
- Because metabolism of propofol is rapid, propofol is relatively safe and effective in animals with liver or kid-ney disease.
- Propofol is an appetite stimulant at low doses.
- Propofol has antiemetic properties.
- Propofol decreases intracranial and intraocular pressure.

> **TECHNICIAN NOTE**   Major effects of propofol are as follows:
> - CNS depression ranging from sedation to general anesthesia
> - Bradycardia, decreased cardiac output, and hypotension
> - Respiratory depression including apnea
> - Muscle twitching during induction
> - Muscle relaxation

### Adverse Effects

#### Central Nervous System

- Transient excitement and muscle tremors are seen occasionally during induction, especially if injection is slow or the animal has not been premedicated. Pad-dling, muscle twitching, **nystagmus,** and opisthotonus (hyperextended head and front legs) can occur and may resemble seizures. This response can be treated with diazepam if persistent.

#### Cardiovascular System

- Hypotension is often of short duration in animals with normal cardiovascular function, but in some patients it may be significant and prolonged. For this reason, propofol should be given cautiously to animals with preexisting hypotension, such as patients in shock or those that have blood loss or dehydration.

#### Respiratory System

- Apnea is sometime seen, particularly after rapid injec-tion or high doses. If apnea lasts more than 1 minute or if pulse oximetry shows oxygen saturation to be less than 95%, the patient should be intubated and venti-lated. The best approach is prevention of hypoxemia by delivering oxygen to the patient (by face mask) for 3 to 5 minutes before inducing anesthesia with propofol.

#### Other Adverse Effects

- Based on experience in people, propofol is known to cause pain on IV injection but does not produce the tissue dam-age after perivascular injection seen with barbiturates.

- When given repeat doses, cats can develop Heinz body production, diarrhea, and anorexia and can experience slow recoveries.
- Animals of some breeds including sighthounds may have prolonged recovery if maintained with propofol for longer than 30 minutes.

*TECHNICIAN NOTE* Major adverse effects of propofol are as follows:
- Transient excitement, muscle tremors, and seizure-like activity during induction
- Significant and prolonged hypotension in some patients
- Apnea after rapid injection or high doses
- Pain from IV injection

## Use of Propofol

Propofol should be given intravenously slowly, over a period of 1 to 2 minutes until the desired anesthetic depth is reached (see Case Studies 3-1 and 3-2). IM injection may cause mild sedation and ataxia but does not induce anesthesia because the drug is metabolized too rapidly.

One effective induction method is to give one quarter of the calculated dose slowly intravenously every 30 seconds until the desired plane of anesthesia is reached. The dose of propofol needed for a patient and the duration of anesthesia depend on the type of premedication used. Do not give propofol too slowly, however, as this can cause paradoxic excitement, making the patient difficult to handle. Propofol is highly protein bound and therefore

should be used with caution in patients with significant hypoproteinemia.

Propofol boluses can be given repeatedly every 3 to 5 minutes or as required to maintain anesthesia in dogs and cats up to 20 minutes. Alternatively, propofol can be delivered by CRI. In this procedure, a low dose of propofol (0.2 to 0.4 mg/kg/min) is continuously administered to the patient with a syringe pump (Figure 3-5) or through an IV line. This method allows the anesthetist to precisely control the depth of anesthesia at a stable plane for up to several hours. Intubation and oxygen administration are advisable for patients unless the period of anesthesia is anticipated to be very brief.

In dogs, recovery from propofol anesthesia is rapid and smooth, even after multiple injections. Because of the rapid recovery seen with this agent, it is useful for patients that need to be released immediately after surgery. Dogs that have received propofol may appear completely recovered within 20 minutes of the final dose. Cats recover within about 30 minutes after a single injection but may experience longer recoveries after multiple injections owing to the fact that they metabolize propofol more slowly.

Administration of tranquilizers decreases the dose of propofol required by as much as 75% and facilitates IV injection in fractious animals. Some premedications, however, may prolong recovery time.

## Handling and Storage

One significant disadvantage of propofol is the poor storage characteristics of this agent. Because the product contains soybean oil, egg lecithin, and glycerol, it will support bacterial growth. Ampules and bottles should be handled in a strictly aseptic manner, and the manufacturer

## CASE 3-1 GIVING AN INJECTABLE IV ANESTHETIC TOO RAPIDLY

Petunia, a 2-year-old, female, 5-kg, intact domestic shorthair cat (DSH) was scheduled to be anesthetized by a student anesthetist. The patient was premedicated with 0.05 mg of hydromorphone per kilogram of body weight by IM injection. Propofol was prepared at a dose of 5 mg/kg, and 25 mg (2.5 mL) was drawn into a syringe. This student was familiar with anesthetic induction using a combination of acepromazine and ketamine intravenously but not propofol, and was used to administering the entire calculated dose quickly. Based on this experience, after approximately 15 minutes, the anesthetist commenced anesthetic induction by injecting the entire dose of propofol over about 30 seconds. The patient immediately became unconscious, hypotensive, and apneic. Heart sounds were nearly inaudible. At this point the student became concerned and summoned the instructor. The patient was quickly assessed and was determined to be in a deep level of anesthesia but stable. The patient was immediately intubated, and manual intermittent positive-pressure ventilation was initiated at a rate of approximately one breath every 15 seconds. The patient remained stable, and gradually over the next 5 minutes began to exhibit

spontaneous respiratory movements, which although weak at first, gradually became stronger and more frequent. The rate of manual ventilation was decreased gradually, and after 15 to 20 minutes, spontaneous respirations were adequate to allow the patient to breathe on its own.

This case illustrates the importance of using an appropriate injection rate when inducing patients with ultra-short IV anesthetics. If these agents are given too quickly, the patient will experience adverse effects, which in the case of propofol include respiratory and cardiovascular depression, apnea, and hypotension. Depending on how much is given, anesthetic depth may become dangerously excessive. For this reason, this agent must be given to effect and must be given slowly in small boluses while the patient is monitored between boluses for signs of readiness for intubation. When ultra–short-acting agents are given, a balance must be struck between injecting the drug slowly enough to minimize apnea and other adverse effects but rapidly enough to bring the patient into a plane of anesthesia sufficient to allow intubation. For these reasons, great care must be given to proper injection technique when these agents are used.

## CASE 3-2 GIVING AN INJECTABLE IV ANESTHETIC TOO SLOWLY

Snoopy, a 1½-year-old, male, 15-kg beagle mix was scheduled to be anesthetized by a student anesthetist. The patient was premedicated with 0.05 mg of acepromazine per kilogram of body weight by IM injection. Propofol was prepared at a dose of 5 mg/kg, and 75 mg (7.5 mL) was drawn into a syringe. After approximately 15 minutes, the anesthetist commenced anesthetic induction. She first injected three consecutive boluses in a total volume of 3.5 mL over 3 minutes in an attempt to bring the patient into a state of readiness for intubation. During this time the patient was unconscious but exhibited muscle tremors, weak spontaneous movements, and swallowing motions. Although the anesthetist continued to inject additional boluses of 0.5 to 1 mL every few minutes, the patient continued to remain at an anesthetic depth inadequate to allow intubation.

The instructor was summoned. He saw no evidence that the drug had been given perivascularly and proceeded to determine why this patient had not reached surgical anesthesia. After assessing the situation, he determined that the patient was in no danger and that the induction agent was simply being given too slowly. He instructed the student to increase the rate of administration. Within 90 seconds at the increased rate, the patient was at an adequate depth to be intubated. The anesthetic procedure was completed with no further complications.

This case also illustrates the importance of using an appropriate injection rate when inducing patients with ultra-short IV anesthetics, but for a different reason than in the previous case. When giving these agents, emphasis is often placed on avoiding rapid injection and overdose, but it is equally important to avoid giving the drug too slowly. If the agent is given too slowly, the patient will remain at an inadequate anesthetic depth. This is very frustrating for the anesthetist and may lead to adverse effects from delayed intubation, epinephrine release, and other issues. Even though these drugs must be given slowly to effect to minimize apnea and other adverse effects, they must be given rapidly enough to produce a depth of anesthesia adequate for intubation within a reasonable period of time. Thus, as in the previous case, a balance must be achieved that results in a smooth and safe induction.

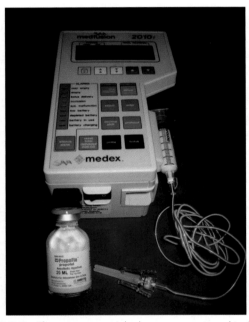

**FIGURE 3-5** This syringe pump (also known as a *syringe driver*) is being used to administer a CRI of propofol from a 5-mL syringe. The syringe is attached to microbore tubing that has been preloaded with propofol.

recommends that unused product be discarded within 6 hours of opening to avoid contamination. (Unopened, the shelf life is approximately 3 years.) Some authorities suggest that unused propofol can be stored up to 24 hours, provided that sterile technique is used for opening, dispensing, and storing the product. Refrigeration may be preferable to storage at room temperature. Unfortunately, detailed studies on the storage characteristics of propofol have not been published, but the incidence of infection from contaminated drug appears to be low.

The cost of propofol induction in dogs is approximately four times that of ketamine-diazepam and two times that of thiopental.

> *TECHNICIAN NOTE* Propofol should be handled in a strictly aseptic manner. The manufacturer recommends that unused product be discarded within 6 hours of opening to avoid contamination.

### Dissociative Anesthetics

In the late 1950s the introduction of the injectable anesthetic phencyclidine made available a new class of injectable anesthetic drugs called the *dissociative anesthetics*. Although phencyclidine is not used in veterinary medicine because of its abuse potential, its derivative, ketamine hydrochloride, is used alone to induce dissociative anesthesia in cats for minor procedures. It is also commonly used in combination with a variety of tranquilizers and opioids to induce general anesthesia in a wide variety of species, and it is given in subanesthetic doses by CRI to provide analgesia. Ketamine may also be given orally in feral cats to facilitate restraint.

Tiletamine hydrochloride, another dissociative agent, is combined with the benzodiazepine zolazepam in a proprietary product called Telazol. This product is administered intravenously or intramuscularly, alone or in combination with other agents, to produce sedation and anesthesia. Both ketamine and Telazol are controlled.

### Mode of Action and Pharmacology

The mechanism of action of the dissociative anesthetics is complex. Unlike most general anesthetics, which cause general CNS depression, dissociative anesthetics cause

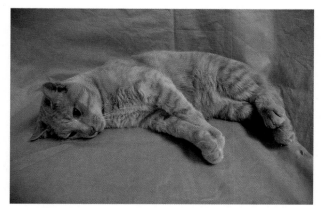

**FIGURE 3-6** A cat in dissociative anesthesia. Note the central, dilated pupils, open eyes, and muscle rigidity. The patient appears awake but unaware of its surroundings.

disruption of nerve transmission in some parts of the brain and selective stimulation in others. Dissociative agents also inhibit NMDA (*N*-methyl-D-aspartate) receptors in the CNS that are responsible for "windup." Windup is an exaggerated response to low-intensity pain stimuli that results in worsening of postoperative pain. This NMDA inhibition is believed to be responsible for the analgesic and many of the other primary effects of these drugs (see Chapter 7).

The unusual combination of actions result in a distinctive trancelike state termed *dissociative anesthesia* (so called because it dissociates various regions of the brain), in which the animal appears awake but immobile and unaware of its surroundings (Figure 3-6). Dissociative anesthesia is described in the section on effects on major organ systems.

Peak action of ketamine is about 1 to 2 minutes after IV injection, and about 10 minutes after IM injection. The duration of effect is about 20 to 30 minutes. A higher dose increases duration but does not increase anesthetic effect. Dissociatives are redistributed and metabolized by the liver; they may also be excreted unchanged in the urine and so should be used cautiously in patients with liver or kidney disease. As with barbiturates, redistribution is largely responsible for the initial decrease in effects.

---

**TECHNICIAN NOTE**    Major effects of dissociatives are as follows:
- Cataleptoid state
- Intact reflexes
- Eyes open, pupils central and dilated
- Normal or increased muscle tone
- Analgesia (primarily somatic)
- Sensitivity to sensory stimuli
- Increased heart rate, cardiac output, and mean arterial pressure (MAP) secondary to SNS stimulation
- Apneustic respiration at higher doses

---

## Effects on Major Organ Systems

### Central Nervous System

- The primary effect on the CNS is dissociative anesthesia. Dissociatives do not induce stage III anesthesia. Characteristics of dissociative anesthesia include the following:
  - *Cataleptoid state.* Catalepsy is a state in which a patient does not respond to external stimuli and has muscle rigidity in which the limbs will remain in the position in which they are placed. In people this state may be drug induced or may occur with conditions including schizophrenia and epilepsy. A cataleptoid state (the suffix *oid* meaning "like") is similar to catalepsy but with a variable degree of muscle rigidity.
  - *Intact reflexes:* Palpebral, corneal, and pedal reflexes, pupillary light reflex (PLR), and laryngeal and swallowing reflexes remain intact. Because reflex activity is preserved even at moderate anesthetic depth, it may be difficult to determine anesthetic depth in patients under dissociative anesthesia. Anesthetic depth in patients that show signs of purposeful movement is likely inadequate, whereas in those with very depressed respiration it is likely excessive. When using these agents, the anesthetist may find it challenging to determine where an individual patient lies between these two extremes.
  - *Ocular effects:* Unlike conventional anesthesia, dissociative anesthesia does not usually result in partial closure of the eyelids or eyeball rotation. The eye normally remains fully open, with a central and dilated pupil. Ophthalmic lubricant should be applied hourly to prevent corneal drying.
  - *Normal or increased muscle tone.* In some animals muscle tone is retained, whereas in others it is increased, almost to the point of rigidity. The animal may assume a stiff posture, with outstretched front limbs and extended neck. During recovery or light anesthesia, spontaneous, random movements of the head and neck may be seen. This is in marked contrast to the muscle relaxation that is seen with most other anesthetics. The concurrent use of a tranquilizing agent such as diazepam, acepromazine, dexmedetomidine, or xylazine helps prevent excessive muscle rigidity, improves ease of intubation, and produces a state more characteristic of general anesthesia.
  - *Analgesia.* Because of inhibition of the NMDA receptor, dissociative agents provide significant analgesia to the skin and limbs (**somatic analgesia**) but limited **visceral analgesia** (that is, involving the organs). A patient given a dissociative anesthetic may be able to perceive pain but is unable to respond to it. It is the veterinarian's obligation to ensure that pain is not perceived, through the use of supplementary anesthetic agents and/or analgesics.

- *Amnesia.* Human patients anesthetized with dissociative agents do not recall the procedure afterward, even though they do not appear unconscious at the time.
- *Sensitivity to sensory stimuli.* Animals anesthetized with these agents may show marked sensitivity to sound, light, and other sensory stimuli. These agents are used in combination with other drugs, particularly diazepam, to avoid excitement and improve muscle relaxation.

### Cardiovascular System
- Unlike most other anesthetics, dissociative anesthetics do not decrease heart rate or decrease cardiac output in patients with normal heart function. In fact, most animals exhibit increased heart rate, cardiac output, and mean arterial blood pressure owing to stimulation of the SNS. These cardiovascular effects are not usually harmful to the animal but can be if the patient has preexisting heart disease (e.g., cats with hyperthyroidism or cardiomyopathy), because cardiac work and oxygen consumption increase.

### Respiratory System
- Dissociative anesthetics do not affect the respiratory system in the same way as most other anesthetics. Respiratory rate and tidal volume may change, but respiratory depression is usually insignificant at usual doses. At higher doses, animals exhibit **apneustic respiration**, a breathing pattern in which there is a pause for several seconds at the end of the inspiratory phase, followed by a short, quick expiratory phase. These animals appear to hold their breath.

---

 *TECHNICIAN NOTE* Major adverse effects of dissociatives are as follows:
- Exaggerated response to touch, light, and sound during recovery
- Seizure-like activity
- Nystagmus
- Decreased inotropy
- Increased salivary and respiratory tract secretions
- Pain after IM injection

---

### Adverse Effects
### Central Nervous System
- Animals recovering from dissociative anesthesia often show an exaggerated response to touch, light, or sound, and seizure-like activity may be observed. Reduction of light, sound, and other stimuli or administration of benzodiazepines may reduce this activity. Because CNS stimulation is seen with dissociatives, these drugs are contraindicated in animals with a history of epilepsy or other seizure disorders. Dissociative anesthetics should be avoided in animals that have ingested strychnine, street drugs, organophosphates, and other toxins that affect the CNS. Dissociative anesthetics should also be used with caution in animals undergoing procedures involving the neurologic system, including cerebrospinal fluid (CSF) taps and myelograms, because such animals are at increased risk for postoperative seizures immediately after these procedures.
- Some animals recovering from dissociative anesthesia may attempt to paw their faces or demonstrate other bizarre behavior, possibly resulting from hallucinations. Recovering patients should be closely monitored in the hospital to prevent self-injury. Personality changes that can persist for several days have been reported in animals after recovery from ketamine anesthesia. Fortunately, these usually resolve spontaneously after a few days or weeks.
- Dissociative anesthetics may induce nystagmus, a repetitive side-to-side motion of the eyeball. Ketamine-induced nystagmus is more commonly seen in cats than in dogs. This condition is harmless and resolves on recovery from anesthesia.

### Cardiovascular System
- Dissociative agents are felt to decrease inotropy—an effect that is normally counteracted by SNS stimulation. This decrease in the strength of heart muscle contraction can become problematic in patients with preexisting heart disease, leading to sudden development of congestive heart failure, even if the heart disease is not evident. For this reason it is important to screen patients for preexisting heart disease (such as hypertrophic cardiomyopathy in cats caused by hyperthyroidism), as these patients are at increased risk for serious complications if given dissociative agents.
- Dissociatives also slightly increase the risk that cardiac arrhythmias will develop in response to epinephrine release.

### Respiratory System
- Although this is not usually a problem at conventional doses, overdoses may cause severe respiratory depression or respiratory arrest.
- Dissociatives also significantly increase salivation and respiratory tract secretions. Care must be taken to ensure that the airway is protected to prevent aspiration. Anticholinergics can be used to control these signs but may further predispose the patient to cardiac arrhythmias.

### Other Adverse Effects
Dissociative anesthetics have many other effects, including the following:
- *Tissue irritation.* Ketamine and tiletamine are irritating to tissues, and many animals show transitory pain after IM injection. However, these agents do not cause tissue necrosis.

- *Increased intracranial and intraocular pressure.* Dissociative anesthetics are contraindicated in patients with cranial trauma, conditions that cause elevated CSF pressure, and some ocular surgeries.

## Use of Dissociative Anesthetics

Unlike barbiturates, propofol, and etomidate, dissociatives may be given by either the IM or IV route. The versatility and wide margin of safety of dissociatives has led to their widespread acceptance in veterinary anesthesia, particularly for use in cats and horses. When given in combination with a tranquilizer (e.g., diazepam, midazolam, xylazine, dexmedetomidine, acepromazine, or zolazepam), they are useful for brief procedures, such as castrations, or as a means of induction before intubation and inhalation anesthesia. They are also useful for chemical restraint of intractable cats, allowing examinations and minor treatments without endangering hospital personnel. In dogs, dissociative-tranquilizer combinations (ketamine-diazepam or tiletamine-zolazepam) are also commonly used as induction agents. These agents are also used in combination with tranquilizers in an extremely wide variety of large animal and exotic species for sedation, immobilization, and anesthesia. In addition to the uses listed above, ketamine is an NMDA antagonist–class analgesic used in combination with other analgesics for pain control.

One limitation of dissociatives is the lack of an effective reversal agent.

### Ketamine

Ketamine is among the most commonly used agents in North American small animal practice and can be used to anesthetize not only cats and dogs but also birds, horses, and exotic species. Currently, ketamine is licensed only for use in cats and subhuman primates.

Ketamine is most commonly supplied as a 100-mg/mL solution. In 1999 ketamine was classified as a Schedule III controlled substance in the United States. It is presently classified as a prescription drug in Canada.

Ketamine has a rapid onset of action after IV or IM administration. This is a result of its high lipid solubility, which allows quick entry into brain tissue. Cats may lose their righting reflex within 90 seconds of IV administration and within 2 to 4 minutes of an IM injection of ketamine. IV administration has several advantages over IM administration, including more rapid induction and recovery and a lower dose. The anesthetist must ensure that the dose of ketamine is correct for the route of administration used: if the IM dose is inadvertently given by the IV route, serious overdose and death could result. Ketamine is given only by the IV route in dogs because IM ketamine may cause excitement and seizure activity. In cats, the primary use of IM injections is for restraint of fractious animals, in which IV injections are problematic. Ketamine can also be administered orally to fractious cats, although this constitutes extra-label use and requires

the owner's informed consent. For a 5-kg cat, 100 mg of ketamine are drawn into a syringe, and an open-ended feline urethral catheter is attached. This is inserted through the cage bars, and the drug is squirted into the cat's mouth. The oral ketamine takes effect in 5 to 10 minutes. If the eyes are accidentally sprayed with ketamine, they should be flushed with saline after the animal is anesthetized.

Although ketamine can be administered repeatedly to maintain anesthesia, this should be done with caution. After repeated injections, large amounts of the drug accumulate in the tissues, increasing the risk of seizure activity during recovery and significantly prolonging recovery.

Recovery from ketamine anesthesia normally occurs within 2 to 6 hours in healthy patients, depending on the dose given and the administration route. Dogs appear to have faster recoveries than cats, probably because of differences in ketamine metabolism and excretion. Elimination of ketamine depends on hepatic metabolism in the dog, but in the cat the drug is primarily excreted through the kidney. It follows that ketamine should be used with caution in dogs with hepatic disease and in cats with compromised renal function or urinary obstruction.

Ketamine is commonly used in combination with acepromazine, benzodiazepines, alpha$_2$-agonists, and other agents to produce a wide variety of mixtures. Although most of these mixtures will be covered in the species chapters, it is fitting to mention diazepam and ketamine, which is one of the most commonly used combinations in small and large animal practice.

> **TECHNICIAN NOTE** Ketamine can be administered orally to cats that cannot be handled, at a dose of 100 mg/5 kg body weight. Squirt the drug into the cat's mouth through the bars of the cage, using an open-ended feline urethral catheter.

### Ketamine-Diazepam Combination

A mixture of ketamine and diazepam is popular for IV induction of cats and dogs (including sighthounds) and is formulated by combining equal volumes of diazepam (5 mg/mL) and ketamine (100 mg/mL). The drugs are commonly mixed in the same syringe, although there is a small risk of precipitate formation. After premedication with an opioid and/or tranquilizer, ketamine-diazepam is given intravenously at a dose of 1 mL/20 lb (9.1 kg). This is equivalent to doses of 0.28 mg of diazepam per kilogram and 5.5 mg of ketamine per kilogram. The animal loses consciousness within 30 to 90 seconds and remains sufficiently deeply anesthetized for intubation or minor surgery for 5 to 10 minutes. This is followed by a 30- to 60-minute recovery period.

This combination of ketamine and diazepam has several advantages, including minimal cardiac depression, good muscle relaxation, superior recovery, and some analgesia. Respiratory depression, however, may be greater than that seen with ketamine alone.

Ketamine-diazepam does not work well when given by the IM route in either cats or dogs, because diazepam is poorly absorbed after IM injection. However, midazolam is well absorbed and may be used in place of diazepam for minor procedures (midazolam 0.28 mg/kg and ketamine 5.5 mg/kg).

## Tiletamine

Tiletamine is a dissociative agent with effects similar to those of ketamine. Tiletamine is sold only in combination with zolazepam, which is a benzodiazepine closely related to diazepam. The use of zolazepam in combination with tiletamine reduces the risk of seizures during recovery and helps promote skeletal muscle relaxation. The product (Telazol) is sold as a powder, which contains 50 mg of each drug per milliliter. It is reconstituted with sterile water and is stable for 4 days at room temperature and 14 days if refrigerated. Telazol is a Class III controlled substance in the United States.

Tiletamine-zolazepam is used alone or in combination with other tranquilizers and with ketamine for immobilization, sedation, restraint, and anesthetic induction in a wide variety of domestic and exotic species. It is useful as an induction agent in healthy dogs and cats, particularly in animals with aggressive temperaments. It can be used alone (after premedication) or supplemented with inhalation anesthetics. The dose used is frequently lower than that recommended by the manufacturer.

The combination of tiletamine and zolazepam is similar in effect to ketamine-diazepam but offers the following advantages:

- Tiletamine appears to cause less pronounced apneustic respiration than ketamine. However, respiratory depression may be significant, particularly if a high dose is used or tiletamine is used in combination with other sedatives or anesthetics.
- Tiletamine-zolazepam may be administered intramuscularly, intravenously, or subcutaneously, although currently in the United States it is approved only for IM use in dogs and cats.
- Tiletamine-zolazepam is effective in many species of wildlife, and in some species it is the drug of choice for capture and immobilization.

Many reflexes are maintained throughout tiletamine-zolazepam anesthesia (including the palpebral, corneal, laryngeal, and pedal reflexes), and depth of anesthesia may be difficult to judge. As with ketamine, there is some analgesia, but visceral analgesia is inadequate for major abdominal surgery unless supplemented with other agents. Tachycardia and cardiac arrhythmias may be present in light anesthesia, and cardiac output is significantly reduced at high doses (more than 20 mg/kg IM). Like ketamine, tiletamine induces a marked increase in salivation and respiratory secretions unless the patient is premedicated with an anticholinergic.

One disadvantage of tiletamine-zolazepam is the long and difficult recoveries seen in some animals. As with ketamine, ataxia and increased sensitivity to stimuli are commonly observed during the recovery period. Tremors, muscle rigidity, seizure activity, and hyperthermia can also be seen, especially in dogs given tiletamine-zolazepam at labeled doses by the IM route. IV diazepam administration may be helpful in affected animals. In cats, recovery may be prolonged (up to 5 hours after IM injection), particularly if high doses are administered. Because the drug is metabolized by the liver and excreted via the kidneys, prolonged recovery should be expected in animals with liver or kidney dysfunction.

Tiletamine-zolazepam should be avoided in patients with an American Society of Anesthesiologists (ASA) physical status class of P3 or greater and in animals with CNS signs, hyperthyroidism, cardiac disease, pancreatic or renal disease, pregnancy, glaucoma, or penetrating eye injuries.

## Etomidate

Etomidate is a noncontrolled, sedative-hypnotic imidazole drug that is occasionally used for induction of anesthesia in dogs, cats, and exotics. Because of its minimal effect on the cardiovascular and respiratory systems, etomidate is very useful in high-risk patients. However, it is not routinely used owing to its high cost and significant adverse effects including pain on IV injection, nausea, and vomiting. This ultra–short-acting nonbarbiturate drug has a wide therapeutic index, is noncumulative, and has a duration of action that is about 3 to 5 minutes but that is somewhat dependent on the dose.

### Mode of Action and Pharmacology

Although the mode of action of etomidate is not completely understood, it appears to augment action of the inhibitory neurotransmitter GABA in a similar manner to barbiturates and propofol. The duration of effect is short because, like propofol, the drug is redistributed away from the brain and rapidly metabolized.

>  **TECHNICIAN NOTE** Major effects of etomidate are as follows:
> - Hypnosis with minimal analgesia
> - Anticonvulsant effect
> - Minimal effect on cardiopulmonary function
> - Good muscle relaxation
> - Spontaneous twitching movements during induction and recovery

### Effects on Major Organ Systems
#### Central Nervous System

- Anesthesia with etomidate is characterized by hypnosis but little analgesia. The drug decreases brain oxygen consumption, maintains brain perfusion better than most other injectable agents, and has anticonvulsant properties. It is therefore a good choice for patients with brain trauma or those undergoing brain or spinal surgery.

## Cardiovascular System

- After a brief period of hypotension, etomidate has little effect on heart rate, rhythm, blood pressure, and cardiac output. It is therefore the induction agent of choice for animals with moderate to severe heart disease or shock.

## Respiratory System

- This drug minimally affects respiratory rate and tidal volume; however, a brief period of apnea may be seen after induction. Although it crosses the placental barrier, it is rapidly eliminated and causes little neonatal respiratory depression and so is a good choice for cesarean sections (C-sections).

## Other Effects

- Etomidate produces good muscle relaxation, but spontaneous muscle twitching and movements may occur during induction and recovery.

 **TECHNICIAN NOTE** Major adverse effects of etomidate are as follows:
- Pain after IV injection
- Hemolysis in cats after rapid injection
- Decreased cortisol levels
- Nausea, vomiting, and excitement during induction and recovery

## Adverse Effects

Although etomidate has a wide margin of safety, it has the following potential adverse effects:

- IV injection is reported to be painful. Some authors recommend administration through a running IV fluid line to decrease pain. Perivascular injection may be associated with the development of sterile abscesses.
- Rapid injection of etomidate may cause RBC hemolysis in cats owing to the propylene glycol vehicle. This is clinically insignificant unless the cat has an extremely low hematocrit or the drug is given repeatedly.
- Adrenal cortical function may be depressed for several hours after etomidate administration, decreasing levels of **cortisol** (a natural cortisone-like hormone). This is not harmful unless the drug is given for several hours or repeated over several days. For this reason, CRI is not recommended to sedate or anesthetize patients with serious illnesses.
- Nausea, vomiting, and involuntary excitement may occur during induction or recovery, particularly in patients that have not been adequately premedicated.

## Use of Etomidate

Etomidate is administered only by the IV route. As with other induction agents, it is given to effect, starting with one quarter to one half of the calculated dose, depending on how rapid an induction is desired. Adverse effects including vomiting and muscle contractions are minimized by premedication with an opioid or diazepam (0.5 mg of diazepam per kilogram given intravenously 30 seconds before etomidate). Some authors also recommend premedication with dexamethasone to counteract suppression of the adrenal gland.

Like propofol, etomidate can be administered in repeated boluses for short-term maintenance of anesthesia.

## Guaifenesin

Guaifenesin (GG) (previously known as *glyceryl guaiacolate ether,* or *GGE*) is a noncontrolled muscle relaxant that is commonly given to large animals to increase muscle relaxation, facilitate intubation, and ease induction and recovery. It is not an anesthetic or analgesic by itself and so is usually given in combination with other agents.

### Mode of Action and Pharmacology

Although the mechanism of action is not fully known, GG is felt to block nerve impulses in the CNS.

 **TECHNICIAN NOTE** Major effects and adverse effects of guaifenesin are as follows:
- Skeletal muscle relaxation
- Minimal cardiopulmonary effects
- Few adverse effects at therapeutic doses
- Thrombophlebitis after IV injection
- Tissue reaction after perivascular injection

### Effects of Guaifenesin

GG causes skeletal muscle relaxation, including the pharyngeal and laryngeal muscles, but minimally affects the diaphragm. It affects the cardiovascular and respiratory systems minimally, causing transient mildly decreased blood pressure and tidal volume and mildly increased respiratory rate and GI motility.

### Adverse Effects

At therapeutic doses, few adverse effects are seen. Excessive doses can cause muscle rigidity and apneustic breathing. GG is irritating to the tissues, so IV injection can cause thrombophlebitis, and perivascular injection may lead to tissue reaction. Concentrated solutions of this agent above 7% in ruminants and above 12% in horses can cause RBC hemolysis. Therefore a 5% or 10% solution in dextrose is preferred, and GG should be used with caution in anemic patients.

## Use of Guaifenesin

GG is usually given as a part of an anesthetic induction protocol in combination with ketamine (after premedication with an alpha$_2$-agonist or acepromazine). GG is also used to maintain anesthesia for short periods of time (less than 1 hour) in horses as part of a total IV anesthetic mixture commonly known as "triple drip" (GG combined with ketamine and an alpha$_2$-agonist, typically xylazine).

It is administered rapidly intravenously after premedication until the patient shows signs of ataxia ("knuckling" at the fetlock in horses; ruminants will sway or even lie down), after which the induction agent is given. Recovery is usually smooth.

Guaifenesin should not be used without premedication or as the sole agent, because excitement is likely to be seen during induction and large doses will be required for recumbency, which increases the risk of side effects. Sedation and analgesia are inadequate for surgery when this agent is used alone.

The 5% solution is prepared by adding 50 g of guaifenesin to 50 g of medical grade dextrose, which is dissolved in 1 L of very hot sterile water. If a precipitate develops, it can be dissolved by rewarming the solution.

## INHALATION ANESTHETICS

As mentioned in Chapter 1, the birth of modern anesthesia can be traced back to the mid 1800s, when inhalant anesthetics were first used clinically (diethyl ether in 1842, nitrous oxide in 1844, and chloroform in 1847). Before that time surgery was performed under extreme and less than ideal conditions. Surgeons often had to work at breakneck speed while the conscious patients were restrained by attendants. Needless to say, surgery at that time involved fear, risk, and pain. Indeed, the introduction of inhalant agents marked one of the most significant advances of medical science by giving surgeons the ability to perform surgery safely and humanely.

The first inhalant anesthetics are no longer used because they have been gradually replaced by the halogenated agents, which continue to be among the safest and most commonly used anesthetics. In fact, their use is so commonplace for such a wide variety of routine veterinary procedures that it is difficult to imagine caring for patients without them.

The inhalation anesthetics in common use at the present time are the halogenated compounds isoflurane and sevoflurane. Desflurane and nitrous oxide are occasionally used in some practices and academic and research settings. Enflurane is not used in veterinary patients owing to problematic adverse effects. Halothane has recently become unavailable in the United States, and methoxyflurane has not been available for two decades. However, as a result of many years of extensive use, methoxyflurane and halothane remain useful points of comparison for the currently used agents isoflurane and sevoflurane. Many other inhalation agents that were used in the past (including diethyl ether, chloroform, divinyl ether, and trichloroethylene) are now of historical interest only.

## Diethyl Ether

Diethyl ether was for many years the most widely used anesthetic because of several desirable characteristics. Animals anesthetized with this agent maintained relatively stable cardiac output, heart rhythm, respirations, and blood pressure. Ether also produced good muscle relaxation and analgesia. Despite these advantages, ether had significant drawbacks that resulted in its eventual replacement by other agents. Ether was very irritating to tracheal and bronchial mucosa, resulting in increased salivation, mucous secretions, and increased risk of laryngospasm and airway blockage. Induction and recovery from ether anesthesia were often prolonged, and postoperative nausea and vomiting were common. In addition, ether is flammable and explosive and requires an explosion-proof refrigerator for safe storage. Devastating operating room fires sometimes resulted from the use of ether in conjunction with oxygen. Ether is of interest to the modern anesthetist because in the early 1900s Dr. Guedel described the classic stages and planes of anesthesia by observing physiological responses to this agent.

## Halogenated Organic Compounds

Isoflurane and sevoflurane, the most commonly used inhalation agents in veterinary practice, are classified as halogenated organic compounds. Other agents in this class include desflurane, halothane, methoxyflurane, and enflurane. Halogenated agents are liquids at room temperature (although the boiling point of desflurane is near room temperature). They are stored inside the vaporizer of the anesthetic machine and evaporate in the oxygen that flows through the vaporizer, with the exception of desflurane, which requires a special injection-type vaporizer. The resulting mixture of oxygen and anesthetic is delivered to the patient through a breathing circuit (discussed in detail in Chapter 4).

### Mode of Action and Pharmacology

The mechanism of action of halogenated anesthetics on the CNS is not fully understood, although it has been suggested that these anesthetics inhibit nerve cell function in the brain and spinal cord.

The uptake, distribution, and elimination of these agents are very different from those of injectable agents. A basic understanding of these differences is necessary if the agents are to be used effectively and safely. What follows is a summary of the movement of these drugs within the body.

Within the anesthetic machine, liquid anesthetic is vaporized, mixed with oxygen, and delivered to the patient by mask or endotracheal tube. The anesthetic travels via the air passages to the lungs, where it diffuses across the alveolar cell membranes and enters the bloodstream. The rate of diffusion is controlled by the concentration gradient between the alveolus and the bloodstream, as well as the lipid solubility of the drug. During the induction period, the concentration of the agent in the alveolus is high, and the concentration in the blood is low. This creates a steep concentration gradient, and diffusion of anesthetic from the alveolus into the blood is rapid during this period.

As with injectable agents, inhalation agents are carried to the body tissues in the blood. Consequently, tissues with greater blood flow (brain, heart, kidney) are more quickly saturated with anesthetic than tissues with lesser blood flow such as skeletal muscle and fat. Because of their relatively high lipid solubility, most inhalation agents readily leave the circulation and enter the brain, inducing anesthesia. The depth of anesthesia is determined by the partial pressure of the anesthetic agent in the brain. This in turn is related to the partial pressure of anesthetic in the blood and alveoli. Anesthesia is maintained as long as sufficient quantities of inhalation agent are delivered to the alveoli so that the blood, alveolar, and brain concentrations are maintained.

When the concentration of the inhalation agent administered is reduced or discontinued by adjustment of the anesthetic machine vaporizer, the amount of anesthetic in the alveolus is reduced. Because the blood level is still high, the concentration gradient now favors the diffusion of anesthetic from the blood into the alveoli. The blood levels of the anesthetic are quickly reduced, provided the animal continues to breathe and eliminate anesthetic from the alveoli. The anesthetist can hasten the elimination of anesthetic by periodically bagging the animal with 100% oxygen. This removes anesthetic from the alveoli and reestablishes a steep concentration gradient between the alveoli and the blood. As the concentration of the anesthetic in the blood falls, the agent leaves the brain and the patient wakes up.

Isoflurane, sevoflurane, and desflurane undergo minimal liver metabolism because they are eliminated from the body chiefly through the lungs. Some of the older halogenated compounds (in particular, methoxyflurane) have very high lipid solubility and accumulate in body fat. Unlike isoflurane, sevoflurane, and desflurane, older agents rely to a significant degree on liver metabolism and renal excretion for their complete elimination from the body.

> TECHNICIAN NOTE Major effects and adverse effects of halogenated inhalation anesthetics are as follows:
> - Dose-related CNS depression
> - Vasodilation, decreased cardiac output and blood pressure
> - Dose-dependent respiratory depression including apnea

## Effects on Major Organ Systems

Although halogenated inhalation agents vary somewhat in their effects, the following characteristics are common to all (see Tables 3-1 to 3-4).

### Central Nervous System
- These anesthetics cause a dose-related, reversible depression of the CNS. These agents also depress the temperature-regulating center, leading to hypothermia.

### Cardiovascular System
- Inhalation agents depress cardiovascular function. Although the effect on heart rate is variable, all of these agents cause vasodilation and decreased cardiac output and may decrease blood pressure and tissue perfusion.

### Respiratory System
- In general, inhalation agents depress ventilation in a dose-dependent manner by decreasing tidal volume and respiratory rate.

## Adverse Effects
### Central Nervous System
- Animals with head trauma or brain tumors may develop dangerously increased intracranial pressure when anesthetized with inhalation agents, especially if carbon dioxide levels in the blood are allowed to increase. However, the currently used halogenated anesthetics are considered safe for animals with a history of epilepsy.

### Cardiovascular System
- Because inhalation anesthetics may decrease blood pressure, they have a potential to decrease renal blood flow. This can be clinically significant in animals with preexisting renal disease or in animals receiving nephrotoxic drugs such as gentamicin or nonsteroidal anti-inflammatory drugs (NSAIDs) (see Chapter 7).

### Respiratory System
- **Hypoventilation** is a possible adverse effect of all inhalation agents. Hypoventilation predisposes the animal to carbon dioxide retention and respiratory acidosis.

Despite this list of potential adverse effects, halogenated anesthetics are considered safe for most patients relative to other anesthetics. However, safety depends to a large degree on the care with which these agents are administered and the vigilance of the anesthetist in monitoring their effect on the patient.

> TECHNICIAN NOTE Halogenated anesthetics are considered safe for most patients relative to other anesthetics. However, safety depends to a large degree on the care with which these agents are administered and the vigilance of the anesthetist in monitoring their effect on the patient.

| TABLE 3-6 | **Physical Properties of the Common Inhalation Anesthetics** | | | | | |
|---|---|---|---|---|---|---|
| | Desflurane | Sevoflurane | Isoflurane | Halothane | Methoxyflurane | Nitrous Oxide |
| Approximate date of first and last clinical use in United States | 1992 In use | 1994 In use | 1981 In use | 1956 to 2008 | 1959 to approximately 1990 | 1845 In use |
| Saturated vapor pressure at 750 mm Hg and 20° C | 700 | 160 | 240 | 243 | 23 | ($N_2O$ is a gas at room temperature) |
| Blood-gas partition coefficient | 0.42 | 0.68 | 1.46 | 2.54 | 15 | 0.47 |
| Fat solubility | 27 | 48 | 45 | 51 | 902 | 1.08 |
| Rubber solubility | 19 | 29 | 49 | 190 | 630 | 1.2 |
| MAC in dogs (%) | 7.2 | 2.34 | 1.3 | 0.87 | 0.23 | 188 |
| MAC in cats (%) | 9.8 | 2.58 | 1.63 | 1.19 | 0.23 | 255 |
| MAC in horses (%) | 7.23 | 2.34 | 1.31 | 0.88 | — | — |
| Metabolism (%) | 0.02 | 2-5 | 0.2 | 20-46 | 50-75 | 0.004 |

Data from Tranquilli WJ, Thurmon JC, Grimm KA: *Lumb and Jones' veterinary anesthesia and analgesia*, ed 4, Ames, Iowa, 2007, Blackwell; except for the MAC values, which are from Muir WW, Hubbell JA, Bednarski RM: *Handbook of veterinary anesthesia*, ed 4, St Louis, 2006, Elsevier. Note that the figures above may not be the same as those published in other sources, as they vary from text to text.
*MAC,* Minimum alveolar concentration.

## Physical and Chemical Properties

Inhalant anesthetics differ considerably in their anesthetic effects, in part because of differences in their physical and chemical properties. The properties of chief importance to the anesthetist include vapor pressure, partition coefficient, minimum alveolar concentration (MAC), and rubber solubility. These agents also vary in their pharmacologic properties, including their effects on the cardiovascular, respiratory, and other vital systems. The physical properties and pharmacology of commonly used inhalation anesthetic agents are summarized in Table 3-6.

> **TECHNICIAN NOTE** Vapor pressure is a measure of the tendency of a liquid anesthetic to evaporate and is significant to the anesthetist because it determines whether a precision or nonprecision vaporizer is used to deliver the agent.

### Vapor Pressure

When a liquid is in a closed container, some of the molecules evaporate from the liquid to form a gas. With time the number of molecules leaving the liquid equals the number of molecules reentering the liquid—a state called *equilibrium.* Vapor pressure is the amount of pressure exerted by the gaseous form of a substance when the gas and liquid states are in equilibrium. In other words, vapor pressure of an inhalation anesthetic is a measure of its tendency to evaporate. Vapor pressure is both agent- and temperature-dependent and is commonly measured at 20° C (68° F), which is considered to be room

temperature. Vapor pressure is significant to the way these agents are used because it determines how readily the anesthetic liquid evaporates in the anesthetic machine vaporizer.

Agents with a high vapor pressure, such as isoflurane, sevoflurane, desflurane, and halothane, are described as volatile because they evaporate readily. For example, the maximum useful level of isoflurane in the fresh gas delivered to a patient is 5%. But because isoflurane evaporates so readily, if not controlled it can reach a concentration of over 30%—a level that would cause a fatal anesthetic overdose. This is why volatile agents must be delivered from a precision vaporizer, which precisely controls the amount of anesthetic delivered and therefore allows them to be used safely.

For this reason, most precision vaporizers intended for use with isoflurane allow a maximum concentration of 5%, a level sufficient for clinical use. Volatile agents generally cannot be used in nonprecision vaporizers because they do not adequately control delivery of the agent, and there is an increased risk of overdose. Isoflurane is an exception, however, as there is a nonprecision vaporizer called the Stevens Vaporizer that is intended for use with this agent. Close monitoring of the patient and anesthetic machine by a skilled anesthetist is required, however, if a nonprecision vaporizer is used (see Chapter 4).

Some agents, such as the discontinued agent methoxyflurane, have relatively low vapor pressure and do not require the use of a precision vaporizer. At 20° C the maximum methoxyflurane concentration attainable in the anesthetic circuit is 4%, a safe level for this agent. Consequently a nonprecision vaporizer, such as a glass jar with a wick (see Figure 4-26), is adequate for vaporizing methoxyflurane. Although precision vaporizers are available for use with methoxyflurane, they are not required to deliver this agent.

All precision vaporizers are designed to deliver one specific halogenated agent (e.g., isoflurane, sevoflurane, or desflurane) because they are designed and calibrated for the vapor pressure unique to that agent. The vapor pressures of isoflurane and halothane are so similar, however, that a recently serviced halothane vaporizer should deliver isoflurane at a concentration within 10% of the dial setting. For this reason, when isoflurane was first introduced it was sometimes used extra-label in halothane vaporizers. Now that isoflurane vaporizers are widely available, this practice is discouraged because of potential liability resulting from either extra-label use or from confusion of or inadvertent mixing of isoflurane and halothane.

Although it is unacceptable to combine agents in the same vaporizer, it is acceptable to switch from one anesthetic to another during the course of surgery if the patient demonstrates an adverse reaction to an anesthetic. In this case, separate vaporizers must be available for each anesthetic, and either the vaporizers must be connected in series or the inlet and outlet hoses must be rapidly changed from one vaporizer to the other when it is time to make the change.

> **TECHNICIAN NOTE** The blood-gas partition coefficient is a measure of the solubility of an inhalant anesthetic in blood as compared with alveolar gas. It is significant because it indicates the speed of induction and recovery one should expect for a given inhalant anesthetic. The lower the blood-gas partition coefficient, the faster the expected induction and recovery.

### Partition Coefficient

Many of the physiologic effects of inhalant anesthetics can be explained by their solubility characteristics in various substances such as air within the alveoli, blood, lipid, and tissue. Solubility is usually expressed as a partition coefficient, which is a ratio of the concentration of an agent in two substances.

The blood-gas partition coefficient is a ratio of the concentration of an inhalation agent in the blood and in the alveolar gas. It is therefore a measure of the solubility of an inhalant anesthetic in blood as compared with alveolar gas. A blood-gas partition coefficient of 0.5 (a low coefficient) indicates that an anesthetic is half as soluble in the blood as it is in the alveolar gas. So at equilibrium, two thirds of the anesthetic are in the alveolar gas and one third is in the blood. In contrast, a blood-gas partition coefficient of 2 (a high coefficient) indicates that the anesthetic is twice as soluble in the blood as in the alveolar gas. In this case, at equilibrium, one third is in the alveolar gas and two thirds are in the blood. So an anesthetic

with a low blood-gas partition coefficient is less soluble in blood than an anesthetic with a high blood-gas partition coefficient.

This is of importance to the anesthetist because the blood-gas partition coefficient indicates the speed of induction and recovery one should expect for a given inhalant anesthetic. The lower the blood-gas partition coefficient for an inhalant anesthetic, the faster the expected induction and recovery. This is because the relative concentration of the agent in the alveoli will remain high, creating a wide concentration gradient between the alveolar gas and the blood. So when the agent enters or leaves the blood, it does so at a rapid rate. An example of an agent with a low blood-gas partition coefficient is sevoflurane, an anesthetic with very rapid induction and recovery characteristics.

In contrast, an agent with a high partition coefficient is highly soluble in the blood and tissues. Because the anesthetic is readily absorbed into the blood and tissues (called the *sponge effect*), high levels of the anesthetic do not build up within the alveoli. This low concentration gradient causes the agent to enter the blood slowly and gradually. As a result, agents with high partition coefficients induce anesthesia less rapidly than do agents with low partition coefficients. Similarly, agents with high partition coefficients are slow to leave tissues, especially fat, and this gradual release results in a slow recovery. Methoxyflurane is an example of an agent with a high partition coefficient and, as expected, demonstrates relatively slow induction and recovery rates.

The blood-gas partition coefficient of an inhalant agent strongly influences the clinical use of the agent in the following ways:

- *Induction.* Agents with a low blood-gas partition coefficient (isoflurane, sevoflurane, desflurane, and halothane) may be used for mask and chamber inductions, because inductions are rapid enough to induce the patient safely and in a reasonable length of time. Methoxyflurane, an agent with a high partition coefficient, cannot be used this way.
- *Maintenance.* Agents with low blood-gas partition coefficients also have the advantage of allowing a rapid patient response to changes in anesthetic concentration during anesthesia. Patients anesthetized with isoflurane or sevoflurane may respond within a few minutes to changes in the vaporizer setting. If an agent with a higher partition coefficient is used (such as methoxyflurane), the anesthetist will observe a slower patient response to changes in the vaporizer setting.
- *Recovery.* Patients anesthetized with agents with low blood-gas partition coefficients have a relatively fast recovery time. Patients anesthetized with sevoflurane or isoflurane are often fully awake within a relatively short time after the vaporizer is turned off. Patients anesthetized with methoxyflurane often sleep quietly for 30 to 60 minutes after anesthesia.

> *TECHNICIAN NOTE*  The MAC of an anesthetic agent is the lowest concentration at which 50% of patients show no response to a painful stimulus. It is significant because it is a measure of the potency of the agent and is used to determine the average setting that must be used to produce surgical anesthesia.

### Minimum Alveolar Concentration

The MAC of an anesthetic agent is the lowest concentration at which 50% of patients show no response to a painful stimulus (e.g., a hemostatic forceps applied to the base of the tail or creation of a surgical incision). For example, isoflurane has a MAC of 1.3% in the dog. This means that if 10 dogs were anesthetized with isoflurane delivered at a setting of 1.3%, five of the dogs would respond to a painful stimulus and five would not. Thus the MAC is used to determine the average setting that must be used to produce surgical anesthesia and is a measure of the potency of the agent. An agent with a low MAC is a more potent anesthetic than an agent with a high MAC. For example, halothane, which has a lower MAC than isoflurane, is more potent than isoflurane. Therefore a higher concentration of isoflurane will be necessary to maintain a similar anesthetic depth.

For any inhalation anesthetic, a vaporizer setting of approximately 1 × MAC will maintain light surgical anesthesia, 1.5 × MAC will maintain moderate surgical anesthesia, and 2 × MAC will maintain deep surgical anesthesia in most patients. These figures are useful only as a rough guide: MAC varies with the age, metabolic activity, and body temperature of the patient. Factors such as disease, pregnancy, obesity, and use of other agents may also alter the potency of an anesthetic agent in a given patient. The anesthetist should also be aware that the response to an anesthetic depends on the concentration of the anesthetic in the patient's brain, which is not necessarily the same as that indicated by the anesthetic machine vaporizer dial setting, particularly early in the induction period (see Chapter 4).

For example, a concentration of approximately 2% isoflurane therefore can be expected to maintain moderate surgical anesthesia in most dogs. Halothane has a slightly lower MAC (0.87%), and a vaporizer setting between 1% and 1.5% is often adequate to maintain anesthesia. Sevoflurane has a high MAC (approximately 2.4), and the maintenance level can be expected to be close to 3.5%. This is only a rough guideline, and the anesthetist must, of course, monitor each animal's response to the anesthetic to determine the optimum setting for that individual.

### Use of Halogenated Organic Compounds

#### Isoflurane

Isoflurane, a halogenated organic compound, is currently the most commonly used inhalant agent for induction and maintenance of general anesthesia in North America. Isoflurane is approved for use only in dogs and horses, although it has gained widespread use in a wide variety of species including exotic and zoo animals and in recent years has gradually replaced its predecessor halothane largely because of fewer cardiovascular adverse effects seen with this agent.

**Physical and chemical properties.**  Isoflurane has a relatively high vapor pressure (240 mm Hg), and therefore a precision vaporizer is normally used to deliver this agent.

The blood-gas partition coefficient of isoflurane is extremely low (1.46). This, combined with the relatively low tissue solubility of this agent, results in extremely rapid induction and recovery. Isoflurane is therefore better suited to mask or chamber induction than are slower-acting agents such as methoxyflurane and halothane. Unfortunately, some animals appear to be irritated by isoflurane vapors and resist mask induction. Recovery from anesthesia is also rapid, and the anesthetist must refrain from turning off the anesthetic machine vaporizer until the end of surgery because return of consciousness may commence as rapidly as a few minutes after isoflurane is discontinued. Because of the low partition coefficient, the anesthetist can change the patient's depth of anesthesia rapidly during the course of anesthesia. An animal under anesthesia that appears too deep or too light usually responds rapidly (within a few to several minutes) after adjustment of the vaporizer dial.

The MAC of isoflurane is 1.3% to 1.63% in the common domestic species. This means that anesthesia is maintained in most patients at a concentration of 1.5% to 2.5%. The rubber solubility of isoflurane is low, and there is little absorption of this anesthetic into rubber components of the anesthetic machine and breathing circuit. Isoflurane is stable at room temperature, and no preservative is necessary. This is an advantage because, unlike with halothane, no preservative residue accumulates in isoflurane vaporizers. However, like all vaporizers, isoflurane vaporizers still require periodic maintenance and calibration.

> *TECHNICIAN NOTE*  Of the volatile anesthetics commonly used in veterinary anesthesia, isoflurane is considered to have the fewest adverse cardiovascular effects and is therefore considered to be the inhalation agent of choice for patients with cardiac disease.

**Effects and adverse effects.**
- When used at normal anesthetic levels, isoflurane maintains cardiac output close to that of preanesthetic levels. It causes some depression of myocardial cells, has little effect on heart rate, and does not sensitize the heart muscle to epinephrine-induced arrhythmias. Of the volatile anesthetics commonly used in veterinary anesthesia, isoflurane is considered to have the fewest

adverse cardiovascular effects and is therefore considered to be the inhalation agent of choice for patients with cardiac disease. Vasodilation and decreased blood pressure may be observed, however, particularly at deeper levels of anesthesia.

- Isoflurane depresses the respiratory system. In patients anesthetized with isoflurane, the respiratory rate decreases over time. A concentration of two to three times the MAC causes respiratory arrest in common domestic species.
- Isoflurane maintains cerebral blood flow and is considered a good anesthetic for animals with head trauma or brain tumors, provided the concentration is 1% or less.
- Nearly all of the isoflurane administered to a patient is eliminated through the lungs once the vaporizer is turned off. Isoflurane has low fat solubility; consequently, little retention in body fat stores, little hepatic metabolism (0.2 %), and very little renal excretion of metabolites occur. For this reason isoflurane is well suited to animals with liver or kidney disease. Isoflurane is also a good anesthetic for use in neonatal and geriatric animals, in which hepatic metabolism and renal excretion mechanisms may be less efficient than in the healthy adult animal.
- Isoflurane induces adequate to good muscle relaxation.
- Isoflurane has little or no analgesic effect in the postanesthetic period. This, combined with the rapid recoveries seen with this agent, may lead to pain and excitement during recovery unless the animal is treated with analgesics.
- When exposed to desiccated $CO_2$ absorbent, isoflurane can produce carbon monoxide, which has over 200 times greater affinity for hemoglobin binding sites than oxygen. Carbon monoxide displaces oxygen from the binding sites, causing hypoxemia. Animals with carbon monoxide poisoning may be asymptomatic, but cherry red blood and mucous membranes suggest carbon monoxide exposure, which must be treated promptly.

### Sevoflurane

Sevoflurane is the second most commonly used inhalant anesthetic for induction and maintenance of general anesthesia (isoflurane being the most commonly used agent). Chemically, it is a halogenated organic compound closely related to isoflurane and shares many of the same characteristics. Sevoflurane is labeled for use in dogs but has been used in a wide variety of species including exotic and zoo animals.

> **TECHNICIAN NOTE** Sevoflurane is the inhalant agent best suited to mask and chamber inductions. The high controllability of anesthetic depth associated with sevoflurane has made this agent popular in equine anesthesia, despite its relatively high cost.

**Physical and chemical properties.** The vapor pressure of sevoflurane, although somewhat lower than that of isoflurane, is relatively high (160 mm Hg). Therefore a precision vaporizer is required to deliver this agent.

The blood-gas partition coefficient is even lower than isoflurane's, allowing even more rapid inductions and recoveries. Observed time to intubation has been reported as 5 to 7 minutes after mask induction (compared with 6 to 8 minutes for isoflurane). Mask induction with sevoflurane is typically associated with less struggling than with isoflurane because this agent is nonirritating and has a more pleasant odor than isoflurane. Because of these characteristics, sevoflurane is the agent best suited to mask and chamber inductions. The high controllability of anesthetic depth associated with sevoflurane has made this agent popular in equine anesthesia, despite its relatively high cost (currently, approximately 10 times that of isoflurane).

The MAC of sevoflurane is 2.34% to 2.58% in common domestic species. Sevoflurane is therefore a less potent agent than isoflurane, and higher concentrations are required to induce and maintain anesthesia. A concentration of 4% to 6% is required for mask induction (compared with 3% to 5% for isoflurane), and 2.5% to 4% is the normal maintenance range (compared with 1.5% to 2.5% for isoflurane).

Sevoflurane can react with the potassium hydroxide (KOH) or sodium hydroxide (NaOH) in desiccated carbon dioxide absorbents to produce a chemical (compound A) that can cause renal damage in rats. This effect is most pronounced in closed-circle systems, in low-flow systems, and at high sevoflurane concentrations. Renal damage has not been reported in dogs or cats anesthetized with sevoflurane, and the potential for nephrotoxicity appears to be low in these species.

**Effects and adverse effects.** The effects of sevoflurane on major organ systems are similar to those of isoflurane.

- Some myocardial depression, vasodilation, and dose-related hypotension are seen with this agent. Like isoflurane, sevoflurane does not sensitize the heart to epinephrine-induced arrhythmias.
- Sevoflurane may depress respiration slightly more than isoflurane. Apnea lasting at least 30 seconds during surgical anesthesia has been reported.
- Like isoflurane, sevoflurane is primarily eliminated by the lungs (with 2% to 5% biotransformed in the liver).
- Sevoflurane does not significantly increase cerebral blood flow and can be used for anesthesia of patients with head trauma or brain tumors.
- Sevoflurane induces adequate muscle relaxation.
- Paddling, excitement, and muscle fasciculations have been reported, primarily during the recovery period.
- Sevoflurane has no analgesic effect at subhypnotic doses. As with isoflurane, an analgesic agent must be administered after any painful procedure, before the patient wakes up.

### Desflurane

Desflurane is a halogenated organic inhalant anesthetic closely related to isoflurane. It can be used for induction and maintenance of anesthesia, although its expense and some adverse effects currently preclude common use in veterinary patients.

**Physical and chemical properties.** Desflurane has the lowest blood-gas partition coefficient (0.42%) of any of the commonly used agents and therefore produces inductions and recoveries that are approximately twice as fast as those of isoflurane (sometimes referred to as "one-breath anesthesia" because it can seem as if a patient is anesthetized or wakes up after taking one breath).

The vapor pressure of desflurane is extremely high (700 mm Hg), and the boiling point is near room temperature (at 23.5° C). Because of these properties, this agent requires a special, electronic, heated vaporizer that keeps the agent under pressure to prevent it from boiling off. The high cost of desflurane and the vaporizer is a significant factor limiting the use of this agent in veterinary medicine.

This agent is the least potent of any of the halogenated agents used in veterinary patients, as evidenced by a MAC of 7.2% to 9.8% in common domestic species. A concentration of 10% to 15% is required for mask induction (compared with 3% to 5% for isoflurane), and 8% to 12% is needed for maintenance (compared with 1.5% to 2.5% for isoflurane).

Like isoflurane, very little of desflurane is metabolized by the liver (0.02%).

> **TECHNICIAN NOTE** Desflurane has the lowest blood-gas partition coefficient of any of the commonly used agents and therefore produces inductions and recoveries that are approximately twice as fast as those of isoflurane. It is sometimes referred to as "one-breath anesthesia" because it can seem as if a patient is anesthetized or wakes up after taking one breath.

**Effects and adverse effects.** Desflurane vapors are very pungent and may induce coughing and breath-holding. This makes mask induction with this agent difficult, unless the patient is premedicated. The effects on the nervous, cardiovascular, and respiratory systems are similar to those of isoflurane with the following exception: desflurane is reported to cause transient increases in heart rate and blood pressure in humans. This phenomenon (called *sympathetic storm*) has not been reported in domestic animals. Desflurane has the greatest tendency of any of the agents to cause the production of carbon monoxide when passed through dry carbon dioxide absorbent.

### Other Halogenated Agents

**Halothane.** Halothane (Fluothane), first introduced in 1956, was until relatively recently one of the most commonly used inhalation agents in veterinary anesthesia. In recent years it has gradually been replaced by isoflurane and sevoflurane.

*Physical and chemical properties.* Many of the physical and chemical properties of halothane are very similar to those of isoflurane. Like isoflurane, halothane has a relatively high vapor pressure (243 mm Hg) and therefore normally requires a precision vaporizer for its safe use. Halothane delivered through a nonprecision vaporizer may readily reach a concentration over 30%, which dangerously exceeds the normal concentration required for anesthesia (0.5% to 4%). Special techniques are required for use of halothane in a nonprecision vaporizer.

Halothane has a moderately low partition coefficient (2.54), producing inductions and recoveries that, although longer than those of isoflurane, are sufficiently rapid to allow the patient to be induced by mask. Mask induction results in unconsciousness and stage III anesthesia within about 10 minutes. Recovery time from anesthesia varies with length of anesthesia, patient condition, and the concurrent use of other agents; however, animals generally assume sternal recumbency in less than 1 hour after the anesthetic is discontinued. Because of halothane's moderate lipid solubility, a portion of the anesthetic is retained within body fat stores rather than being eliminated by the lungs during recovery. About 20% to 46% of halothane is subsequently metabolized by the liver and excreted by the kidneys.

Halothane has a very low MAC (0.87 to 1.19) and so is more potent than any of the commonly used agents. A concentration of 2% to 4% (up to 10% in large animals) is required for mask induction (compared with 3% to 5% for isoflurane), and 0.5% to 1.5% (1% to 2% in large animals) is the normal maintenance range (compared with 1.5% to 2.5% for isoflurane).

Halothane has moderate rubber solubility. This is of concern to the anesthetist because rubber hoses, reservoir bags, and other anesthetic machine parts may absorb halothane during the course of anesthesia. Release of the agent from these machine parts may delay patient recovery after the vaporizer has been turned off.

Halothane is somewhat unstable and for commercial use is mixed with the preservative thymol. The presence of a preservative may cause a buildup of residue within the vaporizer, turning the liquid in the vaporizer yellow. The residue may cause moving parts in some vaporizers to stick, so periodic cleaning and recalibration are recommended.

*Effects and adverse effects.* Halothane is a relatively safe agent for veterinary use; however, it does have the following effects on organ function:

- Halothane sensitizes the heart to the action of catecholamines (such as epinephrine) and thus may induce arrhythmias. Arrhythmias may be treated by increasing oxygen flow and ensuring that anesthetic depth is adequate. If this does not alleviate the arrhythmia, the patient may be given IV lidocaine or switched to another anesthetic, if available.

- Halothane is a myocardial depressant, decreasing myocardial contraction and cardiac output. This effect is dose-dependent (that is, the higher the concentration, the greater the effect).
- Halothane causes vasodilatation. This, along with heart muscle depression, causes a fall in blood pressure that is roughly proportional to anesthetic depth. For this reason, IV fluid support is recommended in hypovolemic or hypotensive patients.
- Halothane is a respiratory depressant, and respiratory rate and tidal volume usually fall if anesthesia is prolonged. Respiratory arrest may occur at high concentrations. Like all inhalant anesthetics, halothane readily crosses the placenta and may depress respiration in the neonates.
- From 20% to 46% of halothane is metabolized; therefore the potential for liver damage exists.
- Halothane may increase cerebral blood flow, which may lead to increased intracranial pressure in patients with head trauma or brain tumors.
- Halothane use is associated with malignant hyperthermia, a rare but often fatal disorder of thermoregulation that occurs in genetically predisposed animals. Affected animals show increased temperature, muscle rigidity, and cardiac arrhythmias and may die. Treatment consists of removal from halothane, cooling, and administration of oxygen and specific drugs such as dantrolene.

**Methoxyflurane.** Although no longer commercially available in North America, methoxyflurane was used extensively for many years, and because of unique physical properties, remains a good point of comparison when learning about currently used agents such as isoflurane and sevoflurane.

The vapor pressure of methoxyflurane is significantly lower (23 mm Hg) than that of isoflurane (240 mm Hg) or sevoflurane (160 mm Hg), and as a result methoxyflurane can be delivered using a nonprecision vaporizer, whereas currently used agents must be delivered from a precision vaporizer.

The blood-gas partition coefficient of methoxyflurane (15) is considerably higher than that of isoflurane (1.46), as is the lipid solubility. These two factors combine to produce slow inductions and recoveries. For this reason, unlike currently used agents, this agent is not useful for mask or chamber inductions.

The MAC of methoxyflurane is considerably lower (0.23%) than that of the other volatile inhalation anesthetics, making this agent more potent than currently used halogenated agents.

Methoxyflurane has a much higher rubber solubility (630) than isoflurane (49) and therefore readily dissolves in reservoir bags, hoses, and rubber endotracheal tubes. This may lead to deterioration of these products unless they are rinsed out immediately after use. This characteristic may also result in considerable release of methoxyflurane gas into the anesthetic circuit even after the vaporizer has been turned off. This is not a significant problem with currently used agents.

Because of its high lipid solubility, methoxyflurane is retained in body fat stores so that approximately 50% to 75% is metabolized and excreted by the liver and kidney. Fluoride ions and other potentially toxic metabolites are produced as a result of hepatic metabolism, and the presence within the kidney of these toxic metabolites may lead to renal damage. The currently used agents isoflurane and sevoflurane are almost entirely (>95%) eliminated by the lungs; consequently liver and kidney damage are not of major concern.

**Enflurane.** Enflurane, a volatile gaseous anesthetic used in human medicine, has not found wide acceptance in veterinary anesthesia because of adverse effects. Induction and recovery are relatively rapid and smooth, with minimal effects on heart rate and minimal sensitization of the myocardium to epinephrine. However, enflurane causes profound respiratory depression, and spontaneous ventilation is poor. In the dog, enflurane also induces significant muscle hyperactivity, and seizure-like muscle spasms may result.

> *TECHNICIAN NOTE* The advantages of nitrous oxide were significant when older agents such as methoxyflurane and halothane were in use. These advantages are much less important with the advent of newer agents such as isoflurane and sevoflurane. Consequently, nitrous oxide is now seldom used in general practice.

### Nitrous Oxide

Nitrous oxide, introduced as an anesthetic more than 150 years ago, is still used in human anesthesia and, to a much lesser extent, in veterinary anesthesia. Unlike other inhalation anesthetics, nitrous oxide is a gas at room temperature, is stored in blue compressed gas cylinders, and does not require a vaporizer. Like oxygen, it is administered with a flow meter, and it is mixed in concentrations of 40% to 67% with oxygen before being delivered to the patient.

When used with other agents, nitrous oxide ($N_2O$) speeds induction and recovery and provides additional analgesia. Nitrous oxide also reduces the MAC (and therefore the vaporizer setting) of other anesthetics by 20% to 30%. This reduces the risk of adverse effects on the cardiovascular, pulmonary, and other systems.

The advantages of nitrous oxide were significant when older agents such as methoxyflurane and halothane were in use. The advantages are much less important since the advent of newer agents such as isoflurane and sevoflurane, however, because of the rapid inductions and recoveries characteristic of these agents and because of the availability of a wide variety of effective injectable analgesics. For these reasons, nitrous oxide is now seldom used in general practice.

There are unique characteristics of nitrous oxide, including adverse effects and other cautions, with which the anesthetist must be familiar if using this agent. The reader is directed to Appendix B for detailed information about its use.

## CENTRAL NERVOUS SYSTEM AND RESPIRATORY STIMULANTS

Most anesthetic agents and many adjuncts are respiratory system depressants, so respiratory depression is commonly seen during anesthesia. This complication is usually managed by precise control of anesthetic depth and, if needed, manual or mechanical-assisted or mechanical-controlled ventilation. In emergency situations, severe respiratory depression associated with opioids and alpha$_2$-agonists can be treated with reversal agents, but the beneficial effects of the corresponding agonist, including sedation, analgesia, and hypnosis, will also be lost. When complete reversal is not desirable or when agents that cannot be reversed are used, the anesthetist may need to use other methods to manage respiratory depression. The pharmacologic agent most commonly used for this purpose is doxapram.

### Doxapram

Doxapram is a noncontrolled injectable **analeptic agent** used in small animals to stimulate respirations and speed awakening during recovery or in emergency situations. It is also commonly used to stimulate respirations in neonates after dystocia or cesarean section. It is most commonly administered intravenously to adult animals. In neonates it is often administered by placing a few drops under the tongue (sublingual administration), although it can be given subcutaneously or in the umbilical vein.

### Mode of Action and Pharmacology

Although the mode of action is not completely known, doxapram stimulates the CNS, including the respiratory centers in the brain stem.

### Effects on Major Organ Systems

Within 2 minutes of IV injection, doxapram will temporarily increase respiratory rate and depth.

### Adverse Effects

Although doxapram has a relatively wide margin of safety, it may cause hyperventilation, hypertension, and arrhythmias in some patients. It must not be used in patients with a history of seizures because the drug lowers the seizure threshold. Doxapram must be used only in the presence of adequate oxygen levels in the brain, otherwise CNS damage may result. Several other cautions are detailed in pharmacology references.

> **TECHNICIAN NOTE**    One drop of doxapram solution contains approximately 1 mg of doxapram. To stimulate respirations, 1 to 5 drops can be dripped under a neonatal puppy's tongue, and 1 to 2 drops under a kitten's tongue, depending on patient size and degree of depression.

### Use of Doxapram

After an initial injection, if CNS and respiratory stimulation is inadequate, a second injection can be given 15 to 20 minutes later. The dose of doxapram varies widely depending on the situation. For instance, in small animals the dose is much lower when used to reverse respiratory depression from inhalant agents (1.1 mg/kg IV) than when used to reverse respiratory depression from barbiturates (5.5 to 11 mg/kg IV).

Because this agent is supplied as a 20-mg/mL solution, and there are approximately 20 drops in 1 mL, 1 drop of the solution contains approximately 1 mg of doxapram. For neonatal puppies, 1 to 5 drops can be dripped under the tongue (1 to 2 drops for kittens), depending on the size and degree of depression, or 1 to 5 mg (1 to 2 mg for kittens) can be given subcutaneously to stimulate respirations.

## KEY POINTS

1. Preanesthetic agents reduce the required dose of general anesthetics, minimize adverse effects, ease induction and recovery, provide muscle relaxation, and reduce patient stress and discomfort.

2. Although not anesthetics, the anticholinergics atropine and glycopyrrolate are used to prevent bradycardia, bronchoconstriction, excessive salivation, and other parasympathetic effects. These agents must be used sparingly, and with caution, as they can produce serious adverse effects.

3. Tranquilizing agents include phenothiazines, benzodiazepines, and alpha-2-agonists. Phenothiazines have a wide margin of safety but may cause hypotension in some patients. Benzodiazepines have a calming effect on geriatric and debilitated animals and are excellent for prevention and treatment of seizures. Alpha$_2$-agonists are potent sedatives and produce excellent muscle relaxation but may cause serious cardiovascular and respiratory complications in some patients.

4. Opioid agonists, partial agonists, and agonist-antagonists may be used as preanesthetic agents, analgesics, and (in combination with tranquilizers) neuroleptanalgesics and induction agents. Many of the best analgesics available are in this group. With few exceptions, their use is subject to government regulation regarding purchase, handling, and dispensing.

5. Opioids, alpha$_2$-agonists, and benzodiazepines have corresponding reversal agents that can be used to sequentially sedate or anesthetize and then wake patients when a procedure or surgery is completed.

6. Although commonly used injectable and inhalation anesthetics have a relatively good safety profile, they have the potential to produce significant cardiovascular, respiratory, and thermoregulatory system depression.

7. Injectable anesthetics include propofol, dissociatives (ketamine and tiletamine), barbiturates (thiopental and methohexital), neuroleptanalgesic combinations, and etomidate.

8. Barbiturates are divided into classes based on duration of action. The ultra–short-acting agents thiopental and methohexital are used for anesthetic induction (and maintenance in the case of methohexital), the short-acting agent pentobarbital is used to stop seizures and for laboratory animal anesthesia, and the long-acting agent phenobarbital is used for seizure control. These classes differ in their lipid solubility, duration of effect, and distribution within the body.

9. Barbiturates show unusual potency in patients that are acidotic, hypoproteinemic, or hypotensive. They may cause prolonged recoveries in sighthounds.

10. Most intravenous (IV) anesthetics are administered by titration (or "to effect") to achieve the minimum effective dose.

11. Injectable anesthetics are eliminated by redistribution, liver metabolism, and renal excretion, whereas commonly used inhalation anesthetics are eliminated primarily by exhalation from the lungs.

12. Dissociatives such as ketamine and tiletamine produce a state of dissociative anesthesia characterized by intact reflexes, central nervous system (CNS) excitement, apneustic respiration, tachycardia, and intact or increased muscle tone. Concurrent use of a tranquilizer is recommended to promote muscle relaxation and to prevent excitement during recovery.

13. Neuroleptanalgesia is a profound hypnotic state produced by the simultaneous administration of an opioid and a tranquilizer. These agents provide relatively safe induction in debilitated patients.

14. Propofol, methohexital, and etomidate are induction agents that can be given by repeat injection to maintain anesthesia.

15. The inhalation agents in common use are isoflurane and sevoflurane. Both agents are administered by means of an anesthetic machine and either a mask or an endotracheal tube.

16. Inhalation anesthetic agents vary in their blood-gas partition coefficient, vapor pressure, and minimum alveolar concentration (MAC). These properties affect the speed of induction and recovery, the type of vaporizer that should be used, and the vaporizer setting that is required for anesthetic induction and maintenance.

17. All inhalation anesthetics may cause respiratory depression and decrease cardiac output and blood pressure. In addition, halothane may potentiate cardiac arrhythmias. Of the commonly used agents, isoflurane and sevoflurane are considered to have the greatest margin of safety and the shortest induction and recovery times.

18. Reversal agents and analeptics may be given after anesthesia to hasten anesthetic recovery. Doxapram is a nonspecific respiratory stimulant that may accelerate arousal from barbiturate or inhalation anesthesia.

## REVIEW QUESTIONS

1. A neuroleptanalgesic is a combination of:
   a. An opioid and an anticholinergic
   b. An anticholinergic and a tranquilizer
   c. An opioid and a tranquilizer
   d. An anticholinergic and a benzodiazepine

2. Most preanesthetics will not cross the placental barrier.
   True    False

3. It is recommended that atropine not be given to an animal that has tachycardia.
   True    False

4. Anticholinergic drugs such as atropine block the release of acetylcholine at the:
   a. Muscarinic receptors of the parasympathetic system
   b. Nicotinic receptors of the parasympathetic system
   c. Muscarinic receptors of the sympathetic system
   d. Nicotinic receptors of the sympathetic system

5. High doses of opioids can cause bradycardia and respiratory depression.
   True    False

6. Severe bradycardia caused by dexmedetomidine is best treated with the following drug:
   a. Atropine
   b. Naloxone
   c. Epinephrine
   d. Atipamezole

7. Opioids may be reversed with:
   a. Atipamezole
   b. Naloxone
   c. Atropine
   d. Yohimbine

8. Which of the following drugs will precipitate out when mixed with other drugs or solutions?
   a. Atropine
   b. Acepromazine
   c. Diazepam
   d. Butorphanol

9. Etomidate is particularly well suited for induction of dogs with which of the following problems?
   a. Severe cardiac disease
   b. Renal failure
   c. Orthopedic disease
   d. Pediatric (younger than 4 weeks)

10. Which of the following is an example of a dissociative anesthetic?
    a. Thiopental sodium
    b. Pentobarbital sodium
    c. Ketamine hydrochloride
    d. Propofol

11. One of the disadvantages of the drug methohexital is that animals that are anesthetized with it may demonstrate excitement during recovery.
    True    False

12. Compared with methoxyflurane, isoflurane is considered to have a:
    a. Higher vapor pressure
    b. Similar vapor pressure
    c. Lower vapor pressure

13. An anesthetic agent that has a low blood-gas partition coefficient will result in _____ induction and recovery time.
    a. Slow
    b. Moderate
    c. Fast

14. Which of the following has the lowest blood-gas partition coefficient?
    a. Halothane
    b. Isoflurane
    c. Methoxyflurane
    d. Sevoflurane

15. As a rough guideline, to safely maintain a surgical plane of anesthesia, the vaporizer should be set at about:
    a. $0.5 \times MAC$
    b. $1 \times MAC$
    c. $1.5 \times MAC$
    d. $2 \times MAC$

16. Propofol sometimes causes transient apnea. To avoid this, the anesthetist should:
    a. Give by infusion only
    b. Premedicate with opioids
    c. Administer intravenously only
    d. Titrate this drug in several boluses

17. One problem frequently associated with recovery from tiletamine-zolazepam in dogs is:
    a. Excitement
    b. Bradycardia
    c. Hypotension
    d. Laryngospasm

For the following questions, more than one answer may be correct.

18. The concentration of barbiturate entering the brain is affected by a variety of factors such as:
    a. Perfusion of the brain
    b. Lipid solubility of the drug
    c. Plasma protein levels
    d. Blood pH

19. Effects that are commonly seen after administration of a dissociative include:
    a. Increased blood pressure
    b. Increased heart rate
    c. Increased CSF pressure
    d. Increased intraocular pressure

20. Adverse effects common with isoflurane include:
    a. Hepatic toxicity
    b. Accumulation in body fat stores
    c. Depression of respiration
    d. Seizures during recovery

21. MAC will vary with:
    a. Body temperature of the patient
    b. Age of the patient
    c. Concurrent use of other drugs
    d. Anesthetic agent

22. Factors that may affect the speed of anesthetic induction with a volatile gaseous anesthetic include:
    a. Partition coefficient of the agent
    b. Vaporizer setting
    c. MAC of the agent
    d. Concurrent use of atropine

23. Which of the following are alpha$_2$-agonists?
    a. Atipamezole
    b. Xylazine
    c. Acepromazine
    d. Dexmedetomidine

24. Effects that atropine may have on the body include:
    a. Decreased salivation
    b. Increased vagal tone
    c. Decreased gastrointestinal motility
    d. Mydriasis

25. Characteristic effects of the benzodiazepines include:
    a. Pronounced sedation in healthy young animals
    b. Muscle relaxation
    c. Significant decrease in respiratory function
    d. Minimal effect on cardiovascular system

## SELECTED READINGS

Bill RL: *Clinical pharmacology and therapeutics for the veterinary technician*, ed 3, St Louis, 2006, Mosby, pp 203-249.

Branson KR, Injectable and alternative anesthetic techniques. In Tranquilli WJ, Thurmon JC, Grimm KA, editors: *Lumb & Jones' veterinary anesthesia and analgesia*, ed 4, Ames, Iowa, 2007, Blackwell Publishing, pp 273-299.

Doherty T, Valverde A: *Manual of equine anesthesia and analgesia*, Ames, 2006, Blackwell Publishing, Ltd, pp 128-174.

El Bahri L: Atipamezole: *Compendium: continuing education for veterinarians* 30(5):256-258, 2008.

Johnson RA, Striler E, Sawyer DC, Brunson DB: Comparison of isoflurane with sevoflurane for anesthesia induction and recovery in adult dogs, *Am J Vet Res* 59(4):478-481, 1998.

Ko JC, Knesl O, Weil AB, et al: Analgesia, sedation, and anesthesia. Making the switch from Medetomidine to Dexmedetomidine, *Supplement to compendium: continuing education for veterinarians* 31(1)A:2-16, 2009.

Lamont LA, Mathews KA: Opioids, Nonsteroidal anti-inflammatories and analgesic adjuvants. In Tranquilli WJ, Thurmon JC, Grimm KA, editors: *Lumb & Jones' veterinary anesthesia and analgesia*, ed 4, Ames, Iowa, 2007, Blackwell Publishing, pp 241-271.

Lemke K, Lin HC, Steffey EP, Cullen LK: Pharmacology. In Thurmon JC, Tranquilli WJ, Benson GJ, editors: *Essentials of small animal anesthesia and analgesia*, Baltimore, 1999, Lippincott Williams & Wilkins, pp 126-191.

Lemke KA: Anticholinergics and sedatives. In Tranquilli WJ, Thurmon JC, Grimm KA, editors: *Lumb & Jones' veterinary anesthesia and analgesia*, ed 4, Ames, Iowa, 2007, Blackwell Publishing, pp 201-239.

Lin HC: Dissociative anesthetics. In Tranquilli WJ, Thurmon JC, Grimm KA, editors: *Lumb & Jones' veterinary anesthesia and analgesia*, ed 4, Ames, Iowa, 2007, Blackwell Publishing, pp 301-353.

Muir WW, Hubbell JA, Bednarski RM: *Handbook of veterinary anesthesia*, ed 4, St Louis, 2006, Elsevier, pp 23-50, 140-194.

Paddleford RR: *Manual of small animal anesthesia*, ed 2, Philadelphia, 1999, WB Saunders Company, pp 12-77.

Plumb DC: *Plumb's veterinary drug handbook*, ed 6, Ames, 2008, Blackwell Publishing Professional, pp 1053-1054.

Steffey EP, Mama KR: Inhalation anesthetics. In Tranquilli WJ, Thurmon JC, Grimm KA, editors: *Lumb & Jones' veterinary anesthesia and analgesia*, ed 4, Ames, Iowa, 2007, Blackwell Publishing, pp 355-393.

# 4

# Anesthetic Equipment

## OUTLINE

Endotracheal Tubes and Associated
  Equipment, 97
  *Endotracheal Tube Parts, 98*
  *Laryngoscopes, 99*
Masks, 99
Anesthetic Chambers, 99
Anesthetic Machines, 100
Components of the Anesthetic Machine, 100
  *Compressed Gas Supply, 101*
  *Anesthetic Vaporizer, 110*
  *Breathing Circuit, 116*
  *Scavenging System, 116*
Rebreathing Systems, 116
  *Rebreathing Circuits, 116*

Non-Rebreathing Systems, 122
  *Non-Rebreathing Circuits, 122*
Operation of the Anesthetic Machine, 125
  *Daily Setup, 125*
  *Choice of Rebreathing Versus Non-
    Rebreathing System, 125*
  *Checking the Low-Pressure System
    for Leaks, 126*
  *Adjusting the Pop-Off Valve, 126*
  *Choice of Carrier Gas Flow Rates, 126*
Care and Maintenance of Anesthetic
  Equipment, 131
  *Routine Maintenance, 131*
  *Disinfecting Anesthetic Equipment, 133*

## LEARNING OBJECTIVES

*After completion of this chapter, the reader will be able to:*

- Identify equipment that is used for anesthetic induction, endotracheal intubation, and anesthetic maintenance.
- Choose and prepare an appropriate endotracheal tube for a dog, cat, horse, or cow.
- List the reasons for and advantages of endotracheal intubation.
- Describe the four basic anesthetic machine systems, and identify the parts of each system.
- Describe the basic operation of an anesthetic machine.
- Trace the flow of oxygen through an anesthetic machine and patient breathing circuit for rebreathing and non-rebreathing systems.
- Describe the function and use of each component of an anesthetic machine, anesthetic masks, and anesthetic chambers.
- Explain the use of oxygen supply of the anesthetic machine, including safety concerns associated with compressed gas cylinders.
- Explain differences between a rebreathing and a non-rebreathing system with regard to equipment, gas flow, advantages, disadvantages, and indications for use.
- Identify the function and use of each component of commonly used rebreathing and non-rebreathing circuits.
- Differentiate between a precision and a nonprecision vaporizer, and recognize the rationale for using each.
- Compare and contrast vaporizer-out-of-circuit (VOC) and vaporizer-in-circuit (VIC) vaporizers in terms of setup, use, and agents administered in each of these systems.
- Identify factors that affect anesthetic vaporizer output.
- Explain the impact of oxygen flow rates on anesthetic concentration within the breathing circuit, changes in anesthetic depth, patient safety, and waste gas production.
- List oxygen flow rates for each common domestic species, breathing system, and period of an anesthetic event.
- Explain the advantages and disadvantages of closed and semiclosed rebreathing systems.
- Explain the procedure that should be followed to prepare an anesthetic machine for use.
- Describe the proper maintenance procedures for anesthetic machines and associated equipment.

## KEY TERMS

Anesthetic chambers
Anesthetic mask
Anesthetic vaporizer
Asphyxiation
Atelectasis
Ayre's T-piece
Bain coaxial circuit
Breathing circuit
Breathing tubes
Carbon dioxide
  absorber canister
Closed rebreathing
  system
Common gas outlet
Compressed gas
  cylinders
Compressed gas supply
Endotracheal tube
Flow meter
Fresh gas inlet
Jackson-Rees circuit
Lack circuit
Laryngoscope
Line pressure gauge
Magill circuit
Mapleson classification
  system
Non-rebreathing
  system
Norman mask elbow
Oxygen flush valve
Pop-off valve
Pressure manometer
Pressure-reducing valve
Rebreathing system
Reservoir bag
Respiratory minute
  volume
Scavenging system
Semiclosed rebreathing
  system
Tank pressure gauge
Tidal volume ($V_T$)
Unidirectional valves
Vaporizer-in-circuit
Vaporizer-out-of-
  circuit

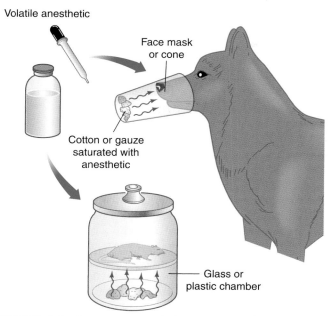

Volatile anesthetic

Face mask
or cone

Cotton or gauze
saturated with
anesthetic

Glass or
plastic chamber

**FIGURE 4-1** Open systems. With the open cone technique, a mask containing liquid anesthetic–soaked gauze is held over the patient's muzzle until the patient is anesthetized. The position of the mask in relationship to the muzzle is altered to change anesthetic depth. The open drop technique is similar, but liquid anesthetic is dripped onto a cloth held over the patient's nose and mouth. Very small patients are anesthetized by dripping liquid anesthetic onto a cloth placed inside a chamber.

Before the introduction of anesthetic machines, administration of inhalant anesthetics was a hazardous undertaking. Up until well into the twentieth century, liquid anesthetics such as ether or chloroform were administered using open systems ("open cone," "open drop," or chamber) (Figure 4-1). When these systems were used, control of anesthetic depth was crude at best and the anesthetist was not able to protect the airway, give supplemental oxygen, or assist ventilation. The development of modern anesthetic equipment greatly increased the safety and effectiveness of inhalation anesthesia by allowing the administration of precise concentrations of anesthetic and oxygen under controlled conditions. This chapter describes the purpose, function, use, and maintenance of equipment used to administer inhalant anesthetics including machines, vaporizers, breathing circuits, endotracheal tubes, masks, and chambers. As anesthetic accidents and complications are frequently associated with machine and equipment malfunctions and misuse, a comprehensive knowledge of and familiarity with this equipment is essential to the anesthetist's ability to deliver anesthetic gases safey.

## ENDOTRACHEAL TUBES AND ASSOCIATED EQUIPMENT

An **endotracheal tube** (ET tube) is a flexible tube, placed inside the trachea of an anesthetized patient, that is used to transfer anesthetic gases directly from the anesthetic machine into the patient's lungs, bypassing the oral and nasal cavities, pharynx, and larynx. ET tubes are commonly used for patients undergoing general anesthesia because they maintain an open airway; decrease anatomic dead space; allow precise administration of inhalant anesthetics and oxygen; prevent pulmonary aspiration of stomach contents, blood, and other material; enable rapid response to respiratory emergencies; and allow the anesthetist to accurately monitor and control patient respirations. Because of these benefits, many veterinarians use ET tubes for most or all patients, even if they are not receiving inhalant anesthetics.

ET tubes are available in several different types and materials and in a wide variety of diameters and lengths. Although the tubes are similar in basic design, this variety in size and type gives the anesthetist the ability to choose a tube uniquely suited to the needs of any particular patient.

There are two basic types of ET tubes. Murphy tubes (Figure 4-2, *A, C, D,* and *E*) have a beveled end and a side hole called the *Murphy eye* and may or may not have a cuff (a balloon-like structure on the patient end of the tube). Cole tubes (Figure 4-2, *B*) have no cuff or side hole but are designed with an abrupt decrease in diameter near the patient end of the tube. Cole tubes are used for species that have complete tracheal rings such as birds and some reptiles to prevent damage to the trachea that would be caused by a cuffed tube. A seal is created by seating the neck of the tube (the point of transition between the larger- and the smaller-diameter portions of the tube) at the tracheal opening.

ET tubes are made of polyvinyl chloride (PVC), red rubber, or silicone. PVC tubes (Figure 4-2, *C* and *E*) are transparent and are somewhat stiffer than other types. This stiffness minimizes the risk of tube collapse but increases the risk of trauma to tracheal mucosa during tube placement, when turning the patient, and during patient transfer. Red rubber tubes (Figure 4-2, *D*) are more flexible and less traumatic but have several disadvantages. They are more prone to kinking or collapsing, especially if small. They may absorb disinfectant solutions, resulting in irritation from contact with the patient's oropharynx or trachea, and tend to dry and crack after prolonged use. Specialized rubber tubes, called *spiral* or *anode tubes,* contain a coil of metal or nylon embedded in the rubber designed to resist kinking or collapse from external pressure. Silicone tubes (Figure 4-2, *A*), although more expensive, combine strength with pliability and are consequently resistant to collapse and less irritating to tissues than either rubber or vinyl tubes.

ET tubes come in standard lengths. On most, with the exception of very small tubes, a scale printed on the side (Figure 4-3, *F*) marks the distance from the patient end in centimeters. Before the tube is placed, this scale can be used to estimate the appropriate distance to advance the tube.

Tube size is most commonly expressed as the internal diameter (ID) in millimeters. The ID of each tube is

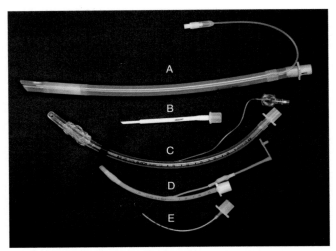

**FIGURE 4-2** Endotracheal tube type, material, and size comparison. *A*, Cuffed 11-mm, silicone rubber Murphy tube. *B*, 2.5-mm Cole tube. *C*, Cuffed 8-mm polyvinyl chloride (PVC) Murphy tube. *D*, Cuffed 4-mm red rubber Murphy tube. *E*, Uncuffed 2 mm PVC Murphy tube.

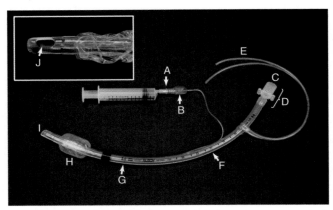

**FIGURE 4-3** Endotracheal tube parts. *A*, Valve with syringe attached. *B*, Pilot balloon. *C*, Machine end. *D*, Connector. *E*, Tie. *F*, Measurement of length from the patient end (cm). *G*, Measurement of internal diameter (mm). *H*, Inflated cuff. *I*, Patient end. *J*, Murphy eye.

written on its surface (Figure 4-3, *G*). ET tubes range in size from as small as 1 mm for exotic animals to 30 mm for mature large domestic animals. (See chapters 8, 9, and, 10 for common sizes used in the common domestic species).

### Endotracheal Tube Parts

The patient end of the tube (Figure 4-3, *I*) is passed through the mouth or nose and into the trachea. The Murphy eye (Figure 4-3, *J*), if present, minimizes the risk of patient **asphyxiation** in the event that the end hole is blocked with mucous. The machine end (Figure 4-3, *C*) protrudes from the mouth or nose and is connected to the breathing circuit of the anesthetic machine via the connector (Figure 4-3, *D*). If present, the cuff (Figure 4-3, *H*) is inflated to create a seal between the tube and trachea. The cuff is connected via a small tube to a pilot balloon (Figure 4-3, *B*)

and a valve (Figure 4-3, *A*) that is used to inflate the cuff. The valve opens to permit air to enter or exit the cuff when a syringe is seated firmly into the valve opening, and automatically closes when the syringe is removed. The pilot balloon allows the anesthetist to monitor cuff inflation visually or manually.

During intubation of mammals, use of a cuffed tube is strongly recommended for the following reasons:

1. The inflated cuff helps prevent leakage of air and gases around the tube and therefore reduces waste gas pollution in the operating room.
2. Use of a cuffed tube minimizes the risk of aspiration of blood, saliva, vomitus, and other material into the lungs.
3. Cuffed tubes prevent the animal from breathing room air, which may otherwise flow around the outside of the tube and dilute anesthetic gases. Adequate depth of anesthesia is difficult to maintain in animals breathing significant amounts of room air.

Despite these advantages, cuffed tubes should be used with caution, especially in small patients. The cuff of the tube may exert significant pressure on the tracheal mucosa and cause local inflammation or necrosis, particularly during long procedures, and in extreme cases can even cause tracheal rupture. Tubes without a cuff or with the cuff not inflated are often used in very small patients to minimize the risk of tracheal damage.

The placement and management of ET tubes is reviewed in detail in Chapters 8, 9, and 10; however, the following points should be noted:

- ET tubes should not bind during placement. Some materials, such as silicon, are naturally slippery, whereas others may require lubrication with water, patient saliva, or commercial water-soluble lubricant.
- When correctly used, ET tubes reduce dead space (see Chapter 8, p. 245). For this to be achieved, the ET tube should be no longer than the distance between the most rostral aspect of the mouth and the thoracic inlet. If longer, there are two possible risks. First, if the tube extends an excessive distance inside the trachea, the patient end may enter one main stem bronchus. Only one lung will be infused with oxygen and anesthetic gas, leading to hypoventilation, hypoxemia, and possibly difficulty keeping the patient anesthetized. Second, if the tube extends beyond the rostral aspect of the mouth, it will increase mechanical dead space, resulting in hypoventilation, especially in small patients. A guideline is that if the tube is more than 2.5 cm longer than the distance between the most rostral aspect of the mouth and the thoracic inlet, it is too long and should be cut shorter or replaced with a shorter tube.
- Special cautions must be observed when ET tubes are used in conjunction with laser surgery. Lasers create intense heat; in a high-oxygen environment such as the trachea, there is a risk of fire, and the ET tube

may ignite. The anesthetist should use special laser-resistant tubes or adapt regular tubes by wrapping them with U.S. Food and Drug Administration (FDA)–approved materials. It may also be advisable to shield the tube with saline-soaked sponges and fill the cuff with saline instead of air.

> *TECHNICIAN NOTE*    The ET tube should be no longer than the distance between the most rostral aspect of the mouth and the thoracic inlet. If longer, there is a risk that only one lung will be infused with oxygen and anesthetic gas or that mechanical dead space will be increased, leading to hypoxemia.

## Laryngoscopes

A **laryngoscope** is a device used to increase visibility of the larynx while placing an ET tube. Laryngoscopes have a handle, a blade, and a light source. The handle contains batteries to power the light source, the blade is used to depress the tongue and epiglottis, and the light source illuminates the throat (Figure 4-4). Small animal blades are available in many sizes ranging from 0 (small) to 5 (large). Custom large animal blades up to 18 inches in length are available for use in swine, small ruminants, camelids, and some exotics. Miller blades are straight (Figure 4-4, *A* and *C*), and McIntosh blades are curved (Figure 4-4, *B* and *D*). Laryngoscopes are often used in small ruminants, camelids, and swine and may be helpful in dogs and cats. They are not generally used in adult cattle, which are intubated by digital palpation, and horses, which are intubated blindly.

## MASKS

**Anesthetic masks** are cone-shaped devices used to administer oxygen and anesthetic gases to nonintubated patients via the nose and mouth (Figure 4-5). Masks may be used for both anesthetic induction and maintenance and are often used exclusively to administer anesthetic gases to very small patients, such as birds, rats, mice, and other laboratory and exotic species, in which intubation is difficult. They may also be used to administer pure oxygen to dyspneic, hypoxic, or other critically ill patients requiring supplemental oxygen.

Masks are usually made of plastic or rubber and come in a variety of diameters and lengths. They have a rubber gasket over the open end, designed to create a seal around the patient's muzzle.

Masks allow the anesthetist to rapidly administer oxygen to a fully conscious patient, sedated patient, or anesthetized patient that cannot be intubated or in which tube placement is delayed. Masks have several disadvantages, however. They do not maintain an open airway as ET tubes do, so airway obstruction is possible, particularly in brachycephalic breed animals and other patients prone to obstruction. There is no protection against pulmonary aspiration as there is with a

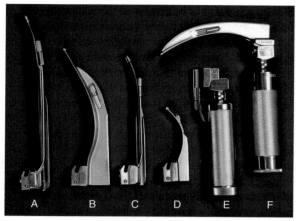

**FIGURE 4-4**  Laryngoscope handles and blades. *A,* Size 4 Miller blade. *B,* Size 4 McIntosh blade. *C,* Size 2 Miller blade. *D,* Size 1 McIntosh blade. *E,* Laryngoscope handle with size 00 Miller blade in unlocked position. *F,* Laryngoscope handle with size 3 McIntosh blade in locked position (note that the light turns on when the blade is locked).

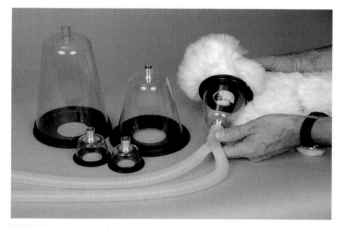

**FIGURE 4-5**  Anesthetic masks. Note the good fit around the patient's muzzle to minimize leakage.

tube, nor is the anesthetist able to ventilate the patient when necessary. The technique for mask induction is described and illustrated in Procedure 8-4.

## ANESTHETIC CHAMBERS

**Anesthetic chambers** are clear, aquarium-like boxes used to induce general anesthesia in small patients that are feral, vicious, or intractable or cannot be handled without undue stress (Figure 4-6).

They are often made of acrylic or Perspex, and have a removable top with two ports, one of which serves as a fresh gas source and the other which allows exit of waste gas.

Chambers are very useful for any patient that would be a danger to the anesthetist or itself if physically restrained. They prevent close monitoring of the patient, however, thus necessitating extreme care when patients are anesthetized using this method. The technique for chamber induction is described in Procedure 8-5.

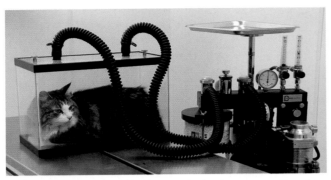

**FIGURE 4-6** Anesthetic chamber attached to the corrugated breathing tubes of a semiclosed rebreathing circuit in place of the Y-piece.

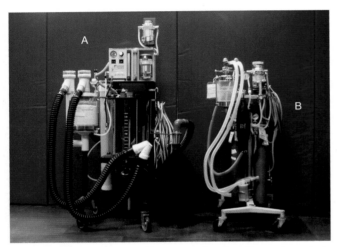

**FIGURE 4-7** Comparison of large animal and small animal anesthetic machines. *A,* Large animal machine with precision isoflurane and sevoflurane vaporizers, a built-in ventilator, and a 30-L rebreathing bag. *B,* Small animal machine with an isoflurane precision vaporizer and a 5-L rebreathing bag. This picture illustrates differences in size and sophistication among anesthetic machines.

## ANESTHETIC MACHINES

The primary function of any anesthetic machine is to deliver precise amounts of oxygen and volatile anesthetic under controlled conditions to patients undergoing general anesthesia. Over the course of a career, the veterinary technician will likely encounter a wide variety of machines in terms of brand, age, size, and sophistication (Figure 4-7). For example, machines in common use may be new or more than 30 years old. New anesthetic machines can cost from $2000 to $5000 for a basic model to more than $100,000 for a machine with state-of-the-art features such as built-in monitors and multiple vaporizers. Despite this diversity, all machines have the same basic design, which has changed surprisingly little over the past several decades, and principles of operation, which are universal. Underlying these similarities, however, is an inherent complexity, which may result in anesthetic accidents if not thoroughly understood. So the technician must devote much study and practice to

achieve the mastery required to use an anesthetic machine safely.

The basic principle of operation of any anesthetic machine can be described as follows: A liquid anesthetic (such as isoflurane or sevoflurane) is vaporized in a carrier gas (oxygen with or without nitrous oxide), which delivers the anesthetic to the patient via a breathing circuit. To achieve this result, the anesthetic machine and breathing circuit must perform several important functions:

- The carrier gases must be delivered at a controlled flow rate. Oxygen ($O_2$) is the primary carrier gas used in all anesthetic machines. Nitrous oxide ($N_2O$) is another carrier gas that was often used with oxygen to deliver older inhalant anesthetics, although it is seldom used with anesthetics in current use.
- A precise concentration of liquid inhalant anesthetic (most commonly isoflurane or sevoflurane) must be vaporized, mixed with the carrier gases, and delivered to the patient.
- Exhaled gases containing carbon dioxide ($CO_2$) must be moved away from the patient and either removed through a scavenging system or recirculated to the patient. If the gases are recirculated, the machine must remove the $CO_2$ before returning them to the patient.

Anesthetic machines are used not only for inhalation anesthesia but also as a means of delivering oxygen to critically ill patients. In these situations the vaporizer (i.e., the anesthetic source) is turned off, and the breathing circuit is used to deliver oxygen directly to the patient via an ET tube or a mask held over the patient's muzzle.

## COMPONENTS OF THE ANESTHETIC MACHINE

The anesthetic machine consists of four distinct systems that can best be understood by following the flow of gases from the oxygen source to the vaporizer, through the breathing circuit to the patient, and finally to the scavenging system (Figures 4-8 and 4-9).

- The **compressed gas supply** supplies carrier gases (oxygen and sometimes nitrous oxide) (Figure 4-10, *A*).
- The **anesthetic vaporizer** vaporizes liquid inhalant anesthetic and mixes it with the carrier gases. Vaporizers are classified as precision or nonprecision, and **vaporizer-out-of-circuit** (VOC) or **vaporizer-in-circuit** (VIC) (Figure 4-10, *B*).
- The **breathing circuit** conveys the carrier gases and inhalant anesthetic to the patient and removes exhaled carbon dioxide. Breathing circuits are classified as rebreathing circuits or non-rebreathing circuits (Figure 4-10, *C*).
- The **scavenging system** disposes of excess and waste anesthetic gases (Figure 4-11).

The parts of each system are listed in Box 4-1.

Anesthetic machines can be configured in several ways. They may have either a precision or a nonprecision vaporizer and may be fitted with a rebreathing or non-rebreathing circuit. The most common machine configuration, used for all but the smallest patients, is one with a precision vaporizer and a rebreathing circuit (Figure 4-10). A machine configured with a precision vaporizer and non-rebreathing circuit is used for patients under 2.5 to 3 kg and may be used for patients up to 7 kg in body weight (Figure 4-12).

## Compressed Gas Supply

Oxygen is necessary to sustain normal cellular metabolism and must be continuously supplied to every patient throughout anesthesia. Room air has an oxygen concentration of about 21%. In a healthy, conscious patient breathing room air with 21% oxygen, the approximate concentration in the alveolus is 13%, in arterial blood 12%, in capillary blood at tissue level 5%, and in the tissues only 2%.

Anesthetized patients breathing room air often have lower tissue oxygen concentrations because most anesthetics decrease both the respiratory rate and **tidal volume** ($V_T$). Consequently the total volume of inspired oxygen is lower. It is therefore desirable to increase the concentration of oxygen in inspired air to at least 30% to compensate for this decrease. Anesthetic machines are designed to provide up to 100% oxygen, thus fulfilling this requirement.

**BOX 4-1 Parts of Anesthetic Machine Systems**

A. Compressed gas supply
- Compressed gas cylinders
- Tank pressure gauge
- Pressure-reducing valve
- Line-pressure gauge
- Flow meter(s)
- Oxygen flush valve

B. Anesthetic vaporizer
- Vaporizer inlet port
- Vaporizer outlet port and common gas outlet

C. Breathing circuit—rebreathing (R) or non-rebreathing (N-R)
- Fresh gas inlet (R and N-R)
- Unidirectional valves (R only)
- Pop-off valve (R and N-R)
- Reservoir bag (R and N-R)
- Carbon dioxide absorber canister (R only)
- Pressure manometer (R only)
- Air intake valve (R only)
- Breathing tubes (R only)
- Y-piece (R only)

D. Scavenging system
- Discharge hose (passive or active system)
- Pressure regulator (active system)
- Outflow pipe (passive or active system)
- Pump (active system)

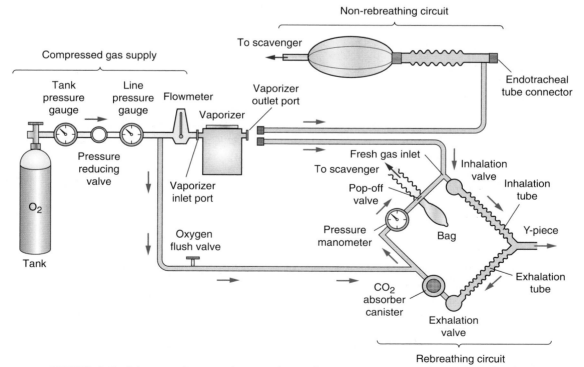

**FIGURE 4-8** Schematic of an anesthetic machine without a common gas outlet, configured with a vaporizer-out-of-circuit (VOC) precision vaporizer. Both rebreathing and non-rebreathing circuits are illustrated.

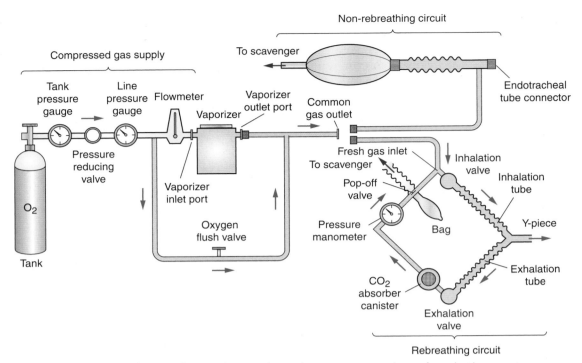

**FIGURE 4-9**  Schematic of an anesthetic machine with a common gas outlet, configured with a vaporizer-out-of-circuit (VOC) precision vaporizer. Both rebreathing and non-rebreathing circuits are illustrated.

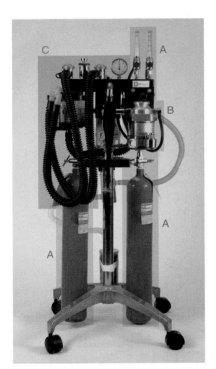

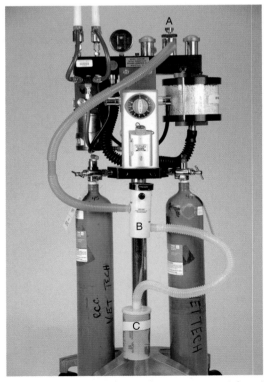

**FIGURE 4-10**  Anesthetic machine systems. *A,* Compressed gas supply: Note the two size E compressed gas oxygen cylinders beside the *A*'s at the bottom of this image. *B,* Precision anesthetic vaporizer. *C,* Breathing circuit. Note that the scavenging system (see Figure 4-11) is not visible in this view.

**FIGURE 4-11**  Scavenging system. The waste gas exits from the pop-off valve *(A)* of this rebreathing system (or the discharge hose of a non-rebreathing system), flows through the vacuum regulator *(B),* and finally flows either into a charcoal canister *(C)* or alternatively into an outlet pipe in the ceiling or wall.

Note that oxygen has a second function. Not only does it meet metabolic requirements, but it also passes through the vaporizer and carries vaporized anesthetic to the patient. Therefore no anesthetic is delivered to the patient unless oxygen is present to act as a carrier gas.

## Compressed Gas Cylinders

### Description and Function

**Compressed gas cylinders** (also called "tanks") contain a large volume of carrier gas in a highly pressurized state (as much as 2200 psi or 15,000 kilopascals [kPa]). This enables large amounts of gas to be stored in a space small enough to be of practical use. Oxygen, nitrous oxide, and medical air are three gases used for anesthesia that are stored in compressed gas cylinders. Nitrous oxide is a carrier gas that, although used in the past in conjunction with older inhalant anesthetics, is seldom used in the current practice of anesthesia. Although medical air is not commonly used in veterinary anesthesia, it is mixed with oxygen in human patients to provide an optimal concentration. Therefore when using a machine originally manufactured for human use, a medical air flow meter, yoke, and/or quick-release connector may be present. In contrast to nitrous oxide and medical air, oxygen is used for all anesthetic procedures involving inhalant anesthetics and therefore will be the focus of the discussion that follows.

Compressed gas cylinders may be either small (E tanks) (Figure 4-13, *B*) or large (H tanks) (Figure 4-13, *A*). E tanks are attached directly to the yoke of an anesthetic machine or may be stored on a cart when not in use (Figure 4-14). H tanks, which are considerably larger than E tanks,

are usually stored on a cart or chained to the wall and attached to a machine remotely by a system of intermediate-pressure gas lines that carry gas to quick-release connectors throughout the hospital (Figure 4-15). Gas lines may take the form of flexible hose, or gas may be carried in pipes mounted within the ceiling or wall. Quick-release connectors join the gas line from the compressed supply to the machine (Figure 4-16). In many hospitals, H tanks are the primary source of oxygen and E tanks are used as a

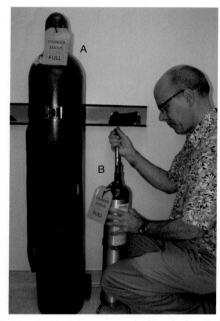

**FIGURE 4-13** *A,* Size H compressed gas cylinder. *B,* Size E compressed gas cylinder.

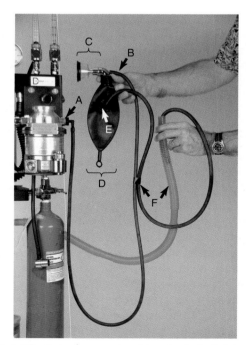

**FIGURE 4-12** Parts of a non-rebreathing circuit. *A,* Outlet port of the vaporizer with keyed fitting. *B,* Fresh gas inlet. *C,* Connector with mask attached. *D,* Reservoir bag. *E,* Pressure relief valve. *F,* Scavenging hose.

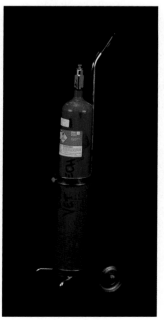

**FIGURE 4-14** E tank in a cart, which is used to store or transport the tank safely.

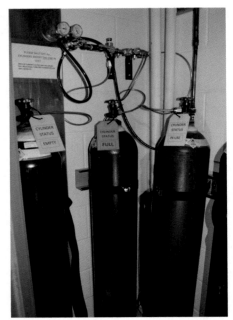

**FIGURE 4-15**    Bank of H tanks used as a primary oxygen supply for the entire hospital via intermediate-pressure gas lines hidden in the ceiling.

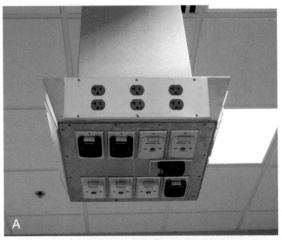

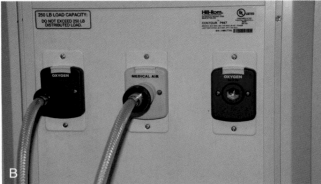

**FIGURE 4-16**    **A,** Ceiling drop with diameter-index safety system (DISS) outlets for oxygen (green), nitrous oxide (blue), medical air (yellow), and vacuum (white). **B,** Quick-release DISS connectors used to couple intermediate-pressure gas lines to the anesthetic machine. Note that the diameter of each outlet port type is unique to prevent attachment of the wrong connector.

backup supply. In locations where piped-in gas is unavailable, E tanks are used as both the primary and the secondary supplies.

The capacities of cylinders are given in Table 4-1. Cylinders often are owned by the company that supplies the oxygen but may be purchased by the user. In either case, empty cylinders are periodically picked up by the oxygen supplier, refilled, and returned to the user.

All compressed gas cylinders have a valve on the top to control the flow of gas. The valve on an H tank has a threaded outlet port through which the gas flows (Figure 4-17). In contrast, the valve on an E tank has three holes—one outlet port, and two pin index safety system holes (Figure 4-18). The outlet port is connected to a pressure-reducing valve (see Figures 4-17, *B* and 4-22, *C*) (directly in the case of an H tank or via the yoke in the case of an E tank), which reduces the outgoing pressure to a usable level before conveying it to the rest of the machine through intermediate-pressure gas lines.

> *TECHNICIAN NOTE*    Check both primary and secondary oxygen supplies at the beginning of the day to be sure they are turned on. A failure to do this may result in a patient not receiving oxygen, a dangerous error that if not recognized may be fatal!

### Use

It is vital that the anesthetist check both primary and secondary oxygen supplies at the beginning of the day to be sure they are turned on. A failure to do this may result in a patient not receiving oxygen, a dangerous error that, if not recognized, may be fatal. Because pressurized gas remains in the high- and intermediate-pressure lines even if the tank is turned off, a failure to turn a tank back on may easily go unnoticed unless double-checked by the technician.

Oxygen flows from the outlet port of the valve when the stem is turned in a counterclockwise direction (i.e., to the left) (see Figure 4-18, *B*). The stem should be turned slowly until it is *fully open.* H-tank valve stems often have a knurled knob (see Figure 4-17, *E*) that is turned by hand. E-tank valve stems are opened and closed with a special wrench or via a lever that can be turned by hand (Figure 4-19). The flow stops when the valve stem is turned completely clockwise until firmly closed (i.e., to the right). The mnemonic "left loose, right tight" (*loose* meaning open and *tight* meaning closed) has been used by several generations of anesthesia students as an aid in remembering the direction to turn the stem. When opening and closing these valves, you should not have to use excessive force. Difficulty in turning the valve stem may indicate a malfunction. In this case the valve should be professionally serviced before use is continued.

After use, the outlet valve of each tank should be closed. Failure to turn off the gas valve can create a danger if anyone attempts to remove the tank while it is open, or over a long period it may result in leakage of gas from the tank.

| TABLE 4-1 | Compressed Gas Cylinder Characteristics, Capacity, and Pressure | | | | | | | |
|---|---|---|---|---|---|---|---|---|
| Gas and Symbol | State within Cylinder | Cylinder Color | Pressure when Full (psi/kPa) at 21° C | Minimum Pressure at Which to Change (psi/kPa) | | Cylinder Dimensions (inches) | Empty Weight (kg) | Capacity (L) |
| Oxygen (O₂) | Gas | White (international) Green (U.S.) | 1900-2200/ 13,000-15,000 | 100-200/ 690-1380 | E | 4.25 OD; 26 High | 6.4 | 660 |
| | | | | | H | 9.25 OD; 51 High | 54 | 6900 |
| Nitrous oxide (N₂O) | Liquid and gas | Blue | 745/5140 | 500/3400 | E | 4.25 OD; 26 High | 6.4 | 1590 |
| | | | | | H | 9.25 OD; 51 High | 54 | 15,800 |

*OD*, Outside diameter.
Modified from Tranquilli WJ, Thurmon JC, Grimm KA: *Lumb and Jones' veterinary anesthesia and analgesia*, ed 4, Ames, Iowa, 2007, Blackwell.

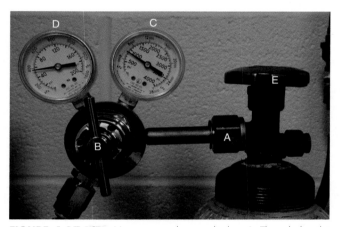

**FIGURE 4-17**  Size H compressed gas cylinder. *A*, Threaded outlet port. *B*, Pressure-reducing valve. *C*, Tank pressure gauge. *D*, Line pressure gauge. *E*, Knurled knob.

Oxygen pressure remaining in the intermediate-pressure lines after the valve is closed (called *line pressure*) should be released by depressing the oxygen flush valve or by turning the flow meter to a high rate of flow until all the gas is vented. Failure to evacuate line pressure may give the anesthetist the false impression that the oxygen is turned on when in fact it is not. (Information on removing

and replacing cylinders may be found in the section on anesthetic machine maintenance found on p. 131).

### Safety

There are four potential risks from compressed gas cylinders, as follows:

1. Both oxygen and nitrous oxide support combustion. Therefore contact with flames, sparks, and other sources of ignition must be avoided.
2. A forceful release of gas from an unprotected outlet port may tear the skin or injure an eye. To avoid this type of injury, turn the tank on *only* when it is attached to a yoke or pressure regulator. The only exception to this rule is when opening the valve to clean dust and dirt from the outlet port before attaching it to a machine or pressure regulator. In this case, turn the valve on *slowly* and only enough to expel the dirt from the port.
3. If a cylinder is dropped and the valve breaks off, the cylinder may cause serious personal injury! High-pressure gas exiting a cylinder through a broken valve will cause the cylinder to fly at high velocity in the opposite direction of the released gas, becoming in effect a "torpedo," the force of which is sufficient to penetrate concrete and injure or kill anyone in its path. Therefore these tanks must be stored *only* attached to a yoke, secured in a cart designed for this purpose, or chained to the wall. *Never drop compressed gas cylinders or leave them standing alone with no support or lying on their side.*
4. If inadvertently attached to a valve, yoke, or hose intended for a different type of gas, the wrong gas will be delivered to a patient. For example, if a nitrous oxide cylinder were attached to an oxygen yoke, the patent would receive nitrous oxide instead of oxygen, resulting in asphyxiation. To safeguard against this, all compressed gas supplies have safety systems and features designed to prevent

*TECHNICIAN NOTE*  When handling compressed gas cylinders:
- Avoid contact with flames, sparks, or other sources of ignition.
- Turn the tank on *only* when it is attached to a yoke or pressure regulator.
- Store tanks *only* attached to a yoke, secured in a cart designed for this purpose, or chained to the wall.
- Never attempt to attach a tank to a yoke that does not fit, and never tamper with the safety system on a tank, line, or pressure-reducing valve.

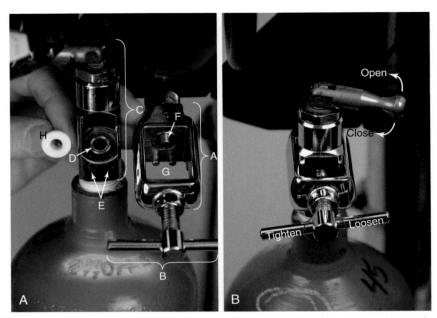

**FIGURE 4-18    A,** Parts of a size E compressed gas cylinder and yoke. *A,* Yoke. *B,* Wing nut. *C,* Outlet valve. *D,* Outlet port. *E,* Pin–index safety system holes. *F,* Nipple of yoke. *G,* Index pins. *H,* Nylon washer. **B,** Opening and closing the outlet valve; loosening and tightening the wing nut.

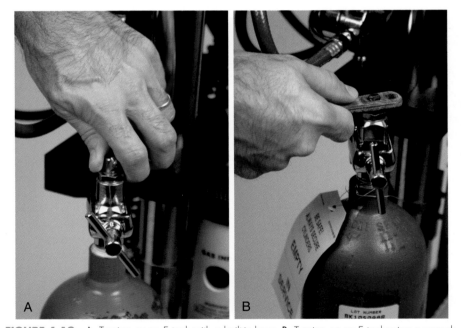

**FIGURE 4-19    A,** Turning on an E tank with a built-in lever. **B,** Turning on an E tank using a wrench.

the wrong type of gas cylinder from being attached to the machine connections. First, all cylinders, flow meters, pressure-reducing valves, gas lines, and quick-release connectors are color-coded to prevent inadvertent use of an incorrect gas. Oxygen cylinders are green (United States) or white (Canada, Europe), nitrous oxide cylinders are blue, and medical air cylinders are yellow (United States) or white and black (Canada, Europe) (see Table 4-1). Carbon dioxide is designated by the color gray. Although not used for anesthesia, carbon dioxide is used as a euthanasia agent for specific applications such as meat packing plants and research facilities.

E-tank yokes are equipped with a pin-index safety system, which, unless tampered with, physically prevents the wrong gas from being connected to the yoke. For example, an oxygen cylinder cannot be put on a nitrous oxide yoke (Figure 4-20). H-tank pressure-reducing valves are threaded to accept only one gas. Quick-release connectors are protected with a diameter-index safety system (DISS). In this system, the diameter of the male and female parts of the connector is specific to one gas (see Figure 4-16).

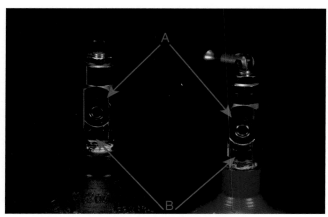

**FIGURE 4-20** *A,* Outlet port. *B,* Pin-index safety system holes. Note that the pin holes on the carbon dioxide tank *(left)* are farther apart than the pin holes on the oxygen tank *(right).* The unique pin hole position for each gas prevents a tank containing the wrong gas from being attached to the yoke.

Attempting to defeat a safety system by removing the pins on a pin-index safety system of an E tank, stacking several washers in a yoke of a machine, or using a thread converter on an H tank will create a life-threatening situation. Never attempt to attach a tank that does not fit or to tamper with the safety system on a tank, line, or pressure-reducing valve.

### Alternate Oxygen Sources

The technician may encounter some situations in which the primary oxygen supply is a bulk tank of liquid oxygen or an oxygen concentrator instead of compressed gas cylinders. This situation is likely to be encountered only in large hospitals.

A bulk tank contains a large quantity of oxygen in liquid form (Figure 4-21). An oxygen concentrator is a device that extracts oxygen from room air, concentrates it, and pressurizes it for medical use. As with any other primary supply, the technician must be sure that a secondary supply is available in the event of a failure of the primary source.

### Tank Pressure Gauge

#### Description and Function

A **tank pressure gauge** is a device attached to the yoke of a machine, or the pressure regulator of an H tank, that indicates the pressure of gas remaining in a compressed gas cylinder measured in pounds per square inch (psi) in the United States or kilopascals in Europe and Canada (Figure 4-22, *B* and Figure 4-17, *C*). See Appendix E for a conversion formula from pounds per square inch to kilopascals.

#### Use

When the tank valve is opened, the gauge indicates the gas pressure inside the tank. This gauge must be checked before commencement of any procedure to ensure that enough gas remains in the tank to safely complete it. The pressure in a full oxygen tank is about 2200 psi (about

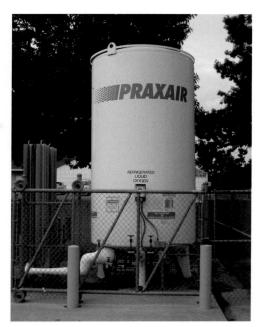

**FIGURE 4-21** A bulk oxygen tank. Used in some large hospitals as a primary oxygen source in place of compressed gas cylinders.

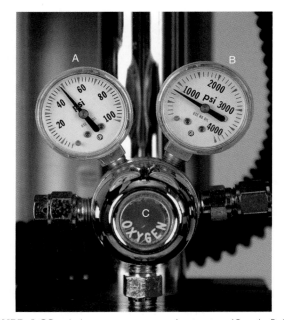

**FIGURE 4-22** *A,* Line pressure gauge (registering 48 psi). *B,* Tank pressure gauge (registering 800 psi). *C,* Pressure-reducing valve.

15,000 kPa). (Note that the pressures in a nitrous oxide tank are different and are discussed in Appendix B). As gas is used, the pressure in the tank will gradually fall, reaching zero when the tank is empty. The gauge also reads zero if the tank is not empty but is turned off and the remaining gas in the intermediate-pressure line has been evacuated (i.e., "bled off") (see p. 108 for a description of this procedure). This gauge functions passively and therefore requires no action on the part of the anesthetist.

> 📎 *TECHNICIAN NOTE*    The volume in liters (L) of oxygen present in a compressed gas cylinder can be calculated by multiplying the pressure (in psi) in an E tank by 0.3 or by multiplying the pressure in an H tank by 3.

The volume in liters (L) of oxygen present in an E tank can be calculated by multiplying the pressure (in psi) by 0.3 (see Table 4-1). For example, a full E tank, at a pressure of 2200 psi, contains about 660 L of oxygen (i.e., 0.3 × 2200 psi). A reading of 1100 psi indicates the tank is approximately half full and therefore contains approximately 330 L of oxygen. The volume in liters for the larger H tank can be calculated by multiplying the pressure (in psi) by 3. For example, a full H tank at a pressure of 2200 psi contains approximately 6600 L of oxygen (i.e., 3 × 2200 psi).

The volume of the oxygen in the tank indicates how much longer the tank can be used. For example, if the anesthetist selects an oxygen flow rate of 1 L per minute (L/min), a full E tank containing 660 L of oxygen will last approximately 11 hours (i.e., 660 minutes), whereas at a flow rate of 2 L/min the same full tank will last approximately 5.5 hours (i.e., 330 minutes). In contrast, a full H tank at a flow rate of 1 L/min contains enough oxygen to last 110 hours (6600 minutes).

Tanks should be marked "full," "in service," or "empty" to indicate their status (Figure 4-23), and a full backup tank must always be kept on the machine as a spare in case the primary tank runs out. The anesthetist may notice a considerable drop in pressure during a lengthy anesthetic procedure. If not detected in time, oxygen flow to the patient will cease, and this will put the patient in danger because veterinary anesthetic machines have no alarm to warn of inadequate flow. Therefore the anesthetist must periodically monitor the oxygen tank pressure gauge during each procedure and change the tank when the gauge indicates that the tank is close to empty. As an example, an E tank with 600 psi should give the anesthetist enough gas to last at least 1 hour, assuming that an oxygen flow of no more than 3 L/min is used and the oxygen flush valve is not activated frequently. In any case, a tank should be changed when the pressure drops below 500 psi (about 3400 kPa), indicating only 150 L of oxygen remaining in the tank.

### Pressure-Reducing Valve (Pressure Regulator)

#### Description and Function
Immediately after exiting the tank, the gas flows through a **pressure-reducing valve** (see Figures 4-17, *B* and 4-22, *C*), which is located near the tank pressure gauge, and then into an intermediate gas line. The pressure-reducing valve reduces the pressure of the gas to a constant safe operating pressure of 40 to 50 psi (about 275 to 345 kPa) regardless of the pressure changes within the tank. Pressure-reducing valves all

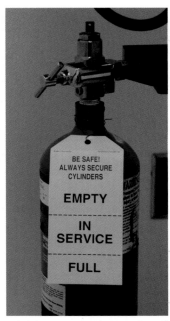

**FIGURE 4-23**   Label for compressed gas tanks. Current status of tank is shown by the wording at the bottom of the label. Label shown is from newly acquired tank and reads "FULL." When the tank is first opened, the lower portion of the label is removed so that the remaining label reads "IN SERVICE." When the tank is empty, the "IN SERVICE" stub is removed, leaving the label that reads "EMPTY."

look slightly different but are usually round and have a color-coded insignia on the outside to identify the gas flowing through them.

#### Use
The pressure-reducing valve functions passively and therefore requires no action on the part of the anesthetist. The line pressure gauge (if present) should be checked before every procedure, however, to verify correct pressure in the intermediate pressure gas lines (40 to 50 psi).

### Line Pressure Gauge

#### Description and Function
The **line pressure gauge** indicates the pressure in the intermediate-pressure gas line between the pressure-reducing valve and the flow meters (see Figures 4-17, *D* and 4-22, *A*). It is not present on all machines, but when present is immediately downstream from the pressure-reducing valve.

#### Use
Like the tank pressure gauge and pressure-reducing valve, this gauge functions passively and so requires no action on the part of the anesthetist. When the oxygen is turned on, this gauge should read 40 to 50 psi. A pressure higher or lower than this indicates a malfunction of or a need to adjust the pressure-reducing valve. After the oxygen tank has been turned off, the line pressure gauge will continue to register line pressure until it is evacuated or "bled

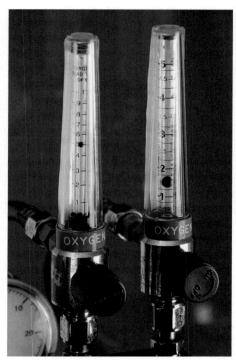

**FIGURE 4-24**   Oxygen flow meters with ball indicators. The flow meter on the left is adjusted to 0.5 L/min, and the flow meter on the right is adjusted to 1.5 L/min for a total oxygen flow of 2 L/min.

off." This is accomplished by depressing the **oxygen flush valve** until the gauge reads 0 psi.

## Flow Meter

### Description and Function

After leaving the pressure-reducing valve, the carrier gas flows through an intermediate-pressure gas line into the **flow meter.** A flow meter is a vertical glass cylinder of graduated diameter with a valve attached to the bottom. When the valve knob is turned, gas enters the cylinder at the bottom and exits at the top. An indicator within the cylinder rises to indicate the gas flow expressed in liters of gas per minute (L/min) (Figure 4-24).

The flow meter also further reduces the pressure of the gas in the intermediate-pressure line from about 50 psi (about 345 kPa) to 15 psi (about 100 kPa). This pressure is only slightly above atmospheric pressure (about 14.7 psi) and is the optimum pressure for entry into the breathing circuit and ultimately the patient's lungs.

If a machine is set up to use both nitrous oxide and oxygen, there will be separate flow meters so that the flow rates of the two gases can be monitored and adjusted separately (Figure 4-25). To prevent the controls for oxygen and nitrous oxide from being confused, they are touch and profile coded (feel and look different), are color coded (green or white for oxygen, blue for nitrous oxide), and are labeled according to the gas they regulate. Some machines provide two flow meters for oxygen: one for flow rates greater than 1 L/min (coarse adjustment) and one to accurately adjust flow rates less than 1 L/min (fine adjustment).

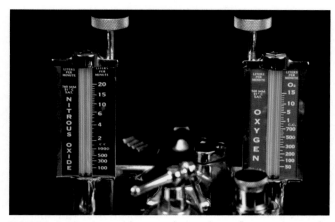

**FIGURE 4-25**   An anesthetic machine with two flow meters, one for nitrous oxide and one for oxygen.

### Use

The flow meter is opened by turning the valve knob to the left, and the flow is then adjusted to the appropriate level for the patient (see p. 126 for a discussion of oxygen flow rates). All flow meters have a ball or rotor indicator that rises to a height proportional to the flow of gas. The scale on the cylinder indicates the gas flow. The meter is read at the center of a ball indicator or the top of a rotor indicator.

Flow meters must be treated gently when turning them off. The valve stem inside the flow meter is delicate and can be damaged by rough handling. Therefore when turning off a flow meter, turn clockwise just until the ball or rotor drops to 0 L/min. Even though the knob can still be turned, do *not* turn it any further to the right. Failure to turn off the flow meter may result in a sudden rush of air into the meter when the oxygen tank is opened, which may jam the rotor or ball at the top of the tube.

*TECHNICIAN NOTE*   When turning off a flow meter, turn clockwise just until the ball or rotor drops to 0 L/min. Even though the knob can still be turned, do *not* turn it any further to the right or you will damage the valve!

### Safety

The flow meter must be turned on if the patient is to receive oxygen. Therefore, a tank pressure gauge or line pressure gauge that registers oxygen pressure does not ensure that the patient is receiving oxygen unless the flow meter is also on.

## Oxygen Flush Valve

### Description and Function

The oxygen flush valve is a button or lever that when activated rapidly delivers a large volume of pure oxygen at a flow rate of 35 to 75 L/min directly from the line exiting the pressure-reducing valve into the common gas outlet or into the breathing circuit of a rebreathing system, bypassing the anesthetic vaporizer and oxygen flow meters. This feature is used to rapidly fill a depleted reservoir bag. It is also used to deliver oxygen to a critically ill patient or at the end of the anesthetic period, to dilute out the anesthetic gas remaining in the circuit (see Figure 4-27, *F*).

### Use

When activating the flush valve, press it briefly, using short bursts while watching the reservoir bag and **pressure manometer** to ensure that the bag does not overfill and the pressure in the circuit does not exceed 2 cm $H_2O$. This will prevent pressurization of the breathing circuit, which could damage the patient's lungs.

When using the oxygen flush valve to fill a collapsed reservoir bag, remember that the gas flowing into the breathing circuit from the valve will contain no inhalant anesthetic. Thus the gas delivered by this valve will dilute the concentration of inhalant anesthetic in the breathing circuit and the patient's lungs.

When using it to deliver fresh oxygen to a critically ill patient or to flush inhalant anesthetic out of the circuit during anesthetic recovery or during a crisis, first turn off the vaporizer. Next force the gases out of the rebreathing bag and into the scavenging system using gentle hand pressure. Finally, press the valve to refill the bag with fresh oxygen.

### Safety

As previously mentioned, the oxygen flush valve should be pressed briefly using only short bursts. Overfilling the bag has the potential of damaging the patient's lungs because of a buildup of pressure. Some anesthetic machines are configured such that the oxygen flush valve discharges into the common gas outlet instead of the rebreathing circuit. In these cases the oxygen flush valve must not be used with a **non-rebreathing system** attached because a high flow rate of oxygen into this type of circuit can seriously damage the animal's lungs.

## Anesthetic Vaporizer
### Description and Function

After exiting the flow meter, oxygen enters the vaporizer through the inlet port (see Figure 4-27, *A*). The function of the vaporizer is to convert a liquid anesthetic such as isoflurane or sevoflurane to a gaseous state and to add controlled amounts of this vaporized anesthetic to the carrier gases ($O_2$ and $N_2O$ if used). After exiting the vaporizer through the outlet port, the oxygen and anesthetic mixture (known as *fresh gas*) enters the breathing circuit through a connection referred to as the *fresh gas inlet*. Most vaporizers are designed for use with only one specific anesthetic agent, which is purchased in liquid form and poured into the vaporizer.

The vaporized anesthetic can exit the vaporizer only by traveling in carrier gas, which transports it from the vaporizer into the breathing circuit. In other words, no anesthetic is delivered to the patient if the flow meter

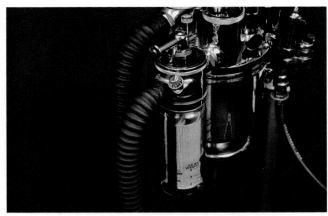

**FIGURE 4-26** Nonprecision vaporizer (Ohio No. 8 vaporizer), designed for delivery of methoxyflurane.

reads zero, because there is no flow of carrier gas to deliver the anesthetic.

Most newer vaporizers are classified as *variable-bypass, flow-over*. This is because they regulate the anesthetic output by routing a portion of the carrier gas through the vaporization chamber where the liquid anesthetic is located, while the remainder of the carrier gas bypasses the vaporization chamber. The portion of the carrier gas that enters the chamber flows over the surface of the liquid anesthetic and picks up vaporized anesthetic. So the more carrier gas that is routed through the chamber, the higher the concentration of the anesthetic delivered to the patient.

### Types of Anesthetic Vaporizers

Anesthetic vaporizers are classified as either precision or nonprecision. This differentiation separates those that allow precise control of the amount of anesthetic delivered to the patient (expressed as the percent of the total gases exiting the vaporizer) from those that allow only estimation of the amount delivered. Nonprecision vaporizers (Figure 4-26) were used in the past to deliver low–vapor pressure anesthetics—such as methoxyflurane—which are no longer available.

Although nonprecision vaporizers can be used to deliver isoflurane or sevoflurane, as long as specific procedures are carefully followed, this practice is uncommon. In contrast, precision vaporizers (Figure 4-27) are used to deliver all commonly used liquid anesthetics including isoflurane, sevoflurane, and desflurane, and so are the main type the technician is likely to encounter in clinical practice. Therefore the discussion that follows refers specifically to precision vaporizers. In the event that the technician is asked to operate a nonprecision vaporizer, more information on their use can be found in Appendix C.

The commonly used liquid anesthetics (isoflurane, sevoflurane, and desflurane) are classified as high–vapor pressure liquids. The designation "high vapor pressure" means that these anesthetics readily evaporate and may reach concentrations of 30% or greater within the anesthetic circuit if the amount of vapor being delivered to the

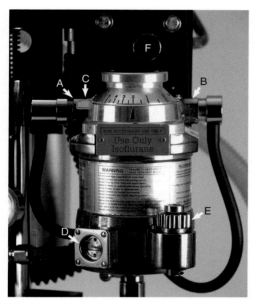

**FIGURE 4-27** *Precision anesthetic vaporizer for isoflurane set on 2%. A, Inlet port with keyed fitting leading from the flow meters. B, Outlet port with keyed fitting leading to the fresh gas inlet or common gas outlet. C, Safety lock. D, Indicator window. E, Fill port. F, Oxygen flush valve (part of the compressed gas supply).*

it. This is because patient respiratory drive during normal breathing is the force that moves gases around the breathing circuit. When resistance to gas flow is high, as is the case with precision vaporizers, respiratory drive is insufficient to push gases through the vaporizer. Consequently, precision vaporizers must be placed outside the breathing circuit. In contrast, nonprecision vaporizers offer little resistance to gas flow and therefore can safely be placed in the breathing circuit.

## Factors Affecting Vaporizer Output

The concentration of anesthetic delivered by any vaporizer depends not only on the vaporizer setting but also on a variety of other factors including temperature, carrier gas flow rate, back pressure, barometric pressure, and respiratory rate and depth. Newer precision vaporizers are compensated and deliver a precise concentration independent of each of these factors with relatively little error or variation. However, older precision vaporizers and nonprecision vaporizers such as the Ohio No. 8 or Stephens vaporizer do not automatically compensate for these factors. Regardless of the type of vaporizer the anesthetist is using, a complete knowledge of proper use requires an understanding of the potential effect of each of these factors on vaporizer output.

### Temperature

Volatile anesthetics, like all liquids, vaporize more readily at high temperatures than at low temperatures. Vaporization directly affects vaporizer output. If a vaporizer is not temperature compensated, vaporization will vary with changes in ambient (room) temperature, because room temperature affects the temperature of the anesthetic. For example, if a noncompensated vaporizer is used in a cold room, vaporization of the gas decreases and the anesthetic output is lower than that indicated on the dial. Conversely, in a warm room the output is greater than the dial setting.

The temperature of the anesthetic is also affected by carrier gas flow. This is because gas exiting a compressed gas cylinder is cold. At high carrier gas flow rates, the temperature of the liquid anesthetic falls, leading to decreased vaporization and lower anesthetic output than that indicated on the dial when a noncompensated vaporizer is used.

Most recently manufactured precision vaporizers are temperature compensated. Older models that are not temperature compensated include an internal thermometer and temperature adjustment scale that the anesthetist can use to adjust the vaporizer setting as needed to compensate for temperature changes.

### Carrier Gas Flow Rate

The amount of carrier gas that flows through the vaporization chamber (primarily controlled by the vaporizer dial setting) determines anesthetic output. In a vaporizer that is not flow compensated, flow through the chamber is also affected by the carrier gas flow rate (determined by the flow meter setting). Higher

breathing circuit is not controlled. Because the maximum useful concentration for isoflurane and sevoflurane is 5% and 8%, respectively, uncontrolled delivery of anesthetic vapor will result in excessively high levels that could be dangerous for the patient. It is therefore necessary to use a precision vaporizer to deliver these agents, affording the anesthetist more exact control of the anesthetic concentration in the circuit.

### VOC versus VIC

The abbreviations *VOC* and *VIC* are used to describe two different ways anesthetic machines are configured based on the location of the vaporizer in relation to the breathing circuit. The letters *VOC* are an abbreviation for *vaporizer-out-of-circuit* (Figure 4-28, *A*) and indicate that the vaporizer is not located within the breathing circuit. In this case, oxygen from the flow meters flows into the vaporizer before entering the breathing circuit. Precision vaporizers are positioned in a VOC configuration.

In contrast, the letters *VIC* are an abbreviation for *vaporizer-in-circuit* (Figure 4-28, *B*). In this type of machine, carrier gases enter the breathing circuit directly from the flow meter without first entering the vaporizer. Instead, the vaporizer is located in the breathing circuit most often between the expiratory breathing tube and the expiratory unidirectional valve. Exhaled gases enter the vaporizer each time the patient breathes. Nonprecision vaporizers (e.g., the Ohio No. 8 or Stephens vaporizer) are positioned this way.

The location in which the vaporizer may be placed in relationship to the breathing circuit (VOC versus VIC) is governed by the resistance to the flow of gases through

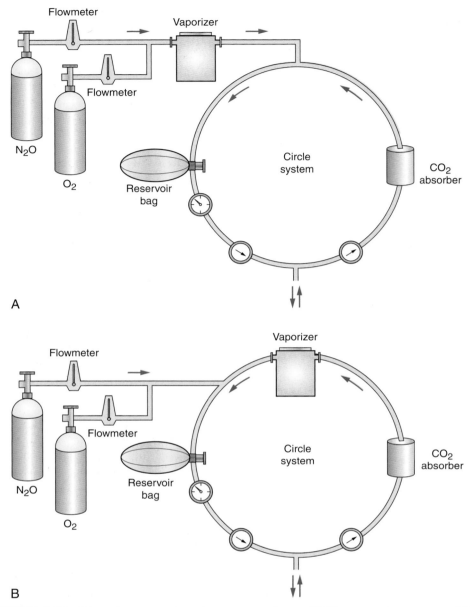

**FIGURE 4-28** Schematic representation of vaporizer-out-of-circuit (VOC) versus vaporizer-in-circuit (VIC) configurations. **A**, VOC. **B**, VIC. (From Warren RG: *Small animal anesthesia*, St Louis, 1983, Mosby.)

flow meter settings result in increased flow through the chamber, and low settings result in decreased flow through the chamber. For example, when a non–flow-compensated vaporizer is used, output is higher at a flow meter setting of 3 L/min than at a flow meter setting of 500 mL/min.

Most modern precision vaporizers compensate for carrier gas flow and will deliver the amount of anesthetic indicated on the dial over a wide range of oxygen flow rates. Even in a flow-compensated vaporizer, compensation is not unlimited, however. Flows that are very high (i.e., in excess of 10 L/min) or very low (i.e., below 250 mL/min) may affect the output of flow-compensated vaporizers. Consequently, the vaporizer setting will not

accurately reflect the concentration of anesthetic released at these extreme flow rates.

In precision vaporizers, whether compensated or non-compensated, carrier gas flow rate also influences the concentration of the anesthetic in the breathing circuit (and consequently in the air that the patient breathes). An oxygen flow rate that approaches the patient's **respiratory minute volume** (RMV) (the total amount of gas a patient inhales or exhales in 1 minute) will produce a concentration in the circuit close to the dialed setting. At a lower flow rate, although the anesthetic concentration in the carrier gas delivered to the circuit does not change, the total amount delivered to the patient is lower, because as anesthetic is absorbed in the patient's lungs and diluted

## BOX 4-2 | Time Constants

The concept of time constants helps explain why a change in the vaporizer dial setting takes time to be reflected in the circuit (and in the patient's lungs), and also gives the anesthetist a rough idea as to how long he or she can expect for a change in anesthetic concentration to occur. *The time constant (in minutes) is calculated by dividing the total volume of the breathing circuit (in L) by the carrier gas flow rate (in L/min).* When the vaporizer dial setting is changed, it takes five time constants to effect a 95% change in circuit concentration.

Consider a circuit that has a total volume of about 5 L (2 L for the reservoir bag, 1.5 L for the carbon dioxide absorber, and 1.5 L in the inspiratory and expiratory hoses). If the fresh gas flow rate is 2 L/min, the time constant is 2.5 minutes (5 L/2 L/min). In this example, if the vaporizer dial setting is changed, it will take 12.5 minutes (2.5 minutes × 5) before the anesthetic concentration in the circuit reaches 95% of the new dial setting. In contrast, if the anesthetist is using a low-flow technique (e.g., an oxygen flow rate of 200 mL or 0.2 L) with a circuit volume of 5 L, then the time constant is 25 minutes (5 L/0.2 L/min). This amounts to a total of 125 minutes (25 minutes × 5) for the anesthetic concentration in the circuit to reach 95% of the new dial setting! This explains why there is such a time lag between making a vaporizer dial change and seeing a change in the anesthetic depth if low flows are used. There are two ways to change the concentration more rapidly: turn up the fresh gas flow rate and shorten the time constant for the circuit being used, or make a big change in the vaporizer dial setting.

by expired gases, the concentration within the circuit decreases. For example, if a 20-kg dog is connected to an anesthetic machine with an oxygen flow rate of 200 mL/kg/min (in this case, 4 L/min) and a vaporizer setting of 2%, the actual concentration of anesthetic being inhaled by the animal is close to 2%. If the oxygen flow rate is reduced to 100 mL/kg/min (in this case, 2 L/min), then to 50 mL/kg/min (1 L/min), and finally to 10 mL/kg/min (200 mL/min), the percent concentration of anesthetic in the circuit may drop to 1.8%, 1.2%, and 0.8%, respectively. In each case the vaporizer is delivering a 2% concentration to the circuit, but the concentration within the circuit varies as a result of dilution and absorption. This is why precision vaporizer settings may need to be increased if low oxygen flow rates are used (Box 4-2).

### Respiratory Rate and Depth

If the anesthetist has occasion to use a VIC nonprecision vaporizer, he or she must be aware that respiratory rate and depth will also affect anesthetic delivery. This is because the respiratory rate and effort affect the flow of carrier gas through the vaporization chamber of a VIC nonprecision vaporizer. Consequently, high and low respiratory rates and depths will have the same effect on vaporizer output as high and low carrier gas flow. This is not an issue with VOC precision vaporizers because in this circumstance the patient's respiratory drive has no influence on the amount of carrier gas passing through the vaporization chamber.

### Back Pressure

*Back pressure* refers to an increase in pressure at the vaporizer outlet port caused by manual ventilation (bagging) or activation of the oxygen flush valve. A vaporizer that is not back pressure compensated will deliver more anesthetic under these circumstances. Most precision vaporizers are pressure compensated so that bagging or flush valve activation does not affect the amount of anesthetic released.

### Use

Each precision vaporizer is designed to be used with a specific inhalant anesthetic such as sevoflurane, isoflurane, halothane, or desflurane and is color-coded (purple, isoflurane; yellow, sevoflurane; red, halothane; and blue, desflurane).

The vaporizer is turned on by depressing the safety lock and turning the dial to the desired level. The safety lock is present as a lever on some vaporizers and is incorporated into the dial on others (Figure 4-29). Inhalant anesthetic levels are measured in percent concentration. For common domestic species, the induction rate of isoflurane is approximately 3% to 5%. The maintenance rate is about 1.5% to 2.5%. The induction rate of sevoflurane is approximately 4% to 6%, and the maintenance rate is about 2.5% to 4%. The induction rate of desflurane is approximately 10% to 15%. The maintenance rate is about 8% to 12%. Patients should receive rates in the lower end of these ranges if preanesthetic medications have been administered.

The dial of a precision vaporizer (see Figure 4-27) is graduated in percent concentration (e.g., 1%, 2%). Throughout any anesthetic procedure, the anesthetist must control the amount of inhalant anesthetic delivered to the patient by periodically adjusting the vaporizer dial. Appropriate and safe use of the vaporizer requires knowledge, experience, and detailed observation. Specifics regarding safe use of the vaporizer are discussed in detail in Chapters 8, 9, and 10.

Vaporizers must be checked before each procedure to make sure that enough anesthetic remains in the vaporization chamber. Most vaporizers have an indicator window at their base that allows the technician to inspect the amount of liquid anesthetic remaining. In order for the vaporizer to function properly, the liquid anesthetic level must be between the upper and lower lines of the window (Figure 4-30). The vaporizer should be refilled as needed but should be kept at least half full at all times. Overfilling a vaporizer will result in anesthetic overdose, and underfilling will result in an inability to keep the patient anesthetized.

> **TECHNICIAN NOTE** Vaporizers must be checked before each procedure to make sure the liquid anesthetic level is between the upper and lower lines of the indicator window. The vaporizer should be refilled as needed but should be kept at least half full at all times.

### Safety

Vaporizers are subject to leakage if the anesthetic machine is tipped over or shaken vigorously. Under these circumstances, liquid anesthetic enters bypass channels of the vaporizer, and a potentially lethal dose of anesthetic may be delivered to the next patient. If an anesthetic machine is tipped or shaken, the anesthetic leak can be remedied by running oxygen through the machine at the maximum flow rate (with the vaporizer dial turned off) for 15 minutes. Emptying anesthetic

> *TECHNICIAN NOTE* If a bottle of liquid inhalant anesthetic accidentally breaks, vacate the room immediately and allow the room to air out until the anesthetic is completely evaporated and evacuated from the room.

machine vaporizers before transport is the best way to avoid this problem.

Volatile anesthetics readily evaporate when exposed to air. Therefore precautions must be taken to avoid inhaling the gas. First, take care not to drop or break the bottle. When refilling the vaporizer, make sure other personnel are not in the immediate vicinity, place a scavenging hose near the bottle while it is open to evacuate evaporated gas, cap the bottle promptly when finished, and close the vaporizer fill chamber immediately after filling. A pouring nozzle designed for use with these bottles is a valuable aid in preventing spills (Figure 4-31).

### Vaporizer Inlet Port

#### Description and Function

The vaporizer inlet port is the point where oxygen and any other carrier gases enter the vaporizer from the flow meters (see Figure 4-27, *A*).

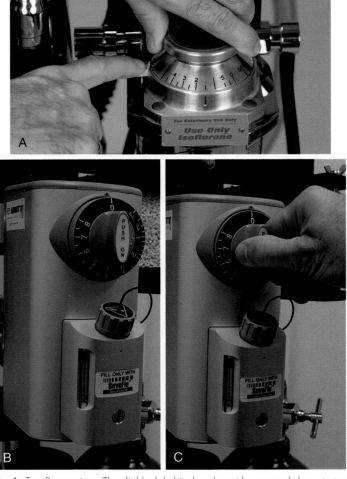

**FIGURE 4-29** *A,* Tec 3 vaporizer. The dial lock (white lever) must be pressed down to turn the vaporizer on. *B,* Penlon Sigma Delta vaporizer. The dial must be pressed in to turn the vaporizer on. *C,* Vaporizer with the dial unlocked.

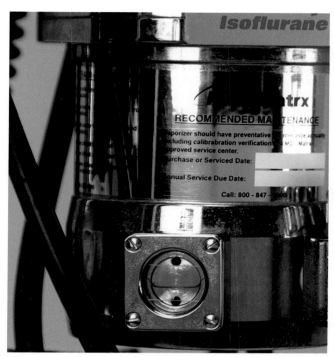

FIGURE 4-30  The indicator window of an anesthetic vaporizer. The level of the liquid anesthetic must be kept between the upper and lower lines.

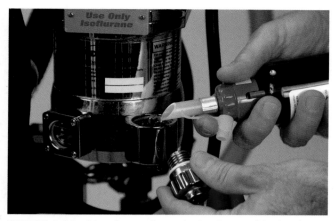

FIGURE 4-31  Note the nozzle attached to the top of the liquid anesthetic bottle. This filling device will only fit on a corresponding bottle (isoflurane device on an isoflurane bottle). It minimizes spillage when the vaporizer is being filled.

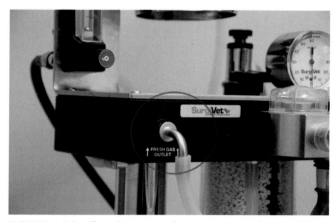

FIGURE 4-32  This 15-mm port is the common gas outlet with the hose leading to the breathing circuit attached. It is present on some machines as an additional connection between the vaporizer outlet port and the fresh gas inlet.

## Use

The vaporizer inlet port is connected to the flow meters by a hose with a female keyed connector. This keyed connector prevents the operator from inadvertently attaching the outlet hose to the inlet port. Check that this connector is securely attached to the vaporizer before commencement of any procedure.

## Vaporizer Outlet Port and Common Gas Outlet (Fresh Gas Outlet)

### Description and Function

Both the vaporizer outlet port and the **common gas outlet** are fittings to which a hose connects. The vaporizer outlet port (see Figure 4-27, *B*) is the point where the oxygen, inhalant anesthetic, and $N_2O$ (if used) exit the vaporizer on the way to the breathing circuit. On some machines this port connects directly to the breathing circuit via a hose. On other machines it connects instead to the common gas outlet. The common gas outlet (Figure 4-32) then connects directly to the breathing circuit via a second hose. So on a machine with a common gas outlet, there are two lengths of hose between the vaporizer outlet port and the breathing circuit instead of one (see Figure 4-9).

### Use

The vaporizer outlet port is connected to the common gas outlet or directly to the breathing circuit by a hose with a male keyed connector. This keyed connector prevents the operator from inadvertently attaching the inlet hose to the outlet port. It is important to check that this fitting is securely attached to the vaporizer before the commencement of any procedure.

### Safety

When a non-rebreathing circuit on a machine without a separate common gas outlet is used, the male keyed connector of the rebreathing circuit is removed from the outlet port and the male keyed connector for the non-rebreathing circuit is attached to the vaporizer outlet port (see Figure 4-8) in its place. When a machine with a separate common gas outlet is used, the connector for the non-rebreathing circuit is attached to the common gas outlet instead. Regardless of which type you are using, after any procedure in which a non-rebreathing circuit is used, the connector of the rebreathing circuit must be reattached to the outlet port or common gas outlet before the next patient is anesthetized. It may, however, be inadvertently left unattached. When this happens, anesthetic gas will discharge into the room instead of into the circuit. This will result in an inability to keep the patient anesthetized and exposure of personnel to anesthetic gas. Checking the machine for leaks before each procedure can prevent this error.

> ▌ *TECHNICIAN NOTE*    After use of a non-rebreathing circuit, the connector of the rebreathing circuit must be reattached to the outlet port or common gas outlet before the next patient is anesthetized. A failure to do this results in an inability to keep the patient anesthetized and exposure of personnel to anesthetic gas.

## Breathing Circuit

The breathing circuit consists of a group of components that carry anesthetic and oxygen from the fresh gas inlet to the patient and convey expired gases away from the patient. The breathing circuit may be incorporated into the anesthetic machine (as is the case with a rebreathing system), or it may be a separate unit (as is the case with a non-rebreathing system).

## Scavenging System

The scavenging system is discussed in detail in chapter 13.

## REBREATHING SYSTEMS

A **rebreathing system** is an anesthetic machine fitted with a rebreathing circuit. Rebreathing systems are also called *circle systems* because exhaled gases minus carbon dioxide are recirculated and rebreathed by the patient, along with variable amounts of fresh oxygen and anesthetic. These systems are appropriate for almost all patients except those that are very small (under 2.5 to 3 kg in body weight).

When a rebreathing system is used, the gases exhaled by the patient travel through the expiratory breathing tube and the expiratory unidirectional valve then enter the $CO_2$ absorber canister. They are then directed past the reservoir bag, **pop-off valve,** and pressure manometer and back toward the patient through the inspiratory unidirectional valve and inspiratory breathing tube. Exhaled gases include $O_2$, anesthetic vapor, $CO_2$, nitrogen, water vapor, and nitrous oxide (if used). Fresh oxygen and anesthetic enter the circuit from the fresh gas inlet and mix with the patient's exhaled gases. The flow of gas through the anesthetic machine therefore is circular (inspiratory unidirectional valve, inspiratory tube, animal, expiratory tube, expiratory unidirectional valve, carbon dioxide canister, past the reservoir bag, pop-off valve, and pressure manometer, and back to the inspiratory unidirectional valve) (see Figure 4-8). When correctly adjusted, the flow meters, vaporizer, reservoir bag, and pop-off valve work in concert to maintain a constant flow of gas to the patient.

Rebreathing systems are further subdivided into **closed rebreathing systems** and **semiclosed rebreathing systems.** The main difference between these systems lies in the amount of carrier gas that is delivered to the breathing circuit (the flow rate) and the position of the pop-off valve. A closed rebreathing system (also called a total rebreathing system) is one in which the pop-off valve is kept nearly or completely closed and the flow of oxygen is relatively low, providing only the volume necessary to meet the patient's metabolic needs. When the system is operating optimally, it is not necessary to vent gases from the circuit because the same volume of gas is added to the circuit as is consumed by the patient. In reality, however, this delicate balance of input and consumption is difficult to achieve and requires constant monitoring and adjustment. For this reason, closed systems are seldom used in practice with the exception of large animal anesthesia.

In contrast, a semiclosed rebreathing system (also called a partial rebreathing system) is one in which the pop-off valve is positioned partially open, and more oxygen is added than the patient requires. In this system, a portion of the gases is recirculated, but the amount beyond the volume that is used by the patient exits through the pop-off valve into the scavenging system. This type of system is relatively easy to use and meets the needs of the majority of patients. For this reason it is the most common machine configuration used in clinical practice.

## Rebreathing Circuits

A rebreathing circuit consists of the following parts:
- Fresh gas inlet
- Unidirectional (or one-way) valves
- Pop-off (or pressure relief) valve
- Reservoir bag
- **Carbon dioxide absorber canister**
- Pressure manometer
- Air intake valve
- Breathing tubes
- Y-piece

A non-rebreathing circuit is less complex and is discussed in the section beginning on p. 122.

### Fresh Gas Inlet

#### *Description and Function*

The **fresh gas inlet** is the point at which the carrier and anesthetic gases enter the breathing circuit. This inlet is usually located near the inspiratory unidirectional valve. The vaporizer outlet port or common gas outlet and the fresh gas inlet are connected by a hose (which is often black or clear) (see Figure 4-27, *B*).

#### *Use*

The fresh gas inlet is permanently attached to the breathing circuit whether rebreathing or non-rebreathing, so no action needs to be taken by the anesthetist.

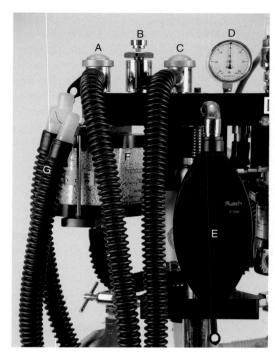

**FIGURE 4-33** Parts of a rebreathing circuit. *A,* Exhalation unidirectional valve. *B,* Pop-off valve. *C,* Inhalation unidirectional valve. *D,* Pressure manometer. *E,* 2 liter reservoir bag. *F,* Carbon dioxide absorber canister. *G,* Small animal corrugated breathing tubes.

## Unidirectional Valves

### Description and Function

The two **unidirectional valves** (Figure 4-33, *A* and *C*) control the direction of gas flow through the rebreathing circuit as the patient breathes. The inspiratory (inhalation) unidirectional valve is the attachment point for the inspiratory breathing tube, and the expiratory (exhalation) unidirectional valve is the attachment point for the expiratory breathing tube. The valves are located inside a housing with a clear, plastic dome on top that allows the anesthetist to observe the action of the valves, which open and close as the patient breathes to allow anesthetic gases to flow past. Sometimes, when the velocity of the gas is very slow, they "flutter" in response to gas flow—thus the alternative name "flutter valves."

When the patient inhales, the inspiratory valve opens, allowing the oxygen and anesthetic gas to enter the inspiratory breathing tube and travel toward the patient. The gases then pass through the Y-piece and into the ET tube or mask. On reaching the patient's lungs, oxygen and anesthetic molecules are absorbed and enter the bloodstream. At the same time, carbon dioxide and anesthetic molecules are released from the bloodstream, enter the alveoli, and are exhaled on the next breath.

Exhaled gases travel through the ET tube or mask and the Y-piece, enter the expiratory breathing tube, pass through the expiratory valve, and pass directly into the carbon dioxide absorber canister (Figure 4-34). This ensures that carbon dioxide is removed from the expired gas before the expired gas returns to the patient. The

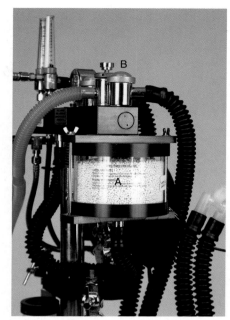

**FIGURE 4-34** *A,* Carbon dioxide absorber canister. Note that exhaled air is directed by the exhalation valve *(B)* directly into the canister.

unidirectional valves thus cause the gases to travel a one-way modified circular path through the breathing circuit.

### Use

The unidirectional valves function passively as the patient breathes and so require no action on the part of the anesthetist. These valves may be used to monitor patient respiratory rate and depth, and as an aid to check for proper placement of the ET tube. If the tube is not properly placed, the valves will move sluggishly or not at all despite normal respiratory volume and rate.

## Pop-off Valve

### Description and Function

The pop-off valve (also known as the *pressure relief valve, exhaust valve, adjustable pressure limiting* [APL] *valve,* or *overflow valve*) is the point of exit of anesthetic gases from the breathing circuit (see Figure 4-33, *B*). Pop-off valves have differing appearances but in all cases have a knob that can be turned to open or close them.

The main function of the pop-off valve is to allow excess carrier and anesthetic gases to exit from the breathing circuit and enter the scavenging system. By venting excess gas, the pop-off valve prevents the buildup of excessive pressure or volume of gases within the circuit. If allowed to occur, this excess pressure could damage the animal's lungs by causing the alveoli to overdistend and rupture. Excess intrathoracic pressure also dramatically decreases return of blood to the heart, resulting in severely decreased cardiac output.

### Use

In a similar way to a water tap, the pop-off valve can be set anywhere from fully closed to fully open, to allow varying

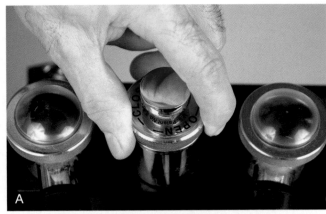

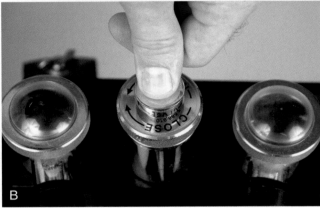

**FIGURE 4-35** **A,** The pop-off valve on any machine can be closed by turning it clockwise, and opened by turning it counterclockwise. **B,** On some machines the pop-off valve can also be closed by pressing it firmly, and opened by releasing pressure.

amounts of gas to exit from the system and to maintain optimum volume in the reservoir bag. When fully open, it releases when the gas pressure in the circuit exceeds 0.5 to 1 cm of water. As the valve is tightened, more pressure is required for release.

When a semiclosed rebreathing system is used, the valve is kept partially open when the patient is spontaneously breathing. It is closed only when providing manual ventilation so that gases may be forced into the patient's lungs using hand pressure. Between each breath provided by manual ventilation, it must be opened again to allow the escape of gases. This rule does not apply to use of a closed rebreathing system. (See Appendix D.)

> *TECHNICIAN NOTE* When manual ventilation is provided, the pop-off valve is closed before the bag is pressed. Between each breath, the pop-off valve *must* be opened again to allow the escape of gases.

Note that most pop-off valves can be closed only by turning the ring clockwise and opened only by turning it counterclockwise (Figure 4-35, *A*). The pop-off valve on some machines may be closed either by turning it as with other valves or by pressing firmly on the top. It is opened again by releasing pressure (Figure 4-35, *B*).

The pop-off valve should be checked for proper operation and adjusted before commencement of any procedure. This should be done at the beginning of every day as a part of the low-pressure system leak test (see Procedure 13-1). It should also be checked periodically during the anesthetic procedure to maintain optimum gas volume within the circuit as indicated by the size of the reservoir bag.

The flow meter setting, the size of the rebreathing bag, and the position of the pop-off valve (open or closed) are related in the following way. The flow meter setting determines the rate at which gas enters the breathing circuit, and the pop-off valve setting determines the rate at which gas leaves the breathing circuit. The size of the bag reflects the net volume of gas in the breathing circuit at any given time. So by adjusting the carrier gas flow rate and pop-off valve setting, the anesthetist can keep the reservoir bag optimally inflated but not pressurized.

### Reservoir Bag

#### Description and Function

The reservoir bag (also called the *rebreathing bag*) is a rubber bag, often black or green (see Figure 4-33, *E*), which serves a number of functions, including the following:

- *It serves as a flexible storage reservoir.* Because the breathing circuit is essentially a system of tubes and parts with a fixed volume, a space is necessary to accept expired air and provide air needed to fill the lungs during inspiration.
- *It allows the anesthetist to observe the animal's respirations.* The bag expands as the patient exhales and contracts as the patient inhales. Both the respiratory rate and the respiratory depth can be determined by observing movement of the bag. A lack of movement of the bag indicates apnea, a disconnected Y-piece, or blockage of the airway. Inadequate movement indicates a leak in the system, a partial airway blockage, or a decreased $V_T$. Either situation will alert the anesthetist to a need for intervention.
- *It may be used to confirm proper ET tube placement.* Movement of the bag in concert with patient respirations indicates that the ET tube is correctly placed within the trachea.
- *It allows delivery of anesthetic gases to the patient.* By application of light pressure to the bag (also known as *manual ventilation* or *bagging*), oxygen with or without anesthetic gas can be forced into the patient's lungs. Manual ventilation is used for a variety of purposes including management of apnea, prevention of atelectasis, and provision of ventilation to patients undergoing any surgical procedure in which the chest cavity is open and to patients given neuromuscular blockers.

There are three reasons why bagging is beneficial for all anesthetized patients:

1. A condition known as **atelectasis** occurs to some degree in many anesthetized patients and compromises gas exchange. Bagging helps to reinflate the

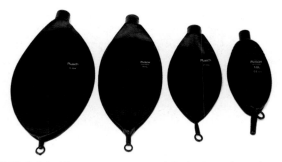

**FIGURE 4-36** The comparative size of 5-, 3-, 2-, and 1-L rebreathing bags.

collapsed alveoli. Many experts recommend bagging all anesthetized patients every 5 to 10 minutes to gently inflate the lungs with fresh oxygen and anesthetic. Use of this technique is further described in Chapter 6.

2. Most anesthetics depress respiratory drive and decrease $V_T$ to as little as 50% of the volume seen in a normal, awake patient. This may lead to hypercarbia and hypoxemia. Bagging forces fresh gas into the alveoli, normalizing gas exchange.

3. Anesthetized patients frequently experience a decreased respiratory rate or apnea. Bagging allows the anesthetist to normalize the respiratory rate.

### Use

Reservoir bags are available in various sizes, from 500 mL (for very small patients) to 30 L (intended for use in adult horses and cattle) (see Figures 4-7 and 4-36). Ideally the bag should hold a volume of at least 60 mL/kg of patient weight (six times the patient's $V_T$), but this is not always practical or necessary. From a practical perspective, the bag should contain enough gas to fill the patient's lungs during an inhalation but should not be so large as to prevent visualization of respiratory movements (Box 4-3).

If the bag is undersized or oversized, a number of complications may arise. If the rebreathing bag is too small, the patient may be unable to fill its lungs completely during inspiration. An undersized bag may also become overinflated during exhalation, increasing air pressure in the patient's airways. On the other hand, movement of an oversized bag is hard to see, impairing the ability of the anesthetist to monitor respirations. It is also more difficult

to judge the amount of gas delivered to the patient when providing manual ventilation with a bag that is too large.

The anesthetist should ensure that the reservoir bag is properly inflated during anesthesia. Inflation is determined by two factors: (1) The rate at which gas is entering the breathing circuit through the fresh gas inlet, which in turn is regulated by the flow meter setting, and (2) the rate at which gas is exiting the breathing circuit through the pop-off valve. During any procedure the bag should be approximately three fourths full at peak expiration. If the fresh gas flow is in excess of the patient's demand (as is most often the case), the bag will tend to remain relatively full. If the bag becomes overfilled, excess gas will be vented through the pop-off valve (see the next section), provided it is left partially open.

> *TECHNICIAN NOTE* During any procedure the bag should be approximately three fourths full at peak expiration.

### Safety

Unless a closed system is being used (which is seldom the case in practice except for large animal patients), the pop-off valve should always be left open when the patient is breathing spontaneously. In the event that it is not left at least partially open, pressure in the breathing circuit will exceed safe limits and make it difficult or impossible for the animal to exhale. When this happens, the reservoir bag will assume the appearance of an inflated beach ball. If not corrected, the pressure will eventually exceed the maximal safe level (see the discussion of pressure manometers on p. 121) and may lead to ruptured alveoli and pneumothorax, a life-threatening complication. Although most commonly caused by a failure to open the pop-off valve adequately, overinflation of the reservoir bag can also be caused by an obstruction in the scavenging system.

On the other hand, the bag should not be allowed to empty completely when the animal inhales, because the patient will be unable to completely fill its lungs with anesthetic gases. Complete emptying of the bag indicates that the fresh gas flow is inadequate, the bag is too small, the pop-off valve is too far open, or the scavenging system is maladjusted.

### Carbon Dioxide Absorber Canister
#### Description and Function

All exhaled gases are directed by the expiratory unidirectional valve to the carbon dioxide absorber canister (see Figure 4-34) before being returned to the patient. Gas may enter the canister through the bottom or the top, depending on the design. The canister contains absorbent granules. The carbon dioxide absorbent and primary ingredient in these products is calcium hydroxide ($Ca[OH]_2$), along with 14% to 19% water and small amounts of sodium hydroxide (NaOH), potassium hydroxide (KOH), calcium chloride (CaCl$_2$), and/or calcium sulfate (CaSO$_4$), which activate the chemical reaction. These substances react with exhaled carbon dioxide to form calcium carbonate (CaCO$_3$) and small amounts of other chemicals. During this reaction, heat and water are produced and the pH decreases.

When significant amounts of carbon dioxide are absorbed, the heat released by this reaction may cause the carbon dioxide absorber canister to become warm during use. The water produced by this reaction may serve to humidify the fresh gas entering the breathing circuit from the fresh gas inlet.

The chemical reaction has several steps and varies slightly depending on the activator but results in the following overall reaction:

$$CO_2 + Ca(OH)_2 \rightarrow CaCO_3 + H_2O + Heat$$

Carbon dioxide absorbents are supplied as loose granules or in a prepackaged cartridge. The granules are of a size (4 to 8 mesh) large enough to allow gases to pass though without excessive resistance, but small enough to provide adequate surface area for absorption of carbon dioxide.

### Use

Carbon dioxide absorbents do not last indefinitely. After absorption of about 26 L of CO$_2$ per 100 g of absorbent, the granules become exhausted. The use of depleted granules will result in rebreathing of carbon dioxide, leading to hypercapnia. There are several ways in which the anesthetist may become aware of granules that are exhausted and must be replaced, including the following:

- Fresh granules, containing mainly calcium hydroxide, can be chipped or crumbled with finger pressure, whereas granules saturated with carbon dioxide (containing mainly calcium carbonate) become hard and brittle.
- Fresh granules are white, whereas exhausted granules are slightly off-white. This difference is subtle but is visible if crystals are examined carefully.
- Most granules contain a pH indicator that will cause the granules to change color when exhausted, from white to violet or, in some cases, from pink to white depending on the brand (Figure 4-37). The color reaction does not always occur, however, especially when smaller patients are anesthetized. In addition, granules that have changed color (indicating saturation with carbon dioxide) may return to the original color after a few hours although they are still saturated with carbon dioxide. Thus it is important that the anesthetist remove granules that have changed color as soon as possible after using an anesthetic machine.
- When a capnograph is used to monitor the patient, the concentration of carbon dioxide during peak inspiration should be at or near 0 mm Hg if the absorbent is working correctly. A higher carbon dioxide level at peak inspiration indicates possible exhaustion of the absorbent (although there are other causes of elevated inspired CO$_2$ such as a nonfunctional expiratory unidirectional valve).

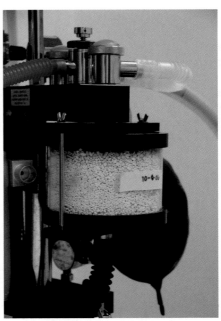

**FIGURE 4-37**  The color change to violet indicates exhaustion of the carbon dioxide absorbent and a need to change the granules. Note that some granules turn from pink to white.

Granules should be discarded when no more than one third to one half have changed color; and regardless of whether or not any of the previously mentioned indicators are evident, the granules should always be changed after 6 to 8 hours of use.

 *TECHNICIAN NOTE*  Signs that CO$_2$ granules must be changed are as follows:
- Hard, brittle granules.
- Granules that are slightly off-white in color.
- Color change of one half to one third of the granules.
- A carbon dioxide (CO$_2$) level greater than 0 during peak inspiration as measured with a capnograph.
- Granules should always be changed after 6 to 8 hours of use.

### Safety

Recent studies have shown that some absorbents containing relatively high concentrations of strong bases such as KOH may react with sevoflurane to produce a potentially nephrotoxic substance known as *compound A*. The production of this substance has been found to have no clinically significant adverse effects in veterinary patients, however.

After use, absorbents may also become desiccated (dried out) and produce a variety of adverse effects. When desiccated, absorbent containing KOH and barium hydroxide (an ingredient found in an older absorbent known as *barium hydroxide lime*) can react with some anesthetics (particularly sevoflurane) to produce excessive heat and carbon monoxide, formaldehyde, and other various toxins that are harmful to the patient. These effects are minimized, however, by using absorbents without barium or potassium hydroxide and with lower concentrations of sodium hydroxide. For this reason, absorbents containing barium hydroxide have recently been discontinued in the United States, and newer agents containing no KOH and lower amounts of NaOH or no NaOH are available (such as KOH-free sodium hydroxide lime or calcium hydroxide lime). In any case, when purchasing an absorbent, be sure that it is compatible with the anesthetic you are using.

## Pressure Manometer

### Description and Function

The pressure manometer (not to be confused with the tank pressure gauge or line pressure gauge) (see Figure 4-33, *D*) indicates the pressure of the gases within the breathing circuit and by extension the pressure in the animal's airways and lungs. This pressure is most often expressed in centimeters of water (cm $H_2O$), although on some machines the pressure may be expressed in millimeters of mercury (mm Hg) or kilopascals.

### Use

The pressure manometer is used when bagging an animal to determine the pressure being exerted on the animal's lungs when the anesthetist squeezes the reservoir bag (Figure 4-38). The pressure manometer should read 0 to 2 cm of water when the patient is breathing spontaneously. It should read no more than 20 cm of water (15 mm Hg) in small animals, or 40 cm of water (30 mm Hg) in large animals, when positive-pressure assisted or controlled ventilation is provided, unless the chest cavity is open, in which case the pressure can be somewhat higher. Excessive pressure in the circuit can result in dyspnea, lung damage, or pneumothorax. Therefore the pressure must be watched closely during any anesthetic procedure.

Higher pressure may be needed in an animal with pulmonary dysfunction, such as a dog with gastric dilatation–volvulus or a colicky, bloated horse. In the case of the dog with gastric dilatation–volvulus, pressures of 30 to 35 cm may be needed to deliver a reasonable tidal breath, and in bloated horses pressures up to 50 to 55 cm may be necessary.

 *TECHNICIAN NOTE*  Maximum safe pressure manometer readings (when the chest is closed) are as follows:
- 0 to 2 cm $H_2O$ when the patient is breathing spontaneously
- 20 cm $H_2O$ in small animals when positive-pressure ventilation is provided
- 40 cm $H_2O$ in large animals when positive-pressure ventilation is provided

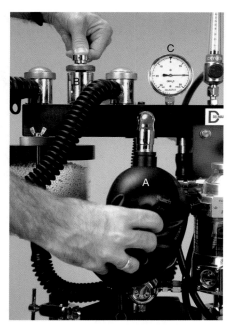

**FIGURE 4-38** *Providing manual ventilation or "bagging" the patient. The pop-off valve (B) is closed, and the bag (A) is squeezed while the pressure manometer (C) is watched to ensure that safe pressure is not exceeded. The pop-off valve is immediately opened as soon as pressure on the bag is released.*

## Air Intake Valve (Negative Pressure Relief Valve)

### Description and Function

An air intake valve is present on some machines either as a separate part or incorporated into the inspiratory unidirectional valve or the pop-off valve. This valve admits room air to the circuit in the event that negative pressure (a partial vacuum) is detected in the breathing circuit, a situation indicated by a collapsed reservoir bag. If a partial vacuum develops, the patient will be unable to fill its lungs and will develop hypoxemia because of inadequate oxygen levels. This may happen when the machine is incorrectly assembled or when an active scavenging system is exerting excessive suction.

Negative pressure may also develop in the circuit if the oxygen flow rate is too low or if the tank runs out of oxygen. The air intake valve ensures that the patient always receives some oxygen by admitting room air (which contains 21% oxygen) into the circuit. Even though this situation is not ideal, it is preferable that the patient breathe room air rather than none at all, as would be the case if the air intake valve were not present.

## Breathing Tubes and Y-piece

### Description and Function

The inspiratory and expiratory breathing tubes (corrugated breathing tubes) complete the breathing circuit by carrying the anesthetic gases to and from the patient. Each tube is connected to a unidirectional valve at one end and to the Y-piece at the other end. They are made of rubber

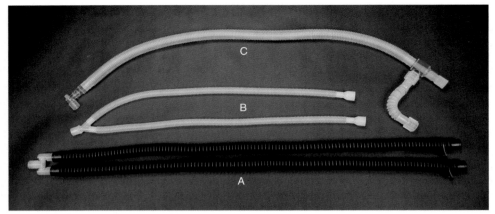

**FIGURE 4-39** Corrugated breathing tubes. **A,** Standard 22-mm small animal breathing tubes; **B,** 15-mm pediatric tubes. **C,** Universal F-circuit.

or plastic and come in three sizes: (1) large animal (50-mm diameter); (2) small animal (22-mm diameter); and (3) small animal pediatric (15-mm diameter) (Figure 4-39, *A* and *B*). An alternative configuration known as a *Universal F-circuit* is a type of breathing tube in which the inspiratory tube is located within the expiratory tube. This arrangement is designed to conserve body heat. As the cold inspired gases travel though the inner turquoise tube, the warm expired gases travel through the outer, transparent tube, warming the inspired gases (Figure 4-39, *C*).

### *Use*

Before using the machine, select the appropriate breathing tubes for the patient. Standard small animal tubes are used on small animal machines for patients over 7 kg body weight, whereas pediatric tubes are recommended for patients weighing 2.5 to 7 kg, to reduce mechanical dead space. Large animal tubes are designed for use only on large animal machines. One end of each tube must be firmly attached to the inspiratory and expiratory unidirectional valves, and the other end of each tube to the Y-piece, which connects the two tubes together. The remaining port of the Y-piece is then connected to a mask or to an ET tube.

> **TECHNICIAN NOTE** Standard small animal tubes are used on small animal machines for patients over 7 kg body weight, whereas pediatric tubes are recommended for patients weighing 2.5 to 7 kg, to reduce mechanical dead space. Large animal tubes are designed for use only on large animal machines.

## NON-REBREATHING SYSTEMS

Although the rebreathing systems just discussed are well suited to many patients, very small patients (those under 2.5 to 3 kg body weight) require the use of an alternative machine configuration called a non-rebreathing (semiopen) system. In a non-rebreathing system, little or no exhaled gases are returned to the patient but are instead evacuated by a scavenger connected to a pop-off or overflow valve, or to an exit port. If no gases are returned to the patient, the system is described as *open;* if some gases return, the system is described as *semiopen.* The characteristics of rebreathing and non-rebreathing systems are compared in Table 4-2.

When a non-rebreathing system is used, the rebreathing circuit is disabled by detaching the fresh gas hose connector from the vaporizer outlet port or the common gas outlet if present. Then a non-rebreathing circuit is attached in its place. As with a rebreathing system, the non-rebreathing system can best be understood by tracing the path of the oxygen from the compressed gas cylinder to the patient and ultimately to the scavenging system.

Just as in a rebreathing system, oxygen (and nitrous oxide gas, if used) flows from the tank, through a flow meter, and into the vaporizer. After exiting the vaporizer, however, the gases follow a different path. Instead of routing the fresh gas into the circle as occurs with a rebreathing system, the fresh gas is routed directly to the patient. Exhaled gases pass through another hose, then in most systems enter a reservoir bag, and ultimately are released into the scavenging system through an overflow valve or other exit port. In this system a carbon dioxide absorbent is not needed, because exhaled gases are vented from the system immediately after exhalation.

### Non-Rebreathing Circuits

Because of the fundamental difference in its structure, several components that are used in a rebreathing circuit are not present in a non-rebreathing circuit. These include the carbon dioxide absorber canister, pressure manometer, and unidirectional valves.

| TABLE 4-2 | Comparison of Rebreathing and Non-Rebreathing Systems | |
| --- | --- | --- |
| Parameters | Non-Rebreathing (Open or Semiopen) | Rebreathing (Semiclosed or Closed System) |
| $CO_2$ absorption | Not required | Must have $CO_2$ absorber canister |
| Changes in depth of anesthesia | Fast | Slow |
| Oxygen flow rates | High flow rates: generally must equal or exceed the respiratory minute volume | Low-flow rates: considerably less than the respiratory minute volume |
| Cost of operation | High because of the amount of oxygen and anesthetic used | Low, because less oxygen and anesthetic used |
| Amount of waste gas produced | High | Low |
| Pop-off valve position | Full open, or no pop-off | Closed (total rebreathing) or partly open (semiclosed rebreathing) |
| Heat and moisture conservation (from exhaled gases) | Poor | Good |
| Vaporizer position | Outside of the breathing circuit (no circle present) | VOC or VIC |
| Size of animal | Any size: limited only by the total gas flow that is delivered; generally recommended for animals under 7 kg | Only for animals over 7 kg (if pediatric hoses used, can be used for animals 2.5-7 kg also) |

*VIC,* Vaporizer-in-circuit; *VOC,* vaporizer-out-of-circuit.

Non-rebreathing circuits are available in several configurations with a confusing variety of names, including (1) **Bain coaxial circuit,** (2) **Ayres T-piece,** (3) **Magill circuit,** (4) **Lack circuit,** (5) **Jackson-Rees circuit,** and (6) **Norman mask elbow.** These circuits are lightweight, are easy to move and position, and are comparatively inexpensive.

Common parts of each of these circuits include an ET tube connector, a fresh gas inlet, a reservoir bag, an overflow valve or exit port, and an associated scavenger tube to connect the overflow valve or exit port to the scavenging system. Most also have a corrugated breathing tube joining the ET tube connector and reservoir bag. The overflow valve may function like an expiratory unidirectional valve or may be opened and closed in a similar manner as the pop-off valve of a rebreathing system. Where these circuits differ is in the position of the fresh gas inlet, reservoir bag, and overflow valve or exit port. Non-rebreathing circuits are grouped using the **Mapleson classification system,** into classes A though F based on the position of these parts (Figure 4-40). Note that only class A, modified A, modified D, E, and F are in common use in veterinary patients.

### Magill Circuit (Mapleson A System).

The Magill circuit (see Figure 4-40, *A*) has an overflow valve at the patient end of the breathing tube. Both the fresh gas inlet and the reservoir bag are located away from the patient at the opposite end of the breathing tube. Fresh gas flow pushes exhaled gases through the overflow valve. The chief advantage of this system is the relatively low fresh gas flow required during spontaneous ventilation (0.7 to 1.0 × the RMV). It is therefore feasible to use this system for medium or large patients. When a patient is manually ventilated, some rebreathing of expired gases may occur with this system, and for that reason it is not recommended for providing controlled ventilation.

### Lack Circuit (Modified Mapleson A System)

The Lack circuit (see Figure 4-40, *B*) is similar to the Magill circuit, except that it has an expiratory tube that runs from the ET tube connector to an overflow valve near the bag. In this system the fresh gas inlet, the overflow valve, and the reservoir bag are located away from the patient at the opposite end of the breathing tube. This system is used in a similar way as the Magill circuit.

### Bain Coaxial Circuit (Modified Mapleson D System)

The Mapleson D system (see Figure 4-40, *C*) has a fresh gas inlet at the patient end of the breathing tube. Both the overflow valve and the reservoir bag are located away from the patient at the opposite end of the breathing tube. The overflow valve may be built into the bag or near the bag. The Bain coaxial circuit (see Figure 4-40, *D*) is a modification of the Mapleson D system in which the tube supplying fresh gas is surrounded by the larger, corrugated tubing (which conducts gas away from the patient). This "tube within a tube" arrangement allows the incoming gases to be warmed slightly by the exhaled gases that surround them, before reaching the patient. This beneficial effect is minimal, however, when high fresh gas flow rates are used.

When this system is used, some rebreathing of waste gases will occur unless an oxygen flow rate of two to three

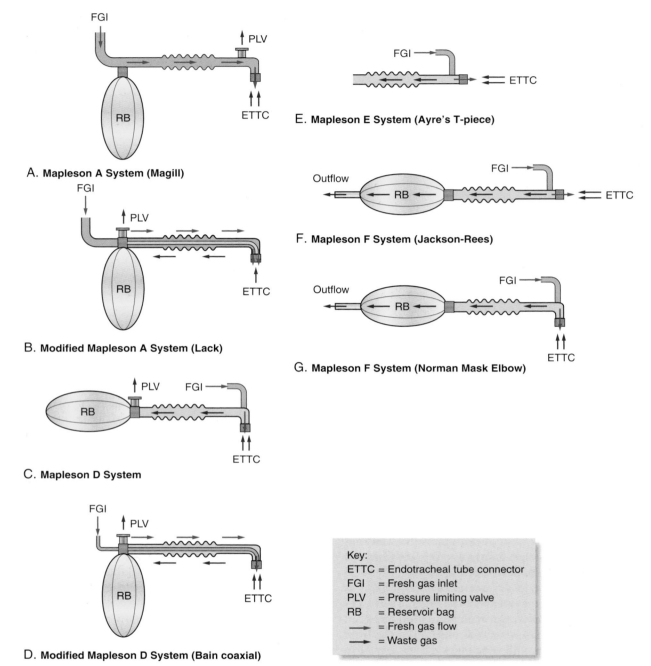

**FIGURE 4-40** A, Mapleson A System (Magill). B, Modified Mapleson A System (Lack). C, Mapleson D System. D, Modified Mapleson D System (Bain coaxial). E, Mapleson E System (Ayre's T-piece). F, Mapleson F System (Jackson-Rees). G, Mapleson F System (Norman mask elbow).

times the RMV is used (up to a maximum of 3 L/min for patients under 7 kg), but when the patient is breathing spontaneously, minimal rebreathing occurs at a flow rate of 0.5 to 1 × the RMV.

## Ayre's T-piece (Mapleson E System)

The Ayre's T-piece (see Figure 4-40, *E*) is a T-shaped tube with a fresh gas inlet entering the patient end of the breathing tube at a 90-degree angle (like the base of the letter *T*). Unlike other circuits, the Ayre's T-piece does

not have a reservoir bag at the opposite end of the breathing tube. The fresh gas flow with this system should be two to three times the RMV.

## Jackson-Rees Circuit and Norman Mask Elbow (Mapleson F Systems)

The Jackson-Rees circuit and the Norman mask elbow (see Figure 4-40, *F* and *G*) have a fresh gas inlet at the patient end of the breathing tube and a reservoir bag at the opposite end. The fresh gas inlet of a Jackson-Rees circuit enters the breathing tube at a 45- to 90-degree angle. The Norman mask elbow is almost identical to a Jackson-Rees circuit, except that the ET tube connector is at right angles to the breathing tube. This circuit may slightly reduce mechanical dead space as compared with an Ayre's T-piece or Jackson-Rees, but otherwise is used in a similar manner as these circuits. The fresh gas flow with both the Norman mask elbow and the Jackson-Rees should be two to three times the RMV.

## OPERATION OF THE ANESTHETIC MACHINE

### Daily Setup

At the beginning of each day, before using an anesthetic machine, the anesthetist must assemble the machine or machines to be used, check the oxygen and liquid anesthetic levels, check the low pressure system for leaks (see Procedure 13-1), and set the pop-off or overflow valve (Procedure 4-1, p. 135). Before each case the anesthetist must also choose between a small animal and a large animal machine, determine what type of breathing circuit to use (rebreathing or non-rebreathing), and choose carrier gas flow rates. (Procedure 4-2, p. 135, is a checklist to be followed when setting up anesthetic equipment.)

> TECHNICIAN NOTE    The appropriate choice of a machine (large animal versus small animal), reservoir bag, breathing tubes, oxygen flow rates, and breathing circuit type is based on patient body weight.

### Choosing a Machine

The decision of whether to use a small animal or large animal machine is based on patient weight. A small animal machine is intended for patients under 150 kg (about 350 lb), and a large animal machine is intended for patients weighing 150 kg or more.

### Machine Assembly

Before assembling the machine, choose the breathing circuit, and, if using a rebreathing circuit, choose appropriately sized breathing tubes and rebreathing bag. These decisions are based on patient weight. Once the equipment has been chosen, connect all necessary parts including the vaporizer inlet and outlet port hoses, the breathing circuit if using a non-rebreathing system, and the rebreathing bag and breathing tubes if using a rebreathing system. Finally, connect the scavenging system hoses and any other parts required for the machine you are using, such as the common gas outlet.

### Checking Oxygen and Anesthetic Levels

The oxygen supply must be checked to be sure enough oxygen remains to complete the procedure. Guidelines regarding oxygen supply may be found in the discussion of the tank pressure gauge on p. 107.

Anesthetic vaporizers must also be checked to make sure that enough anesthetic remains in the vaporization chamber. Most vaporizers have an indicator window at their base that allows the technician to inspect the amount of liquid anesthetic remaining. In order for the vaporizer to function properly, the liquid anesthetic must be between the full and empty lines of the window. The vaporizer should be refilled as needed but should be kept at least half full at all times. A keyed filling device should be used for this purpose (see Figure 4-31). Overfilling a vaporizer will result in anesthetic overdose, and underfilling will result in an inability to keep the patient anesthetized. The vaporizer should also be turned off when the machine is not in use.

### Choice of Rebreathing Versus Non-Rebreathing System

The decision of whether to use a rebreathing system or a non-rebreathing system is generally made on the basis of patient size. This is because the patient's respiratory drive—the force generated by the respiratory muscles during breathing—is directly related to body weight. The respiratory drive in very small patients is insufficient to move gas through areas of resistance to air movement (primarily the unidirectional valves, carbon dioxide canister, and breathing tubes).* In contrast, non-rebreathing systems offer little resistance to air movement, a significant advantage for these patients. The choice of system to be used is important in terms of machine setup and use because it will determine the following:

- The type of equipment required (a conventional anesthetic machine with or without a non-rebreathing system such as a Bain coaxial circuit)
- Position of the pop-off valve (closed, partially open, or open)
- Carrier gas flow rates (oxygen and nitrous oxide, if used)

Rebreathing systems may be safely used on all larger patients but, as mentioned, are not safe for very small patients. For this reason, most anesthetists recommend a rebreathing system for patients weighing 7 kg (15 lb) or over, unless the system is fitted with pediatric hoses (and assuming the unidirectional valves are of a lightweight and nonstick design), in which case it may also be used on patients as small as 2.5 to 3 kg. Patients smaller than 2.5 to 3 kg should be placed on a non-rebreathing system.

Although patient weight is the primary determining factor in making a decision concerning which system to use, other advantages and disadvantages of each of these systems must be considered, including the following:

- *Cost:* Closed rebreathing (total) systems are most economical because the very low gas flow rates used

---

*The size of the endotracheal tube has a greater effect on resistance than does the type of circuit used. The use of an endotracheal tube that is too small results in far greater resistance to air passage than that offered by the remainder of the anesthetic circuit, even in a rebreathing setup.

with these systems conserve carrier and anesthetic gases. Semiclosed rebreathing (partial) systems use higher gas flow rates and so are not as economical as closed rebreathing systems. Non-rebreathing systems are the least economical because they use the highest gas flow of all the systems and consequently use more carrier and anesthetic gas per unit body weight.

- *Control of anesthetic depth:* The speed at which the anesthetist can change anesthetic depth depends in part on the type of system used. Changes take longer with a rebreathing system because the flow of fresh oxygen and anesthetic into the system is low compared with the volume of the circuit (Box 4-2). Therefore when the vaporizer setting is changed, it will take longer for the anesthetic concentration in the breathing circuit to reach the desired level. A non-rebreathing system allows a much faster turnover of gases because flow rates of fresh gas are higher relative to the volume of the circuit. Because of this higher flow and because the fresh gas is often delivered very close to the patient, changes in the anesthetic concentration breathed in by the patient occur more rapidly. This means that the anesthetic concentration breathed by the patient is very close to that indicated by the dial with a non-rebreathing system. In contrast, with a rebreathing system, the concentration of anesthetic breathed in by the patient will not be the same as that indicated on the dial for several to many minutes after the setting has been changed.*

- *Conservation of heat and moisture:* Fresh gas entering a breathing system from the vaporizer is relatively cool and dry, compared with the patient's exhaled gases, which are warm and moist. Inspired fresh anesthetic gases have a relative humidity close to 0% and a temperature of approximately 16° C (61° F), whereas exhaled gases have a relative humidity of almost 100% and a temperature close to 25° C (77° F). Rebreathing systems automatically warm and humidify fresh gas that enters the circuit as it mixes with the patient's expired gases. In non-rebreathing systems, the warmed and humidified gases exhaled by the patient exit through the scavenger, and the patient breathes only the cool, dry fresh gas. Non-rebreathing systems are therefore associated with significant heat and water loss from the patient. In addition, the dry anesthetic gases may impair tracheobronchial ciliary function and dry the airways.

- *Production of waste gas:* Closed rebreathing systems release little waste anesthetic gas because oxygen flow rates are low and exhaled gases are recirculated

rather than vented through the pop-off valve. Semiclosed rebreathing systems vent some waste anesthetic gas, which varies depending on the carrier gas flow rates used. In contrast, non-rebreathing systems vent nearly all exhaled gas.

## Checking the Low-Pressure System for Leaks

The low-pressure system includes the breathing circuit, the vaporizer, and all the tubing between the flow meters and the fresh gas inlet. Checking this system for leaks helps to ensure that the machine is properly assembled and has no damaged or missing parts (Case Study 4-1 illustrates the importance of leak testing any anesthetic machine before use.). The procedure for performing a low-pressure system leak test can be found in Procedure 13-1.

## Adjusting the Pop-off Valve

With a semiclosed rebreathing system, the pop-off valve should be adjusted immediately after the leak test is performed. The action ensures that the pop-off valve has not been inadvertently left closed and is set at the right level for the patient. The procedure for adjusting the pop-off valve can be found in Procedure 4-1, p. 135.

## Choosing Carrier Gas Flow Rates

At various times during any anesthetic procedure, the anesthetist must determine the appropriate carrier gas flow. Usually oxygen is used alone, but if both oxygen and nitrous oxide are used, flow rate determinations must take into consideration the total flow of both gases as well as the individual flow rates of each gas. (More information on the use of nitrous oxide can be found in Appendix B.)

The flow rates for each anesthetic procedure are calculated using the patient body weight and the $V_T$ or RMV. The $V_T$ is considered to be approximately 10 mL/kg/min in most anesthetized animals. The RMV is $V_T$ multiplied by the respiratory rate in breaths per minute (an average of 20 breaths/min in most patients). Therefore the RMV is considered to be about 200 mL/kg/min.

Flow rates also depend on the type of breathing system (closed rebreathing, semiclosed rebreathing, or non-rebreathing) and the period of anesthesia (i.e., induction, maintenance, or recovery or when changing the anesthetic depth). Relatively high rates are used for non-rebreathing systems at all times regardless of the period of anesthesia. With closed rebreathing systems, flow rates are very low (only enough to meet the metabolic needs of the patient). With semiclosed rebreathing systems, flow rates vary from relatively low rates when maintaining a patient at a desired anesthetic depth to relatively high rates during induction and recovery and when changing anesthetic depth. This is because higher flows cause the anesthetic concentration within the breathing circuit to

---

*The type of volatile anesthetic used will also determine how quickly anesthetic depth can be changed, regardless of oxygen flow rates or the type of circuit used. (See discussion of blood-gas solubility coefficients in Chapter 3.)

## CASE 4-1 THE IMPORTANCE OF MACHINE TESTING

Molly, a 1-year-old, female, 3.5-kg domestic shorthair (DSH), was anesthetized in preparation for a routine ovariohysterectomy. Based on preanesthetic assessment, she was classified as a physical status class P1 patient. Molly was premedicated with 0.01 mg of dexmedetomidine per kilogram intramuscularly (IM) 15 minutes before anesthetic induction and was induced with a mixture of 5.5 mg of ketamine per kilogram and 0.28 mg of diazepam per kilogram intravenously (IV). She was intubated, connected to a Bain coaxial non-rebreathing circuit, placed on isoflurane, and prepared for surgery. During preparation of the surgical site, she was in a surgical plane of anesthesia and remained stable.

After being transferred to the operating room, Molly was connected to a different machine, and maintained with 1.5% isoflurane and 1 L/min oxygen. The final surgical preparation was completed, the patient was draped, and preparations were made to make the incision. At this point, the veterinarian noticed that Molly's respiratory efforts seemed somewhat labored, and she was in a light plane of anesthesia. She asked the circulating nurse to lift the drapes and assess Molly more closely. The circulating nurse determined that the lung sounds were normal, but the mucous membrane color seemed somewhat darker than expected. In addition, the heart and respiratory rates were elevated, but other vital signs were normal. The oxygen was on at the desired flow rate, and the endotracheal tube was correctly placed. The oxygen flow was increased to 2 L/min.

During this time the patient's color deteriorated, at which point, the veterinarian ordered that the patient be removed from the breathing circuit. The color improved immediately after removal. In view of this change in status, the veterinarian suspected a machine malfunction and ordered that another machine be used for the rest of the procedure until the problem could be identified. After this change was made, the patient continued to improve.

For the remainder of the procedure, the patient was continuously monitored. A pulse oximeter probe was placed on the tongue to monitor oxygen saturation. The patient was bagged as needed and kept on an oxygen flow of 2 L/min until vital signs were completely stable.

Later examination of the machine revealed the problem. The machine had both an isoflurane and a sevoflurane vaporizer. The day before, the previous user had used sevoflurane to anesthetize a bird but had not reconnected the inlet and outlet hoses to the isoflurane vaporizer after the procedure. The machine had not been leak tested before this procedure, and therefore the error in machine assembly was not identified. Because a non-rebreathing system was attached to the outlet port of the isoflurane vaporizer, but the carrier gas supply line was attached to the sevoflurane vaporizer inlet port instead of the isoflurane vaporizer inlet port, no oxygen was being delivered to the patient, and the patient was attempting to breathe against a partial vacuum in the breathing circuit.

This case illustrates the importance of careful examination of the machine before use. Anesthetic machines are complex and subject to a variety of malfunctions that must be identified and corrected before use. If this machine had been leak tested, the error in machine assembly would have been identified. Although this patient was not harmed, if rapid action had not been taken, this error could have resulted in a variety of serious complications including permanent central nervous system (CNS) damage, or even an anesthetic fatality.

---

change more rapidly and consequently cause the patient's anesthetic depth to change more quickly. This is desirable when a rapid change in anesthetic depth is necessary, such as during induction and when the patient's anesthetic level is excessive. See Box 4-4 for recommended flow rates, Box 4-5 for examples of flow rate calculations, and Tables 4-3 and 4-4 for quick look-up charts for rebreathing and non-rebreathing systems respectively.

> **TECHNICIAN NOTE** With semiclosed rebreathing systems, flow rates vary from relatively low when maintaining a patient at a desired anesthetic depth to relatively high during induction and recovery and when changing anesthetic depth. This is because higher flows cause the patient's anesthetic depth to change more quickly.

### Flow Rates during Mask or Chamber Induction

During mask and chamber induction, very high flow rates are required. Use of high flow rates in the induction period saturates the anesthetic circuit with carrier gas and anesthetic vapor, and dilutes the expired gases of the patient. Otherwise, expired nitrogen gas ($N_2$), which comprises almost 80% of the air in patient's lungs and bloodstream at the start of the anesthetic period, will enter the circuit and dilute out the anesthetic vapor and oxygen. If high flow rates are used, the nitrogen will be flushed out of the breathing circuit by fresh gas within a few minutes. The flow rate can be decreased to a maintenance level once the patient reaches the desired plane of anesthesia.

For mask induction it is generally agreed that the flow rate per minute should equal 30 times the $V_T$ (approximately 300 mL/kg/min) for cats and small dogs, and somewhat less for larger dogs. This works out to a recommended total flow rate of 1 to 3 L/min for animals less than or equal to 10 kg, and 3 to 5 L/min for animals over 10 kg. A flow rate of 5 L/min is recommended for chamber induction regardless of patient body weight.

In large animal anesthesia, mask induction is rarely used, with the exception of neonates, in which case rates similar to those in cats and dogs can be used, and pigs, because of the difficulty in gaining venous access in conscious swine. Small to medium pigs (less than

| BOX 4-4 | Oxygen Flow Rates |
|---|---|

**Oxygen Flow Rates for Small Animals, Foals, Calves, and Small Ruminants (<150 kg [350 lb])**
*Chamber and Mask Inductions*
Chamber induction: 5 L/min
Mask induction: 300 mL/kg/min or 30 times the tidal volume
- 1 to 3 L/min for patients ≤10 kg
- 3 to 5 L/min for patients >10 kg

*Rebreathing Systems*
Semiclosed system after induction, during a change in anesthetic depth, or during recovery: 50 to 100 mL/kg/min with a maximum of 5 L/min. Flows in the higher end of this range will result in faster changes in anesthetic depth.
- Approximately 0.5 to 1 L/10 kg body weight per minute up to a maximum of 5 L/min. (This guideline represents approximately one quarter to one half of the respiratory minute volume.)
Semiclosed system during maintenance: 20 to 40 mL/kg/min
- Approximately 0.2 to 0.4 L (200 to 400 mL)/10 kg body weight per minute with a minimum of 250 mL/min regardless of patient size. (Note: The use of a maintenance rate of 0.2 L/10 kg/min is sometimes referred to as "low flow.")
Semiclosed system during maintenance with minimal rebreathing: 200 to 300 mL/kg/min
- Approximately 2 to 3 L/10 kg body weight per minute up to a maximum of 5 L/min. (Note: At this flow rate, the machine functions in a manner similar to that of a non-rebreathing system.)
Closed system during maintenance: 5 to 10 mL/kg/min
- Approximately 0.05 to 0.1 L (50 to 100 mL)/10 kg body weight per minute. (Note: Oxygen flow rates below 0.25 L/min may decrease the accuracy of vaporizer output, making the use of a closed system more challenging in patients weighing less than 25 kg.)

*Non-Rebreathing Systems*
Mapleson A (Magill), modified Mapleson A (Lack), and modified Mapleson D (Bain) systems (150 to 200 mL/kg/min—approximately 0.75 to 1.0 × the respiratory minute volume)
- Approximately 0.5 to 1.5 L/min (used only for patients 7 kg or under)
Modified Mapleson D systems (Bain coaxial circuit) with no rebreathing, Mapleson E systems (Ayre's T-piece), and Mapleson F systems (Jackson-Rees and Norman mask elbow circuits) (400 to 600 mL/kg/min—approximately 2 to 3 × the respiratory minute volume)
- Approximately 1 to 3 L/min (used only for patients 7 kg or under)

**Oxygen Flow Rates for Large Animals (≥150 kg [350 lb])**
*Rebreathing Systems (Note: Only rebreathing systems are used in large animal patients.)*
Semiclosed system after induction, during a change in anesthetic depth, or during recovery:
- Approximately 8 to 10 L/min. (This guideline represents approximately 20 mL/kg/min with a maximum of 10 L/min.)
Semiclosed system during maintenance:
- Approximately 3 to 5 L/min. (This guideline represents approximately 10 mL/kg/min with a maximum of 5 L/min.)
Closed system during maintenance:
- Approximately 1 to 2.5 L/min. (This guideline represents approximately 3 to 5 mL/kg/min.)

50 kg) require oxygen flow rates of 3 to 5 L/min during mask induction. A flow rate of 5 L/min is rarely exceeded when larger pigs are masked in order to decrease pollution of the induction area with anesthetic gases, as masks for this size of pig are custom made and may leak. Induction will, however, be much slower, so if faster induction time is required, then flow rates of up to 10 L/min can be used.

## Flow Rates When Using a Semiclosed Rebreathing System

### After Induction with an Injectable Agent
For animals induced with an injectable anesthetic and subsequently intubated and connected to an anesthetic machine, the flow rate should be relatively high (50 to 100 mL/kg/min). This results in a flow rate of about

500 mL to 5 L/min for small animals, or for large animal patients connected to a small animal anesthetic machine, depending on the patient body weight. Initial flow rates for large animal patients on a large animal machine range from 8 to 10 L/min.

### Flow Rates When Making Changes in Anesthetic Depth
It is also desirable to use a higher oxygen flow rate (50 to 100 mL/kg/min) when the patient's level of anesthesia is too deep or too light and a change in anesthetic depth is desired. Although not absolutely required, use of flows at the higher end of this range will result in more rapid changes in the desired anesthetic concentration within the breathing circuit, and ultimately in the patient's anesthetic depth.

| BOX 4-5 | Examples of Flow Rate Calculations |
| --- | --- |

1. Given a 5-kg cat and a conventional machine with a vaporizer-out-of-circuit (VOC) precision vaporizer, what type of circuit and flow rate would normally be used? Calculate the flow rates for oxygen alone and for oxygen and nitrous oxide used together (maintenance).

   *Answer:* Because the cat weighs less than 7 kg, a Bain coaxial circuit or other non-rebreathing system is preferred, although a rebreathing system with pediatric hoses could also be used for this patient. The flow rate recommended for the Bain system is at least 150 to 200 mL/kg/min, with 400 to 600 mL/kg/min to prevent any rebreathing. Thus the anesthetist could select 200 mL × 5 kg = 1000 mL or 1 L of gas flow per minute, or 2 L/min if no rebreathing is desired. If nitrous oxide is used for this animal, a 2:1 ratio of $N_2O/O_2$ should be provided. For a 2-L total flow of gas, this is equal to:

   Oxygen: One third of 2 L/min = Approximately 667 mL/min

   Nitrous oxide: Two thirds of 2 L/min = Approximately 1333 mL/min

   If nitrous oxide is used, the anesthetist must ensure that the animal receives adequate oxygen (30 mL/kg/min). For this cat the minimum is 30 mL of oxygen per minute × 5 kg = 150 mL of oxygen per minute. (Therefore 667 mL is safe.)

2. Given a 25-kg dog and a conventional machine with a VOC precision vaporizer, what type of circuit and flow rate would be preferred during the maintenance period?

   *Answer:* For economic reasons, the type of circuit used would most likely be a circle system. If a semiclosed rebreathing system is used, the oxygen flow rate is 20 – 40 mL/kg/min. 20 mL/kg/min × 25 kg = 500 mL/min; and 40 mL/kg/min × 25 kg = 1000 mL/min or 1 L/min.

   If a closed rebreathing system is used, the flow rate should be 5 to 10 mL/kg/min. For this animal, the flow rate would therefore be about 250 mL of oxygen per minute.

   If the anesthetist wishes to increase the flow rate to minimize rebreathing, the flow rate would be calculated as 200 to 300 mL/kg/min, which is 5 L/min in this patient.

   When using a semiclosed system, the oxygen flow rate therefore can be set at a minimum of 500 mL/min and at a maximum of 5 L/min (with the pop-off valve completely open and the animal minimally rebreathing expired gases). Many anesthetists would choose a flow rate midway between these two extremes, approximately 1 to 2 L/min.

3. Given a 15-kg dog and a conventional machine with a VOC precision vaporizer, what would be the recommended flow rate if the patient's anesthetic depth is inadequate and needs to be increased?

   *Answer:* For practical reasons, this patient is most likely to be on a semiclosed rebreathing system, and the flow rate can be anywhere from 50 to 100 mL/kg/min. For this animal, the flow rate therefore would be 750 mL to 1.5 L/min. Although any flow in this range may be used, the higher the flow, the more rapidly the anesthetic depth will change. So if it is important that the anesthetic depth change quickly, it is always preferable to choose a higher rate, even though more gas will be used. If the change can be more gradual, a lower rate (for instance 750 mL/min) can be used to conserve gases. These rates are appropriate any time the anesthetic depth needs to be changed, including the induction and recovery periods.

## Flow Rates during Maintenance

Once the animal achieves a satisfactory level of anesthetic depth, the flow rate may be safely reduced to a maintenance level. Rebreathing systems require relatively low flow rates compared with non-rebreathing systems during this period because carbon dioxide is removed from the expired gases, which are then returned to the patient. Provided the carbon dioxide absorbent is effective and there are no leaks in the system, the carrier gas and anesthetic can be recycled continuously, and only a small amount of fresh gas is required. During this period flow rates of 20 to 40 mL/kg/min are recommended for small animals (SA) and 3 to 5 L/min for adult large animals (LA).

## Flow Rates during Anesthetic Recovery

When the vaporizer is turned off, the patient enters the recovery period. During this time, even though the vaporizer is turned off, anesthetic gas is exhaled by the recovering patient and remains in the circuit until replaced by fresh oxygen. Recovery will be delayed if this waste anesthetic gas is allowed to remain in the circuit. So it is to the patient's advantage to remove this waste gas as quickly as possible by taking the following actions.

Immediately after the vaporizer is turned off, increase the flow to the same rate used during induction (50 to 100 mL/kg/min). Then, with the pop-off valve open, use gentle pressure to evacuate the reservoir bag and refill it using short bursts from the oxygen flush valve. These actions will flush out waste anesthetic gas, increase the oxygen concentration in the breathing circuit, and hasten patient recovery. Maintain this higher flow for 5 minutes or until the patient must be extubated.

This same procedure can be followed for patients connected to a large animal anesthetic machine, using flow rates of up to 10 L/min to "flush" the system.

## Flow Rates When Minimal Rebreathing of Anesthetic Gases Is Desired

Note that when the oxygen flow rate matches or exceeds the patient's RMV (at least 200 to 300 mL/kg/min), a rebreathing system can be made to function in a manner similar to a non-rebreathing system. In emergency situations, such as exhaustion of the carbon dioxide absorbent, these rates help to flush exhaled gases from the breathing circuit through the pop-off valve and may be necessary until the problem is rectified.

| TABLE 4-3 | Oxygen Flow Rate Quick Look-up Chart for Rebreathing Systems | | | |
|---|---|---|---|---|
| | Guideline Oxygen Flows (L/min) | | | |
| Weight (kg) | Closed System* (5-10 mL/kg/min, SA) | Semiclosed during Maintenance (20-40 mL/kg/min, SA) | Semiclosed during Induction, Recovery, and Changes (50-100 mL/kg/min, SA) | Semiclosed with Minimal Rebreathing† (200-300 mL/kg/min) |
| 2.5 | 0.1 | 0.25 | 0.25-0.3 | 0.5-0.8 |
| 5 | 0.1 | 0.25 | 0.3-0.5 | 1-1.5 |
| 10 | 0.1 | 0.25-0.4 | 0.5-1 | 2-3 |
| 15 | 0.1-0.15 | 0.3-0.6 | 0.8-1.5 | 3-4.5 |
| 20 | 0.1-0.2 | 0.4-0.8 | 1-2 | 4-5 |
| 25 | 0.13-0.25 | 0.5-1 | 1.3-2.5 | 5 |
| 30 | 0.15-0.3 | 0.6-1.2 | 1.5-3 | 5 |
| 40 | 0.2-0.4 | 0.8-1.6 | 2-4 | 5 |
| 50 | 0.25-0.5 | 1-2 | 2.5-5 | 5 |
| 60 | 0.3-0.6 | 1.2-2.4 | 3-5 | 5 |
| 70 | 0.35-0.7 | 1.4-2.8 | 3.5-5 | 5 |
| 80 | 0.4-0.8 | 1.6-3.2 | 4-5 | 5 |
| 90 | 0.45-0.9 | 1.8-3.6 | 4.5-5 | 5 |
| 100 | 0.5-1 | 2-4 | 5 | 5 |
| 150 | 0.75-1.5 | 3-5 | 5 | 5 |

SWITCH TO LA MACHINE

| | (3-5 mL/kg/min, LA) | (10 mL/kg/min, LA) | (20 mL/kg/min, LA) | |
|---|---|---|---|---|
| 300 | 1-1.5 | 3-5 | 8-10 | 10 |
| 450 | 1.4-2.3 | 3-5 | 8-10 | 10 |
| 600 | 1.8-3 | 3-5 | 8-10 | 10 |
| 750 | 2.3-3.8 | 3-5 | 8-10 | 10 |
| 900 | 2.7-4.5 | 3-5 | 8-10 | 10 |

*LA*, Large animal; *SA*, small animal.

*At flow rates less than 250 mL/min, vaporizer output may not be accurate.

†Minimal rebreathing occurs only when the oxygen flow is greater than or equal to the RMV.

| TABLE 4-4 | Oxygen Flow Rate Quick Look-up Chart for Non-Rebreathing Systems | |
|---|---|---|
| | Guideline Oxygen Flows (L/min) | |
| Wt. (kg) | Mapleson A (Magill)* Modified Mapleson A (Lack)* Modified Mapleson D (Bain Coaxial)†(0.75-1.0 × RMV) | Modified Mapleson D (Bain Coaxial with No Rebreathing) Mapleson E (Ayre's T-piece) Mapleson F (Norman Mask Elbow and Jackson-Rees) (2-3 × RMV) |
| 1-2.5 | 0.25-0.5 | 0.5-1.5 |
| 2.5-5 | 0.5-1 | 1.5-2.5 |
| 5-7 | 1-1.5 | 2-3 |

*Controlled ventilation is not recommended with these systems.

†Flows listed in this column are believed to result in minimal rebreathing with this system during spontaneous ventilation.

## Flow Rates When Using a Closed Rebreathing System

Closed rebreathing systems are normally used only during anesthetic maintenance. When these systems are used, the oxygen flow must equal only the oxygen requirements of the animal. The minimum metabolic oxygen requirement for the anesthetized animal is 5 to 10 mL/kg/min. (See Appendix D). The anesthetist should be aware that when flow rates of less than 250 mL/min are used, some precision vaporizers and flow meters might not accurately deliver the dialed vaporizer concentration and oxygen flow. Large animal patients, particularly adult horses and cattle, have lower metabolic oxygen requirements, and it is possible that oxygen flow rates as low as 3 to 5 mL/kg/min may be used during maintenance with a closed rebreathing system.

### Safety Concerns with a Closed Rebreathing System

Although closed rebreathing systems are more economical than semiclosed rebreathing systems, there are serious safety concerns that must be addressed when a closed rebreathing system is used:

- *Carbon dioxide accumulation.* If the carbon dioxide absorber in a closed system is not operating efficiently, exhaled carbon dioxide will build up within the circuit. This is less likely to happen in a semiclosed rebreathing system, in which some $CO_2$ is vented to the scavenger.
- *Increased pressure in the anesthetic circuit.* In a closed rebreathing system, the volume of gas in the system may increase as fresh gas enters the circuit, particularly if the fresh gas flow exceeds the patient's uptake of oxygen and anesthetic and the pop-off valve is closed. As a result, excessive pressure may build up in the circuit, making it difficult for the animal to exhale. This risk is lessened with a semiclosed rebreathing system because the pop-off valve is partially to fully open and excessive gas is vented.
- These disadvantages must be balanced against the economic advantages of a closed rebreathing system and the fact that little or no waste anesthetic gas is produced when flow rates are low. In most situations (e.g., where continuous monitoring of the patient and the anesthetic machine is not possible) the anesthetist may prefer to use a semiclosed rather than a closed rebreathing system for the safety reasons just outlined. The anesthetist may choose to err on the side of wasting some gas by using higher gas flow rates rather than risk accumulation of carbon dioxide and depletion of oxygen within the circuit. A closed rebreathing system can easily be converted to a semiclosed rebreathing system by opening the pop-off valve (except when bagging the patient) and increasing the oxygen flow rate.

Procedures used in the operation of a closed rebreathing system are listed in Appendix D.

### Flow Rates When Using a Non-Rebreathing System

Non-rebreathing systems require relatively high flow rates per unit body weight during all periods of general anesthesia (induction, maintenance, and recovery) because the removal of carbon dioxide from the circuit is dependent on fresh gas flow, which must be sufficient to ensure that there is minimal rebreathing of exhaled gases. Therefore close attention must be given to the selection of an appropriate flow rate. Recommended rates are based on body weight and the Mapleson classification of the circuit. Because these systems are generally used for patients weighing less than 7 kg, maximum rates listed are based on this body weight.

With Mapleson A systems (Magill circuit), Modified Mapleson A systems (Lack circuit), and modified Mapleson D systems (Bain coaxial circuit), carrier gas flow should be near the RMV (200 mL/kg/min). This equals about 0.5 to 1.5 L/min depending on patient size.

Modified Mapleson D systems (Bain coaxial circuit) with no rebreathing, Mapleson E systems (Ayre's T-piece), and Mapleson F systems (Jackson-Rees circuit or Norman Mask Elbow circuit) require an oxygen flow rate of two to three times the RMV (400 to 600 mL/kg/min) with a maximum flow of 3 L/min for patients under 7 kg. This equals about 1 to 3 L/min depending on patient size.

These recommended flow rates are high enough to prevent most exhaled gases from being rebreathed by the patient. Some rebreathing of gas can occur, however, particularly during peak inspiration, if the respiratory rate is rapid, or if the volume of the circuit is lower than it should be for the size of the patient. The anesthetist can partially control the amount of gas rebreathed by adjusting the oxygen flow rate. For example, when using a Bain coaxial circuit, if the anesthetist selects a high oxygen flow rate (e.g., 2 L/min for a 4-kg cat), there is little return of exhaled gases to the patient. The system is therefore truly non-rebreathing. At lower flow rates (e.g., 500 mL of oxygen per minute for the same 4-kg cat), significant rebreathing of exhaled gases may occur. So even though these systems are technically classified as non-rebreathing, the way they function is somewhat dependent on carrier gas flow.

### Summary

Within the aforementioned guidelines, there is considerable leeway for the anesthetist's own judgment in determining the flow rate for any particular procedure. (See Boxes 4-4 and 4-5 for a summary of currently recommended flow rates and examples of flow rate calculations.) In many cases the ultimate decision is based on both economic factors and the needs of the patient. For instance, low gas flow rates are more economical than high flow rates because less carrier gas and anesthetic are used, but higher rates may be necessary at certain times (such as induction, recovery, and change in anesthetic levels) or during management of a crisis. On the other hand, if the patient is small, the cost of anesthetic gases is less significant.

## CARE AND MAINTENANCE OF ANESTHETIC EQUIPMENT

### Routine Maintenance

As with any piece of equipment, the anesthetic machine requires periodic maintenance to ensure proper performance. In addition to routine maintenance procedures performed by hospital staff, a qualified repair professional should be contracted to examine and test all parts of each anesthetic machine on an annual basis.

> 📎 *TECHNICIAN NOTE* In addition to routine maintenance procedures performed by hospital staff, a qualified repair professional should be contracted to examine and test all parts of each anesthetic machine on an annual basis.

## Compressed Gas Cylinders

Usually, compressed gas cylinders are regularly inspected and maintained by the company that fills them, and they require no regular maintenance by hospital staff. At times, however, tank valve stems become difficult to turn. If excessive force is needed, the tank should not be used again until it is sent in for inspection and maintenance. Petroleum products (e.g., grease and kerosene) should not be used to lubricate oxygen tanks or their connections because an explosion could occur when these materials contact oxygen released from the tank. Silicon or Teflon-based lubricants are generally safe for this use. When empty, compressed gas cylinders must be removed, refilled, and replaced as described in the following paragraphs.

### Removing and Replacing E Tanks

When viewed from the front face, the E-tank valve has three holes — one outlet port, through which the gas exits the cylinder, and two receiving holes for the pin-index safety system. The outlet port fits on the nipple of the yoke with a single washer placed in between to prevent leakage. The pin-index holes fit onto the pins of the yoke (see Figure 4-18). To remove an E tank from the machine, be sure the tank valve is closed and the oxygen is purged from the system. Place your shoe under the tank to support it. Loosen the wing nut, and back the valve port off of the yoke. Carefully remove your shoe and lower the tank until the valve clears the yoke. The tank should be stored in an upright position, on a cart or chained to the wall, until it is picked up by the company for refilling.

When replacing a tank on a machine, first inspect the valve port for cleanliness, then place a single washer between the valve port and the nipple. There are two types of washers. Flanged washers have a flange on one side that fits inside the outlet port. A flat washer, which has no flange, fits on the nipple of the yoke (see Figure 4-18). Either type may be used as long as it is clean, undamaged, and smooth with no surface defects. After either a flanged or flat washer has been placed, gently raise the tank into place, lining up the valve port and the pin holes with the corresponding structures on the yoke. Tighten the wing nut as securely as you are able to by hand. Open the tank slowly and listen for leaks. If the tank leaks, recheck the holes for proper alignment, tighten the wing nut further,

or use a new washer. One of these maneuvers should resolve the problem.

### Detaching and Reattaching H Tanks

Most remote oxygen sources have a bank of two or more H tanks next to one another (see Figure 4-15). One or more of the tanks is attached to a pressure-reducing valve and a series of lines that pipe the gas to DISS connectors throughout the hospital (see Figure 4-16). First, be sure that no patients are currently receiving oxygen. Then turn the tank off before attempting to remove the valve. Remove the pressure-reducing valve by using a hex wrench to loosen the nut connecting the valve and outlet port, and then remove the valve by hand. Immediately attach the pressure-reducing valve to another full H tank.

### Tank and Line Pressure Gauges, Pressure Manometer, and the Oxygen Flush Valve

Some parts of the anesthetic machine including the tank pressure gauge, line pressure gauge, pressure manometer, and oxygen flush valve require no regular maintenance. A repair professional should check these parts for proper function during an annual maintenance visit or when a problem is suspected.

### Pressure-Reducing Valve

The pressure-reducing valve may need to be adjusted if the line pressure is not correct (40 to 50 psi). Many valves have an external adjusting screw that is turned left or right to increase or decrease the pressure. Consult the owner's manual for specific directions.

### Flow Meters

Although flow meters require no regular maintenance, always treat them gently by not overtightening the valve when turning them off. If excessive hand pressure is necessary to stop oxygen flow, the valve is damaged and needs to be replaced.

Flow meter accuracy can be assessed easily by performing the following test:
- Empty the reservoir bag completely.
- Close the pop-off or overflow valve.
- Occlude the Y-piece or ET tube connector.
- Choose a flow setting that corresponds to the size of the reservoir bag in liters (e.g., 2 L/min for a 2-L bag or 3 L/min for a 3-L bag).

The flow meter is accurate if the bag fills completely in 1 minute.

### Vaporizer

Precision vaporizers must be serviced and maintained regularly to ensure accurate output. Because they are the most complex part of the anesthetic machine, they should be cleaned, tested, and recalibrated by the manufacturer or other qualified personnel every year or as indicated by the manufacturer. It may be necessary to remove the vaporizer from the anesthetic machine and send it away for servicing. Many companies provide a "loaner" replacement during the servicing period.

Precision vaporizers designed for halothane or methoxyflurane should be emptied of anesthetic every 6 to 12 months to help remove the buildup of preservative within the vaporizer. Despite periodic emptying, a halothane precision vaporizer may eventually become clogged with preservative and other residue and should be serviced if the anesthetic is discolored, dial movement is sticky, or the patient can no longer be maintained at a satisfactory anesthetic depth even at high vaporizer settings. Isoflurane and sevoflurane are supplied without a preservative, so periodic emptying is not usually necessary.

### Vaporizer Inlet Port, Outlet Port, Common Gas Outlet, and Fresh Gas Inlet

The vaporizer inlet port, outlet port, common gas outlet, and fresh gas inlet are all components of the low-pressure system. The hose commonly attached to these parts is subject to damage, so check all hoses for holes or defects and replace them as necessary. A routine low-pressure leak test of the machine will usually uncover any damage.

### Unidirectional Valves

Periodically the unidirectional flow valves should be disassembled, cleaned, and inspected to prevent a buildup of water vapor, mucus, and dust from the carbon dioxide absorbent and other material. Valves that are not cleaned may become sticky and adhere to the machine housing, impeding airflow through the circuit or preventing closure.

To clean these valves, unscrew the valve collar and remove the valve parts. Clean the dome, collar, valve, valve seat, and gaskets with alcohol or mild disinfectant like chlorhexidine gluconate. After drying the parts, inspect the valve and valve seat to be sure they are not damaged or warped. An incompetent valve will allow reinhalation of expired carbon dioxide—a serious or potentially fatal complication. Finally, reassemble the valve, being sure that it is properly positioned on the valve seat.

The integrity of the unidirectional valves can be tested as follows:
- Put on a surgical mask.
- Detach the *expiratory* breathing tube from the Y-piece.
- Place the end of the tube up to your mouth with the surgical mask in between, so that the air will pass through the mask.
- Attempt to *inhale* through the tube.
- Now detach the *inspiratory* breathing tube from the Y-piece and place the end up to your mouth as before.
- Attempt to *exhale* through the tube.

Any air movement through either tube indicates an incompetent valve, which must be serviced before the machine is used again.

### Pop-off Valve

Although the pop-off valve does not require regular maintenance, it should be checked for proper operation and adjusted (Procedure 4-1, p. 135) before commencement of any procedure. This should be done at the beginning of every day immediately after the low-pressure system leak test. The valve should also be checked periodically during the anesthetic procedure to maintain optimum gas volume within the circuit.

### Reservoir Bag, Breathing Tubes, and Y-Piece

Between each case, the reservoir bag, the breathing tubes, and the Y-piece or the non-rebreathing system should be removed and cleaned to prevent interpatient transfer of infectious agents that collect inside. Wash each part with a mild soapy disinfectant such as chlorhexidine gluconate, then rinse thoroughly. A surgical scrub brush or bottle brush is useful in cleaning equipment surfaces. Hang these parts in a vertical position until completely dry. Before reattaching them, check each part for integrity. The neck of the bag is especially vulnerable, and holes commonly develop in this location.

### Carbon Dioxide Absorber Canister

The carbon dioxide absorbent must be changed according to the guidelines indicated on p. 120. To change the absorbent, you must first remove the absorber canister and dispose of the absorbent granules. Next disassemble the canister, clean each part with mild soapy disinfectant, and rinse each part thoroughly. Dry each part, check all gaskets for integrity, and reassemble the canister. Fill the clean canister loosely with fresh granules but leave at least 1 cm or ½" of air space at the top to allow unimpeded airflow. Gently shake the canister to distribute the granules evenly. This helps prevent channels from forming in the granules, which could reduce the efficiency of the absorbent. Following reassembly, the canister must be airtight. An airtight seal may be prevented if any granules inadvertently become lodged in a seal or gasket.

Absorbent granules should not be handled without gloves, and dust from the absorbent granules should not be allowed to enter the tubing or hoses of the machine or be breathed in by the technician, because it is irritating to skin and corrosive to mucous membranes. Also, some machines have a water trap below the absorber canister. Any water that collects in this trap should be periodically drained.

### Disinfecting Anesthetic Equipment

Some anesthetic equipment components including ET tubes, laryngoscope blades, and face masks will require more thorough disinfection because this equipment directly contacts the patient's airway or oral cavity. Otherwise, equipment used on a patient harboring certain viruses or bacteria (e.g., feline upper respiratory viruses,

*Bordetella,* and other respiratory pathogens) may transmit infectious agents to the next patient.

First disassemble any parts that can be removed such as laryngoscope blades and mask gaskets; then wash the parts thoroughly with disinfectant, rinse, dry, and reassemble. Unfortunately, there is no ideal agent for disinfection, but several can be used. Chlorhexidine gluconate is relatively harmless to tissues but is not effective against all microorganisms and spores. Glutaraldehyde solutions (2%) are effective against many microorganisms but are stable for only 2 to 4 weeks and so must be periodically replaced. Ethylene oxide gas is an effective sterilizing agent but requires special equipment for safe use. Both glutaraldehyde and ethylene oxide are potentially toxic and may cause severe tissue injury to hospital personnel and to the patient if the anesthetic equipment or supplies are not properly handled. Personnel who work with these chemicals must have special training in their safe use.

All items exposed to any chemical solution should be thoroughly rinsed with water after cleaning and dried before use. Rubber may absorb some chemicals, which, if not completely removed by rinsing, may cause burns on contact with the patient's airway or skin. Ethylene oxide is particularly well absorbed by materials being sterilized, and ET tubes exposed to this substance or glutaraldehyde have been known to cause tracheal necrosis.

Autoclaving causes rubber surfaces to become brittle and crack, and prolonged exposure to disinfectants may cause rubber surfaces to deteriorate. Therefore, damaged masks and reservoir bags, as well as ET tubes that are damaged or have leaking or nonfunctional cuffs, should be discarded.

## KEY POINTS

1. Endotracheal tube placement offers many advantages and increases patient safety for both injectable and inhalant anesthetic techniques.
2. Proper endotracheal tube selection, preparation, placement, and monitoring are of primary importance in any general anesthetic procedure.
3. Anesthetic machines deliver precise amounts of carrier and anesthetic gases, remove carbon dioxide, and permit manual ventilation of anesthetized patients.
4. An anesthetic machine can be used as a source of oxygen in emergencies.
5. Compressed oxygen cylinders store carrier gases under high pressure. Cylinders come in various sizes and capacities, and the gas contained within is identified by the color of the cylinder.
6. The pressure-reducing valve decreases carrier gas pressure to a safe operating pressure of 40 to 50 psi before the gas enters the flow meters.
7. The flow rate of each carrier gas is set by its respective flow meter. Flows are generally expressed in liters per minute. The flow rate indicates to the anesthetist how much gas is being delivered to the patient at any given time.
8. Liquid anesthetic is vaporized and added to the carrier gas in the vaporizer. The combination of anesthetic vapor, oxygen, and nitrous oxide (if present) is called *fresh gas.*
9. Vaporizers may be precision or nonprecision, based on their construction. Precision vaporizers are commonly used for anesthetics with high vapor pressures and provide compensation for variations in temperature, gas flow rate, and back pressure.
10. Precision vaporizers are found outside of the anesthetic circuit (VOC), whereas nonprecision vaporizers are found inside the anesthetic circuit (VIC).
11. The reservoir bag (rebreathing bag) serves as a reservoir to receive and provide gas during the respiratory cycle. It can be used to monitor the animal's ventilation and to deliver oxygen (with or without anesthetic) to the patient by a process called *bagging.*
12. Inhalation and exhalation unidirectional valves permit only one-way flow of gas through the breathing circuit and prevent rebreathing of $CO_2$.
13. Waste gas exits the machine at the pop-off valve and is removed by the scavenging system.
14. Carbon dioxide is removed from a rebreathing circuit by absorbent granules. These granules must be replaced when saturated, or at least every 6 to 8 hours, to prevent rebreathing of carbon dioxide.
15. The pressure manometer measures the pressure of gases within the breathing circuit and the patient's lungs.
16. Anesthetic circuits may be classified as rebreathing (either closed or semiclosed) or non-rebreathing. Rebreathing systems use lower oxygen flow rates but must provide for carbon dioxide absorption. Non-rebreathing systems, such as the Bain system, require relatively high flow rates and are commonly used in small patients.
17. Carrier gas flow rates vary with the period of anesthesia and type of anesthetic circuit used (i.e., rebreathing or non-rebreathing). With a rebreathing system, high flow rates are used during induction, recovery, and changing of anesthetic depth, and lower rates are used during maintenance. When a non-rebreathing system is used, high flow rates are used at all times.
18. Anesthetic equipment requires routine cleaning, inspection, and maintenance.

## PROCEDURE 4-1 Setting the Pop-off or Overflow Valve

### When Using a Semiclosed Rebreathing System

Set the pop-off valve immediately after checking the low-pressure system for leaks.

1. Keep the pop-off valve closed.
2. Occlude the Y-piece with your thumb or hand.
3. Turn the oxygen flow on to the anticipated maximum for that procedure (about 1 to 3 L/min for patients <30 kg, about 3 to 5 L/min for small animal patients ≥30 kg, and 10 L/min for large animal patients).
4. Fill the bag until the pressure manometer indicates a pressure of 25 cm $H_2O$.
5. Open the pop-off valve gradually until the pressure manometer indicates a pressure of 1 to 2 cm $H_2O$.
6. During the anesthetic procedure periodically check that the bag is not collapsed or too full and readjust the pop-off valve accordingly. (The goal is for the bag to remain about three-quarters full at peak expiration.)

### When Using a Non-Rebreathing System

The pop-off (overflow) valve should be open when this system is used, unless positive-pressure manual ventilation is being provided.

## PROCEDURE 4-2 Equipment and Machine Setup Checklist

1. Assemble all needed supplies.
2. If using an active scavenging system, turn on the scavenging system exhaust fan.
3. Identify and weigh the patient.
4. Choose appropriately sized endotracheal tubes based on patient signalment and body weight.
5. Check the endotracheal tubes for integrity, and inflate the endotracheal tube cuffs to check for leaks
6. If a laryngoscope is used, choose an appropriately sized blade and check the light.
7. Choose an appropriate machine (large animal [LA] versus small animal [SA]) based on the patient body weight.
8. Choose an appropriate breathing circuit based on patient body weight.
9. If using a rebreathing system, choose appropriate corrugated breathing tubes (LA, SA, or pediatric) and rebreathing bag based on patient body weight.
10. Assemble the machine(s):
    a. Connect the vaporizer inlet port hose.
    b. Connect the fresh gas inlet hose of the breathing circuit to the vaporizer outlet port or common gas outlet if present.
    c. If using a rebreathing system, attach an appropriately sized rebreathing bag and breathing tubes.
    d. Connect the scavenging system hoses.
11. Check that all compressed gas cylinders are correctly mounted in the yokes (E tanks) or connected to pressure-reducing valves (H tanks).
12. Turn on oxygen supply, check the primary and secondary oxygen supply pressure, and replace empty tanks as necessary.
13. Check the flow meter controls to ensure proper function.
14. Check the amount of anesthetic in the vaporizer, and replenish as necessary. Ensure that the vaporizer and flow meter are off before filling the vaporizer.
15. Rotate the vaporizer dial to ensure smooth function. Turn to "off."
16. Check the carbon dioxide absorbent, and change if necessary.
17. Check the low-pressure system for leaks (see Procedure 13-1).
18. Set the pop-off or overflow valve (see Procedure 4-1).

## REVIEW QUESTIONS

1. When the oxygen tank is half full, the tank pressure gauge will read approximately:
   a. 1100 psi
   b. 2000 psi
   c. 500 psi
   d. 2200 psi

2. Nitrous oxide is present in the tank as a:
   a. Liquid
   b. Gas
   c. Liquid and a gas

3. The amount of oxygen an animal is receiving is indicated by the:
   a. Oxygen tank pressure gauge
   b. Flow meter
   c. Pressure manometer
   d. Vaporizer setting

4. Flow meters that have a ball for reading the gauge should be read from the _____ of the ball.
   a. Top
   b. Bottom
   c. Middle

5. The most commonly recommended ratio for nitrous oxide and oxygen flow rates is:
   a. 50% oxygen and 50% nitrous oxide
   b. 80% oxygen and 20% nitrous oxide
   c. 23% oxygen and 77% nitrous oxide
   d. 77% oxygen and 23% nitrous oxide
   e. 33% oxygen and 67% nitrous oxide

6. The minimum size for the reservoir bag can be calculated as:
   a. 20 mL/kg
   b. 60 mL/kg
   c. 80 mL/kg
   d. 100 mL/kg

7. The flutter valves on an anesthetic machine help:
   a. Control the direction of movement of gases
   b. Maintain a full reservoir bag
   c. Regulate pressure
   d. Vaporize the liquid anesthetic

8. The pop-off valve is part of the anesthetic machine and helps:
   a. Vaporize the liquid anesthetic
   b. Prevent excess gas pressure from building up within the breathing circuit
   c. Keep the oxygen flowing in one direction only
   d. Prevent waste gases from reentering the vaporizer

9. In small animal anesthesia, when the patient is bagged, the pressure manometer reading should not exceed:
   a. 5 cm $H_2O$
   b. 10 cm $H_2O$
   c. 15 cm $H_2O$
   d. 20 cm $H_2O$

10. Rebreathing systems, when used with standard small animal corrugated breathing tubes, are best reserved for animals weighing more than 7 kg.
    True    False

11. Rebreathing is determined primarily by the:
    a. Fresh gas flow
    b. Type of anesthetic
    c. Presence of a reservoir bag
    d. Open or shut pop-off valve

12. Non-rebreathing systems should have maintenance flow rates that are:
    a. Very low (5 to 10 mL/kg/min)
    b. Low (20 to 40 mL/kg/min)
    c. Moderate (50 to 100 mL/kg/min)
    d. Very high (at least 200 mL/kg/min)

13. The negative pressure relief valve is particularly important when:
    a. Nitrous oxide is being used
    b. There is no scavenging system
    c. There is a failure of oxygen flow through the system
    d. The carbon dioxide absorber is no longer functioning

14. The tidal volume of an anesthesized animal is considered to be _____ mL/kg of body weight.
    a. 5
    b. 10
    c. 15
    d. 20

15. A scavenging system is generally attached to:
    a. The pressure-reducing valve
    b. The exhalation unidirectional valve
    c. The pop-off valve
    d. The negative pressure-relief valve

For the following questions, more than one answer may be correct.

16. A reservoir bag that is not moving well may indicate that:
    a. The endotracheal tube is not in the trachea
    b. The animal has a decreased tidal volume
    c. There is a leak around the endotracheal tube
    d. The vaporizer is empty

17. The anesthetist will know when the granules in the carbon dioxide absorber have been depleted because the:
    a. Anesthetist will smell waste carbon dioxide
    b. Granules will be brittle
    c. Granules may change color
    d. Granules may be hard

18. An increase in the depth of anesthesia can be achieved quickly by:
    a. Having high oxygen flow rates
    b. Having high vaporizer settings
    c. Using a closed anesthetic system
    d. Bagging the animal with the precision vaporizer on

19. The concentration of anesthetic delivered from a nonprecision vaporizer may depend on the:
    a. Temperature of the liquid anesthetic
    b. Flow of the carrier gas through the vaporizer
    c. Back pressure
    d. Type of anesthetic in the vaporizer

20. When an anesthetic machine is operating correctly, the pressures in the machine are always:
    a. 40 to 50 psi between the pressure-reducing valve and the flow meters
    b. 15 psi between the flow meters and the breathing circuit
    c. 2200 psi between the compressed gas cylinder and the pressure-reducing valve
    d. 15 psi entering a VOC vaporizer

## SELECTED READINGS

Doherty T, Valverde A: *Manual of equine anesthesia and analgesia*, Ames, Iowa, 2006, Blackwell, pp 175-182.

Hartsfield SM: Airway Management and Ventilation. In Tranquilli WJ, Thurmon JC, Grimm KA, editors: *Lumb & Jones' veterinary anesthesia and analgesia*, ed 4, Ames, Iowa, 2007, Blackwell, pp 495-510.

Hartsfield SM: Equipment. In Thurmon JC, Tranquilli WJ, Benson GJ, editors: *Essentials of small animal anesthesia and analgesia*, Baltimore, 1999, Lippincott Williams & Wilkins, pp 225-269.

Hartsfield SM: Anesthetic Equipment. In Paddleford RR, editor: *Manual of small animal anesthesia*, ed 2, Philadelphia, 1999, Saunders, pp 89-109.

Hartsfield SM: Anesthetic Machines and Breathing Systems. In Tranquilli WJ, Thurmon JC, Grimm KA, editors: *Lumb & Jones' veterinary anesthesia and analgesia*, ed 4, Ames, Iowa, 2007, Blackwell, pp 453-493.

Lerche P, Muir W, Bednarski RM: Rebreathing anesthetic systems in small animal practice, *J Am Vet Med Assoc* 217(4):485-492, 2000.

Muir WW, Hubbell JA, Bednarski RM: *Handbook of veterinary anesthesia*, ed 4, St Louis, 2006, Elsevier, pp. 226-248.

Thurmon JC, Tranquilli WJ, Benson JG: *Essentials of small animal anesthesia and analgesia*, Baltimore, 1999, Lippincott Williams & Wilkins, pp 225-269.

# 5

# Anesthetic Monitoring

**OUTLINE**

Introduction to Monitoring, 139
Stages and Planes of Anesthesia, 140
   *Overview of Anesthetic Stages*
     *and Planes, 141*
   *Finding the Optimum Depth, 142*
Determining Whether or Not the Patient Is
   Safe, 143
   *Indicators of Circulation, 143*
   *Indicators of Oxygenation, 157*

   *Indicators of Ventilation, 163*
   *Indicators of Body Temperature, 169*
Assessment of Anesthetic Depth, 170
   *Reflexes and Other Indicators of*
     *Anesthetic Depth, 170*
   *Judging Anesthetic Depth, 176*
Recording Information during
   Anesthesia, 176

**LEARNING OBJECTIVES**

*After completion of this chapter, the reader will be able to:*
- Explain the principles of anesthetic monitoring, including the reasons for and goals of monitoring.
- List the physical monitoring parameters, and classify each in one of the following categories: (1) vital signs; (2) reflexes; (3) other indicators of anesthetic depth.
- List and describe each of the classic stages and planes of anesthesia.
- List the monitoring parameters used primarily to determine whether or not the patient is safe, and group them according to whether they primarily assess circulation, oxygenation, or ventilation.
- Explain and demonstrate assessment of each of the vital signs, reflexes, and other indicators of anesthetic depth.
- List normal values for each physical monitoring parameter, and identify values that should be reported to the veterinarian-in-charge (VIC).
- Explain setup, operation, care, maintenance, and troubleshooting of an esophageal stethoscope, electrocardiograph, Doppler monitor, oscillometric blood pressure monitor, pulse oximeter, apnea monitor, and capnograph.
- Interpret output and data from an esophageal stethoscope, electrocardiograph, Doppler monitor, oscillometric blood pressure monitor, pulse oximeter, apnea monitor, and capnograph.
- Describe how to determine the blood pressure using a Doppler monitor, oscillometric blood pressure monitor, or arterial catheter and transducer.
- Identify the following rhythms on an electrocardiographic tracing: normal sinus rhythm (NSR); sinus arrhythmia (SA); sinus bradycardia and tachycardia; first-, second-, and third-degree atrioventricular (AV) heart block; supraventricular premature complexes (SPCs) and ventricular premature complexes (VPCs); supraventricular and ventricular tachycardia; atrial and ventricular fibrillation; and QRS and T-wave configuration changes.
- Identify machine-generated data that should be reported to the VIC.
- Identify abnormal monitoring parameters, and list common causes of abnormal monitoring parameters.
- Use monitoring parameters to determine anesthetic depth.
- Explain adverse consequences of hypothermia, and identify strategies to prevent hypothermia.

**KEY TERMS**

Apnea monitor
Atelectasis
Blood gas analysis
Blood pressure
Calculated oxygen
  content
Capnogram
Capnograph
Cardiac arrhythmias
Central venous
  pressure
Circulation
Diastolic blood
  pressure
Doppler blood flow
  detector
Esophageal stethoscope
Flaccid
Icterus
Mean arterial pressure
Monitor
Oscillometer
Oxygenation
Partial pressure of
  oxygen
Percent oxygen
  saturation
Pressure transducer
Pulmonary
  thromboembolism
Pulse oximeter
Respiration
Respirometer
Sphygmomanometer
Systolic blood pressure
Tachypnea
Ventilation

## INTRODUCTION TO MONITORING

The word **monitor** comes from the Latin word *monere*, which means "to warn." This is a fitting definition for this aspect of anesthesia, as the main purpose of monitoring is to warn the anesthetist of changes in anesthetic depth and patient condition in enough time to permit intervention before they become dangerous.

Throughout any anesthetic event, a delicate balance must be maintained. There must be sufficient central nervous system (CNS) depression, analgesia, muscle relaxation, and immobility for the procedure to be performed, yet cardiopulmonary function must not be dangerously compromised. Monitoring is therefore necessary for two reasons. First, it is necessary to keep the patient safe; and second, it is necessary to regulate anesthetic depth. To keep the patient safe, the anesthetist must monitor the patient at many points in time to ensure that vital signs remain within acceptable limits. Failure to monitor and maintain vital signs within acceptable limits may lead to devastating consequences such as permanent brain damage or even death. The anesthetist also must maintain the animal at an appropriate anesthetic depth (i.e., one that is neither too light nor too deep) by monitoring reflexes and other indicators. Failure to maintain an adequate depth of anesthesia may result in perception of pain and premature arousal from anesthesia. On the other hand, maintaining an animal at an excessive depth of anesthesia may lead to anesthetic overdose or slow recovery.

> **TECHNICIAN NOTE** Monitoring is necessary for two reasons. First, it is necessary to keep the patient safe; and second, it is necessary to regulate anesthetic depth.

When monitoring, the anesthetist must observe various parameters that can be separated into three classifications: (1) vital signs, (2) reflexes, and (3) other indicators of anesthetic depth. Although information from all these monitoring parameters is used to determine the depth of anesthesia and patient well-being, some are more helpful in determining anesthetic depth, and others are more helpful in determining whether the patient is safe.

The term *vital signs* refers to those variables that indicate the response of the animal's homeostatic mechanisms to anesthesia, including heart rate (HR), heart rhythm, respiratory rate (RR) and depth, mucous membrane color, capillary refill time (CRT), pulse strength, **blood pressure** (BP), and temperature. The patient's vital signs indicate how well the patient is maintaining basic circulatory and respiratory function during anesthesia and therefore are the best indicators of patient well-being. Although vital signs also generally reflect the anesthetic stage and plane, they are not reliable indicators of anesthetic depth.

The term *reflex* refers to an involuntary response to a stimulus (such as an eye blink in response to touching the skin at the corner of the eye or a kick in response to a tap on the patellar tendon). Reflexes used in veterinary anesthesia include the palpebral, corneal, pedal, swallowing, and laryngeal reflexes as well as the pupillary light reflex (PLR). *Other indicators of anesthetic depth* include spontaneous movement, eye position, pupil size, muscle tone, nystagmus, salivary and lacrimal secretions, and response to surgical stimulation. Both reflexes and other indicators are useful for determining anesthetic depth but are not useful for assessing cardiopulmonary function or homeostasis.

In 1995 the American College of Veterinary Anesthesiologists (ACVA) published guidelines for anesthetic monitoring in the *Journal of the American Veterinary Medical Association,* intended to maximize quality of care and assist veterinary professionals in making sound anesthetic monitoring decisions. In 2009 these guidelines were substantially updated to reflect important changes in the profession (see Appendix A). In this document, the ACVA indicates that, when compared with the status of the profession at the time of the original publication of these guidelines, the general standard of care has increased, client expectations are higher, and equipment is more widely available that permits earlier detection of adverse effects such as hypotension, hypoxemia, and severe hypercapnia. These changes supported a shift from a model centered on minimizing the risk of anesthetic deaths to one centered on decreasing anesthetic complications of all types. In the revised document the ACVA offers recommendations in each of the following categories:
- Assessment of circulation, oxygenation, ventilation, and body temperature
- Monitoring of patients under, and recovering from, neuromuscular blockade
- Record-keeping
- Monitoring during the recovery period
- Recommendations regarding personnel
- Monitoring sedated patients

The focus of these recommendations is assessment of vital signs, and therefore the recommendations address the problem of keeping the patient safe. Determining the depth of anesthesia is accomplished primarily by monitoring reflexes and other indicators of depth listed previously and is covered later in this chapter.

For monitoring to be effective, the patient must be evaluated frequently during any anesthetic procedure. Although continuous monitoring of any anesthetized patient by a veterinary technician is ideal, it is not practical in many veterinary clinics. Therefore, in lieu of continuous monitoring of all patients, the ACVA recommends that class P1 and P2 patients should be monitored at least once every 5 minutes. In contrast, class P3, P4, and P5 patients, as well as horses receiving inhalant anesthetics or that have been anesthetized for more than 45 minutes, should be monitored continuously.

Anesthetic monitoring is based on the principle that in the average patient, each monitoring parameter is expected to show a predictable response at any given anesthetic depth. For instance, swallowing and pedal reflexes are expected to be present when the patient's anesthesia level is too light but are absent during surgical anesthesia. Muscle tone, HR, and RR are expected to be high during light anesthesia and to gradually decrease as anesthetic depth increases. Eyes are in a central position during light anesthesia, generally rotate into a ventromedial position during surgical anesthesia, and return to a central position as anesthetic depth increases.

Interpretation of these indicators is quite challenging in practice, however, because a number of factors including drugs, disease, and individual variation may alter expected responses, producing contradictory evidence. In other words, a patient may show some signs that indicate one stage of anesthesia and other signs that indicate another. For instance, a dog that received an opioid agonist may have a smaller than expected pupil size while in surgical anesthesia. A patient with preexisting heart failure may have a higher HR than expected at a given depth. A patient given an alpha$_2$-agonist such as dexmedetomidine may have significant hypotension and bradycardia, whereas another given atropine may have tachycardia, even though both are in the same plane. Therefore is it important to observe multiple parameters and make decisions based on the predominant evidence. This requires careful observation, rapid decision-making, and safe and appropriate action. (See p. 177 for examples of depth assessment.)

## STAGES AND PLANES OF ANESTHESIA

During World War I, Arthur Guedel, MD, a U.S. army doctor, developed a classification system of stages and planes of anesthesia based on observation of patient responses to the inhalant anesthetic diethyl ether. Under this system, general anesthesia was divided into four stages (I to IV), and stage III was subdivided into four planes (1 to 4) (Figure 5-1). Development of this system gave anesthetists a basis to accurately assess depth of anesthesia based on detailed observation. Although responses to modern general anesthetics differ somewhat from responses to ether, this system is still used today in a slightly altered form.

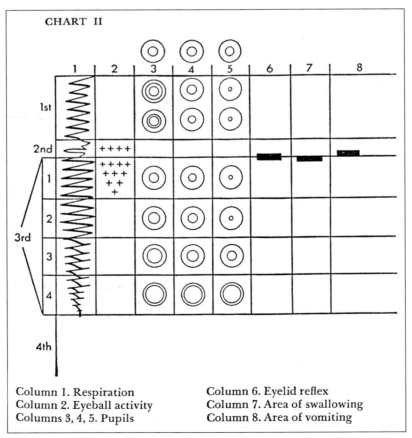

Column 1. Respiration
Column 2. Eyeball activity
Columns 3, 4, 5. Pupils
Column 6. Eyelid reflex
Column 7. Area of swallowing
Column 8. Area of vomiting

**FIGURE 5-1**   Guedel's stages and planes of anesthesia. (From Arthur E. Guedel Commemorative Issue of the California Society of Anesthesiologists Bulletin, 1975. Used with permission of the Guedel Anesthesia Center, Health Sciences Library, California Pacific Medical Center.)

| TABLE 5-1 | Expected Responses of Selected Monitoring Parameters | | |
|---|---|---|---|
| Stage of Anesthesia | Behavior | Respiration | Cardiovascular Function |
| I | Disorientation, struggling, fear | Respiratory rate increased; dogs may pant | Heart rate increased |
| II Excitement stage | Excitement: reflex struggling, vocalization, paddling, chewing | Irregular, may hold breath or hyperventilate | Heart rate often increased |
| III/Plane 1 Light anesthesia | Unconscious | Regular; rate—high normal | Pulse strong; heart rate high normal |
| III/Plane 2 Medium (surgical) anesthesia | | Regular (may be shallow); rate—moderate | Heart rate moderate |
| III/Plane 3 Deep anesthesia | | Shallow; rate—low or below normal | Heart rate low normal; capillary refill time (CRT) increased; pulse less strong |
| III/Plane 4 | | Jerky | Heart rate below normal; prolonged CRT; pale mucous membranes |
| IV | Moribund | Apnea | Cardiovascular collapse |

## Overview of Anesthetic Stages and Planes

As an induction agent is given, the patient passes through stage I; and as it loses consciousness, it enters stage II. The loss of consciousness marks the border between these stages. As the anesthetic depth increases, the patient then enters stage III, the period of surgical anesthesia. The loss of spontaneous muscle movement marks the border between stages II and III. If the depth continues to increase, the patient will enter stage IV. The loss of all reflexes, widely dilated, unresponsive pupils, **flaccid** muscle tone, and cardiopulmonary collapse mark this stage, which, if not aggressively managed, is closely followed by cardiopulmonary arrest and death of the patient. As the animal passes through each stage, there is a progressive decrease in pain perception, motor coordination, consciousness, reflex responses, muscle tone, and eventually cardiopulmonary function. Expected responses of selected monitoring parameters during each stage and plane are summarized in Table 5-1.

### TECHNICIAN NOTE

- Loss of consciousness marks the border between stages I and II.
- Loss of spontaneous muscle movement marks the border between stages II and III.
- Loss of all reflexes, widely dilated pupils, flaccid muscle tone, and cardiopulmonary collapse mark stage IV.

## Stage I—Period of Voluntary Movement

During stage I, the patient begins to lose consciousness. This stage is usually characterized by fear, excitement, disorientation, and struggling. The HR and RR increase, and the patient may pant, urinate, or defecate. A patient in stage I is typically difficult to handle. Near the end of stage I, the patient loses the ability to stand and becomes recumbent.

## Stage II—Period of Involuntary Movement

During stage II, also known as the *excitement stage,* the patient loses voluntary control and breathing becomes irregular. This stage is usually characterized by involuntary reactions in the form of vocalizing, struggling, or paddling. The HR and RR are often elevated, pupils are dilated, muscle tone is marked, and reflexes are present and in fact may appear exaggerated. Although animals in stage II may appear to be "fighting" the anesthesia, the actions are not under conscious control. Rather, they are thought to occur because the anesthetic selectively depresses neurons in the brain and spinal cord that normally inhibit and control the function of motor neurons. Stage II ends when the animal shows signs of muscle relaxation, slower RR, and decreased reflex activity.

This stage is unpleasant and potentially hazardous for both the animal and hospital personnel. There is a risk of epinephrine release and the possibility of cardiac arrhythmias or arrest. The struggling patient may injure itself, the restrainer, or the anesthetist. Therefore it is desirable to plan the procedure such that the patient passes through this stage as quickly as possible, by additional administration of anesthetic until stage III is reached.

Premedicated animals in which anesthesia is rapidly induced with an injectable anesthetic often appear to pass from consciousness directly to stage III. Although these patients pass through stages I and II, they are not clinically evident. In contrast, stages I and II are often very pronounced in animals in which anesthesia is mask or chamber induced without premedication, sometimes creating a challenging and unpleasant situation for the anesthetist and patient.

- Stage III, plane 1 is inadequate to perform surgery.
- Stage III, plane 2 is suitable for most surgical procedures.
- Stage III, plane 3 is considered to be excessively deep for most surgical procedures.
- Stage III, plane 4 indicates anesthetic overdose.

## Stage III—Period of Surgical Anesthesia

During stage III, which is subdivided into four planes, the patient is unconscious and progresses gradually from light to deep surgical anesthesia. It is characterized by progressive muscle relaxation, decreasing HR and RR, and loss of reflexes. The pupils gradually dilate, tear production decreases, and the PLR is lost. The increase in HR, BP, and RR seen in response to surgical stimulation during light anesthesia is also gradually lost.

In plane 1, the respiratory pattern becomes regular, and involuntary limb movements cease. The eyeballs often start to rotate ventrally, the pupils may become partially constricted, and the pupillary response to bright light is diminished. The gagging and swallowing reflexes are depressed such that an endotracheal tube may be successfully passed, allowing the patient to be connected to a gas anesthetic machine. Other reflexes (such as the pedal and palpebral reflexes) are present; however, responses are less brisk than in stage II. Although unconscious, the patient will not tolerate surgical procedures at this light plane of anesthesia and will move and exhibit increased HR, RR and respiratory depth, and BP, in response to painful stimuli. This plane is inadequate for surgery.

Plane 2 is suitable for most surgical procedures. Surgical stimulation may evoke a mildly increased HR, or RR, but the patient remains unconscious and immobile. The PLR is sluggish, and the pupil size is moderate. The respirations are regular but shallow, and the RR, HR, and BP are mildly decreased. The skeletal muscle tone is more relaxed, pedal and swallowing reflexes are absent, and laryngeal and palpebral reflexes are diminished or lost. So loss of the pedal and swallowing reflexes marks entry into plane 2, and ventromedial eye rotation also generally occurs at this time.

In plane 3, the patient is deeply anesthetized. Significant depression of circulation and respiration is often present, and for this reason plane 3 is considered to be excessively deep for most surgical procedures. In the dog or cat, the HR and RR are low and the tidal volume ($V_T$) is decreased. Manual or mechanical ventilation may be necessary in some small animal patients and most large animal patients. HR is also notably reduced even in the presence of surgical stimulation. Pulse strength may be reduced because of a fall in BP. The CRT may be increased to 1.5 to 2 seconds. The PLR is poor throughout this plane and may be absent. The eyeballs are often central, and the pupils are moderately dilated. Reflex activity is often

totally absent. Skeletal muscle tone is so relaxed that no resistance occurs when the mouth is opened (i.e., jaw tone is flaccid or slack).

Plane 4 is the period of early anesthetic overdose. It is characterized by abdominal breathing, which occurs as the thoracic muscles progressively become less active and abdominal muscles are increasingly responsible for ventilation. Abdominal breathing is recognized by a "rocking" motion, in which the abdomen expands and contracts in an attempt to move air into and out of the lungs. Plane 4 is also characterized by fully dilated pupils and the absence of all reflexes. The eyes may be dry because of an absence of lacrimal secretions. Muscle tone is flaccid. The cardiovascular system is markedly depressed, with a dramatic drop in HR and BP, accompanied by pale mucous membranes and a prolonged CRT. The patient in this plane is too deeply anesthetized and is in danger of respiratory and cardiac arrest.

*TECHNICIAN NOTE* Many authors now divide stage III into three planes:
- *Light surgical anesthesia* indicates an inadequate depth.
- *Medium surgical anesthesia* indicates the optimum depth for most procedures.
- *Deep surgical anesthesia* indicates an excessive depth.

## Stage IV—Stage of Anesthetic Overdose

If anesthetic depth is increased past stage III, plane 4, the animal enters stage IV anesthesia. At this stage there is a cessation of respiration, which may be followed by circulatory collapse and death. Immediate resuscitation is necessary to save the patient's life.

This system can be somewhat confusing, because not all anesthetic agents produce signs that fit into these classic stages and planes. Consequently, many authors now divide stage III into three planes called *light, medium,* and *deep surgical anesthesia,* with light surgical anesthesia indicating an inadequate depth, medium surgical anesthesia indicating the optimum depth for most procedures, and deep surgical anesthesia indicating an excessive depth. These levels correspond to the classic planes as follows: light roughly corresponds to stage III, plane 1; medium to stage III, plane 2 and early plane 3; and deep to stage III, later in plane 3, and plane 4.

## Finding the Optimum Depth

So what is the optimum depth of anesthesia? This question has no easy answer, because what is "optimum" differs for every patient depending on the procedure it is undergoing and the interaction of a complex set of factors. The anesthetist may be guided in discovering an optimum depth for each patient, however, by seeing that the objectives of surgical anesthesia are fulfilled.

The objectives of surgical anesthesia are that the patient does not move, is not aware, does not feel pain, and has no memory of the procedure afterward. At the same time, the anesthetist must avoid excessive anesthetic depth, which will result in a dangerous depression of the cardiovascular and respiratory systems.

Studies in human patients suggest that with increasing depth of anesthesia, most patients lose memory of the procedure first, awareness during the procedure second, unconscious movement in response to a painful stimulus third, and an increase in BP, HR, or RR in response to a painful stimulus fourth. So although a patient that moves in response to a painful stimulus such as a surgical incision (in light surgical anesthesia) may or may not feel pain depending on the anesthetic depth, these studies support the assumption that a patient that does not move in response to a painful stimulus (in medium surgical anesthesia) is not aware, does not perceive pain, and will have no memory of the procedure afterward. Therefore a lack of unconscious movement is evidence of sufficient depth to fulfill the objectives of surgical anesthesia. Although a lack of increase in the HR, RR, or BP in response to a painful stimulus is further evidence that these objectives are fulfilled, some patients will have adverse cardiopulmonary effects that prevent this depth from being maintained. Thus some reflex increase in these vital signs is not uncommon, and is even expected when the patient is at optimal depth.

Maintaining the delicate balance required to fulfill the objectives of surgical anesthesia can be challenging. There are times in any procedure that even the experienced anesthetist will feel unsure. When in doubt, it is usually safer to err on the side of caution and to maintain the patient at the least depth required to fulfill the objectives. In any case, gauging anesthetic depth is a dynamic process that requires frequent reassessment with subsequent adjustments in the rate of anesthetic administration throughout the procedure.

> *TECHNICIAN NOTE* The objectives of surgical anesthesia are that the patient does not move, is not aware, does not feel pain, has no memory of the procedure afterward, and does not have dangerous depression of the cardiovascular and respiratory systems.

## DETERMINING WHETHER OR NOT THE PATIENT IS SAFE

Determining whether or not the patient is safe during any anesthetic procedure is accomplished primarily by assessing vital signs. Vital signs may be assessed either by physical means (i.e., touch, hearing, and vision) or through the use of various instrumentation and machines such as an electrocardiograph, BP monitor, **capnograph, Doppler blood flow detector,** or **pulse oximeter.** These vital signs can be grouped according to whether they reflect

**circulation** (HR and heart rhythm, pulse strength, CRT, mucous membrane color, and BP); **oxygenation** (mucous membrane color, hemoglobin saturation, measurement of inspired oxygen, measurement of arterial blood oxygen [$Pao_2$]; or **ventilation** (RR and respiratory depth, breath sounds, end-expired $CO_2$ levels, arterial carbon dioxide [$Paco_2$], and blood pH).

Although a competent technician can safely monitor most patients without the use of specialized instruments, the use of monitoring devices may be of significant benefit. Instruments offer continuous monitoring, whereas the technician in a busy veterinary practice is seldom able to sit with the patient constantly. Instruments also allow precise measurement of variables that are impossible to determine by observation alone, such as BP and the percent oxygen saturation of the hemoglobin.

On the other hand, monitoring instruments are subject to malfunction, failure, and artifacts and are not able to completely capture the full range of information that is required for safe and effective monitoring. No matter how sophisticated, expensive, convenient, or complex, instruments cannot replace a skilled and conscientious anesthetist.

This section describes indicators of circulation, oxygenation, and ventilation, including vital signs, and instruments that can be used to monitor the following variables: BP (Doppler blood flow detector, **oscillometer,** and transducer with arterial line), **central venous pressure** (CVP) (manometer), heart rhythm (electrocardiograph), HR **(esophageal stethoscope),** $Pao_2$ and $Paco_2$ (blood gases), oxygen saturation (pulse oximeter), and expired carbon dioxide (capnograph). Note that electrocardiographs, BP monitors, and pulse oximeters also measure HR, and the capnograph also measures RR.

### Indicators of Circulation

The objective of the ACVA monitoring guidelines for circulation is "to ensure adequate circulatory function." To meet this objective, the ACVA makes the following recommendations:

"Continuous awareness of heart rate and rhythm during anesthesia, along with gross assessment of peripheral perfusion (pulse quality, [mucous membrane] color and CRT) are mandatory. Arterial blood pressure and ECG should also be monitored. There may be some situations where these may be temporarily impractical, e.g., movement of an anesthetized patient to a different area of the hospital."

### Heart Rate

HR may be physically assessed by palpation of the apical pulse through the thoracic wall, palpation of a peripheral pulse, or auscultation with a stethoscope or with the assistance of an esophageal stethoscope, which is a device that amplifies the heart sounds. It may be measured mechanically with an electrocardiograph, a BP monitor (Doppler blood flow detector or oscillometric monitor), or an

| TABLE 5-2 | **Normal Vital Signs during Anesthesia** | | | |
|---|---|---|---|---|
| Species | Heart Rate (bpm) | Heart Rhythm | Respiratory Rate (breaths/min), $V_T$, and Effort* | Body Temperature (° F [° C]) |
| Dog | 60-150[†] | NSR or SA | 8-20 | 97°-100° F (36.1°-37.8° C) |
| Report to VIC if: | <60 or >140 (lg) <70 or >160 (sm) | Any other rhythm is present | <6 or >20 | >103.5° F (39.7° C) or <97° F (36.1° C) |
| Cat | 120-180 | NSR | 8-20 | 97°-100° F (36.1°-37.8° C) |
| Report to VIC if: | <100 or >200 | Any other rhythm is present | <6 or >20 | >103.5° F (39.7° C) or <97° F (36.1° C) |
| Horse | 28-40 | NSR, SA, or first- or second-degree AV heart block | 6-12 | 97° -100° F (36.1°-37.8° C) |
| Report to VIC if: | <25 or >60 | Any other rhythm is present | <6 or >20 | >101.5° F (38.6° C) or <97° F (36.1° C) |
| Cattle | 50-80 | NSR or SA | 6-12, although rapid shallow breathing is very common | 97°-100° F (36.1°-37.8° C) |
| Report to VIC if: | <40 or >100 | Any other rhythm is present | <6 or >20 | >103.5° F (39.7° C) or <97° F (36.1° C) |

*AV*, Atrioventricular; *lg*, large; *NSR*, normal sinus rhythm; *SA*, sinus arrhythmia; *sm*, small; *VIC*, veterinarian-in-charge; $V_T$, tidal volume.
*Respiratory effort should be normal, and $V_T$ is typically decreased approximately 25%. Any increase in effort or >25% decrease in $V_T$ should be reported to the VIC.
†Owing to the extreme variability of size, large dogs tend to have lower rates, whereas small dogs and puppies have higher rates.

intraarterial line attached to a transducer. Most mechanical monitors generate an audible beep, flashing light, or other visual indicator to make each heartbeat detectable from a distance. Many also show a digital readout of the HR in beats per minute (bpm). Some monitors can be adjusted to sound an alarm when the HR moves above or below limits set by the anesthetist.

When assessing the HR with a stethoscope during anesthesia, be aware that the heartbeat can be harder to hear than when the patient is awake for two reasons: first, because of a decreased strength of contraction often associated with anesthesia, and second, because the heart will gravitate to the lowest aspect of the thoracic cavity, making the heartbeat hard to hear if the stethoscope is placed in the customary locations. For instance, if the patient is in dorsal recumbency, as are many anesthetized patients, the heartbeat is often difficult to hear at all through the chest wall, especially in cats or obese patients. If the patient is lying in lateral recumbency, the heartbeat can generally be heard but is often audible only on the dependent side because of the effect of gravity on the position of the heart.

HRs are typically decreased in anesthetized animals owing to the depressant effect of most anesthetics. Alpha$_2$-agonists and opioids are particularly likely to cause bradycardia. Some drugs (e.g., anticholinergics, cyclohexamines) have the opposite effect and can elevate HRs. The minimum acceptable, maximum acceptable, and typical HRs for anesthetized patients are listed in Table 5-2. Bradycardia is commonly caused by excessive anesthetic depth or adverse effects of drugs, and common causes of tachycardia are inadequate anesthetic depth, pain during light surgical anesthesia, hypotension, blood loss, shock, hypoxemia, and hypercapnia.

### Heart Rhythm

The heart rhythm is assessed along with the HR. During anesthesia, normal sinus rhythm (NSR) is the most common rhythm in normal dogs, cats, and other small animals. Some normal dogs, however, especially if young and fit, have an SA that can at times be quite pronounced and that can easily be mistaken for a cardiac arrhythmia. The anesthetist can usually differentiate SA from an abnormal rhythm by looking for the cyclic decrease in rate during expiration and increase in rate during inspiration characteristic of SA. Large animals typically have an NSR but may also have an SA. First- or second-degree block is also considered to be normal in the athletic horse, provided that when the patient is conscious the rhythm returns to SA or NSR after gentle exercise or stimulation.

The anesthetist can generally develop a high degree of suspicion of a cardiac arrhythmia by its irregular sound, but some, such as first-degree heart block, defy detection this way. The only certain way to absolutely identify this and other abnormal rhythms is by using an electrocardiographic monitor, which reveals the electrical activity

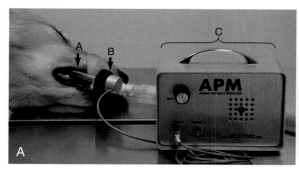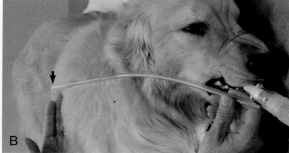

**FIGURE 5-2**   **A,** Esophageal stethoscope—*A,* catheter; *B,* sensor; *C,* base unit. **B,** Measurement of the catheter to the level of the fifth rib or the caudal border of the scapula *(arrow).*

of the heart. Cardiac arrhythmias are not uncommon during anesthesia and are commonly caused by anticholinergics, alpha$_2$-agonists, barbiturates, and cyclohexamines, but they are also caused by a number of states and disease conditions including hypoxia, hypercarbia, heart disease, trauma, and gastric dilatation–volvulus. Disturbances in cardiac rhythm should always be brought to the attention of the veterinarian for assessment because benign arrhythmias can quickly degenerate into dangerous rhythms if not recognized and managed.

> *TECHNICIAN NOTE* Disturbances in cardiac rhythm should always be brought to the attention of the veterinarian for assessment because benign arrhythmias can quickly degenerate into dangerous rhythms if not recognized and managed.

### Instruments used to Monitor Heart Rate and Rhythm

**Esophageal stethoscope.** An esophageal stethoscope (Figure 5-2) permits auscultation of the heart from a distance even when the patient's chest is covered with surgical drapes and conventional auscultation is difficult. The esophageal stethoscope consists of a thin, flexible catheter attached to an audio monitor that electronically amplifies the heart sounds. The catheters come in various sizes (small, medium, and large) to fit small animal patients of varying sizes. There are multiple holes near the patient end, which is covered with a plastic sheath. The opposite end has a hole that fits into a sensor, which in turn transfers the heart sounds to the monitor. A conventional stethoscope tube can also be attached to the catheter as an alternative.

For an esophageal stethoscope to be used, the catheter tube is lubricated with a small amount of water or lubricating jelly and the patient end is inserted through the oral cavity into the patient's esophagus to about the level of the fifth rib. The position of the catheter is changed a little at a time, and the volume on the monitor is adjusted until the heartbeat is audible. Although it does not give quantitative information, this relatively simple, reliable, and inexpensive instrument allows the anesthetist or surgeon to easily hear the heart sounds anywhere in the surgical suite.

Esophageal stethoscopes require relatively little maintenance. Catheters must be cleaned with chlorhexidine or other disinfectant after each use. When cleansing, do not immerse the catheter or allow water to enter the hole in the end of the catheter. Some audio monitors use nonrechargeable batteries, which periodically must be changed.

**Electrocardiography.** **Cardiac arrhythmias** occur commonly in anesthetized animals. The term *cardiac arrhythmia* (also known as *cardiac dysrhythmia*) may be defined as any pattern of cardiac electrical activity that differs from that of the healthy awake animal. Arrhythmias vary in significance from innocuous to life-threatening depending on the cause and the patient's general condition. Therefore the anesthetist must assess the patient's heart rhythm at many points during any anesthetic procedure to keep the patient safe.

Only a veterinarian can make an electrocardiographic diagnosis, but as a monitor the technician must be able to differentiate normal from abnormal, and dangerous from nondangerous rhythms. Although an alert anesthetist may strongly suspect an arrhythmia based on careful auscultation and palpation of the pulse, electrocardiography is the only monitoring tool that allows definitive identification of the heart rhythm. Electrocardiography not only is used to monitor anesthetized animals, but is also used to guide treatment of cardiac arrest (see p. 341 in Chapter 12).

The normal electrocardiographic tracing (electrocardiogram [ECG]) is a graphic representation of the electrical activity of the heart as it travels through the cardiac conduction system (Figure 5-3) and heart muscle. The wave of electrical activity starts in the sinoatrial node and travels through the internodal tracts, causing atrial contraction. Next it is conducted to the atrioventricular (AV) node, where it briefly slows down to allow the ventricles to fill with blood. It then travels to the ventricles via the bundle of His, bundle branches, and Purkinje fibers, causing ventricular contraction. Although the precise appearance of the ECG varies according to the lead, the patient position, the species, and other factors, it always has the same general pattern of waveforms, intervals, and segments

(Figure 5-4). Box 5-1 reviews electrode placement for both small animal and large animal patients.

> **TECHNICIAN NOTE**    Only a veterinarian can make an electrocardiographic diagnosis, but as a monitor the technician must be able to differentiate normal from abnormal, and dangerous from nondangerous rhythms.

The P wave, the first waveform, represents contraction of the atria. It is normally small, rounded, and positive and is often "double-humped" (also known as *bifid*) in adult large animals. It is separated from the QRS complex by the PR interval, which represents the time required for the impulse to move from the sinoatrial node to the Purkinje fibers. In normal patients, the PR interval must be within a range of 0.6 to 0.13 seconds in a dog, 0.05 to 0.09 seconds in a cat, and 0.22 to 0.56 seconds in a horse (see Figure 5-4). The QRS complex represents contraction of the ventricles and follows the PR interval. It is the largest waveform, is pointed (peaked), and is primarily positive in small animals when lead II is used and negative in large animals when the base apex lead is used. The T wave, which follows the QRS complex, represents repolarization of the ventricles in preparation for the next contraction. It is variable in appearance but is normally no more than one fourth the size of the QRS complex.

Although detailed interpretation of ECGs is complex and beyond the scope of this text, the anesthetist should be familiar with the following rhythms, which are commonly encountered in anesthetized patients.

- *Normal sinus rhythm.* NSR is a regular rhythm in which the HR is normal and the distance between each heartbeat (each QRS complex) is approximately equal (Figure 5-5). NSR is normal in anesthetized dogs, cats, horses, and cattle.
- *Sinus arrhythmia.* SA is a cyclic change in the HR coordinated with respirations, in which the HR decreases (recognized by an increased distance between QRS complexes) during expiration and increases (recognized by a decreased distance between QRS complexes) during inspiration (Figure 5-6). SA is normal in dogs, especially if young and healthy, is normal in horses and cattle, but is not normal in cats.
- *Sinus bradycardia.* Sinus bradycardia (an abnormally slow HR) is common during anesthesia and has a variety of causes including excessive anesthetic depth and drug reactions (see Chapter 12, p. 337). Treatment, if necessary, may include administration of appropriate reversal agents or anticholinergics.

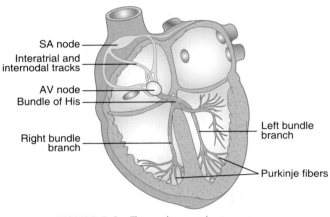

**FIGURE 5-3**    The cardiac conduction system.

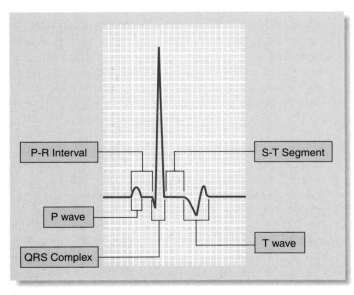

A

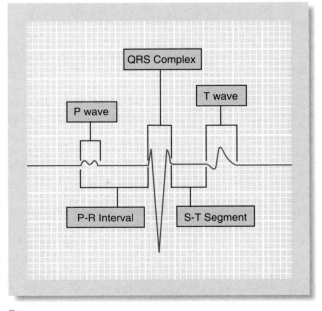

B

**FIGURE 5-4**    Appearance of the normal waveforms, intervals, and segments in **A**, the dog and **B**, the horse.

## BOX 5-1 Standard Electrode Placement for Electrocardiography

### General Principles
- The patient should be on a nonconductive surface.
- Wet the skin-electrode contact points with a small amount of alcohol or saline.

### Small Animals (Figure 1)
- Place the patient in right lateral recumbency if obtaining a full diagnostic electrocardiogram (ECG).
- If monitoring patients undergoing procedures, position does not matter.
- Place the electrodes on the following locations:
  - White electrode on right forelimb
  - Black electrode on left forelimb
  - Green electrode on right hind limb
  - Red electrode on left hind limb
  - Forelimb electrodes should be placed slightly proximal to the elbows
  - Rear limb electrodes should be placed slightly proximal to the knees

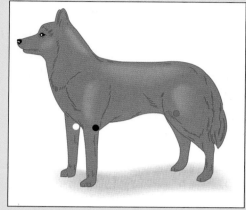

**FIGURE 1**

### Large Animals (Figure 2)
- Obtain ECG before anesthesia with the patient in a standing position, as long as the patient is cooperative.
- If monitoring for patients undergoing procedures, position does not matter.
- Place the electrodes on the following locations:
  - White electrode on the right jugular furrow
  - Black electrode on the right jugular furrow a few centimeters away from the white electrode

- Red electrode at the apex of the heart (left lateral thorax)
  - Monitor ECG using lead II

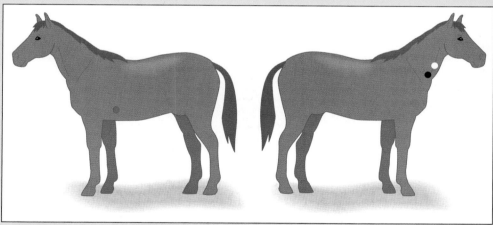

**FIGURE 2**

- *Sinus tachycardia.* Sinus tachycardia (an abnormally fast HR) is less common than bradycardia during anesthesia. It has a variety of causes including inadequate anesthetic depth, drug reactions, and surgical stimulation (see Chapter 12, p. 336). Treatment depends on the underlying cause.
- *AV heart block.* AV heart block involves a delay or interruption in conduction of the electrical impulse through the AV node. There are three types

(first-degree, second-degree, and third-degree), which vary in appearance, but all involve a change in the relationship between the P wave and QRS complex (in other words, a changed PR interval).
- *First-degree AV block* is recognized by a prolonged PR interval (Figure 5-7). It is often abnormal but is seen in normal resting horses.
- *Second-degree AV block* appears as occasional missing QRS complexes. In other words, not all

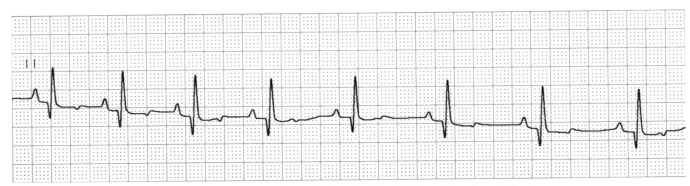

**FIGURE 5-5**    Normal sinus rhythm (dog—lead II; 50 mm/sec; 1 cm/mV).

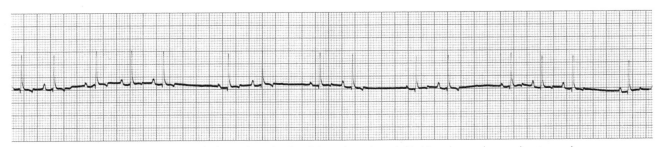

**FIGURE 5-6**    Sinus arrhythmia (dog—lead II; 25 mm/sec; 1 cm/mV). Note the regular acceleration and slowing of the heart rate. This waxing and waning correlate with breathing.

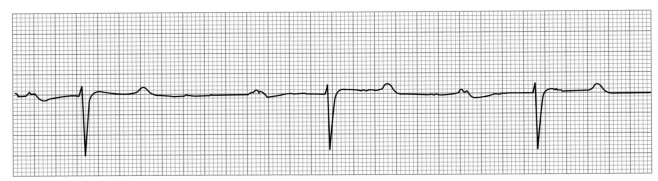

**FIGURE 5-7**    First-degree atrioventricular heart block (horse—base apex lead; 25 mm/sec; 1 cm/mV). This tracing was recorded at 25 mm/sec. Therefore each box = 0.04 seconds. Note the wide PR interval at approximately 0.72 seconds (normal 0.22 to 0.56 seconds).

P waves are followed by QRS complexes (Figure 5-8). Like first-degree AV block, it is often abnormal but is also seen in normal resting horses as long as no more than one beat is skipped in a row, and it resolves with exercise or stimulation. It decreases cardiac output but may or may not require treatment, depending on how severe it is. Both first- and second-degree AV heart block are commonly seen after the administration of alpha$_2$-agonists such as dexmedetomidine. Other causes include high vagal tone, hyperkalemia, and cardiac disease.

- *Third-degree AV block* is an abnormal rhythm in which the atrial and ventricular contractions occur independently. It is recognized by a complete loss

of the normal relationship between the P waves and QRS complexes and is characterized by randomly irregular PR intervals (Figure 5-9). This rhythm indicates cardiac disease and is infrequently seen in anesthetized patients, but when present, decreases cardiac output and requires treatment.

- *Premature complexes.* A premature complex is one that occurs too early. If the premature complex is associated with a heartbeat or pulse it may be referred to as a *premature contraction.*
- *Supraventricular premature complexes* (SPCs) appear as one or more normal QRS complexes that closely follow the previous QRS, interrupting an otherwise regular rhythm (Figure 5-10). P waves may or may not be present, but if present

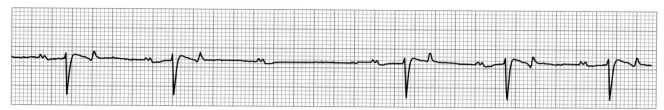

**FIGURE 5-8** Second-degree AV heart block (horse—base apex lead; 25 mm/sec; 1 cm/mV). Note that there is a missing QRS complex after the third P wave from the left.

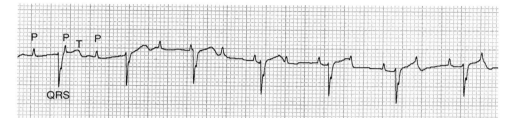

**FIGURE 5-9** Third-degree AV heart block (cat—25 mm/sec; 1 cm/mV). Note that the P waves are regular and are occurring independently of the QRS complexes. (From Bonagura JD, Twedt DC: *Kirk's current veterinary therapy XIV*, St Louis, 2009, Elsevier.)

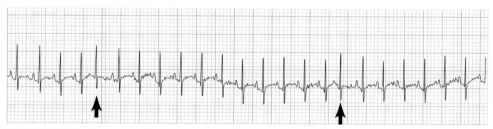

**FIGURE 5-10** Supraventricular premature complexes (cat—25 mm/sec; 1 cm/mV). Note the early complexes with normal QRS morphology. (From Bonagura JD, Twedt DC: *Kirk's current veterinary therapy XIV*, St Louis, 2009, Elsevier.)

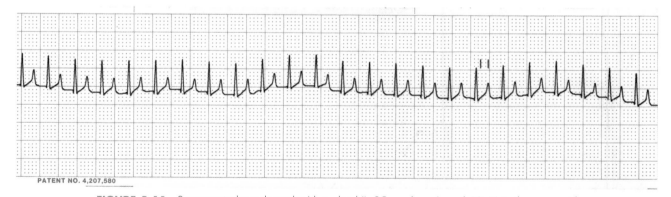

**FIGURE 5-11** Supraventricular tachycardia (dog—lead II; 25 mm/sec; 1 cm/mV). Note the very rapid heart rate with normal QRS complexes. P waves are superimposed over the T waves and so are not easily visualized.

are almost always different from normal P waves. Atrial premature complexes (APCs) are a specific type of SPC.

- *Supraventricular tachycardia* (Figure 5-11) is a series of three or more SPCs in a row. SPCs are abnormal but may or may not require treatment, depending on the frequency.

- *Ventricular premature complexes* (VPCs) appear as one or more wide and bizarre QRS complexes that closely follow the previous QRS, interrupting an otherwise regular rhythm (Figure 5-12). So like SPCs they are early, but unlike SPCs they appear different from normal QRS complexes. Isolated VPCs are commonly seen in anesthetized

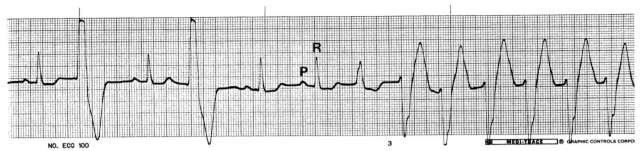

**FIGURE 5-12** Ventricular premature complexes (dog—lead II; 50 mm/sec; 1 cm/mV). Note the early wide, bizarre QRS complexes, second and fourth from the left (ventricular premature complexes [VPCs]), and the last six complexes (which represent an episode of ventricular tachycardia). (From Birchard SJ, Sherding RG: *Saunders manual of small animal practice*, ed 3, St Louis, 2006, Elsevier.)

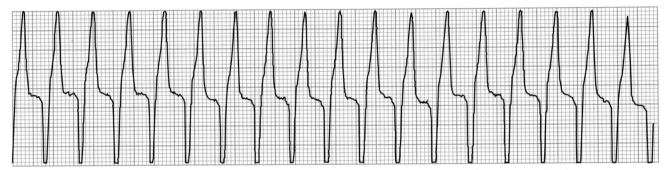

**FIGURE 5-13** Ventricular tachycardia (dog—lead II; 25 mm/sec; 1.6 cm/mV). This is a series of wide, bizarre QRS complexes followed by T waves.

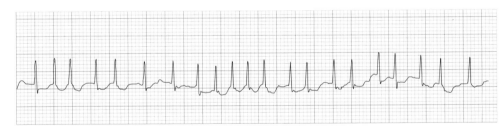

**FIGURE 5-14** Atrial fibrillation (cat—25 mm/sec; 1 cm/mV). Note the absence of P waves, the undulating baseline (f waves), and the irregular ventricular rate. (From Bonagura JD, Twedt DC: *Kirk's current veterinary therapy XIV*, St Louis, 2009, Elsevier.)

animals. They have a variety of causes including heart disease, drugs, hypoxia, and acid-base or electrolyte disorders. Epinephrine release in fearful patients is also a potent stimulus of VPCs. This is one reason why it is unwise to forcibly restrain a struggling animal during induction, as release of epinephrine may potentiate severe and even fatal arrhythmias (particularly in patients given arrhythmogenic agents). VPCs may or may not require treatment, depending on the frequency.

- *Ventricular tachycardia* (Figure 5-13) is a series of three or more VPCs in a row. It is a dangerous rhythm that significantly compromises cardiac output and requires intervention. Intravenous (IV) lidocaine is the most common treatment for severe VPCs.

- *Fibrillation.* Fibrillation is the chaotic, uncoordinated contraction of small muscle bundles within the atria or ventricles that appears as an undulating baseline with or without QRS complexes.
  - *Atrial fibrillation* appears as fine undulations of the baseline (often referred to as f waves), an absence of P waves, a high HR, and normal QRS complexes with irregular intervals between them (Figure 5-14). This rhythm, which is usually caused by heart disease, decreases cardiac output and requires treatment.
  - *Ventricular fibrillation* appears as an irregular undulating baseline, with complete absence of recognizable QRS complexes (Figure 5-15). Ventricular fibrillation is associated with cardiac arrest and requires emergency treatment.

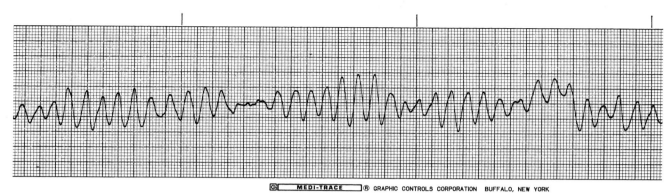

**FIGURE 5-15** Ventricular fibrillation (dog—lead II; 50 mm/sec; 1 cm/mV). This is a chaotic electrical activity unassociated with organized contraction of the heart muscle. (From Birchard SJ, Sherding RG: *Saunders manual of small animal practice,* ed 3, St Louis, 2006, Elsevier.)

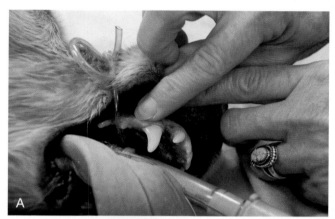

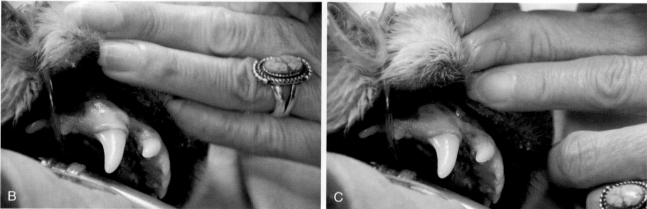

**FIGURE 5-16** Capillary refill time. **A,** Application of digital pressure. **B,** Blanching of the mucous membranes. **C,** Return of color, which in a normal patient should occur in 2 seconds or less.

A change in the configuration of the QRS complex or T wave over time indicates hypoxia of the cardiac muscle, is dangerous, and requires immediate intervention.

Pulseless electrical activity (PEA) is the cessation of heart contractions and/or palpable pulses in the presence of a normal or nearly normal ECG and is associated with cardiac arrest. As the ECG is not a sure indicator of mechanical activity of the heart, electrocardiographic monitoring must always be accompanied by physical monitoring of the heartbeat, apical pulse, and arterial pulses.

## Capillary Refill Time

The CRT is the rate of return of color to oral mucous membranes after the application of gentle digital pressure (Figure 5-16) and is indicative of the perfusion of the peripheral tissues with blood. The pressure applied to the mucous membranes compresses the small capillaries and temporarily blocks blood flow to that area. When the pressure is released, the capillaries rapidly refill with blood and the color returns, provided perfusion is adequate. Normal capillary refill is not always a reliable indicator of adequate circulation, however (e.g., CRT may appear normal shortly after euthanasia in some animals).

A prolonged CRT (greater than 2 seconds) indicates that tissues in the area tested have reduced blood perfusion. This may be a result of vasoconstriction caused by epinephrine release. Poor perfusion may also be a result of low BP caused by anesthetic drugs (including acepromazine, alpha$_2$-agonists, propofol, and inhalation agents), hypothermia, cardiac failure, excessive anesthetic depth, blood loss, or shock. Poor perfusion will also result in reduced temperature of the affected part.

## Blood Pressure

BP is the force exerted by flowing blood on arterial walls. This monitoring parameter is used during anesthesia to evaluate tissue perfusion. BP is determined by complex interactions among HR, stroke volume (the volume of blood ejected by the heart on each beat), vascular resistance (the diameter of the vessels), arterial compliance (elasticity), and blood volume. Therefore it is altered by anything that affects these factors, including drugs, disease, surgical stimulation, and hydration status.

Normal BP varies throughout the cardiac cycle as the ventricles contract and relax. **Systolic blood pressure** is produced by the contraction of the left ventricle as it propels blood through the systemic arteries. **Diastolic blood pressure** is the pressure that remains in the arteries when the heart is in its resting phase, between contractions. **Mean arterial pressure** (MAP) is the average pressure through the cardiac cycle and is the most important value from the anesthetist's standpoint because it is the best indicator of blood perfusion of the internal organs. MAP is automatically calculated by some instruments or can be mathematically calculated as follows:

$$MAP = \text{Diastolic pressure} + \frac{1}{3}(\text{Systolic pressure} - \text{Diastolic pressure})$$

> **TECHNICIAN NOTE**  MAP is the average pressure through the cardiac cycle and is the most important value from the anesthetist's standpoint because it is the best indicator of blood perfusion of the internal organs.

All BP monitoring instruments are able to measure systolic BP, and some are able to measure diastolic

| BOX 5-2 | **Common Causes of Hypotension** |

- Anesthetic agents (especially acepromazine, alpha$_2$-agonists, barbiturates, propofol, and inhalant agents)
- Excessive anesthetic depth
- Vasodilatation secondary to allergic reactions or endotoxic shock
- Blood loss
- Dehydration
- Cardiac arrhythmias
- Preexisting heart disease
- Positive-pressure ventilation
- Gastric distention

pressure and MAP as well (transducers and oscillometric BP monitors). Because BP can be difficult to measure accurately, changes rapidly, and is subject to many influences, it is best to monitor trends rather than a single value. BP that is below normal limits is called *hypotension*, and BP that is above normal limits is termed *hypertension*. BP may be decreased by anything that decreases HR, stroke volume, vascular resistance, or blood volume and increased by anything that increases these parameters. Box 5-2 lists common causes of hypotension in anesthetized patients. Because of the complexity of the interactions among these parameters, interpretation of the significance of BP changes is not always straightforward. For example, under normal circumstances, the body compensates for MAP values between 60 and 150 mm Hg by changing vascular resistance to maintain blood flow. So the MAP can fall to as low as 60 mm Hg without a significant change in tissue perfusion. In contrast, in situations when vascular resistance is high and cardiac output is low, BP may remain normal even though perfusion is poor. So under normal circumstances, in an awake animal, BP does not always reflect tissue perfusion.

During anesthesia, however, BP is a good indicator of tissue perfusion. This is because when inhalant anesthetics are used, the body's ability to compensate decreases as anesthetic depth increases, so that tissue perfusion is essentially directly determined by MAP. If MAP falls below 60 mm Hg, blood flow to internal organs is reduced, and tissues may become hypoxic. The kidneys are particularly sensitive to reduced perfusion and can fail postoperatively if the MAP is

> **TECHNICIAN NOTE**  During anesthesia MAP is a good indicator of tissue perfusion. If MAP falls below 60 mm Hg, blood flow to internal organs is reduced, and tissues may become hypoxic. Every effort should be made to maintain a MAP of 60 mm Hg or greater in small animals and ruminants, and 70 mm Hg or greater in horses.

**Strategies to Prevent Hypotension**

- Avoid excessive anesthetic depth.
- Provide adequate analgesia.
- Use preanesthetic medications to decrease the amount of anesthetic required.
- Administer drugs that decrease cardiac output, induce bradycardia, or cause vasodilatation cautiously.
- Administer IV fluids at a rate sufficient to maintain blood pressure.
- Some patients may require medication to maintain blood pressure (such as ephedrine, dobutamine, or dopamine).

inadequate during anesthesia. This risk is increased by preexisting disease and by some drugs including nonsteroidal antiinflammatory drugs (NSAIDs). In horses, a MAP below 70 mm Hg decreases blood flow to the muscle, predisposing the patient to postanesthetic myopathy.

Hypotension is common during anesthesia because most anesthetic drugs, with the exception of dissociatives, decrease BP, and because many common complications of anesthesia and surgery, including blood loss, also decrease it. Although a modest drop in BP is acceptable during anesthesia, every effort should be made to maintain a MAP of 60 mm Hg or greater (70 mm Hg or greater in horses). Changes in BP over the course of an anesthetic procedure give the anesthetist valuable information that can be used to warn of situations that may endanger the patient, including excessive blood loss, excessive anesthetic depth, decreased heart function, or changes in blood vessel tone. BP lower than minimum safe levels signals the need for intervention to support perfusion of vital tissues. Box 5-3 lists strategies to prevent hypotension.

### Pulse Strength

Pulse strength is a physical parameter that can be used as a rough indicator of BP. It is assessed by palpating a peripheral artery in one of several locations. Peripheral arteries appropriate to assess pulse strength include the lingual (dogs only), (Figure 5-17, *A*) dorsal pedal (Figure 5-17, *C*), femoral (small animals and small ruminants only) (Figure 5-17, *B*), carotid, facial (horses only), and aural (large animals only). A normal pulse should be strong and should occur shortly after each apical beat or S1 heart sound. During anesthesia in most cases the pulse strength naturally decreases, but the pulse should still be palpable during all stages.

Caution must be used when interpreting pulse strength because interpretation is subjective and normal pulse strength among healthy animals varies widely. Also, pulse strength does not always correlate well with BP because pulse strength is determined by the difference between systolic and diastolic BP, vessel diameter, and

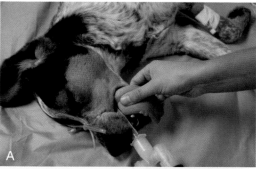
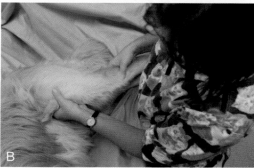
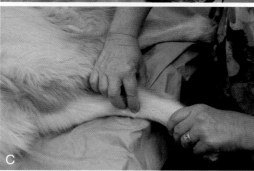

**FIGURE 5-17**  Assessment of pulse strength. **A,** Lingual artery (dog). Place the forefinger firmly but gently over the ventral aspect of the midline of the tongue. **B,** Femoral artery (dog). Cup the hand under the thigh from a cranial approach. Place the forefinger or second finger firmly but gently over the caudomedial aspect of the proximal femur. **C,** Dorsal pedal artery (dog). Place the forefinger over the dorsomedial aspect of the tarsus.

other factors that do not always correlate with MAP or with tissue perfusion.

For example, the pressure difference between a systolic BP of 100 mm Hg and a diastolic pressure of 30 mm Hg is 70 mm Hg. This relatively large difference will produce a strong pulse that will be subjectively interpreted as normal, even though the MAP in this patient is approximately 55 mm Hg, which is inadequate. In contrast, the pressure difference between a systolic pressure of 100 mm Hg and a diastolic pressure of 70 mm Hg is 30 mm Hg, which will feel weak and will be interpreted as indicative of hypotension even though the MAP is about 80 mm Hg, which is within the normal range.

Despite these inaccuracies, by comparing pulse strength during the preanesthetic period with the pulse strength throughout the anesthetic period, many relative changes in BP can be detected that may indicate a problem and require further assessment by instrumentation.

### Instruments Used to Monitor Blood Pressure

There are two general types of BP monitors; direct and indirect. When BP is monitored directly, the reading is obtained by means of a catheter inserted into an artery and attached to a **pressure transducer** (sensor) and monitor. In the case of indirect BP monitoring, the reading is obtained by using an external sensor and cuff.

Direct BP monitoring is infrequently performed in small animal veterinary practice but is used commonly in equine practice and in research and referral institutions. An indwelling catheter is placed in the femoral or dorsal pedal artery (small animals) or the facial or auricular arteries (large animals) by means of a surgical cutdown or percutaneous insertion technique. The catheter is connected by a length of fluid-filled tubing to a manometer or pressure transducer, which displays the pressure as directly measured from within the artery. Direct BP monitoring gives the anesthetist a continuous reading of the BP throughout the cardiac cycle and is more accurate than indirect methods. More detail concerning direct BP monitoring may be found in Chapter 9. In general practice, BP is more commonly determined by indirect methods, which are noninvasive and technically less demanding than direct monitoring. There are two basic types of indirect methods (Doppler and oscillometric), both of which use a cuff to sequentially occlude and release blood flow in a major artery of a limb or the tail. These systems differ in the way the pressure is measured.

> **TECHNICIAN NOTE** In general practice, indirect monitors are most commonly used to measure BP. There are two basic types of indirect monitors (Doppler and oscillometric), both of which use a cuff to sequentially occlude and release blood flow in a major artery of a limb or the tail. These systems differ in the way the pressure is measured.

The photoplethysmograph is another method used to provide indirect BP measurements. This method uses infrared light to measure changes in volume caused by pulse pressure. This instrument, designed for humans, is not in common use in veterinary patients but may be especially useful for dogs and cats weighing less than 10 kg. It creates a continuous waveform tracing in real time, and so is able to display systolic, diastolic, and mean pressures.

In human patients BP is routinely determined by using a stethoscope to listen for blood flow in a peripheral artery, as a cuff is sequentially inflated until

flow stops, and deflated until the flow resumes. As the cuff is slowly deflated, the point at which flow is first audible (because of turbulent blood flow through a partially occluded artery) represents the systolic BP, and the point at which it is no longer audible (because of restoration of normal flow) represents the diastolic pressure. This method is not practical in domestic animals because arterial flow is not audible with a stethoscope.

**Doppler blood flow detector.** The Doppler blood flow detector is a monitoring device that consists of an ultrasonic probe and an electronic monitor. The Doppler probe contains a crystal that emits ultrasound frequency waves and another crystal that receives the returning echoes. Outgoing waves bounce off red blood cells (RBCs) traveling inside a pulsating artery and return to the probe, where they are sent to an electronic monitor for processing. The monitor converts the returning echoes into a "whooshing" sound audible to the attendant via a speaker or earphones. The frequency (or pitch) of the sound changes in proportion to the velocity of the RBCs, and the intensity changes in proportion to the number of RBCs detected. This device can be used to continuously monitor HR and heart rhythm or can be used with a conventional cuff and sphygmomanometer to determine the systolic BP. Diastolic pressure and MAP cannot be measured by most Doppler systems.

*Use and operation.* Choose a location to place the probe over a peripheral artery. In small animal patients, the ventral surface of a paw just proximal to the metacarpal or metatarsal pad (over the median palmar or median plantar artery), the dorsomedial surface of the tarsus (over the dorsal pedal artery), the ventral surface of the tail base (over the coccygeal artery), or over the medial surface of the thigh in patients weighing under 5 kg (over the femoral artery) are all possible locations. In large animal patients the ventral tail is the most frequently used site. Figure 5-18 shows common locations for placement of the probe.

After choosing the location, clip a 1- to 2-cm square patch of hair over the artery, gently cleanse the skin, and apply a generous amount of ultrasonic gel. Avoid lubricating jelly and gels containing electrolytic substances such as those used for electrocardiographic leads. The concave surface of the probe must be oriented parallel to and precisely over the artery and must make firm but not excessive contact. Acquiring a good signal requires very fine changes in position of the probe, sometimes of only a millimeter or two. This can be a challenge, so the technician must be prepared to persevere until an audible signal is found. Once a signal has been found, the probe can be manually held in place by the technician if it is going to be used for only a short time (Figure 5-19), but if it is to be used as a heart monitor for the duration of an entire procedure, it may be carefully taped in place.

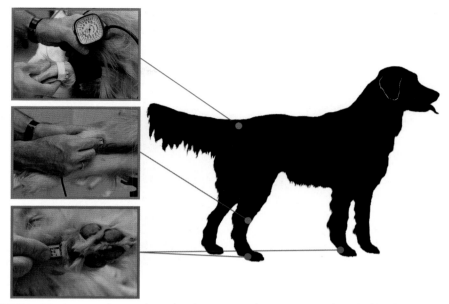

**FIGURE 5-18** Locations for Doppler probe placement. *Red,* Determination of systolic blood pressure by use of a sphygmomanometer with the cuff placed around the tail base and the probe placed on the ventral surface of the tail distal to the cuff. *Green,* Probe over the dorsomedial surface of the hock. *Blue,* Probe proximal to the metatarsal pad or metacarpal pad.

Doppler probes are expensive and can easily be damaged. They must therefore be handled gingerly. After use, clean the probe by wiping it gently with a gauze sponge. Gentle cleaning with tap water is acceptable, but the probe must not be immersed, scrubbed, or autoclaved. It should be stored in a protective case.

*Determining the blood pressure.* When used with a cuff and **sphygmomanometer,** the Doppler monitor can be used to determine BP (see Figure 5-18). A sphygmomanometer is an instrument, much like the pressure manometer on an anesthetic machine, which measures pressure within a cuff. The principle by which this system operates is as follows: When the cuff is inflated with a rubber bulb, an artery lying beneath the cuff is compressed. When the cuff pressure exceeds the systolic BP, blood flow through the artery stops and the sound is no longer audible. When the cuff pressure is slowly released, blood flow resumes and is again audible when the cuff pressure equals the systolic BP.

> TECHNICIAN NOTE When the BP is measured, the width of the cuff should be 30% to 50% of the circumference of the extremity, and the cuff should be placed firmly but not too tightly over a peripheral artery. The cuff should be wrapped slightly more tightly in large animals than in small animals and should ideally be at the same horizontal plane as the heart.

To determine the systolic pressure, fit a cuff to the extremity. The width of the cuff should be 30% to 50%

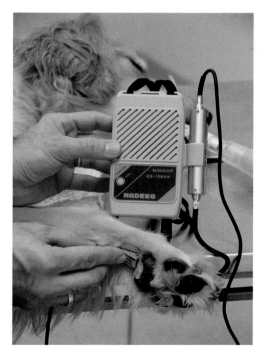

**FIGURE 5-19** Doppler monitor base unit with the probe positioned over the ventral surface of the metacarpus proximal to the metacarpal pad.

of the circumference of the extremity (Figure 5-20, *inset*). Place the cuff firmly, but not too tightly, proximal to the site where the probe is positioned. The cuff should be wrapped slightly more tightly in large animals than in small animals and should ideally be at the same horizontal plane as the heart (the level of the sternum when in lateral

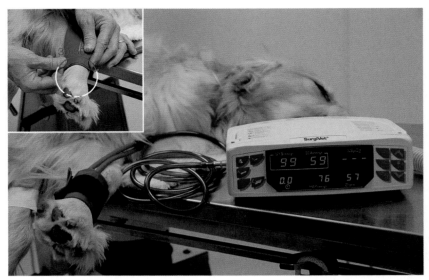

**FIGURE 5-20** Oscillometric blood pressure (BP) monitor with a cuff placed on the metacarpus. The following measurements are indicated: systolic BP, 99 mm Hg; diastolic BP, 59 mm Hg; mean arterial pressure (MAP), 76 mm Hg; heart rate 57 bpm. *Inset,* Selecting an appropriately sized blood pressure cuff, the width of which should be 30% to 50% of the circumference of the extremity.

recumbency or the shoulder when in dorsal recumbency). All cuffs contain a balloon inside that inflates as the cuff is pressurized. Some cuffs require that the balloon be centered over the artery, but others do not, as specified in the manufacturer's equipment manual. After establishing a good Doppler signal, use the bulb to inflate the cuff until the signal can no longer be heard. While reading the manometer, gradually decrease the pressure until the pulsing signal first returns. This represents the systolic pressure. Diastolic pressure is the pressure indicated just before the sound becomes continuous, but is difficult to determine reliably with this instrument. Procedure 5-1 (p 180) describes the technique for measuring BP with a Doppler device.

Specific locations in which adequate superficial arteries are located include the medial aspect of the proximal forelimb (radial artery), over the palmar aspect of the metacarpus (median palmar artery—Figure 5-21, blue), proximal to the tarsus over the dorsomedial aspect of the limb (cranial tibial artery), below the tarsus over the dorsomedial aspect of the limb (dorsal pedal artery—Figure 5-21, green), and over the ventral aspect of the tail base (coccygeal artery—Figure 5-21, red).

Doppler systems are accurate over a wide range of pressures and are the preferred instrument for cats and small dogs. They are labor-intensive instruments, however, because there is no automatic readout, and like most instruments they are subject to various unique technical problems and artifacts, including the following:

- Doppler monitors underestimate the systolic BP in cats by about 15 mm Hg but are fairly accurate in dogs and large animals. Therefore when taking a cat's BP, add 15 mm Hg to the pressure indicated on the manometer.

- Values are affected by patient position in relationship to the probe and blood flow to the extremity and can be altered by ropes used to tie the patient to the table as well as many other factors. Therefore several readings should be taken and averaged.
- The signal is difficult to maintain over time and is commonly lost if the patient is moved, the patient is shivering, the probe shifts, or the contact pressure is not exactly right.
- Finding the right location and tightness for the cuff can be challenging and requires experience.
- The use of a cuff that is too narrow will give falsely high readings, and a cuff that is too wide will give falsely low readings.

**Oscillometric blood pressure monitors.** An oscillometric BP monitor (oscillometer) consists of a cuff with an internal pressure-sensing bladder, connected to a computerized monitor (see Figure 5-20). The machine inflates and deflates the cuff, and the computer measures the oscillations in intracuff pressure caused by the subtle volume changes of the extremity resulting from pulsations of the artery beneath the cuff. It then calculates the systolic, mean, and diastolic pressures, and the HR from the pressure changes.

Oscillometers are more expensive than Doppler devices but offer two significant advantages: they work automatically, and they determine the diastolic pressure and MAP in addition to systolic pressure.

*Use and operation.* The cuff is selected in the same way, and placed in the same locations, as a Doppler cuff. Currently available machines are technologically sophisticated and will automatically inflate the cuff at preprogrammed intervals (such as every 5 minutes) or on demand (when a button is pushed). Alarm limits

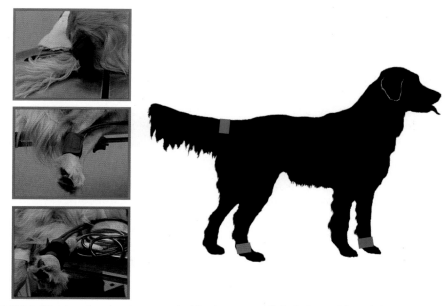

**FIGURE 5-21**    Locations for placement of a blood pressure cuff. Red—base of the tail. Green—metatarsus. Blue—metacarpus.

can be programmed for any of the parameters, and the computer often can store or print patient data. These machines contain rechargeable batteries and require very little maintenance other than cleansing and periodic recharging.

As with Doppler detectors, oscillometers are subject to artifacts and technical problems, as follows:

- These instruments are relatively accurate in animals weighing over 7 kg in body weight but may have difficulty detecting pulsations in cats and other animals with small superficial arteries.
- They tend to underestimate high pressures and overestimate low pressures.
- They are also inaccurate in animals with significant hypotension, arrhythmias, or fast HRs.
- Systolic pressures measured by these instruments are generally 10 to 15 mm Hg lower than those obtained by direct BP monitoring in dogs.
- The instrument may not work if the patient moves, if the patient is shivering, or if the cuff slips.
- If the cuff is too loose the machine may be unable to measure the pressure. If too tight, the values will be inaccurate.

### Central Venous Pressure

CVP is the BP in a large central vein such as the anterior vena cava. This value allows the veterinarian to assess blood return to the heart and heart function. This value is especially helpful in monitoring animals for right-sided heart failure because it can detect the increased pressure in the vena cava that results from this condition. It is also useful in preventing overhydration in animals receiving IV fluids, because CVP values rise when blood volume is excessive.

CVP can be directly measured by inserting a long catheter percutaneously into the jugular vein or by cutting down into the jugular vein. The catheter is advanced into the anterior vena cava and toward the heart so that the tip of the catheter lies close to the right atrium. The catheter is connected to a water manometer to obtain a measurement. The manometer should be positioned so that "0" on the manometer is at the same horizontal plane as the right atrium (halfway between shoulder and sternum in sternally recumbent patients, level with the sternum in laterally recumbent patients, and level with the shoulder in dorsally recumbent patients). If the catheter is correctly positioned, the meniscus of the fluid in the manometer should rise and fall with each breath. Normal CVP in dogs and cats is less than 8 cm $H_2O$. Pressures over 12 to 15 cm $H_2O$ (taken during exhalation) are considered elevated. As with arterial BP, it is usually more valuable to monitor trends over time rather than base an assessment on a single reading.

### Indicators of Oxygenation

The objective of the ACVA monitoring guidelines for oxygenation is "to ensure adequate oxygenation of the patient's arterial blood." To meet this objective, the ACVA makes the following recommendation: "Assessment of oxygenation should be done whenever possible by pulse oximetry, with **blood gas analysis** being employed when necessary for more critically ill patients."

### Mucous Membrane Color

Mucous membrane color is most commonly assessed by observing the gingiva (see Figure 5-16, *C*). Normal mucous membrane color is sometimes referred to as "bubblegum pink," although the color varies from patient to patient. For this reason, mucous membrane color should be assessed before each procedure so that the anesthetist knows what is normal for the patient and can use this as a point of comparison. This parameter gives the anesthetist a crude assessment of both oxygenation and tissue perfusion. In patients with pigmented gums, alternative sites may be used to assess mucous membrane color, including the tongue, the conjunctiva of the lower eyelid, or the mucous membrane lining the prepuce or vulva.

Pale mucous membranes indicate intraoperative blood loss, anemia from any cause, or poor capillary perfusion (as may occur with vasoconstriction, excessive anesthetic depth, or prolonged anesthesia). Cyanosis (purple or blue discoloration of the mucous membranes or skin) indicates very low blood oxygen concentration (a partial pressure [$PaO_2$] of approximately 35 to 45 mm Hg) in patients with a normal packed cell volume (PCV). Some common causes of cyanosis are respiratory arrest, oxygen deprivation (such as when the oxygen tank is empty or the flow meters are inadvertently turned off), and severe pulmonary disease.

Mucous membrane color is not a reliable indicator of perfusion because many other factors affect it including body temperature, vascular resistance, and gum disease. It is a crude indicator of oxygenation for two reasons. First, in animals with a normal PCV the blood oxygen concentration is so low by the time cyanosis occurs that the situation is already a medical emergency. Second, there must be a minimum concentration of deoxygenated hemoglobin for cyanosis to occur. Consequently animals with severe anemia may not have enough hemoglobin to reach this threshold and may not become cyanotic even though tissues are hypoxic.

Before examination of the ways in which oxygen is measured, it is important to understand how oxygen is carried in the bloodstream.

> **TECHNICIAN NOTE** Pale mucous membranes indicate intraoperative blood loss, anemia from any cause, or poor capillary perfusion. Cyanosis indicates very low blood oxygen concentration.

## Physiology of Oxygen Transport

As discussed previously, tissues must have adequate oxygen at all times to perform metabolic processes. This need is paramount in the brain and heart, which use the highest proportion of oxygen, and which will be damaged within seconds or minutes when oxygen levels are decreased. Consequently, assessment of blood oxygen levels is a critical component of patient monitoring.

The total oxygen content of the blood is carried in two forms: as free, unbound $O_2$ molecules dissolved in plasma, and as oxygen that is chemically bound to the hemoglobin contained in RBCs. Each hemoglobin molecule has four oxygen binding sites, each of which can bind one molecule of $O_2$. Thus each hemoglobin molecule can carry four oxygen molecules if all the binding sites are full. When all available binding sites are occupied with oxygen, the hemoglobin is said to be 100% saturated.

In healthy patients, dissolved oxygen in plasma represents a small amount of the total blood oxygen content, whereas bound oxygen represents the majority. For example, in a healthy animal breathing room air (with approximately 21% oxygen), the amount of oxygen dissolved in arterial blood is about 1.5% of the total content, and the remaining 98.5% is bound to hemoglobin. Thus the majority of oxygen necessary for normal cell function is carried by hemoglobin. That is why PCV is such an important determinant of oxygen available to the tissues.

Blood oxygen is measured in one of three ways.

1. **Calculated oxygen content** measures the total volume of oxygen in the blood, including both dissolved and bound forms, expressed in milliliters per deciliter (mL/dL). This system of measurement accurately measures total oxygen available to the tissues. Arterial oxygen content is calculated by using the following formula: $CaO_2 = (Hb \times 1.39 \times SaO_2/100) + (PaO_2 \times 0.003)$, where Hb = hemoglobin in grams per deciliter (g/dL), $SaO_2$ = oxygen saturation, and $PaO_2$ = partial pressure of oxygen in arterial blood.

   In a healthy animal breathing room air (with approximately 21% oxygen), with 15 g/dL of hemoglobin that is 100% saturated, each deciliter of arterial blood contains about 21.15 mL of oxygen (0.3 mL dissolved in plasma and 20.85 mL bound to hemoglobin). So in this situation oxygen availability is largely dependent on hemoglobin concentration and saturation. Therefore in nonanemic animals (with normal hemoglobin concentration), saturation alone gives the anesthetist a good estimate of oxygen available to the tissues. In contrast, a patient with anemia may have severely decreased oxygen availability even though saturation is normal.

2. **Partial pressure of oxygen** ($PO_2$), measures the unbound $O_2$ molecules dissolved in the plasma and is expressed in millimeters of mercury (mm Hg). Partial pressure differs depending on whether arterial, capillary, or venous blood is measured. Oxygen content is the highest after oxygen is picked up by blood in the lungs, decreases as it is consumed by the tissues, and is lowest as the blood travels back to the heart before reoxygenation in the lungs. Normal partial pressure of oxygen in arterial blood ($PaO_2$) in an animal breathing room air is about 90 to 110 mm Hg (100 mm Hg for practical purposes). In contrast, the partial pressure of oxygen in venous blood ($PvO_2$) is about 40 mm Hg owing to extraction of the difference (60 mm Hg) by the tissues. Partial pressure represents only a small portion of the total amount of oxygen available to tissues (1.5%), because it does not measure bound oxygen at all.

3. **Percent oxygen saturation** ($So_2$) measures the percentage of the total number of hemoglobin binding sites occupied by oxygen molecules. Like partial pressure, oxygen saturation varies depending on whether it is sampled in the arterial blood, capillary blood, or venous blood. Normal arterial oxygen saturation ($Sao_2$) is 97% or above. Normal venous saturation ($Svo_2$) is about 75%. Unlike partial pressure, percent oxygen saturation measures the majority of oxygen available to tissues (98.5%).

### The Relationship between Partial Pressure and Oxygen Saturation

The partial pressure of oxygen in the plasma is dependent almost exclusively on the amount of oxygen in the alveoli and the health of the lungs. Decreased inspired oxygen or lung disease will decrease partial pressure. Partial pressure in turn influences saturation of the hemoglobin because there must be an adequate level of dissolved oxygen in the blood for binding to occur. Thus, partial pressure and oxygen saturation are directly related (when one goes up, the other does also). This relationship is relatively predictable in healthy patients, so knowing one allows the anesthetist to estimate the other.

However, this direct relationship between the two is not linear, but looks rather more like the first big hill on a roller coaster. This means that as the partial pressure decreases, the saturation decreases very slowly at first, but the decrease gradually accelerates. For example when a patient is breathing 100% oxygen, the $Pao_2$ is about 500 mm Hg and hemoglobin is nearly 100% saturated (Box 5-4, Figure 1). When the $Pao_2$ drops from 500 mm Hg to 100 mm Hg (a drop of 400 mm Hg), as for a patient breathing room air, saturation drops only from 100% to about 98% (Box 5-4, Figure 2). As $Pao_2$ drops from 100 to 80 mm Hg (a drop of 20 mm Hg), the saturation decreases from 98% to 95% (Box 5-4, Figure 3). Below this point, the saturation drops more quickly. As $Pao_2$ drops from 80 to 60 mm Hg (also a drop of 20 mm Hg), the saturation drops from 95% to 90% (Box 5-4, Figure 4). When $Pao_2$ drops from 60 to 40 mm Hg (again, a drop of 20 mm Hg), the saturation drops much more quickly from 90% to 75% (Box 5-4, Figure 5). So in animals with normal hemoglobin, total oxygen available to the tissue decreases very little at partial pressures above 80 mm Hg (saturation above 95%), whereas total oxygen available to the tissues decreases much more rapidly below this level.

In contrast, when hemoglobin is low (the patient is anemic), neither of these parameters gives an accurate measure of oxygen availability. This is because even if the partial pressure and/or saturation are normal, the carrying capacity of the blood is severely decreased owing to the decrease in the number of hemoglobin binding sites. For example, a patient with a hemoglobin of 5 g/dL (equivalent to a very anemic patient with a PCV of about 15%) breathing room air or 100% oxygen will have a total blood oxygen content of only slightly more than one third

of the normal level, even though percent saturation and partial pressure are both normal. So with anemic patients, the value of these parameters in predicting patient tissue oxygenation is limited.

> *TECHNICIAN NOTE* When a patient is anemic, neither $Pao_2$ nor $Spo_2$ gives an accurate measure of oxygen availability. This is because even if the $Pao_2$ and/or $Spo_2$ are normal, the carrying capacity of the blood is severely decreased owing to the decrease in the number of hemoglobin binding sites.

Once hemoglobin is 100% saturated, as occurs when the partial pressure is near 120 mm Hg, any further increase in inspired oxygen will have almost no effect on the oxygen-carrying capacity of the blood, and thus will be of little benefit to the patient. When the partial pressure of oxygen decreases to values lower than about 80 mm Hg, as could occur with lung disease, lack of oxygen, inadequate ventilation, or shunting, the saturation begins to decrease more quickly. Saturation is therefore an early warning system that can alert the anesthetist to a potentially devastating decrease in the oxygen content of the blood.

When patients are breathing pure oxygen from an anesthetic machine, the amount of dissolved oxygen ($Pao_2$) can increase markedly (up to about 500 mm Hg). But as dissolved oxygen represents only a very small proportion of the total oxygen content, and because hemoglobin is already nearly 100% saturated when the patient is breathing room air, this extra oxygen contributes only about a 10% increase in the total oxygen content of the blood.

Both $Po_2$ and $So_2$ can be measured, although by different instruments. Blood gas analyzers measure $Pao_2$; pulse oximeters measure $Spo_2$. Both values reflect inspired oxygen and how well the lungs deliver oxygen to the blood. Most anesthetized animals show a greatly elevated $Pao_2$ (up to 500 mm Hg compared with the normal 90 to 110 mm Hg for an awake patient breathing room air) because they are breathing almost 100% oxygen from the anesthetic machine, whereas the conscious animal breathes approximately 21% oxygen in room air. Similarly, $Spo_2$ readings on anesthetized animals breathing pure oxygen are usually high (97% to 99%).

Low $Pao_2$ and $Spo_2$ values are sometimes observed during anesthesia. A $Pao_2$ value below 80 mm Hg ($Spo_2$ 95%) indicates hypoxemia, and a value below 60 mm Hg ($Spo_2$ 90%) indicates the need for oxygen supplementation and possibly assisted ventilation.

### Pulse Oximeter

A pulse oximeter estimates the saturation of hemoglobin ($So_2$), expressed as a percentage of the total binding sites. Pulse oximeters are readily available, relatively inexpensive, noninvasive, portable, and relatively easy to use.

## BOX 5-4   How to Read Oxygen Dissociation Curves

At the top of each figure is the oxygen dissociation curve, which illustrates the relationship between partial pressure of oxygen and oxygen saturation (with $P_{O_2}$ on the x-axis and $S_{O_2}$ on the y-axis).

When the amount of dissolved oxygen ($P_{O_2}$) is above 100 mm Hg (after oxygenation in the lungs), nearly all (at least 98%) of the binding sites on the hemoglobin molecules are occupied. But as the blood reaches the systemic capillaries, oxygen diffuses into the tissues causing the $P_{O_2}$ to decrease. As the $P_{O_2}$ decreases, oxygen separates or "dissociates" from the hemoglobin to meet tissue needs.

The red rectangle represents a blood vessel containing dissolved $O_2$ and $O_2$ bound to hemoglobin. Each $O_2$ floating in the plasma represents 10 mm Hg of dissolved, unbound oxygen, with the exception of Figure 1 in which each $O_2$ represents 20 mm Hg of dissolved, unbound oxygen. Each "leg" of an "H" represents 2.5% of the available binding sites. So the relative proportion of binding sites occupied represents the $S_{O_2}$. Thus if all available site are occupied with $O_2$, the $S_{O_2}$ is 100%. If nine out of ten of the available sites are occupied, the $S_{O_2}$ is 90%, and so on. Note that as the number of sites occupied decreases, the color of the hemoglobin and the blood gradually changes (representing the change in light absorption associated with decreased saturation). Although exaggerated in these illustrations, a change in color actually occurs in live non-anemic patients, leading to visible cyanosis in patients with dangerously decreased saturation.

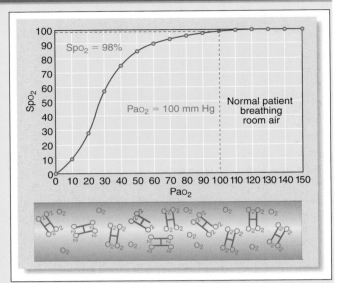

**FIGURE 2**   Oxygen dissociation curve for a normal patient breathing room air. Generally accepted values for $Pa_{O_2}$ (100 mm Hg) and $Sp_{O_2}$ (98%) in a normal patient breathing 21% oxygen. Note that one out of 40 (approximately 2%) of the available binding sites is unoccupied, and the color is subtly changed.

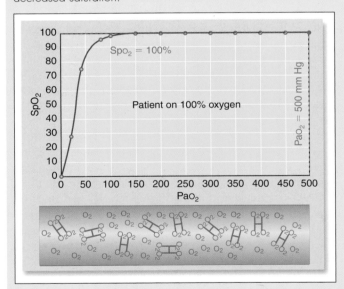

**FIGURE 1**   Oxygen dissociation curve for a normal patient breathing 100% oxygen. Generally accepted values for $Pa_{O_2}$ (500 mm Hg) and $Sp_{O_2}$ (100%) in a normal patient when breathing 100% oxygen. Note that all binding sites are occupied, and the blood is bright red.

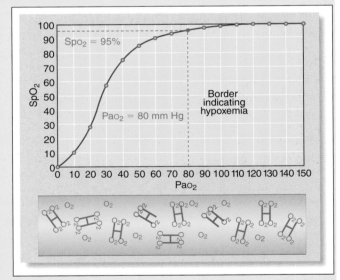

**FIGURE 3**   Oxygen dissociation curve for a patient with early hypoxemia. Generally accepted values for $Pa_{O_2}$ (80 mm Hg) and $Sp_{O_2}$ (95%) in a patient with early hypoxemia. Note that two out of 40 (5%) of the available binding sites are unoccupied, and the color is changed to a slightly greater degree.

A pulse oximeter is equipped with a probe, which is sensitive to both the absorption of light by hemoglobin and to blood pulsations in the small arterioles (Figure 5-22).

Red- and infrared-wavelength light emitted by the probe is passed through or reflected off the tissue bed, and the frequency of the emergent light is read by a sensor and analyzed. The machine determines the oxygen saturation

($Sp_{O_2}$) by calculating the difference between levels of oxygenated and deoxygenated hemoglobin based on subtle differences in absorption of light. The HR is determined by detecting pulsations in the small arterioles. Both the HR and the oxygen saturation are digitally displayed.

Normally when pure oxygen is breathed, hemoglobin in the lungs is at least 97% saturated with oxygen.

## BOX 5-4  How to Read Oxygen Dissociation Curves—cont'd

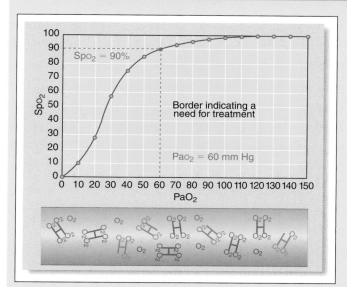

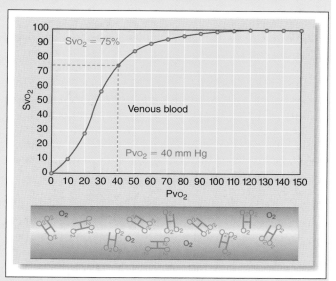

**FIGURE 4** Oxygen dissociation curve for a patient requiring treatment. Generally accepted values for PaO2 (60 mm Hg) and SpO2 (90%) in a patient requiring treatment. Note that four out of 40 (10%) of the available binding sites are unoccupied, and the color is noticeably changed.

**FIGURE 5** Oxygen dissociation curve for venous blood. Generally accepted values for PvO2 (40 mm Hg) and SvO2 (75%) in venous blood. Note that 10 out of 40 (25%) of the available binding sites are unoccupied, and the color is significantly changed. If the oxygen content of arterial blood decreases approximately to this level in a patient with a normal packed cell volume (PCV), cyanosis will occur, indicating a critically low oxygen level, which will rapidly lead to death if not immediately corrected.

Therefore during oxygen administration the oxygen saturation should be greater than 95%. A pulse oximeter reading of 90% to 95% must be investigated, because it indicates that the patient's hemoglobin is not fully saturated and the patient is hypoxemic. Saturation less than 90% indicates a need for therapy. Saturation less than 85% for longer than 30 seconds is a medical emergency.

 *TECHNICIAN NOTE*

- During oxygen administration the oxygen saturation should be greater than 95%.
- A pulse oximeter reading of 90% to 95% must be investigated because it indicates that the patient is hypoxemic.
- Saturation less than 90% indicates a need for therapy.
- Saturation less than 85% for longer than 30 seconds is a medical emergency.

### Use and Operation
Pulse oximeters usually come with a variety of probes, each of which analyzes light either passed through or reflected off a tissue bed. The probes are classified as transmission or reflective. Transmission probes are constructed in a "clothespin" type configuration. One of the jaws houses a light source, and the other houses a sensor that detects the transmitted light. Transmission

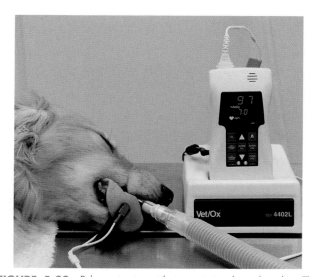

**FIGURE 5-22** Pulse oximeter with transmission lingual probe. The upper number (97) represents the percent oxygen saturation (SpO2). The lower number (70) represents the heart rate in beats per minute.

probes must be applied over a nonpigmented tissue bed that is thin enough to allow light transmission through the tissue. In anesthetized animals the tongue is commonly used, but the probe may also be applied to the pinna, toe web, vulvar fold, prepuce, Achilles tendon, lip, or any other area that is thin, relatively hairless, and nonpigmented. Although these probes are able to function through a thin hair coat, excessive hair will prevent operation. Figure 5-23 shows examples of probe types and placement.

Reflective probes reflect light off a tissue bed. The light source and sensor are located next to each other on one side of the probe. These probes are placed inside a hollow organ such as the esophagus or rectum, or against the ventral surface of the tail with the light source and sensor in contact with a tissue bed. During placement of a reflective probe in the rectum, care must be taken to digitally displace the feces from the wall of the rectum and place the side of the probe that houses the light source and sensor against the tissue.

Pulse oximeter probes can be frustrating to work with because the probes are temperamental and often give inaccurate readings or lose the signal altogether. When this happens, values will no longer appear on the display, the numbers will be incorrect, or an alarm may sound. Tissue pigmentation, motion, excessive pressure, orientation in relation to ambient light, and patient conditions such as anemia, **icterus**, vasoconstriction, or edema will all decrease accuracy or result in signal loss. Box 5-5 contains suggestions for troubleshooting signal loss.

Pulse oximeters require little maintenance but must be handled with care. Transmission probes should be cleaned with alcohol or other mild disinfectant after use. Reflective probes should be covered with a plastic sleeve supplied by the manufacturer before insertion into the rectum or esophagus. None of the probes can be immersed, scrubbed, or autoclaved.

If pulse oximeter readings are abnormally low during anesthesia, the anesthetist should consider the following questions:

- Is the instrument working correctly? Readings may be affected by factors such as probe placement, external light sources, and motion.

---

**BOX 5-5** | **Suggestions for Troubleshooting Pulse Oximeter Signal Loss**

**Transmission Probes**
- Make sure the patient is stable by assessing vital signs.
- Remove and replace the probe.
- When using a lingual probe, if the tongue is dry, rewet it.
- Be sure there is not excessive or inadequate pressure on the tissue.
- When possible, the jaw with the sensor should be oriented toward the ceiling to avoid interference from ambient light.
- Choose a different area that is not pigmented, covered with excessive hair, icteric, or edematous.
- If the area is heavily haired, clip and gently cleanse the area.

**Reflective Probes**
- Make sure the patient is stable by assessing vital signs.
- Be sure the side with the light source and sensor is oriented toward the tissue.
- Check for adequate tissue contact.
- When the probe is placed in the rectum, be sure that feces are not between the probe and the tissue.

---

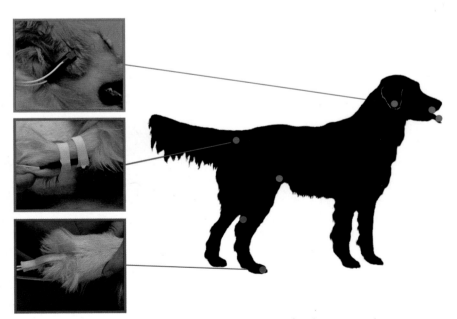

**FIGURE 5-23** Examples of pulse oximeter probes and locations for placement. Red—transmission probe on the ear flap. Additional red dots show alternate placement locations for this probe (tongue, lip, and flank fold). Green—reflective probe taped to the ventral surface of the tail base. Blue—"C-probe" (a transmission probe) on the toe web. The other blue dot shows an alternate placement location for this probe (the skin fold between the Achilles tendon and the tibia).

- Does the agent cause vasoconstriction? Some anesthetic agents (especially alpha$_2$-agonists such as dexmedetomidine) cause vasoconstriction and decreased peripheral perfusion, which may significantly lower $SpO_2$ values.
- Is the tissue under the probe adequately perfused? Regardless of the anesthetic agents used, perfusion of an extremity such as the tongue may decrease gradually with time and give artificially reduced $SpO_2$ readings. If this is the case, readings may improve if the probe is moved to a different location. If higher readings cannot be obtained, the patient should be evaluated for hypothermia, hypotension, blood loss, and other causes of reduced perfusion.
- Is adequate oxygen being delivered to the patient? Inadequate oxygen delivery may result from esophageal intubation, an oxygen flow rate that is too low, an empty oxygen tank, endotracheal tube blockage or disconnection, or respiratory failure.
- Is oxygen being transferred from the alveoli to the blood? This process may be impeded by inadequate ventilation or preexisting lung disease.
- Is circulation adequate? Heart disease, bradycardia, severe arrhythmias, or pulmonary embolism may decrease oxygenation.

Regardless of the cause, patients with subnormal $PaO_2$ or $SpO_2$ readings may require supplemental oxygen delivery, or ventilation through bagging or use of a ventilator.

Pulse oximeters can be used not only on anesthetized patients but also on animals that are in intensive care because of trauma, heart failure, respiratory difficulty, or unconsciousness. Their chief limitation is the difficulty of finding a suitable probe site in alert and mobile patients.

## Blood Gas Analysis

Blood gas analysis is an alternative method used to evaluate oxygenation. This monitoring tool is discussed in detail in the next section (indicators of ventilation).

## Indicators of Ventilation

The objective of the ACVA monitoring guidelines for ventilation is "to ensure that the patient's ventilation is adequately maintained." To meet this objective, the ACVA makes the following recommendations:

"Qualitative assessment of ventilation is essential as outlined in either [of the following statements:] (1) Observation of thoracic wall movement or observation of breathing bag movement when thoracic wall movement cannot be assessed... [or] (2) Auscultation of breath sounds with an external stethoscope, an esophageal stethoscope, or an audible respiratory monitor; and capnography is recommended, with blood gas analysis as necessary."

The term *ventilation* refers to the movement of gases in and out of the alveoli, whereas **respiration** is a more general term that means the processes by which oxygen is supplied to and used by the tissues, and carbon dioxide is eliminated from the tissues. The following monitoring parameters and indicators give the anesthetist information about ventilation.

### Respiratory Rate

RR is the number of breaths per minute (breaths/min). It is most often monitored by watching the chest wall. In situations in which the chest excursions are not visible, such as when the patient is covered by a surgical drape, it may also be monitored by observing movements of the reservoir bag. Auscultation of breath sounds is not a particularly good way to determine the RR because the low $V_T$ typically seen during anesthesia renders respiratory sounds inaudible or nearly so in many anesthetized patients. RR may also be monitored mechanically with an apnea monitor or capnograph. The apnea monitor generates an audible beep with each breath, and a capnograph displays a digital readout of the RR in breaths per minute. The minimum acceptable, maximum acceptable, and typical RR for anesthetized patients are listed in Table 5-2. During anesthesia, there is normally a decrease in the RR. Inhalant anesthetics, opioids, and alpha$_2$-agonists are particularly likely to cause respiratory depression. Propofol and thiopental sodium typically cause bradypnea or apnea during induction, especially if given quickly or at higher doses.

An increase in RR is called **tachypnea.** Tachypnea must be differentiated from panting, in which breaths are rapid but shallow and air is taken in through an open mouth. Panting (only seen in conscious, nonintubated patients) is a common side effect of neuroleptanalgesia. True tachypnea has many possible causes including hypercapnia, pulmonary disease, or a response to a mild surgical stimulus. For example, tachypnea is often apparent when the surgeon pulls on the suspensory ligament of the ovary during an ovariohysterectomy. An elevated RR may also indicate a progression from moderate to light anesthesia and is one of the first signs of arousal from anesthesia. Some patients (particularly obese dogs) breathe rapidly even at a moderate depth of anesthesia.

### Tidal Volume

$V_T$ is the amount of air inhaled during a breath. As with RR, $V_T$ is monitored by watching the chest wall or movement of the reservoir bag. Normal $V_T$ is generally considered to be 10 to 15 mL/kg but decreases by at least 25% in most anesthetized animals, largely because most preanesthetic and general anesthetic drugs decrease the contraction of the intercostal muscles on inspiration. As the animal's breaths become more shallow (i.e., as $V_T$ decreases), some alveoli in the lungs may not receive amounts of air adequate for normal gas exchange. As a result the alveoli will partially collapse (a condition called **atelectasis**). This is most pronounced in the "down" lung (also called the dependent lung) of a patient that is lying on its side and in the dorsal lung fields of a patient lying on its back. In its early stages atelectasis can be reversed by gentle inflation of the lungs by the anesthetist. In this procedure, called *bagging* or *sighing* the patient, the reservoir bag of the anesthetic machine is carefully squeezed, forcing air into the patient's breathing passages. When bagging a patient, the anesthetist should closely observe the animal's chest to ensure that it rises only slightly, as with a normal breath, to prevent overinflation of the lungs. Some anesthetists routinely bag every patient under inhalation anesthesia once every 5 to 10 minutes. Alternatively, hypoventilation and atelectasis may be prevented by use of a mechanical ventilator (see Chapter 6).

Anesthetized patients may occasionally have increased $V_T$ (hyperventilation). As with tachypnea, hyperventilation may result from hypercapnia or surgical stimulation.

$V_T$ can be measured by using a **respirometer,** which is placed between the expiratory hose of a rebreathing circuit and the anesthetic machine. When the patient breathes out, vanes within the respirometer turn small dials on the front of the device. One dial (one complete circuit of the needle) turns with every breath and is noncumulative. The other dial is cumulative, so the patient's minute volume (breaths/min × $V_T$) can be monitored. The respirometer dials are easily reset to zero by depressing the buttons at the top, much like a stopwatch.

> **TECHNICIAN NOTE** In its early stages, atelectasis can be reversed by gentle inflation of the lungs. In this procedure, called *bagging* or *sighing* the patient, the reservoir bag of the anesthetic machine is carefully squeezed, forcing air into the patient's breathing passages, until the animal's chest rises as with a normal breath.

## Respiratory Character

*Respiratory character* refers to the effort required to breathe, the relative length of inhalation and exhalation, and regularity. Respiratory character is monitored by watching the chest wall.

The anesthetized animal's breathing should be smooth and regular, with both thoracic and diaphragmatic components (i.e., the chest wall and the diaphragm should move). Gasping, difficult, or labored breathing (dyspnea) indicates a problem requiring intervention, including airway blockage, respiratory disease, pressure buildup in the breathing circuit, or hypoxemia, and must be brought to the veterinarian's attention.

The time relationship between inspiration and expiration may vary also. Normal inspiration lasts 1 to 1.5 seconds, and expiration lasts at least 2 to 3 seconds. Expiration is usually followed by a pause before the next inspiration begins. Animals anesthetized with ketamine may exhibit an apneustic respiratory pattern in which there is a prolonged pause between inspiration and expiration.

Auscultation of the chest is useful to assess respiratory function. Normal respiratory sounds are almost inaudible in the dog and cat. Harsh noises, crackles, gurgling, whistles, or squeaks may indicate narrow or obstructed airways or the presence of fluid in the airways or alveoli and should be brought to the veterinarian's attention.

## Apnea Monitor

The **apnea monitor** (Figure 5-24) monitors respirations and warns the anesthetist when the patient has not taken a breath. The sensor, which is placed between the endotracheal tube connector and the breathing circuit, detects temperature changes between the cool inspired and warm expired air in the breathing circuit. The base unit emits an audible beep each time the patient breathes and will sound an alarm when no breath is detected for a preset time period.

The sensor increases mechanical dead space, which can be significant, especially in small patients. For this reason, special endotracheal tube connectors are available that accommodate the sensor and minimize dead space. Although apnea monitors do not warn of inadequate respiratory depth, they may have difficulty detecting respirations if the patient's $V_T$ is significantly decreased or the patient becomes hypothermic, and will sound the apnea alarm. Consequently, as with any monitor, alarm signals must be confirmed by physical examination of the patient.

## Capnograph (End-Tidal CO₂ Monitor)

A capnograph measures the amount of $CO_2$ in the air that is breathed in and out by the patient. Capnography is a noninvasive, continuous, and practical method of monitoring $CO_2$ levels in anesthetized patients without the need to catheterize an artery, as is necessary with blood gas analysis. Although this monitoring device does not measure blood $CO_2$ directly, expired $CO_2$ closely mirrors arterial $CO_2$ ($Paco_2$). Specifically, end-tidal $CO_2$ ($ETco_2$) is about 2 to 5 mm Hg less than $Paco_2$.

A capnograph consists of a sensor and a computerized monitor with a digital readout (Figure 5-25). The sensor measures infrared light absorption, which is directly proportional to the $CO_2$ level. Sensors are of two general

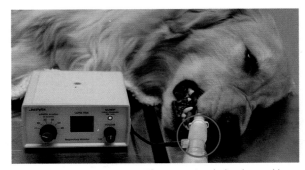

**FIGURE 5-24** Apnea monitor. The sensor (circled) is located between the breathing circuit and the endotracheal tube connector. The lapse time indicates the time in seconds since the previous breath. This alarm is set to sound if the interval between breaths exceeds 10 seconds.

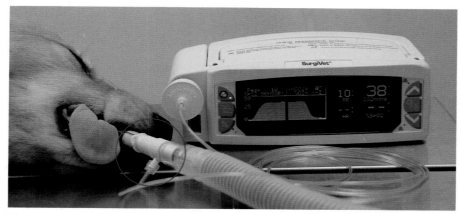

**FIGURE 5-25**   A sidestream capnograph registering an end-tidal $CO_2$ level of 38 mm Hg and a respiratory rate of 10 *(upper right)*. The fitting (circled) is located between the breathing circuit and the endotracheal tube connector. The graph indicates the carbon dioxide levels throughout the respiratory cycle, which in normal anesthetized patients is 35 to 55 mm Hg during expiration and 0 mm Hg during inspiration.

types. A mainstream capnograph is an instrument in which the sensor chamber is placed directly between the endotracheal tube and the breathing circuit. A sidestream capnograph is one in which the sensor chamber is located in the computerized monitor and air is pulled into it through a tube attached to a fitting placed between the endotracheal tube and breathing circuit. Both systems measure the $CO_2$ in the air that passes into and out of the endotracheal tube on both inspiration and expiration and display this information as a waveform (called the **capnogram**) and as a numeric display of the $ET_{CO_2}$.

The fitting on sidestream samplers (placed between the endotracheal tube and breathing circuit) is very lightweight and small, adding relatively little mechanical dead space to the circuit. These units often come with special endotracheal-tube connectors for very small patients, which, when used in place of the regular endotracheal-tube connector, effectively produce no increase in dead space. There is a 2- to 3-second delay in the display of $CO_2$ levels with these units, however. Also, these units sample 50 to over 400 mL of air per minute from the circuit, which may cause a significant loss of gas and false readings when very low oxygen flow rates are used.

Mainstream samplers produce an immediate reading with no delay. But the sensor chamber, which is placed between the endotracheal tube and the breathing circuit, is relatively large and heavy and is heated to prevent condensation. This results in increased dead space, a greater risk that the endotracheal tube will kink, and a risk that the patient may be burned.

> **TECHNICIAN NOTE**   Blood $CO_2$ levels are determined by the following three factors:
> 1. The rate of production by the cells
> 2. The rate of transport to the lungs
> 3. The rate of elimination from the lungs

### Generation of the Capnogram

Carbon dioxide is produced in the cells as a byproduct of cellular metabolism. After diffusing into venous blood, $CO_2$ is transported from the cells to the lungs, where it is eliminated on expiration. Blood $CO_2$ levels are determined by the following three factors:

1. The rate of production by the cells (determined by cellular metabolism)
2. The rate of transport to the lungs (determined by cardiovascular output and pulmonary perfusion)
3. The rate of elimination from the lungs (determined by respiratory system health, RR, and $V_T$)

The $ET_{CO_2}$ level as well as the configuration of the waveform are thus influenced by the interaction among all three of these factors (metabolism, perfusion, and ventilation), as well as equipment function. Interpretation of a capnogram requires knowledge of normal and abnormal $ET_{CO_2}$ values, common abnormal waveform configurations, and causes of each abnormality. Therefore, interpretation is somewhat complex and may be confusing until the anesthetist acquires some experience. Once mastered however, the capnogram is an extremely valuable tool that can alert the anesthetist to a wide variety of anesthetic problems.

### Appearance of a Normal Capnogram

On the capnogram, the x-axis displays time, and the y-axis displays the $CO_2$ level (Figure 5-26). The configuration of the waveform is determined by the levels of $CO_2$ passing through the machine end of the endotracheal tube. Provided the anesthetic machine is working correctly and appropriate oxygen flow rates are used, during inspiration the inspired $CO_2$ is 0 mm Hg. This period during which the $CO_2$ level is 0 is called the *baseline*. During expiration, the $CO_2$ level abruptly increases to about 40 mm Hg (35 to 45 mm Hg is considered normal in a non-anesthesized patient), increases slightly until the end of the expiratory effort, then abruptly decreases back to 0 at the beginning of the subsequent inspiratory effort.

## CASE 5-1 THE BENEFITS OF CAPNOGRAPHY

Cooper, a 1-year-old, male, 17-kg beagle mix, was anesthetized in preparation for a routine castration. Based on preanesthetic assessment, he was classified as a physical status class P1 patient. Cooper was premedicated with 0.1 mg of acepromazine per kilogram by intramuscular (IM) injection 15 minutes before anesthetic induction and was induced with a mixture of 5.5 mg of ketamine per kilogram and 0.28 mg of diazepam per kilogram intravenously. He was intubated and placed on a semiclosed rebreathing system. After reaching surgical anesthesia, he was maintained with isoflurane at a rate of 1.5% to 2.0% and oxygen at a rate of 0.5 L/min. Pulse oximetry was used to monitor Cooper via a transmission probe placed on the tongue.

During surgical preparation, the anesthetist noticed that Cooper's anesthetic depth was stage III, plane 2, but he had a slightly increased respiratory rate (at 22 breaths/min) and tidal volume. An investigation ensued to determine the cause of the hyperventilation, but an immediate cause was not identified. Oxygen saturation ($SpO_2$) was in the range of 97% to 98%, and all other vital signs were normal.

A decision was made to use a capnograph to assess carbon dioxide levels. It was immediately noted that the $ETCO_2$ was 62 mm Hg (normal 35 to 55), and the carbon dioxide level on inspiration was about 25 mm Hg (normal 0 mm Hg). Knowing that these levels suggested rebreathing of $CO_2$, the anesthetist immediately examined the carbon dioxide absorber canister and the unidirectional valves. The absorbent granules had not changed in color or appearance and had been recently changed. The unidirectional valves were difficult to evaluate because of the presence of a large amount of condensation inside the domes. Careful examination revealed that the expiratory valve leaflet had temporarily become stuck to the top of the dome because of the presence of the moisture within the valve. The patient was immediately disconnected from the breathing circuit and another machine was used for the duration of the procedure. Within a short time of placement on the new machine, Cooper's respirations and capnogram returned to normal and the procedure was completed without further incident.

Later, the valve was disassembled, cleaned, and reassembled. Although there was nothing wrong with the valve, it appeared that a combination of factors caused the valve to malfunction. Apparently during a particularly forceful exhalation, the valve leaflet was momentarily forced to the top of the dome, where it adhered to the inner surface of the dome because of the presence of the excess moisture, preventing proper closure.

This case illustrates the importance of vigilant monitoring, shows how monitoring equipment can provide vital information not available from physical monitoring parameters, and underscores the importance of monitoring multiple parameters whenever possible. Although the anesthetist initially identified the problem by observation of physical signs, the capnograph allowed her to identify, isolate, and correct the problem rapidly and efficiently, before the patient was seriously affected.

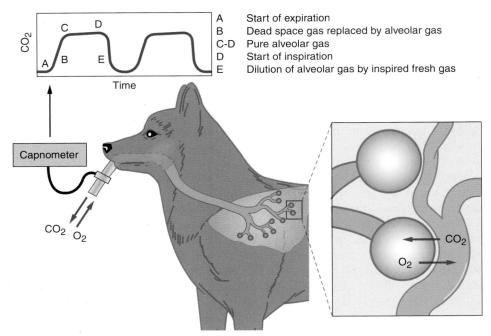

| | |
|---|---|
| A | Start of expiration |
| B | Dead space gas replaced by alveolar gas |
| C-D | Pure alveolar gas |
| D | Start of inspiration |
| E | Dilution of alveolar gas by inspired fresh gas |

**FIGURE 5-26** Normal capnogram. The capnograph measures the partial pressure of the $CO_2$ in the air moving between the endotracheal tube and the breathing circuit. As long as the patient is not rebreathing expired gases, and the $CO_2$ absorbent is not exhausted, $CO_2$ is 0 mm Hg during inhalation. Shortly after the beginning of exhalation (point A), $CO_2$ rapidly increases to about 40 mm Hg (point C), then continues to increase slightly until immediately before the next inhalation (point D). This represents the $ETCO_2$. Immediately after the beginning of the next inhalation, the $CO_2$ again rapidly decreases to 0 mm Hg.

The shape of the resulting waveform can be described as a modified rectangle. It is called an "end-tidal" monitor because the displayed $CO_2$ value at the end of the expiration is most reflective of arterial $CO_2$ levels.

Effective interpretation requires evaluation of four distinct aspects of the capnogram:

1. The baseline value
2. The $ETCO_2$ value
3. The waveform shape
4. The rate at which changes occur (suddenly, rapidly, or gradually)

> **TECHNICIAN NOTE**  Effective interpretation of the capnogram requires evaluation of four distinct aspects:
> 1. The baseline value
> 2. The $ETCO_2$ value
> 3. The waveform shape
> 4. The rate at which changes occur (suddenly, rapidly, or gradually)

### Appearance of an Abnormal Capnogram

A change in metabolism, perfusion, or ventilation, as well as equipment malfunction, will affect $ETCO_2$ levels and/or the waveform configuration. In most normal patients, provided metabolism and perfusion are normal, abnormal $CO_2$ levels are most commonly a result of changes in ventilation (hyperventilation, hypoventilation, apnea) or equipment problems. Following are some common abnormalities:

- Hyperventilation caused by increased RR or $V_T$ or overzealous mechanical or manual ventilation will cause $CO_2$ to be exhaled more quickly than it is produced and will consequently cause a gradual decrease in the $ETCO_2$ (a shorter rectangle).
- Hypoventilation (decreased RR or $V_T$ or inadequate mechanical or manual ventilation) will cause a gradual increase in $ETCO_2$ (a taller rectangle).
- Detachment of the endotracheal tube from the sensor fitting, esophageal intubation, a blocked endotracheal tube, or apnea will cause a sudden loss of the waveform (a flat line), because in each of these circumstances, no $CO_2$ will reach the sensor.
- A malfunctioning exhalation unidirectional valve or exhausted $CO_2$ absorbent will cause the baseline to rise above 0, reflecting rebreathing of $CO_2$ in the inspired air (a failure of the baseline to return to 0 during inspiration) and increased $ETCO_2$.
- A leaky cuff or partially kinked endotracheal tube will cause a sloppy up-stroke and down-stroke (rounding of the edges of the rectangle).

Many other conditions not related to ventilation or equipment can also cause abnormal $ETCO_2$ values or waveforms, including pulmonary or heart disease, shock, changes in BP and body temperature, cardiac arrest, blood loss, and **pulmonary thromboembolism.**

Following are examples of these abnormalities:

- Cardiac arrest will cause a rapid loss of the waveform because $CO_2$ is no longer circulated to the lungs, and the waveform will rapidly reappear with the return of spontaneous circulation (ROSC) if cardiopulmonary cerebrovascular resuscitation (CPCR) is successful.
- Hypotension or a sudden decrease in cardiac output will cause a rapid decrease in the $ETCO_2$ (a shorter rectangle).
- Hypothermia will cause a gradual decrease in the $ETCO_2$ because of a decrease in the metabolic rate and subsequent $CO_2$ production (a shorter rectangle). Hyperthermia will cause a gradual increase (a taller rectangle).

Other, subtler changes in the configuration of the waveform may occur as a result of high or low gas flow, the type of breathing circuit used, the amount of dead space, and other factors. Also, capnograph malfunctions will affect the waveform, including excess moisture in the sampling line, blockage of the line, or a leak in the system. Table 5-3 shows common changes in the capnogram and associated causes.

### Blood Gas Analysis

Blood gas analysis refers to the measurement of blood pH, and dissolved oxygen and carbon dioxide gas in arterial ($PaO_2$ and $PaCO_2$) or venous ($PvO_2$ and $PvCO_2$) blood. It is therefore an indicator of both oxygenation and ventilation as well as acid-base status. Each of these variables is influenced by respiratory function, which can be roughly evaluated by observation of the rate, depth, and character of the patient's respirations. However, physical monitoring may give an inaccurate impression of the patient's status because although respirations may appear normal, oxygenation and ventilation may in fact be abnormal.

Blood gas monitoring is most commonly used for large animal patients and is seldom used in small animal practice outside of specialty practices for several reasons. First, sample collection may be difficult because blood intended for blood gas analysis is most often obtained from an artery (as opposed to routine blood samples, which are taken from a vein). In certain situations, a venous sample may be used. For example, the lingual vein has extensive anastomoses with arteries in the tongue, the blood gas values obtained from lingual vein samples are close to arterial values, and the head is often easily accessed by the anesthetist during surgery. Second, sample handling is labor-intensive. Once obtained, the blood sample must be stored on ice, and values should be measured within 2 hours. Many veterinary reference laboratories and some veterinary hospitals are equipped to perform these tests, and some human hospital laboratories may be willing to accept samples from nonhuman patients. Portable analyzers have recently been introduced to the veterinary market.

Carbon dioxide ($CO_2$) is transported through the blood in three ways. About 20% to 30% is bound to hemoglobin in the RBCs. About 5% to 10% is dissolved in plasma and is measurable as $PCO_2$ (the $CO_2$ partial pressure in the vessels). The remainder (about 60% to 70%) reacts with

| TABLE 5-3 | Common Changes in the Capnogram and Associated Causes | |
|---|---|---|
| Changes | Causes | Capnogram Readout |
| No waveform | Esophageal intubation<br>Machine malfunction<br>Sensor not properly connected | |
| Sudden loss of waveform | Apnea<br>Cardiac arrest<br>ET-tube disconnected<br>Accidental extubation<br>Complete ET tube–circuit obstruction<br>Machine malfunction<br>Ventilator malfunction (if using one) | |
| Gradual decrease in $ET_{CO_2}$ | Hypothermia<br>Hyperventilation | |
| Rapid decrease in $ET_{CO_2}$ | Cardiac arrest<br>Severe blood loss<br>Pulmonary embolism<br>Sudden hypotension | |
| Gradual increase in $ET_{CO_2}$ | Hypoventilation<br>Malignant hyperthermia<br>Fever<br>Muscle tremors, shivering | |
| Rapid increase in $ET_{CO_2}$ | Return of spontaneous circulation after successful CPCR | |
| Increase in baseline $CO_2$ (usually with gradual increase in $ET_{CO_2}$) | Malfunction of expiratory unidirectional valve<br>Saturation of $CO_2$ absorbent<br>Contamination of sensor with secretions | |
| Sudden, temporary increase in $ET_{CO_2}$ | Release of a tourniquet<br>Administration of sodium bicarbonate | |
| Increased angle of the plateau | Asthma or other obstructive lung disease | |
| Slow upward stroke | Asthma or other obstructive lung disease<br>Obstructed breathing circuit | |
| Sloppy upstroke and downstroke | Leaky cuff<br>Partially kinked endotracheal tube | |

$CO_2$, Carbon dioxide; *CPCR*, cardiopulmonary cerebrovascular resuscitation; *ET*, endotracheal; $ET_{CO_2}$, end-tidal $CO_2$.

water to form carbonic acid, which is quickly converted into bicarbonate and hydrogen ions according to the following reaction:

$$CO_2 + H_2O = H_2CO_3 = HCO_3^- + H^+$$

The anesthetist can evaluate how well the patient is eliminating $CO_2$ by measuring $Pa_{CO_2}$ through blood gas determination. $Pa_{CO_2}$ is often elevated during anesthesia (45 to 60 mm Hg compared with less than 45 mm Hg in the awake patient) because the respiratory depression produced by most anesthetics causes the body to retain $CO_2$. In other words, the patient does not breathe often enough or deeply enough to eliminate the normal amount of $CO_2$.

A $Pa_{CO_2}$ greater than 60 mm Hg indicates that the patient is hypoventilating. If this happens, the anesthetist needs to determine if the patient is in trouble by assessing the oxygenation, cardiac rhythm, BP, and anesthetic depth. It may be necessary to assist ventilation by compressing the reservoir bag or using a ventilator (see Chapter 6).

*TECHNICIAN NOTE*   $Pa_{CO_2}$ is often 45 to 60 mm Hg during anesthesia because the respiratory depression produced by most anesthetics causes the body to retain $CO_2$. A $Pa_{CO_2}$ greater than 60 mm Hg indicates that the patient is hypoventilating.

Because of high $CO_2$ levels, anesthetized patients may also become mildly acidotic (i.e., excess hydrogen ions are produced from $CO_2$ according to the previous equation). Blood pH in anesthetized animals usually reflects this mild respiratory acidosis and is commonly 7.2 to 7.3, compared with the normal animal's blood pH of 7.35 to 7.45. Cellular enzymes do not work well outside certain pH ranges, so when acid-base disturbances are suspected or present, maintaining pH between 7.2 and 7.5 is advisable. The correction of the underlying cause often results in improvement of acid-base status, thus treatment should be discussed with the veterinarian-in-charge (VIC). Blood pH measurement can be performed at the same time blood gas determinations are made, to help the anesthetist determine the acid-base status of the body and the adequacy of the patient's respiration. In the absence of elevated $Pa_{CO_2}$, a decreased pH is evidence of metabolic acidosis, which should be brought to the attention of the VIC. Blood pH that is elevated (greater than 7.45) when $Pa_{CO_2}$ is decreased (less than 35 mm Hg) indicates hyperventilation, which may be caused by light anesthetic depth, overzealous ventilation, pain, or hypoxemia. Blood pH that is elevated with a normal $Pa_{CO_2}$ indicates metabolic alkalosis, which may be caused by obstruction of outflow from the pylorus of the stomach or by excessive administration of $NaHCO_3$.

$Pa_{O_2}$ is the partial pressure of dissolved oxygen in arterial blood. This should be approximately five times the inspired concentration of oxygen. Therefore when a patient is breathing room air, which is approximately 21% $O_2$, $Pa_{O_2}$ is approximately 100 mm Hg, and when it is breathing 100% $O_2$ under general anesthesia, $Pa_{O_2}$ is approximately 500 mm Hg. Clinically significant hypoxemia is present if $Pa_{O_2}$ is below 80 mm Hg, and $Pa_{O_2}$ below 60 mm Hg requires intervention such as mechanical ventilation (see Chapter 6). Causes of hypoxemia are hypoventilation, decreased fraction inspired oxygen, shunting of blood flow (blood bypasses the lungs and is returned, unoxygenated, to the systemic arteries), and decreased ability of oxygen to diffuse from the lung into the bloodstream (diseases such as pneumonia or pulmonary edema). In the absence of disease, small animals and ruminants are rarely hypoxemic during anesthesia. Anesthetized horses are commonly hypoxemic, regardless of health status (see Chapter 9).

## Indicators of Body Temperature

The objective of the ACVA monitoring guidelines for body temperature is "to ensure that patients do not encounter serious deviations from normal body temperature." To meet this objective, the ACVA makes the following recommendations: "Temperature should be measured periodically during anesthesia and recovery and if possible checked within a few hours after return to the wards."

Core body temperature is another vital sign that, although not an indicator of circulation, oxygenation, or ventilation, is nonetheless important for reasons indicated

below. Body temperature should be monitored at least every 15 to 30 minutes during anesthesia, using a rectal thermometer or an esophageal or rectal probe attached to a continuous display monitor.

Body temperature is regulated by a physiologic process called *thermoregulation,* in which changes in a variety of physiologic processes including shivering, metabolic rate, and peripheral blood flow keep the temperature within the normal range. The hypothalamus of the brain is the "control center" for thermoregulation. With few exceptions, anesthetics decrease the body temperature by depressing the hypothalamus, reducing muscular activity, and slowing the metabolic rate. For this reason, hypothermia is a frequent and even an expected response to general anesthesia that if not prevented, recognized, and controlled will cause a variety of adverse effects including prolonged recovery. In severe cases of hypothermia, depressed CNS and heart function will endanger the patient. Temperature loss is greatest in the first 20 minutes, and can be 3° C or more during the course of a prolonged procedure. (See Table 5-2 for common body temperatures during anesthetic procedures.) Several factors contribute to this effect:

- Animals are routinely shaved before surgery, and the skin is often prepared with antiseptic and alcohol solutions that cool the skin by evaporation.
- An anesthetized animal is incapable of generating heat by shivering or muscular activity.
- The metabolic rate of an anesthetized animal is less than that of a conscious animal, resulting in less heat generation.
- During the course of surgery, a body cavity may be opened and the viscera exposed to air at room temperature.
- Some preanesthetic and general anesthetic agents cause peripheral vasodilation, resulting in an increased rate of heat loss.
- Pediatric and geriatric animals are less able to maintain thermoregulation and are therefore even more predisposed to hypothermia then adult animals.
- Small patients lose heat faster because the body surface area is proportionately greater than the surface area of larger patients.
- Administration of room temperature IV fluids will further decrease body temperature.
- Patients placed on non-rebreathing systems constantly breathe fresh gas, which is cold and dry; they therefore expend energy warming and humidifying this gas.

*TECHNICIAN NOTE* During anesthesia, body temperature loss is greatest in the first 20 minutes. Body temperatures in the range of 32° to 34° C (89.6° to 93.2° F) prolong anesthetic recovery and significantly decrease the dose of anesthetic agents required. Temperatures below 32° C (89.6° F) cause dangerous CNS depression and changes in heart function.

The magnitude of hypothermia determines the effects, but temperatures as low as 36° C (96.8° F) do not cause significant harm.

There are several potential problems associated with hypothermia during the maintenance and recovery periods. Body temperatures in the range of 32° to 34° C (89.6° to 93.2° F) prolong anesthetic recovery and significantly decrease the dose of anesthetic agents required to maintain surgical anesthesia by slowing the rate at which liver enzymes metabolize the drugs. This predisposes the patient to anesthetic overdose if the rate of administration is not reduced. Shivering during recovery will increase the patient's oxygen demands by as much as six times. This can cause significant complications when the patient is unable to respond to this increase in demand (as may be the case in a patient not receiving adequate oxygen or with cardiopulmonary disease). Temperatures below 32° C (89.6° F) cause dangerous CNS depression and changes in heart function. To avoid these problems the anesthetist should endeavor to monitor the patient's temperature and to maintain it as much as possible within the normal range. A variety of techniques can be used to minimize heat loss.

- Avoid excessively cold temperatures in the surgery suite or treatment room.
- Always place a barrier between the patient and tabletops, especially those made of stainless steel.
- Warm IV fluids to 37.5° C (approximately 100° F) before administration, or place a segment of the fluid line in a bowl of warm (37.5° C [approximately 100° F]) water to warm the fluids as they travel through the IV line. Realize that warming fluids in a microwave can result in excessively hot regions or can easily overheat the fluids. Fluids over 42° C (107.6° F) cause hemolysis and damage to the vascular endothelium and organs. For this reason, fluids must be mixed and the temperature always checked before they are administered to the patient.
- Place a circulating warm water blanket between the patient and the table. These quilted, vinyl blankets are attached to a unit that circulates warm water through the blanket.
- Place the patient on a forced warm-air blanket. These devices consist of a quilted plastic blanket (similar to a pool floater) that is placed under and sometimes over the patient. A device is attached that circulates warm air through the blanket.

The same techniques can be used to manage hypothermic patients. Additional rewarming techniques include the following:

- Place warm water bottles containing 37.5° C (approximately 100° F) water next to the patient. These bottles will lose heat quickly, however, and if left near the patient too long will worsen the hypothermia. Consequently, they must be checked and reheated on a regular basis.
- Place the patient under infrared heating lamps at a distance of 75 cm (30 inches).
- Flush the abdominal cavity with warmed fluids.

Never use electric heating pads, because they are not usually temperature regulated and often exceed the maximum safe operating temperature of 42° C (107.6° F). Thus, severe burns can result from their use. Also, avoid rapid warming of very cold patients because dilatation of the peripheral vasculature may decrease BP and release cardiotoxic substances that may accumulate in hypoxic tissues.

Hyperthermia (increased body temperature) is occasionally seen in anesthetized animals. Hyperthermia may occur for several reasons, including excessive administration of external heat, drug-induced reactions (e.g., opioid administration in some cats, excessive muscular activity after drugs such as ketamine), inability to dissipate heat (e.g., large dogs with thick coats under surgical drapes and/or placed on low-flow or closed system anesthesia in which the rebreathed gases are warmer). Hyperthermia in these cases is often noted during or just before recovery. Cooling methods should be applied, such as administering cold fluids intravenously, intraperitoneally, or rectally and performing surface cooling with fans and ice or alcohol. When opioids have been given to cats, administration of acepromazine (0.03 to 0.05 mg/kg) or reversal using naloxone should be considered. If the patient is still anesthetized, increasing the flow rate of oxygen to nonrebreathing levels will also help.

One particular type of hyperthermia, malignant hyperthermia (MH), is most commonly seen in pigs, although there are reports of susceptible individuals in other species. In pigs this is caused by a genetic defect that results in excess muscle metabolism in the presence of some anesthetic drugs such as halothane and the muscle relaxant succinylcholine. Restraint can also precipitate this syndrome, so stress should be minimized during handling of susceptible swine. Clinically, the anesthetized pig will become hot and stiff to the touch, pink pigs will turn red, large amounts of $CO_2$ are produced, and tachyarrhythmias occur. Anesthesia should be halted immediately, 100% oxygen administered, and cooling methods applied. The only medical treatment for MH is dantrolene, which is typically available only at large veterinary or human hospitals.

## ASSESSMENT OF ANESTHETIC DEPTH

### Reflexes and Other Indicators of Anesthetic Depth

At all times during an anesthetic procedure, the anesthetist must accurately assess the patient's anesthetic depth. Like many things, this is more complex than it first seems and requires detailed observation and interpretation of subtle changes in physical signs. In practice, the subtleties of anesthetic monitoring are all too often neglected for a variety of reasons including a lack of adequate skill, a sense of complacency borne of past experience with many successful anesthetic procedures (and a subsequent attitude that can be summarized by the statement "it's not a big deal—my patients never have any problems"), or more job demands than the technician can reasonably handle. When not given due attention, monitoring is turned into a crude and alarmingly simplified system consisting of the following three stages of anesthesia: "awake," "asleep," and "dead."

Obviously the anesthetist needs considerably more detail than that. The goal of monitoring is to ensure throughout the entire procedure that the patient is at a depth that provides immobility, unconsciousness, and lack of awareness of pain while avoiding conditions that endanger the patient such as hypoventilation, hypoxemia, hypotension, and hypothermia. Achieving this balance is not always easy and requires timely and effective response to changes in monitoring parameters. Although vital signs provide some help, reflexes, muscle tone, pupil size, eye position, and response to surgical stimulation are the best indicators of anesthetic depth (Table 5-4).

> **TECHNICIAN NOTE** In practice, the subtleties of anesthetic monitoring are all too often neglected for a variety of reasons. When not given due attention, monitoring is turned into a crude and alarmingly simplified system consisting of the following three stages of anesthesia: "awake," "asleep," and "dead."

## Reflexes

A reflex is an unconscious response to a stimulus. All healthy, conscious animals demonstrate predictable reflex responses. One example is the cough reflex, which is a response to the presence of foreign material in the airways. Reflex responses help protect the animal from injury (in the case of the cough reflex, by clearing upper airway obstructions and preventing aspiration of harmful material). These protective reflexes gradually decrease in response to an increasing depth of anesthesia, such that by stage III, plane 3, few to no reflex responses remain. The reflexes most commonly monitored in veterinary anesthesia include the swallowing, laryngeal, pedal, palpebral, and corneal reflexes as well as the PLR. When describing the status of these reflexes verbally to other surgical team members, or in written records, the terms "present," "decreased" or "depressed," and "absent" are often used.

### Swallowing Reflex

The swallowing reflex is a response to the presence of saliva or food in the pharynx. This reflex is monitored by watching for swallowing motions in the ventral neck region. The swallowing reflex is present in light surgical anesthesia, is lost in medium surgical anesthesia, and returns during recovery just before the patient regains consciousness. The return of the swallowing reflex during recovery is the main indicator used to determine when it is safe to remove the endotracheal

---

## TABLE 5-4 Indicators of Anesthetic Depth

| Parameter | Light | Medium | Deep |
|---|---|---|---|
| | | Indicators of Anesthetic Depth | |
| Swallowing | Maybe | No | No |
| Vaporizer setting | Low (approximately 1 × MAC) | Medium (approximately 1.5 × MAC) | High (approximately 2 × MAC) |
| Palpebral reflex | Present | Decreased or absent | Absent |
| Pedal reflex | Present | Absent | Absent |
| Corneal reflex[†] | Present | Present | Absent |
| Pupillary light reflex | Present | May be present | Absent |
| Spontaneous movement | Maybe | No | No |
| Muscle tone[‡] | Marked | Moderate | Flaccid |
| Eyeball position | Usually central | Usually ventromedial | Central |
| Pupil size[‡] | Midrange to constricted | Usually midrange | Dilated |
| Heart rate | Often high or high normal | Often moderate | Often decreased |
| Respiratory rate | Often high or high normal | Often moderate | Often decreased |
| Nystagmus (horses) | Fast | Slow | Absent |
| Salivation, lacrimation | Normal | Decreased | Absent |
| Response to surgical stimulation | Marked | Moderate | None |

Modified from Haskins SC: General guidelines for judging anesthetic depth, *Vet Clin North Am Small Anim Pract* 22:432-434, 1992.
*MAC,* Minimum alveolar concentration.
[†]The corneal reflex is not reliable in small animals.
[‡]Strongly influenced by anesthetic protocol and signalment.

tube. Animals that vomit after this point usually will swallow rather than aspirate the vomited material, and the endotracheal tube is therefore no longer needed to protect the airway. In fact, if the endotracheal tube is not removed at this point, the patient will begin to chew on it.

> ⬚ TECHNICIAN NOTE   The return of the swallowing reflex during recovery is the main indicator used to determine when it is safe to remove the endotracheal tube.

### Laryngeal Reflex

The laryngeal reflex is an immediate closure of the epiglottis and vocal cords when the larynx is touched by any object. This reflex protects the animal from tracheal aspiration. The laryngeal reflex may be observed during intubation, is present if the animal is in a lighter plane of anesthesia, and can make it difficult to pass the endotracheal tube. It is strong in cats, pigs, and small ruminants. A sustained or exaggerated laryngeal reflex, referred to as *laryngospasm,* is most commonly seen in these species and is a complication of endotracheal intubation.

> ⬚ TECHNICIAN NOTE   The palpebral reflex should be absent during surgical anesthesia in small animals maintained with isoflurane or sevoflurane. In most horses a very slight response indicates a surgical plane of anesthesia. Ruminants tend to have a slightly stronger reflex than horses, although spontaneous blinking is almost always associated with a plane of anesthesia that is too light.

### Palpebral Reflex

The palpebral reflex (blink reflex) is a blink in response to a light tap on the medial or lateral canthus of the eye (Figure 5-27). In the conscious animal, this reflex helps protect the eye from injury. When eliciting this reflex, it is important to use a "light touch," because vigorous tapping may artificially cause the eyelid to move, giving the anesthetist a false-positive response. Some anesthetists prefer to test this reflex by lightly stroking the hairs of the upper eyelid. As with most reflexes, the palpebral reflex is gradually lost as anesthetic depth increases. Most animals retain the palpebral reflex in light anesthesia and lose it during medium anesthesia, although the exact point at which it is lost varies among individuals, species, and agents. In small animals maintained with isoflurane or sevoflurane, this reflex should be absent during optimum and deep levels of anesthesia. Therefore when gas anesthetics are used in small animal patients, the presence of this reflex indicates that the anesthetic depth is inadequate, although the absence of the reflex cannot be used to determine if the anesthetic depth is excessive. In most horses a very slight palpebral response (very slow closure of the eyelid) indicates a surgical plane of anesthesia. Ruminants tend to have a slightly stronger eyelid reflex than horses, although spontaneous blinking is almost always associated with a plane of anesthesia that is too light. During recovery, return of the reflex usually indicates impending arousal.

> ⬚ TECHNICIAN NOTE   The pedal reflex is present during light anesthesia and is lost during optimum anesthesia. It is particularly important in animals undergoing mask inductions, in which the presence of a mask makes assessment of other reflexes or jaw tone somewhat difficult.

### Pedal Reflex

The pedal reflex is flexion or withdrawal of the limb in response to vigorous squeezing and twisting or pinching of a digit or pad (Figure 5-28). This reflex is useful only in small animal patients. The pedal reflex varies

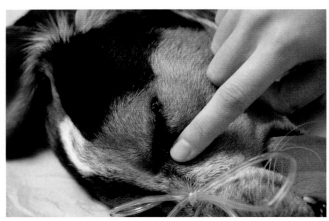

**FIGURE 5-27**   Assessing the palpebral reflex by lightly tapping the medial or lateral canthus.

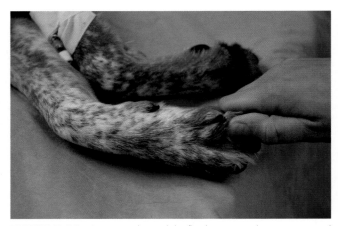

**FIGURE 5-28**   Assessing the pedal reflex by vigorously squeezing and twisting or pinching a digit or pad.

depending on the anesthetic depth, from a very subtle contraction of muscles to a full withdrawal of the limb. Because false-negative responses are common, accurate assessment of this reflex requires a stimulus of a surprisingly high intensity (a really hard squeeze and twist), although obviously it must not be so forceful as to injure the patient. This is an important point when learning to elicit this reflex, because many novices are often surprised at how much force is required to obtain an accurate response.

This reflex is present during light anesthesia, is lost during optimum anesthesia, and is particularly important in animals undergoing mask inductions, in which the presence of a mask makes assessment of other reflexes or jaw tone somewhat difficult. Once the patient is in medium surgical anesthesia, this reflex is not useful in detecting the onset of excessive anesthetic depth, because the reflex is absent in both optimum and deep anesthesia.

> **TECHNICIAN NOTE**  The corneal reflex should be present in light and medium planes of anesthesia and is lost when the anesthetic depth is excessive, but it is unreliable in small animals. It is therefore used primarily to tell the anesthetist when a large animal patient is anesthetized too deeply.

### Corneal Reflex

The corneal reflex is a retraction of the eyeball within the orbit and/or a blink in response to stimulation of the cornea. It is tested by touching the cornea with a sterile object (a drop of saline or artificial tear solution is commonly used) (Figure 5-29). This reflex is most useful in large animals but is very difficult to elicit in small animals, except when the patient is in very light anesthesia. Retraction of the eye is often subtle and best seen by positioning oneself so that the line of sight is near the same horizontal plane as the cornea.

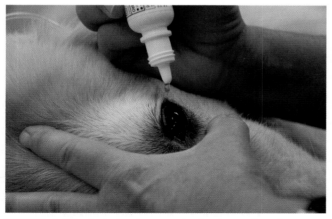

**FIGURE 5-29**  Assessing the corneal reflex by touching the cornea with a drop of sterile artificial tears.

This reflex should be present in light and medium planes of anesthesia and is lost when the anesthetic depth is excessive but is unreliable in small animals. It is therefore used primarily to tell the anesthetist when a large animal patient is too deeply anesthetized and should be reserved for this purpose only so that damage to the cornea is avoided.

### Pupillary Light Reflex

The PLR is a constriction of the pupils in response to a bright light shined on one of the retinas. It is elicited by following the steps described on p. 19 in Chapter 2. This reflex gradually diminishes with increasing anesthetic depth, should be present in light and medium surgical anesthesia, but is lost during deep surgical anesthesia.

### Dazzle Reflex

The dazzle reflex is a blink in response to a bright light shined on the retinas. It has the same significance as the PLR but is generally lost very early.

## Other Indicators of Anesthetic Depth
### Spontaneous Movement

Spontaneous movement in an unconscious patient indicates a very light plane of anesthesia and often indicates imminent arousal. This may manifest as shivering, alternating flexion and extension of the limbs, muscle twitching, or tremors. However some drugs, including etomidate, propofol, and opioids, may be associated with focal muscle twitching even in a medium plane of anesthesia.

> **TECHNICIAN NOTE**  When assessing jaw tone, it is important to avoid opening the patient's mouth too wide, because when the mouth is open to the maximum extent the anesthetist will feel resistance regardless of the muscle tone and will thus falsely interpret the muscle tone as being greater than it actually is.

### Muscle Tone

Assessment of muscle tone gives the anesthetist an indication of the degree of skeletal muscle relaxation. Muscle tone is usually assessed by attempting to open the jaws from a closed position and estimating the amount of passive resistance (referred to as *jaw tone*) (Figure 5-30). When assessing jaw tone, it is important to avoid opening the patient's mouth too wide, because when the mouth is open to the maximum extent the anesthetist will feel resistance regardless of the muscle tone and will thus falsely interpret the muscle tone as being greater than it actually is. If the anesthetist does not have access to the mouth, muscle tone can also be assessed by noting the size of the anal orifice (referred to as *anal tone*).

With increasing depth of anesthesia, the resistance to movement of the jaw will progressively decrease and the anal orifice will progressively increase in size. Tone generally is "marked" in light anesthesia, "moderate" in medium anesthesia, and "flaccid" in deep anesthesia.

The degree of muscle relaxation observed in the patient depends not only on anesthetic depth but also on the patient signalment and the agents used. For example, dogs with very strong muscles of mastication (such as Rottweilers) will have higher tone than dogs with smaller jaw muscles. This reflex is unreliable in pediatric patients (which normally have little tone regardless of the plane). Tone is generally decreased in patients receiving benzodiazepines, alpha$_2$-agonists, and other muscle relaxants, absent in patients receiving neuromuscular blockers, and increased in patients receiving cyclohexamines.

Jaw tone is not useful in large animal patients as their large masseter muscles (for chewing and grinding plant material) and relatively small mouth opening make it impossible to detect changes in muscle tone.

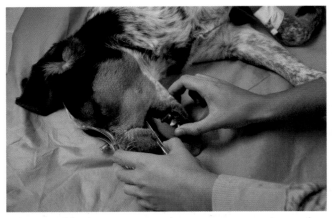

**FIGURE 5-30** Assessing jaw tone by attempting to open the jaws from a closed position and estimating the amount of passive resistance.

> **TECHNICIAN NOTE** In small animals and ruminants the eye is generally central during light anesthesia, ventromedial during medium anesthesia, and central during deep anesthesia. In horses the eye can rotate in any direction, and sometimes the eyes will rotate in opposite directions. Generally rotation of one or both eyes indicates adequate anesthetic depth for surgery.

### Eye Position

Eye position refers to the orientation of the cornea in relation to the palpebral fissure. Eye position changes from central to ventromedial (the patient appears to be looking toward its chin) and back to central with increasing anesthetic depth, although there is considerable variation among individuals in exactly when these changes occur (Figure 5-31). When the eye is ventromedial, only the sclera and conjunctiva are visible, which precludes assessment of the pupil size and the PLR. In small animals the eye is generally central during light anesthesia, ventromedial during medium anesthesia, and central during deep anesthesia. Some anesthetics (e.g., ketamine) do not cause eye rotation, even at moderate anesthetic depth. Eye position in ruminants is often similar to that in dogs, and the eyes rotate ventromedially during surgical anesthesia. In horses the eye can rotate in any direction, and sometimes the eyes will rotate in opposite directions. Generally rotation of one or both eyes indicates adequate anesthetic depth for surgery. The eyes of swine are quite sunken and are often unhelpful when trying to determine depth of anesthesia in pigs.

### Pupil Size

The size of the pupil also varies with anesthetic depth; pupils are dilated (mydriatic) during stage II anesthesia, are normal or constricted (miotic) during light surgical anesthesia, progressively dilate as anesthetic depth increases, and are widely dilated during deep anesthesia (Figure 5-32). This indicator is influenced by drugs, however, including opioids, cyclohexamines, and parasympatholytics.

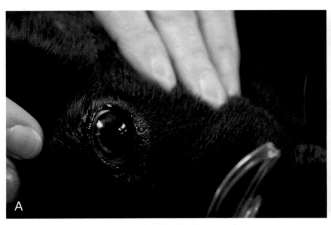 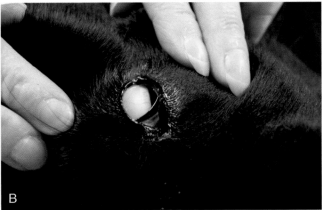

**FIGURE 5-31** Eye position. **A,** Central position. **B,** Ventromedial position.

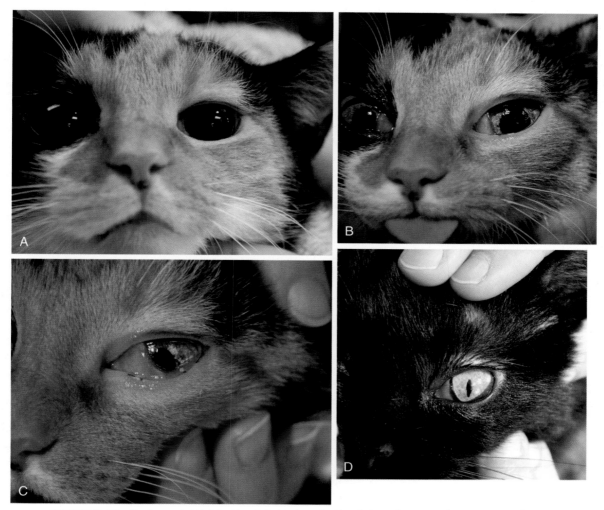

**FIGURE 5-32** Pupil size. **A,** Widely dilated. **B,** Moderately dilated. **C,** Midrange pupils. **D,** Constricted pupils.

> **TECHNICIAN NOTE** Nystagmus is commonly seen in horses during certain planes of anesthesia. Fast nystagmus occurs in very light anesthesia and gradually slows as the anesthetic depth increases. Very slow nystagmus may still be present as a "roving eye" during medium anesthesia.

### Nystagmus

Nystagmus is an oscillation of the eyeballs that is commonly seen in horses during certain planes of anesthesia. Fast nystagmus occurs in very light anesthesia (including recovery) and gradually slows as the anesthetic depth increases (or once anesthesia wears off at the end of the procedure). Very slow nystagmus may still be present as a "roving eye" during medium anesthesia. In horses in which this occurs, one eye is rotated either rostrally or caudally, and the other eye remains central or rotated in the opposite direction ("divergent eye signs"). After a period of time the eyes will then very slowly rotate to the alternate position. This eye movement pattern is typically associated with an adequate plane of anesthesia for surgery.

Ruminants and small animals rarely show nystagmus under anesthesia.

### Salivary and Lacrimal Secretions

The presence or absence of salivary and lacrimal secretions may give clues about anesthetic depth, particularly in an animal that has not received anticholinergics. Normal production of tears and saliva diminishes with increasing anesthetic depth and is totally absent in deep surgical anesthesia. A lack of production is recognized as a dry appearance to the cornea, in which it loses its glistening appearance, and tacky mucous membranes. Because of the relative absence of tears, the use of ophthalmic artificial tear drops or ointment every hour is advised for all animals undergoing general anesthesia. Note that application of ointment may decrease the ability to test the corneal reflex. Atropine ointment should not be used because it causes significant pupil dilation. In horses, increased lacrimation and salivation indicate light anesthesia.

## Heart and Respiratory Rates

Although not reliable indicators of anesthetic depth, HR and RR can be used to supplement other data. Both values tend to decrease as anesthetic depth increases, and increase as anesthetic depth decreases. Caution should be used in interpreting both HR and RR because each is subject to many influences in addition to anesthetic depth. For example, HR increases in response to a fall in BP. HR and RR may also increase in response to surgical stimulation or to a painful stimulus.

Some anesthetic drugs and adjuncts (e.g., cyclohexamines and parasympatholytics) increase HR, whereas most other agents decrease HR. Bradycardia may be induced by endotracheal intubation or manipulation of the eye as would occur during ocular surgery. Hypercarbia (high $PaCO_2$) and hypoxemia (low $PaO_2$) can also increase RR.

> *TECHNICIAN NOTE*  An increase in HR, RR, or BP in response to surgical stimulation does not usually reflect a conscious perception of pain. The anesthetist should not necessarily interpret these signs as an indication that the animal's anesthetic depth is inadequate unless other evidence supports this conclusion.

## Response to Surgical Stimulation

Surgical stimulation (e.g., incising the tissue, manipulating viscera, manipulating bones during fracture repair, or pulling on the suspensory ligament of the ovary may cause an increase in HR, RR, or BP. These responses do not usually reflect a conscious perception of pain. The anesthetist should not necessarily interpret these signs as an indication that the animal's anesthetic depth is inadequate unless this conclusion is supported by other evidence. Minor changes in HR during surgery are considered normal, and in fact are absent when anesthetic depth is excessive.

## Judging Anesthetic Depth

During the course of anesthesia, the anesthetist should monitor as many variables as possible and weigh all available evidence before judging the anesthetic depth of the patient. No one piece of information is unfailingly reliable, and it is unwise to determine the anesthetic plane by monitoring only one or two reflexes or vital signs. In addition, each animal is unique and has an individual response to increasing anesthetic depth. For example, many animals develop bradypnea and hypoventilation shortly after induction with injectable general anesthetics, while still in a light plane of anesthesia. If RR is used as the sole criterion for judging anesthetic depth, the animal that develops respiratory depression may be incorrectly

judged to be too deeply anesthetized. Decreasing the concentration of anesthetic delivered to such a patient might easily result in the patient's becoming dangerously lightly anesthetized. Observation of the other indicators of anesthetic depth would likely give the anesthetist a more balanced view of the situation and a more accurate assessment of true anesthetic depth. Examples of the use of judgment in interpreting anesthetic depth are given in Box 5-6.

Similarly, observation of the amount of anesthetic being delivered to the patient (e.g., the vaporizer setting) does not in itself indicate the patient's anesthetic depth. Although high vaporizer settings result in increased delivery of anesthetic to the patient and, subsequently, an increase in anesthetic depth, there is tremendous variation in patient response. This variation results in part from the patient's response to the anesthetic and in part from the influence of other drugs given to the animal. One animal may be maintained at stable surgical anesthesia with a vaporizer setting of 3% isoflurane, whereas another animal may require 2%, and still another may be satisfactorily maintained at 1.5%. The concentration of anesthetic gas received by the animal also is not necessarily the concentration indicated by the vaporizer setting; it may vary with the oxygen flow rate, the quality of respirations, and other factors (see Chapter 4). Nevertheless, the vaporizer setting and the length of time for which the animal has been anesthetized are additional evidence that must be considered. The basic rule is that if there is doubt about the level of anesthesia in a particular patient, one should decrease the vaporizer setting and continue to monitor the animal closely.

## RECORDING INFORMATION DURING ANESTHESIA

The objectives of the ACVA monitoring guidelines for record keeping are as follows:

"1. To maintain a legal record of significant events related to the anesthetic period.
2. To enhance recognition of significant trends or unusual values for physiologic parameters and to allow assessment of the response to intervention."

To meet these objectives, the ACVA makes the following recommendations:

"1. Record all drugs administered to each patient in the perianesthetic period and in early recovery, noting the dose, time, and route of administration, as well as any adverse reaction to a drug or drug combination.
2. Record monitored variables on a regular basis (minimum every 5 to 10 minutes) during anesthesia. The minimum variables that should be recorded are heart rate and respiratory rate, as well as oxygenation status and blood pressure if these were monitored.

## BOX 5-6  Examples of Depth Assessment

1. A mature cat has been anesthetized with propofol given intravenously. The anesthetist notes that the cat appears unconscious and relaxed. The pulse is strong, and the heart rate is 144 bpm. The respirations are regular, and the rate is 20 breaths/min. The pupils are centrally positioned. The palpebral reflex is brisk, but no pedal or swallowing reflex is present. The anesthetist wishes to intubate the animal. At this depth of anesthesia, is it possible? What other tests could the anesthetist perform to determine anesthetic depth?

   *Answer:* The cat appears to be in stage III, plane 1 anesthesia and may be deeply anesthetized enough to intubate. The anesthetist should assess the jaw tone and observe whether there is any resistance when the tongue is gently pulled before assuming that intubation is possible.

2. A 13-year-old dog has been anesthetized by mask induction with isoflurane. After intubation, it is maintained on 2% isoflurane. The anesthetist wishes to ensure that the dog is sufficiently anesthetized to allow removal of a large skin tumor. The dog's respirations are shallow, with a rate of 8 breaths/min. The heart rate is 90 bpm. There is no response to surgery, and all reflexes are absent. The pupils are central; the jaw tone is flaccid. Is the animal adequately anesthetized for this procedure?

   *Answer:* The animal is indeed adequately anesthetized and in fact may be at an excessive anesthetic depth. The respiratory rate and tidal volume are low. The absence of all reflexes, the central pupils, and the flaccid jaw tone all indicate that the animal may be in stage III, plane 3 anesthesia. At this point, the anesthetist should consider reducing the isoflurane setting to 1.5% and monitoring the animal for signs of decreased depth. After doing this, the anesthetist should carefully monitor the animal for signs that may be indicative of pain perception (e.g., increased respiratory rate, increased blood pressure, or voluntary movement) to ensure that the vaporizer setting is high enough for adequate analgesia. In animals at adequate anesthetic depth, the heart rate and respiratory rate will commonly increase slightly in response to surgical stimulation.

3. An 8-year-old dog has been anesthetized with glycopyrrolate and intravenous (IV) ketamine and diazepam and is now under sevoflurane anesthesia. The dog's heart rate is 100 bpm, and the respirations are 8 breaths/min. The jaw tone appears moderate, but the pupils are central and show no response to light. No reflexes are present. Is the anesthetic depth appropriate?

   *Answer:* The anesthetist cannot be sure whether the anesthetic depth is appropriate or too deep because some parameters indicate stage III, plane 2 (heart rate, jaw tone) but others indicate stage III, plane 3 (respiratory rate, reflexes, pupil position, and response to light). The patient has been given glycopyrrolate and ketamine, which may have elevated the heart rate. At this point, the anesthetist should assume the patient is excessively deeply anesthetized and should reduce the concentration of sevoflurane. At the same time the anesthetist should monitor the patient for signs of arousal.

---

3. Record heart rate, repiratory rate, and temperature in the early recovery phase.
4. Any untoward events or unusual circumstances should be recorded for legal reasons, and for reference should the patient require anesthesia in the future."

Complete and accurate medical records are a legal requirement in veterinary practice. Most jurisdictions require that some form of anesthetic record be maintained during anesthesia. In many cases this record can be in the form of a logbook in which information is listed, such as the date, client and patient identification, preoperative physical status, nature of the procedure performed with the patient under anesthesia, and the anesthetic protocol. A brief description of the animal's response to anesthesia should also be given. Records of this type allow the veterinarian to review the total number of anesthetic procedures that have been carried out in a given period and determine the frequency and nature of complications. This information may be helpful in assessing the anesthetic protocols. Controlled substance logs must be meticulously maintained to document use of benzodiazepines, opioids, cyclohexamines, barbiturates, and other controlled drugs.

In addition, medical information regarding the anesthetic procedure must be written in the patient's record. This allows the veterinarian to quickly review the animal's anesthetic history and may be helpful in determining the best anesthetic protocol to use for future procedures. For example, if the record indicates that the animal was anesthetized with a barbiturate agent and experienced a lengthy recovery, the veterinarian may choose to anesthetize the patient with an alternative agent in the future. On the other hand, if a patient with a preexisting disease was recently anesthetized without incident with a particular agent, the veterinarian would be justified in using the same agent for the next anesthesia.

In some practices, an anesthesia form such as shown in Figure 5-33 is used to record a detailed description of an anesthetic procedure. This type of record contains information on the patient's preoperative status (e.g., vital signs and the results of diagnostic tests), the anesthetic protocol used (including fluids administered and the amounts of drugs given), the patient's vital signs throughout anesthesia (e.g., pulse, respiration, BP, temperature, and laboratory results), the time at which anesthesia commenced and was terminated, the beginning and end of surgery, and the time required for recovery. Typically, the information is recorded chronologically to allow an overview of the patient's responses at every point throughout the procedure. Figure 5-34 is an example of a completed record. Detailed records of this type are not commonly used in veterinary practice; however, they are common in teaching, referral, or research institutions.

# ANESTHESIA RECORD

Date: _____          Monitor: _____

Patient Name: _____ Wt: _____ Species: _____ Breed: _____ Sex: _____ Age: _____

| Premedications: | Amount Given: | Route: | Time: |
|---|---|---|---|
| | | | |
| | | | |
| | | | |

**NOTES:**
Physical Status Class:
Procedure:
Anesthetist/Surgeon:

| Induction Agents: | Amount Given: | Route: | Time: |
|---|---|---|---|
| | | | |
| | | | |

Pre-op/Post-op data:

| Maintenance: | % Range/Total: | Route: |
|---|---|---|
| | | |

| Reversal Agents: | Amount Given: | Route: | Time: |
|---|---|---|---|
| | | | |
| | | | |

**TIME**    00   15   30   45   00   15   30   45   00   15   30   45     Comments

Oxygen Flow (L/min)    10 8 6 4 2 1 0

Inhalant Agent:    8 7 6 5 4 3 2 1 0

Vaporizer Setting (%)

**CODE:**

● HR *(monitor q5 min)*    **200**

○ RR *(monitor q5 min)*    **180**

v  Systolic BP    **160**
ʌ  Diastolic BP
–  Mean BP    **140**
X  SpO2
□  CO2    **120**
S -Ⓢ (begin-end surgery)
P -Ⓟ (begin-end procedure)
Ⓘ-Ⓔ (intubate-extubate)    **100**

   **80**

**Monitoring:**
❑ Esophageal stethoscope
❑ ECG monitor    **60**
❑ Doppler monitor
❑ Oscillometric BP    **40**
❑ Direct BP monitoring    **35**
❑ Pulse Oximeter    **30**
❑ Capnograph    **25**
❑ Apnea monitor    **20**
❑ Temperature probe    **15**
   **10**

**Anesthetic System:**    **8**
Machine: SA❑; LA❑; Ventilator ❑    **6**
Non-rebreathing ❑; Rebreathing ❑    **4**
ET tube size _____ Bag size _____    **2**

| Temperature *(monitor q 15 min)* | |
|---|---|
| Line # | |

| Meds/Fluids: | 1 | |
|---|---|---|
| | 2 | |
| | 3 | |
| | 4 | |
| | 5 | |

**FIGURE 5-33** Anesthesia record. This is an example of an anesthesia record used to document the anesthetic procedure.

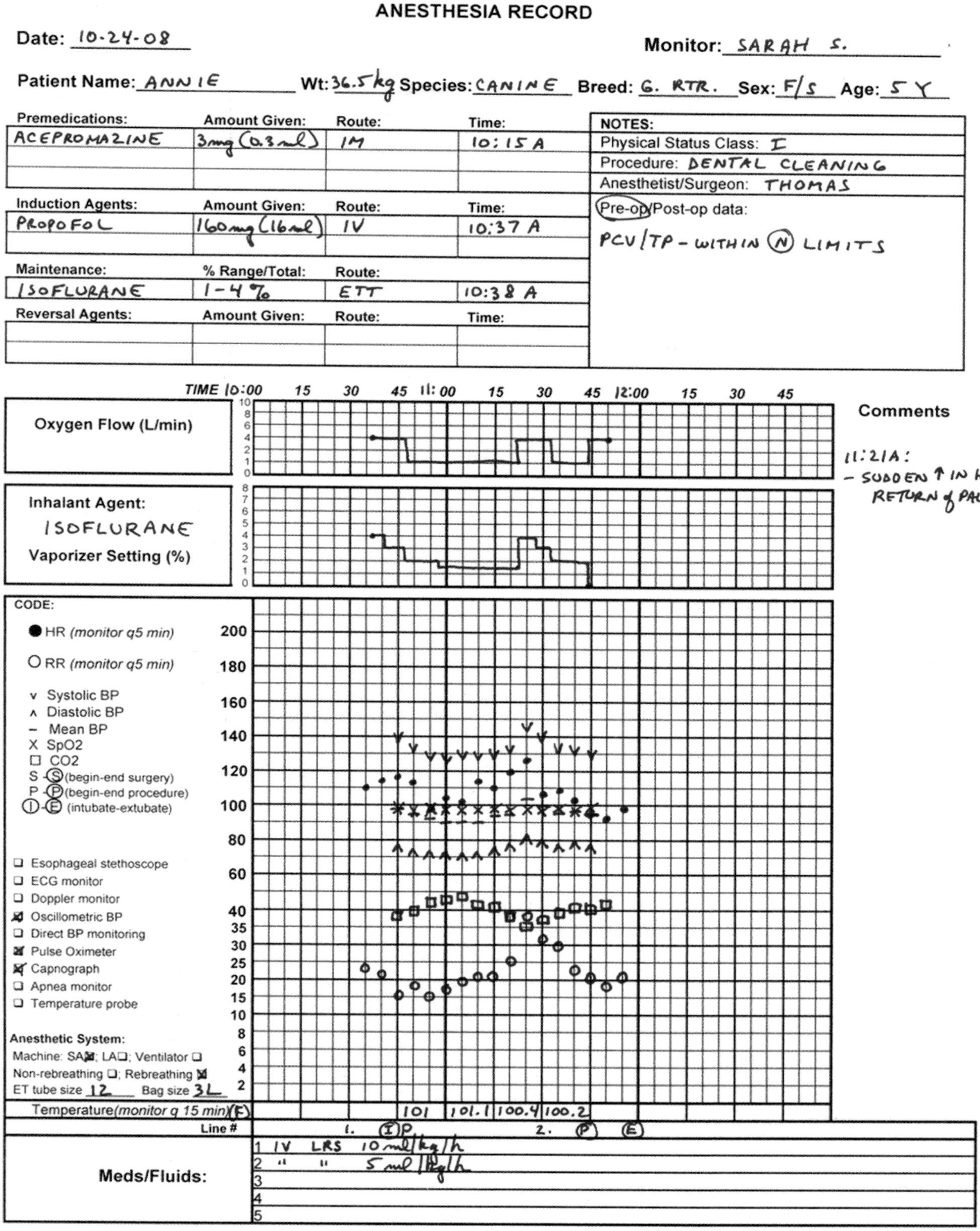

## ANESTHESIA RECORD

Date: 10-24-08

Monitor: SARAH S.

Patient Name: ANNIE    Wt: 36.5 kg  Species: CANINE  Breed: G. RTR.  Sex: F/S  Age: 5 Y

| Premedications: | Amount Given: | Route: | Time: |
|---|---|---|---|
| ACEPROMAZINE | 3 mg (0.3 ml) | IM | 10:15 A |
| | | | |

| Induction Agents: | Amount Given: | Route: | Time: |
|---|---|---|---|
| PROPOFOL | 160 mg (16 ml) | IV | 10:37 A |

| Maintenance: | % Range/Total: | Route: | |
|---|---|---|---|
| ISOFLURANE | 1-4 % | ETT | 10:38 A |

| Reversal Agents: | Amount Given: | Route: | Time: |
|---|---|---|---|
| | | | |

**NOTES:**
Physical Status Class: I
Procedure: DENTAL CLEANING
Anesthetist/Surgeon: THOMAS
Pre-op/Post-op data:
PCV/TP - WITHIN (N) LIMITS

**Comments**

11:21A:
- SUDDEN ↑ IN HR + RR
  RETURN OF PALPEBRAL

TIME 10:00  15  30  45  11:00  15  30  45  12:00  15  30  45

Oxygen Flow (L/min)

Inhalant Agent: ISOFLURANE
Vaporizer Setting (%)

CODE:
- ● HR (monitor q5 min)
- ○ RR (monitor q5 min)
- v Systolic BP
- ∧ Diastolic BP
- − Mean BP
- X SpO2
- ☐ CO2
- S - Ⓢ (begin-end surgery)
- P - Ⓟ (begin-end procedure)
- Ⓘ - Ⓔ (intubate-extubate)

- ☐ Esophageal stethoscope
- ☐ ECG monitor
- ☐ Doppler monitor
- ☒ Oscillometric BP
- ☐ Direct BP monitoring
- ☒ Pulse Oximeter
- ☒ Capnograph
- ☐ Apnea monitor
- ☐ Temperature probe

Anesthetic System:
Machine: SA☒; LA☐; Ventilator ☐
Non-rebreathing ☐; Rebreathing ☒
ET tube size 12    Bag size 3 L

| Temperature (monitor q 15 min)(F) | | | 101 | 101.1 | 100.4 | 100.2 | | | | |

| Line # | 1. Ⓘ Ⓟ | 2. Ⓟ Ⓔ |
|---|---|---|

| Meds/Fluids: | 1 | IV | LRS | 10 ml/kg/h |
|---|---|---|---|---|
| | 2 | " | " | 5 ml/kg/h |
| | 3 | | | |
| | 4 | | | |
| | 5 | | | |

**FIGURE 5-34** Completed anesthesia record. Looking at this finished record permits all details of this procedure to be easily reviewed, including patient data; doses, times, and routes of administration of all agents, adjuncts, and fluids; physical and machine-generated monitoring parameters; and detailed observations about the procedure.

pre-meds → help recover

## KEY POINTS

1. The American College of Veterinary Anesthesiologists (ACVA) has published guidelines for anesthetic monitoring intended to help veterinary anesthetists make sound monitoring decisions.

2. During any anesthetic procedure, the anesthetist must monitor the animal closely to ensure that the patient is safe and that the degree of central nervous system (CNS) depression or anesthetic depth is appropriate.

3. Effective monitoring is based on the principle that at any given anesthetic depth, monitoring parameters show predictable responses. Much discernment is required on the part of the anesthetist to interpret the significance of these parameters, however.

4. Knowledge of the anesthetic stages and planes give the anesthetist a framework for meaningful interpretation of monitoring parameters.

5. The objectives of surgical anesthesia are that the patient does not move, is not aware, does not feel pain, has no memory of the procedure afterwards, and has stable cardiopulmonary function.

6. Physical monitoring parameters can be grouped into one of the following three classifications: 1, vital signs; 2, reflexes; and 3, other indicators of anesthetic depth.

7. Vital signs (including heart rate and rhythm, pulse strength, capillary refill time, mucous membrane color, respiration rate and depth, and temperature) are most helpful to determine if the patient is safe.

8. Reflexes (including the laryngeal, swallowing, pedal, palpebral, corneal, and pupillary light reflex) and other indicators (including spontaneous movement, muscle tone, eye position, pupil size, response to surgical stimulation, lacrimation, salivation, and nystagmus) are most helpful to determine if the anesthetic depth is appropriate.

9. Physical and machine monitoring parameters can be grouped according to whether they assess circulation, oxygenation, ventilation, or anesthetic depth.

10. Monitoring equipment, although not mandatory for effective patient monitoring, generates data (including oxygen saturation, arterial blood pressure, cardiac electrical activity, inspired and expired $CO_2$ levels, blood gases, heart rate [HR], respiratory rate [RR], and tidal volume [$V_T$]) that help the anesthetist accurately assess patient status. This equipment often warns of impending problems early, so that the anesthetist can take action before they reach crisis level.

11. Effective monitoring requires the anesthetist to memorize normal monitoring parameters and to know what levels signal a need to inform the veterinarian-in-charge (VIC).

12. The anesthetist must keep accurate and complete records of anesthetic procedures, the nature of which will vary depending on the clinical situation.

## PROCEDURE 5-1 Measuring Blood Pressure with a Doppler Probe

1. Clip any hair from the area where the probe will be placed.
2. Apply ultrasound gel to the concave portion of the probe.
3. Select a cuff that has a width 30% to 50% of the circumference of the extremity used for the reading (wrap intravenous [IV] tubing around the limb to measure). Place the cuff snugly over the limb or tail, proximal to where the probe will be placed.
4. Place the probe over the appropriate artery distal to the cuff (coccygeal, median palmar, median plantar, or dorsal pedal artery).
5. Turn on the amplifier. Adjust the position of the probe until a signal is acquired.
6. Attach the manometer and bulb to the cuff tubing.
7. You may tape the probe in place, but do not apply the tape tightly or the artery will be occluded and no readings will be possible.
8. Inflate the cuff until the sound stops.
9. Slowly release pressure from the cuff until the first "whooshing" sound is heard. This represents the systolic pressure.
10. Take five readings. Discard the highest and lowest values and average the remaining values to determine the systolic pressure.

## REVIEW QUESTIONS

1. With most injectable and inhalant anesthetics, there is generally a progressive depression of cardiovascular and respiratory function as the depth of anesthesia increases.

   True          False

2. The plane of anesthesia most suitable for surgical procedures is generally considered to be:
   a. Stage III, plane 1
   b. Stage III, plane 2
   c. Stage III, plane 3
   d. Stage III, plane 4

3. Breath holding, vocalization, and involuntary movement of the limbs are most likely an indication that the animal is in what stage or plane of anesthesia?
   a. Stage I
   b. Stage II
   c. Stage III, plane 1
   d. Stage III, plane 2

4. Anatomic dead space is considered to be the:
   a. Air within the breathing circuit
   b. Air within the digestive tract
   c. Air within the trachea, pharynx, larynx, bronchi, and nasal passages
   d. Air within the alveoli

5. The minimum acceptable heart rate for an anesthetized large breed dog is _____ bpm.
   a. 60
   b. 70
   c. 80
   d. 100

6. If the ECG is normal, the heart must be beating normally.

   True          False

7. In general, a respiratory rate of less than _____ breaths/min in an anesthetized dog should be reported to the veterinarian.
   a. 4
   b. 6
   c. 10
   d. 15

8. Tachypnea is:
   a. An increase in respiratory depth (tidal volume)
   b. An increase in respiratory rate
   c. A decrease in respiratory depth (tidal volume)
   d. A decrease in respiratory rate

9. A patient that has been anesthetized will often have a:
   a. Mild metabolic acidosis
   b. Mild metabolic alkalosis
   c. Mild respiratory acidosis
   d. Mild respiratory alkalosis

10. An animal that is in a surgical plane of anesthesia should not respond in any way to any procedure that is being done to it (e.g., pulling on viscera should not change heart rate).

    True          False

11. A 20-kg dog has been anesthetized by mask induction with isoflurane and after intubation is maintained on 2% isoflurane with a flow rate of 2 L of oxygen per minute. The heart rate is 80 bpm, respiratory rate is 8 breaths/min and shallow, the jaw tone is relaxed, and all reflexes are absent. This animal is most likely in what stage of anesthesia?
    a. Stage III, plane 1
    b. Stage III, plane 2
    c. Stage III, plane 3
    d. Stage III, plane 4

12. Pulse oximetry allows accurate estimation of:
    a. Arterial blood pressure
    b. Pulse pressure
    c. $Pa_{O_2}$
    d. Percent saturation of hemoglobin with oxygen
    e. Blood gas values

13. During anesthesia, a mean arterial blood pressure of less than 60 mm Hg indicates:
    a. Inadequate tissue perfusion
    b. Imminent cardiac arrest
    c. A normal expected value during anesthesia
    d. This value is not indicative of patient condition

14. A pulse oximeter reading of 89% indicates:
    a. A normal value
    b. A need for supportive therapy
    c. A state of hypoxemia, but no need for therapy
    d. A medical emergency

15. An $ET_{CO_2}$ level of 65 would commonly be caused by:
    a. Hyperventilation
    b. Detachment of the endotracheal tube from the connector
    c. Decreased tidal volume
    d. Hypothermia

16. Regarding oxygen transport:
    a. Most oxygen travels in the blood dissolved in plasma.
    b. $SpO_2$ is an accurate indicator of oxygen available to the tissues even in anemic animals.
    c. $PaO_2$ is closely related to $SpO_2$ (as one goes up, the other does also).
    d. When a patient is breathing 100% oxygen, the $PaO_2$ is expected to be in the range of 100 to 120 mm Hg.

For the following questions, more than one answer may be correct.

17. Which of the following statements about body temperature is/are correct?
    a. Body temperatures of 32° to 34° C (89.6° to 93.2° F) cause prolonged anesthetic recovery.
    b. Dangerous CNS depression and changes in cardiac function may be seen at body temperatures less than 32° C (89.6° F).
    c. Ideally, IV fluids should be warmed to about 37.5° C (approximately 100° F) before administration to surgery patients.
    d. Circulating warm water blankets should be set at 45° C (approximately 111° F).

18. Which of the following statements about nystagmus as a monitoring tool is/are accurate?
    a. Nystagmus is commonly seen in horses in very light anesthesia.
    b. Nystagmus is not a useful indicator of anesthetic depth in small animals.
    c. In a horse, a "divergent eye sign" is typically associated with an adequate plane of anesthesia for surgery.
    d. Ruminants rarely show nystagmus under anesthesia.

19. Pale mucous membranes commonly indicate:
    a. Blood loss
    b. Anemia
    c. Decreased perfusion
    d. Hypertension

20. An animal under stage III, plane 2, anesthesia would exhibit which of the following signs?
    a. Very brisk palpebral reflex
    b. Regular respiration
    c. Relaxed skeletal muscle tone
    d. Very dilated pupils

## SELECTED READINGS

American College of Veterinary Anesthesiologists: *Suggestions for monitoring anesthetized veterinary patients.* Accessed June 2009 at www.acva.org.

Baetge C: Monitoring the anesthetized patient, *Vet Tech* 28(1):31-38, 2007.

Bill RL: *Clinical pharmacology and therapeutics for the veterinary technician,* ed 3, St Louis, 2006, Elsevier, pp 124-132.

Egger CM: Detection & correction of hypoxia during anesthesia, *Clin Brief* 6(9):55-59, 2008.

Gordon AM, Wagner AE: Anesthesia-related hypotension in a small animal practice, *Vet Med* 101(1):22-26, 2006.

Grosenbaugh DA, Muir WW: Blood pressure monitoring, *Vet Med* 93(1):48-59, 1998.

Grosenbaugh DA, Muir WW: Pulse oximetry: a practical efficient monitoring method, *Vet Med* 93(1):60-66, 1998.

Grosenbaugh DA, Muir WW: Using end-tidal carbon dioxide to monitor patients, *Vet Med* 93(1):67-74, 1998.

Haskins SC: Monitoring. In Thurmon JC, Tranquilli WJ, Benson GJ, editors: *Essentials of small animal anesthesia and analgesia,* Baltimore, 1999, Lippincott Williams & Wilkins, pp 269-291.

Haskins SC: Perioperative monitoring. In Paddleford RR, editor: *Manual of small animal anesthesia,* ed 2, Philadelphia, 1999, WB Saunders Company, pp 123-146.

Haskins SC: Monitoring anesthetized patients. In Tranquilli WJ, Thurmon JC, Grimm KA, editors: *Lumb & Jones' veterinary anesthesia and analgesia,* ed 4, Ames, Iowa, 2007, Blackwell, pp 533-558.

Love L, Harvey R: Arterial blood pressure measurement: physiology, tools, and techniques, *Compendium* 28(6):450-462, 2006.

Mama K: Anesthesia monitoring and pulse oximeters, *Clin Brief* 6(9):35-37, 2008.

Marshall M: Capnography in dogs, *Compendium* 26(10):761-778, 2004.

Mazzaferro E, Wagner A: Hypotension during anesthesia in dogs and cats: recognition, causes and treatment, *Compendium* 23(8): 728-737, 2001.

Muir WW, Hubbell JA, Bednarski RM: *Handbook of veterinary anesthesia,* ed 4, St. Louis, 2006, Elsevier, pp 269-303.

Murrell JC: Monitoring the anesthetized horse. In Doherty T, Valverde A, editors: *Manual of equine anesthesia and analgesia,* Ames, Iowa, 2006, Blackwell, pp 187-205.

Reeder D: Arterial blood pressure monitoring, *Vet Tech* 29(8):478-483, 2008.

# Special Techniques

6

## OUTLINE

Local Anesthesia, 183
  Local Anesthetic Agents, 184
  Characteristics of Local Anesthetics, 184
  Mechanism of Action, 184
  Route of Administration of Local
    Anesthetics, 185
  Adverse Effects of Local Anesthetics, 189
Assisted and Controlled Ventilation, 190
  Ventilation in the Awake Animal, 191

Ventilation in the Anesthetized Animal,
  191
Types of Controlled Ventilation, 192
Technical Consideration for Intermittent
  Mandatory Ventilation of
  Anesthetized Patients, 194
Risks of Controlled Ventilation, 194
Neuromuscular Blocking Agents, 194

## KEY TERMS

Assisted ventilation
Atelectasis
Bagging
Cauda equina
Controlled ventilation
Epidural anesthesia
Eutectic mixture
Infiltration
Intermittent mandatory
  ventilation
Line block
Local anesthesia
Manual ventilation
Mechanical ventilation
Motor neurons
Nerve block
Paralysis
Paresis
Respiratory minute
  volume
Ring block
Scoliosis
Sensory neurons
Splash block
Sympathetic blockade
Tidal volume

## LEARNING OBJECTIVES

*After completion of this chapter, the reader will be able to:*
- Define or explain the terms local anesthesia, sensory neuron, motor neuron, infiltration, line block, nerve block, ring block, splash block, epidural anesthesia, cauda equina, tidal volume, respiratory minute volume, atelectasis, controlled ventilation, assisted ventilation, manual ventilation, mechanical ventilation, and sympathetic blockade.
- List the advantages and disadvantages associated with the use of local anesthetic agents.
- Describe the ways in which local anesthetic agents may be used, including topical, infiltration, regional, intraarticular, epidural, and intravenous administration.
- Outline the methods for performing a nerve block and a line block, and list clinical situations in veterinary practice in which these blocks are used.
- Describe the technique for performing an epidural block, and give examples of clinical situations in which this block could be used.
- Explain the risks involved and the adverse effects that may be seen with the use of local anesthetic agents.
- Explain the difference between assisted and controlled ventilation.
- Describe the techniques of manual, mechanical, periodic, and intermittent mandatory ventilation and their application to anesthesia.
- List the indications for the use of neuromuscular blocking agents and the hazards associated with their use.
- Describe the differences between the two classes of neuromuscular blocking agents, including mode of action and reversibility.

The anesthetic agents and techniques used for routine procedures on most veterinary patients are described in Chapters 8, 9, and 10. In addition, one or more specialized techniques such as **local anesthesia,** mechanical ventilation, and/or the use of neuromuscular blocking agents may be indicated for a patient. This chapter describes these techniques and indicates the circumstances in which they may be useful.

## LOCAL ANESTHESIA

The term *local anesthesia* (also referred to as *local analgesia,* because local anesthesia blocks pain transmission) can be defined as the use of a chemical agent on **sensory neurons** to produce a disruption of nerve impulse transmission, leading to a temporary loss of sensation.

Local anesthesia is an effective, practical, and inexpensive means of producing anesthesia when the patient is tractable, when general anesthesia is undesirable or of high risk, or when the means to deliver it safely are unavailable. The advantages of local anesthesia include low cardiovascular toxicity, low cost, excellent pain control in the immediate postoperative period, and minimal patient recovery time. Local anesthetics are therefore commonly used in ruminants for obstetric and abdominal procedures, often without sedation. Local anesthesia is frequently used to complement standing sedation in horses. Although local anesthesia is less commonly used than general anesthesia in canine and feline patients, it may be a viable alternative in some patients. The choice between local anesthesia and general anesthesia is made by the veterinarian on the basis of such factors as the temperament, age, species, and physical status of the patient; cost; the nature of the operation to be performed; and the anesthetist's skill in performing the local anesthesia procedure.

Local anesthetics are also used in conjunction with general anesthesia to enhance pain control during and after surgery. The dose of the general anesthetic required may be significantly reduced because of the excellent analgesia provided by the local anesthetic.

> *TECHNICIAN NOTE*  Local anesthetics can be used in conjunction with general anesthesia to enhance pain control during and after surgery. The dose of the general anesthetic required may be significantly reduced because of the excellent analgesia provided by the local anesthetic.

## Local Anesthetic Agents

Many local anesthetic agents are available. These agents vary in strength, duration of effect, and method of use (Table 6-1). Lidocaine, bupivacaine, mepivacaine, and procaine are the agents most commonly used for skin **infiltration** and application to mucous membranes. Tetracaine and proparacaine are reserved chiefly for ophthalmic use.

Of the various local anesthetic agents available, lidocaine and bupivacaine are most commonly used in veterinary medicine. Lidocaine is administered at a concentration of 0.5% to 2%, and bupivacaine as a 0.25% or 0.5% solution. Both agents can be diluted with sterile saline (not water) if a lower concentration is desired. Bupivacaine has a slower onset of action (20 minutes) and a longer duration (6 hours) compared with lidocaine (almost immediate onset, duration 1 to 2 hours).

## Characteristics of Local Anesthetics

Local anesthetics differ from general anesthetics in several important respects:
- Local anesthetics are not general anesthetics. The term *general anesthetic* is reserved for those drugs such as inhalation anesthetics, propofol, ketamine, or barbiturates that primarily affect neurons in the brain. Like general anesthetics, local anesthetics exert their effect on neurons, but the target is the peripheral nervous system and spinal cord. Because local anesthetics normally do not affect the brain, they have no sedative effect. The patient remains fully conscious unless other agents such as tranquilizers, neuroleptanalgesics, or general anesthetics are used.
- If the appropriate dose and route of administration are used, local anesthetics have relatively few effects on the cardiovascular or respiratory systems. In contrast, preanesthetics and general anesthetics may have significant cardiovascular and respiratory effects. For this reason, local anesthesia may be preferable to general anesthesia in certain high-risk patients. However, local anesthetics are not without risk of toxicity, and the anesthetist should use caution to avoid overdosage, especially in small patients.
- Whereas general anesthetics are widely distributed throughout the body, local anesthetics primarily exert their effects in the area closest to the site of injection. Effective use of local anesthetics requires precise placement of the drug immediately adjacent to the target nerve. The veterinarian or technician performing the procedure must be familiar with the technique involved for each type of **nerve block.** For example, it is possible to block the sensory nerve of a tooth in a dog to perform a dental procedure; however, accurate and detailed knowledge of the neuroanatomy of the oral cavity is necessary. Local anesthetics are relatively ineffective in areas where drug diffusion is impeded by fat, bone, cartilage, fascia, tendon, and other connective tissues, as well as the presence of inflammation and infection.
- Unlike general anesthetics, local anesthetics are not normally transferred across the placenta to the fetus. For this reason, local anesthesia is used for cesarean sections and obstetric manipulations, particularly in ruminants, and also in small animal patients when general anesthesia is considered high risk.

> *TECHNICIAN NOTE*  Local anesthetics do not cross the placenta to the fetus. They are therefore useful for cesarean section and obstetric manipulation, particularly in ruminants.

## Mechanism of Action

The peripheral nervous system and spinal cord are made up of many types of neurons. The primary targets of local anesthetic drugs are the neurons that convey sensations (i.e., pain, heat, cold, and pressure) from the skin,

| TABLE 6-1 | Local Analgesics | | | |
|---|---|---|---|---|
| Agent (Generic Name) | Agent (Trade Name) | Potency (Procaine = 1) | Dose | Onset and Duration of Action |
| Lidocaine* | Xylocaine | 2 | 0.5%-2% for injection<br>2%-4% for topical use<br>Do not exceed 10 mg/kg SC or<br>2 mg/kg IV in dogs; do not exceed<br>4 mg/kg SC or 0.5 mg/kg IV in cats | Immediate onset; duration 1-2 hr with epinephrine, 1 hr without |
| Mepivacaine | Carbocaine | 2.5 | 1%-2% for injection<br>Do not exceed 5 mg/kg in dogs or<br>2.5 mg/kg in cats | Immediate onset; duration 90-180 minutes |
| Tetracaine | Pontocaine | 12 | 0.1% for injection<br>0.2% for topical use | Onset 5-10 minutes; duration 2 hr |
| Bupivacaine | Marcaine | 8 | 0.25%-0.5% for injection<br>Give SC only<br>Do not exceed 2 mg/kg in dogs or<br>1 mg/kg in cats | Onset 20 minutes; duration 4-6 hr |
| Procaine | Novocain | 1 | 1%, 2%, 10% | Immediate onset, 1-hr duration |

*Sodium bicarbonate (8.4%, 1 mEq/mL) is used as follows: add 0.8 mL bicarbonate to 10 mL of 2% lidocaine or 0.08 mL of bicarbonate to 20 mL of 0.5% bupivacaine.

*IV*, Intravenously; *SC*, subcutaneously.

From Skarda RT: Local and regional analgesia. In Short CE: *Principles and practices of veterinary anesthesia*, Baltimore, 1987, Williams & Wilkins.

muscles, and other peripheral tissues to the brain. These neurons (called *sensory neurons*) are affected by even small amounts of local anesthetic, provided the drug is deposited in proximity to the neuron. Local anesthetics result in antagonism, or blockade, of sodium channels. When the sodium channels of a neuron are blocked, the neuron cannot generate electrical impulses. A local anesthetic drug therefore acts as a membrane stabilizer, stopping the process of nerve depolarization. The result is a loss of nerve conduction. Reversal of this effect occurs as the drug is absorbed into the local circulation. Local anesthetics are then redistributed to the liver, where they are metabolized.

Another type of neuron (called a *motor neuron*) conveys impulses from the brain to muscle fibers and is responsible for initiating and controlling voluntary movements. **Motor neurons** are also sensitive to the effect of local anesthetics, and administration of a local anesthetic may cause temporary **paresis** (weakness) or **paralysis** (loss of voluntary movement) in the area served by the affected motor neurons.

Loss of sensation and loss of motor ability are seen concurrently. For example, use of a local anesthetic near the terminal end of the spinal cord (called an *epidural block*) will result in loss of sensation and voluntary movement to all areas innervated by the affected sensory and motor neurons. The patient sensations that are lost include (in order of loss) pain, cold, warmth, touch, joint sensation, and deep pressure in the caudal abdomen and pelvic limbs. After an epidural block, the patient will be unable to move the pelvic limbs, and the muscles will appear relaxed.

Local anesthetics also affect the neurons of the autonomic nervous system. These neurons convey impulses between the brain and the blood vessels and internal organs (including the heart). If these neurons are exposed to local anesthetics, there may be a temporary loss of function. This is most important in the sympathetic nervous system, and the loss of function of these neurons is called a **sympathetic blockade.** The main effect in the peripheral tissues is vasodilation, resulting in flushing and increased skin temperature of the affected area. If severe, vasodilation may cause blood pressure to fall, leading to hypotension. Sympathetic blockade can also be seen after epidural blocks with lidocaine and other local anesthetics, because sympathetic ganglia adjacent to the vertebrae are affected. If sympathetic blockade occurs within the thoracic spinal cord (as may occur if local anesthetic is allowed to diffuse into the thoracic spinal canal), sympathetic innervation to the heart may be blocked, resulting in bradycardia and impaired ventricular contractions, which are undesirable.

## Route of Administration of Local Anesthetics

Local anesthetic techniques are often used in conjunction with neuroleptanalgesics, tranquilizers, or other injectable medications. This helps to ensure adequate restraint, allowing accurate and safe injection of the local anesthetic and preventing patient movement during the surgical procedure.

Local anesthetics can be administered by a variety of routes, including topical application, infiltration (injection), or introduction into a joint, nerve plexus, vein, or the epidural space.

## Topical Use

Local anesthetics such as lidocaine are usually ineffective when applied directly to intact skin because the drug molecules are unable to penetrate the epidermis and reach the dermis, where the peripheral nerves are located. However, local anesthetics can be used for topical analgesia in some clinical situations:

- Ethyl chloride sprayed on intact skin provides partial, short-term (less than 3 minutes) analgesia by significantly cooling the skin. It is occasionally used for skin biopsies and other superficial procedures. There is some risk of frostbite if a large area is sprayed.
- A cream formulation containing a **eutectic mixture** of 2.5% lidocaine and 2.5% prilocaine (EMLA cream) can be used to desensitize intact skin for superficial minor procedures such as catheterization. A thick layer of cream is applied to intact shaved skin in the area to be anesthetized and covered with an occlusive dressing for 10 minutes. Duration of effect is 1 to 2 hours. EMLA cream is available in 5-g or 30-g tubes and in single-dose anesthetic discs. It should not be applied to the eyes or to inflamed or broken skin. The patient should be prevented from licking treated areas.
- Wounds or open surgical sites (e.g., lateral ear resections, dewclaw removals) can be treated with topical anesthetic sprays such as 10% lidocaine, or by direct application of 0.25% bupivacaine. Sterile gauze sponges soaked with a mixture of local anesthetic and saline can also be placed on an open surgery site. The use of sprays or soaked gauze sponges is called a **splash block.** The efficacy of this technique has not been well established, but it appears to be most effective if the surgical field is relatively dry, with minimal bleeding. Care must be taken to avoid local anesthetic overdose, which is a particular concern with small patients. The dose of lidocaine given by this route should not exceed 4 mg/kg for the dog (2 mg/kg for the cat). For bupivacaine the dose should not exceed 2 mg/kg in dogs and 0.5 mg/kg in cats.
- Bupivacaine can be instilled through a chest tube placed during thoracic surgery. Local anesthetic administration should be delayed until the patient is awake, because instillation of bupivacaine into the chest cavity of an anesthetized patient may cause cardiac arrhythmias.
- Local anesthetics can be absorbed by mucous membranes, including the conjunctiva, nose, mouth, larynx, and lining of the urethra. They can be administered as topical sprays, drops, or ointment applied to these areas. For example, lidocaine spray is used to desensitize the larynx and prevent laryngospasm in cats. Another example of topical use of local anesthetics is the application of 0.5% proparacaine or tetracaine to the surface of the eye. This procedure desensitizes the cornea and conjunctiva, allowing procedures such as conjunctival scraping or tonometry. Gel containing local anesthetic (lidocaine, tetracaine, or amethocaine) can be applied to a urinary catheter to ease the catheterization process. In each case, analgesia of the mucous membrane results within 60 to 90 seconds and allows procedures to be performed with less discomfort to the patient. Analgesia lasts for 10 to 15 minutes.

Although topical anesthetics are useful in some situations, they generally offer less pain relief and shorter duration of effect than local anesthetics given by infiltration. Lidocaine patches are available that are applied to the skin and are effective for management of wound or incisional pain.

## Infiltration

Local anesthetics may be infiltrated (injected) into tissues, preferably in proximity to the target nerve. The local anesthetic can be given intradermally, subcutaneously, or between muscle planes. Infiltration techniques are used to provide analgesia for surgery involving superficial tissues, including skin biopsies, removal of small skin tumors, and repair of minor lacerations.

The procedure used for infiltration of local anesthetics is relatively simple. The area must be clipped and a skin antiseptic applied in a manner similar to surgical preparation. This prevents inadvertent contamination of the tissues with skin bacteria when the local anesthetic is injected. A small needle (23 or 25 gauge in small animal and equine patients, 20 or 22 gauge in ruminants) is often used to prevent tissue damage and allow for more precise placement of the drug. The amount of the drug to be injected varies with the location and procedure used and may be as little as 0.1 mL or as much as several milliliters in a dog, or several to tens of milliliters in large animal patients. The onset of analgesia is usually 3 to 5 minutes after the injection of lidocaine.

Before surgery commences it is advisable to test the effectiveness of the block by gently pricking the skin with a 22-gauge needle. If sensation is still present, the anesthetist should wait several minutes longer and consider repeating the injection or using another anesthetic protocol if the block does not take effect.

The infiltration of local anesthetics is not universally effective. Deep tissues such as muscles are unlikely to be affected when only superficial neurons are blocked. In addition, obstacles such as scar tissue or fibrous tissue, fat, edema, and hemorrhage impede diffusion of local anesthetic. Local anesthetics are also relatively ineffective when injected into inflamed or infected areas. In areas of active inflammation, tissue pH is acidic, resulting in rapid inactivation of the drug. For this reason and also for the prevention of contamination of other tissue, local anesthetics should not be infiltrated into infected tissues.

Once the local anesthetic reaches the neuron, the duration of effect depends on the type of drug being used and the rate of absorption by local blood vessels (see Table 6-1). This in turn depends on whether epinephrine is used with the local anesthetic. Lidocaine, the drug most commonly used for local injection, may be purchased with or without epinephrine. The concentration of epinephrine used is 0.01 mg/mL of lidocaine.

Epinephrine is added to lidocaine for the following two reasons:

1. Epinephrine causes constriction of blood vessels in the area of the injection. This decreases the rate of drug absorption and thereby prolongs the effect of the lidocaine by approximately 50%.
2. By causing vasoconstriction, epinephrine reduces the concentration of local anesthetic that enters the circulation at any given time, thereby reducing toxicity of the drug. This is most effective for short-acting drugs such as lidocaine and less helpful for long-acting drugs such as bupivacaine.

Lidocaine without epinephrine may be preferred to lidocaine with epinephrine in some situations. A solution containing epinephrine should not be used at an incision site because it may impair tissue perfusion and healing. Lidocaine with epinephrine should not be used on the ears, tail, or digits, because circulation to these areas may be compromised. Epinephrine also increases the risk of ventricular arrhythmias (particularly in animals anesthetized with halothane) and should be used with caution in animals with known cardiac disease. Lidocaine without epinephrine is used for intravenous techniques.

> **TECHNICIAN NOTE** Local anesthetics with epinephrine should not be administered intravenously and should be avoided when blocks of extremities are performed, as circulation to these areas may become compromised.

Local anesthetic injections may be painful in the awake patient. Some anesthetists add sodium bicarbonate (one tenth the volume of local anesthetic) to decrease pain on injection.

Two techniques are commonly used for infiltration of local anesthetics: nerve blocks and **line blocks.**

### Nerve Blocks

A nerve block is achieved by injecting local anesthetic in proximity to a nerve to desensitize a particular anatomic site. One familiar example is the use of Novocain in human dentistry. Nerve blocks are used commonly in anesthesia of large animals and also may be used in small animals provided the location of the target nerve is known exactly. Reference texts contain illustrations that indicate the location of nerve blocks for different species and particular areas of the body. Before a nerve block is performed, the nerve is palpated to determine its location, although this may not always be possible if the nerve is small.

Once the location of the nerve supplying the surgical site is known, the procedure is straightforward. After the skin is clipped and prepared for surgery, a small amount of local anesthetic is injected immediately adjacent to the nerve. Lidocaine, bupivacaine, or a 1:1 mixture of the two can be used to take advantage of the shorter onset of action of lidocaine and the longer duration of action of bupivacaine. The drug diffuses through the tissues to reach the target nerve. Caution should be used to avoid injecting directly into the nerve because temporary or permanent loss of nerve function can occur. Also, avoid intravenous injection of the local anesthetic, which may cause unwanted central nervous system and cardiovascular effects. To avoid intravenous injection, aspirate before injecting a local anesthetic. If blood appears in the syringe, the needle should be withdrawn and the location of the injection changed.

Clinical situations in which nerve blocks can be used include the following:

- Lameness examinations in horses
- Cornual blocks for dehorning cattle
- Paravertebral blocks for abdominal surgery or cesarean sections in cattle (Procedure 6-1, p. 197)
- Dental blocks in dogs and cats (infraorbital, mental, mandibular, and maxillary nerve blocks)
- Intercostal nerve blocks in animals undergoing chest surgery
- Infiltration of nerves during amputation of a limb (0.5 mL of 0.5% bupivacaine, injected into and around the nerve during the operation)
- Nerve block to provide analgesia for declawing cats (Procedure 6-2, p. 199)

Specialty textbooks and journal articles provide complete descriptions of these and other nerve blocks. Regardless of the technique used, it is important to allow sufficient time for the tissues to absorb the drug (15 to 20 minutes) before the surgical or dental procedure is started. When properly performed, these blocks not only decrease the amount of general anesthetic required, but also provide excellent short-term analgesia after the procedure.

**Line blocks.** Often the veterinarian will perform an operation on an area of tissue that is served by numerous small nerves. In this situation, a line block consisting of a continuous line of local anesthetic can be placed in the subcutaneous or subcuticular tissues immediately proximal to the target area (Figure 6-1, *A*). If the line of local anesthetic completely encircles an anatomic part, such as a digit or teat, it is called a **ring block.**

Line blocks should be positioned between the target area and the spinal cord because this will block the sensory neurons most effectively. As with nerve blocks, the area is

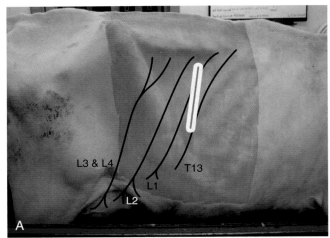

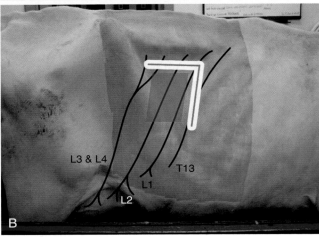

**FIGURE 6-1** Location for performing a line block or L-block in a cow for standing flank laparotomy. **A,** Line for infiltrating local anesthetic. The surgical incision is made along the line where anesthesia has been infiltrated. **B,** The line can be extended in an inverted L shape to anesthetize the caudal part of the surgical field. The surgical incision is made anywhere in the box outlined to the right of the L.

clipped and the skin prepared. A line block is placed by inserting the needle along the proposed line of infiltration, then gradually withdrawing the needle while simultaneously injecting a small amount of local anesthetic. If several injections are made, the needle should be inserted into a desensitized area of skin to avoid patient discomfort. Care should be taken to avoid inserting the needle into contaminated tissue (e.g., an infected wound).

Line blocks and ring blocks are used extensively in food animal and equine surgery, particularly in cattle. Examples include teat surgery and wound repair. A particular type of line block, called an *L-block,* is used for laparotomy in ruminants (see Figure 6-1, *B*).

## Intraarticular Administration

In certain circumstances, local anesthetics can be injected directly into a joint. For example, bupivacaine has been shown to provide significant analgesia when injected into the stifle joint at the conclusion of stifle arthroscopy and

surgery. A dose of 0.4 mL of 0.5% bupivacaine per kilogram, diluted with sterile saline (not water) to a volume sufficient to fill the joint, has been recommended. The drug is injected immediately after closure of the joint capsule.

### Regional Anesthesia

Regional anesthesia is a technique whereby a local anesthetic is injected into a major nerve plexus or in proximity to the spinal cord. This results in the blockage of nervous impulses to and from a relatively large area, such as an entire limb or the caudal portion of the body. Examples of regional anesthesia in veterinary medicine include paravertebral, epidural, spinal (intrathecal), and brachial plexus blocks.

### Paravertebral Anesthesia (Ruminants Only)

This is an alternative to a line block for standing laparotomy in cattle. The dorsal and ventral branches of spinal nerves T13-L2 are blocked, along with L3-L4 if anesthesia of the paralumbar fossa is required (e.g., for flank cesarean section) (see Procedure 6-1).

Advantages include provision of a wide, uniform area of anesthesia and a shorter time required to perform the block. Disadvantages include the increase in technical difficulty, hindlimb weakness if L3 and L4 are blocked, and the **scoliosis** (lateral curvature of the spine) commonly seen with this technique, which may make closure of the incision more challenging.

### Epidural Anesthesia

**Epidural anesthesia** is a regional anesthesia technique that is commonly used in both large and small animal patients. The procedure is not difficult (Procedure 6-3, p. 200) and, once mastered, allows the anesthetist to reliably block sensation and motor control of the rear, abdomen, pelvis, tail, pelvic limbs, and perineum. The technique is useful for tail amputation, anal sac removal, perianal surgery, urethrostomies, obstetric manipulations, cesarean sections, and some rear limb operations. Epidural anesthesia is most commonly used in three classes of patients:

1. Ruminants, in which procedures such as replacement of a vaginal prolapse can be undertaken with epidural anesthesia alone or in combination with a sedative. Epidural procedures are also useful to prevent straining during obstetric procedures, including cesarean sections.
2. Debilitated small animal patients in which general anesthesia is problematic but that may tolerate sedation and a lidocaine or bupivacaine epidural block. One common example is cesarean sections.
3. Patients requiring profound pain control after surgical procedures involving the hind limbs, pelvis, or caudal abdomen. For example, morphine or lidocaine epidural blocks are useful for animals undergoing surgical repair of a fractured femur.

The choice of drug used for epidural anesthesia is governed by the reason for the epidural: if immobility and anesthesia for surgery are required, a local anesthetic such as 2% lidocaine or 0.5% bupivacaine can be used at a dose of 1 mL/5 kg of body weight. Duration of effect is 1 to 2 hours for lidocaine and up to 6 hours for bupivacaine. If the main objective is epidural analgesia to ensure postoperative pain control, an opioid such as morphine is used instead (see Chapter 7). Opioids and local anesthetics such as lidocaine can also be mixed together and delivered epidurally. Opioids are generally associated with fewer unwanted side effects than lidocaine or bupivacaine (less risk of sympathetic blockade and hypotension, unlikely to cause motor blockade, and therefore less ataxia) but may cause pruritus and urinary retention in some patients. Opioids may also be combined with alpha$_2$-agonists for epidural analgesia in horses and cattle.

**Anatomic considerations.** To understand the technique used for epidural anesthesia, the anesthetist must be familiar with the anatomy of the terminal spinal cord region (see Procedure 6-3, Figure 5). The spinal cord is made up of sensory, motor, and autonomic neurons and is surrounded by three membrane layers: the pia mater, arachnoid, and dura mater. The subarachnoid space, which is the area between the arachnoid and the pia mater, is filled with cerebrospinal fluid. This fluid surrounds the entire spinal cord and communicates with the cerebrospinal fluid in the ventricles of the brain. The spinal cord and its membrane layers are encased within the spinal canal. This canal consists of bony vertebrae (cervical, thoracic, lumbar, sacral, and coccygeal) that protect the spinal cord from injury. Several ligaments also protect the vertebral canal, including the supraspinous ligament (which lies directly under the skin), the ligamentum flavum (also called the *ligamentum interarcuatum*), and the interspinous ligament (see Procedure 6-3, Figure 5). The neurons that supply the tissues exit from the spinal cord at regular intervals, emerging between the vertebrae and ultimately ending in the skin and other tissues. The spinal cord itself terminates in a group of neurons collectively called the **cauda equina.**

When epidural anesthesia is performed, local anesthetic is deposited in the epidural space, between the dura mater and the vertebrae. This is a potential space that is often filled with fat. Spinal nerves pass through the epidural space as they exit through the intervertebral foramina and are affected by local anesthetics and other drugs deposited in this space. In dogs the location of the block is between the last lumbar vertebra (L7) and the sacrum (see Procedure 6-3, Figure 5). When properly performed, injection of local anesthetic into this area is unlikely to damage the spinal cord because the cord normally ends at the sixth or seventh lumbar vertebra (L6 or L7). In cats the spinal cord extends farther caudally (as far as S1), and there is a slight risk of entering the subarachnoid space when performing epidural anesthesia.

Epidural anesthesia must be differentiated from spinal anesthesia, which is commonly performed in human patients. In spinal anesthesia the local anesthetic is injected into the subarachnoid space, where it mixes with the cerebrospinal fluid. Inadvertent injection of local anesthetic into the subarachnoid space is more common in the cat than in the dog.

Because local anesthetics block not only sensory nerves (including those that transmit pain sensation) but also motor neurons, an animal that has undergone epidural anesthesia may be unable to walk until the block wears off. Opioids, on the other hand, have minimal effect on motor neurons, and movement of the legs and tail is usually unimpaired after morphine epidural analgesia.

### Intravenous Regional Anesthesia (Bier Block)

Intravenous regional anesthesia is used to provide short-term (less than 1 hour) of local anesthesia to an extremity. When a Bier block is performed, a calculated amount of lidocaine (bupivacaine is not used, as it is more cardiotoxic when given intravenously) is injected into the distal segment of a superficial vein after a tourniquet has been applied proximal to the vein (Procedure 6-4, p. 203).

> *TECHNICIAN NOTE* Bupivacaine should not be used for intravenous regional anesthesia as cardiotoxicity is likely after release of the tourniquet.

### Systemic Administration

Lidocaine can also be administered by constant rate infusion to healthy anesthetized animals to reduce the dose of general anesthetic or analgesic required for painful operations and to prevent cardiac arrhythmias. The dose used is 50 to 75 mcg/kg/min in dogs and horses, and 25 mcg/kg/min in cats.

### Adverse Effects of Local Anesthetics

The use of local anesthetics is not without risk, and several adverse effects have been reported, including the following:

1. Motor neurons may also be affected, and the patient may lose voluntary motor control of the affected body part. The loss of motor function to the limbs typically results in recumbency. This may be inconvenient (e.g., for a standing procedure in a cow) or undesirable and dangerous (e.g., a horse that falls and thrashes as it repeatedly tries unsuccessfully to stand).
2. If local anesthetic is injected into a nerve, temporary or permanent loss of function may result. Direct injection into a nerve should be avoided, except for animals undergoing an amputation.
3. Tissue irritation may occur after the injection of some local anesthetics. Some veterinarians prefer

mepivacaine instead of other local anesthetics because it appears to cause less tissue irritation.

4. Paresthesia, an abnormal sensation of tingling, pain, or irritation, may be apparent during recovery from local anesthesia. (Human patients also experience this tingling sensation—for example, during recovery from "numbing" of the oral cavity with Novocain.) Animals should be monitored during recovery because they may chew or otherwise traumatize affected areas and may require chemical or physical restraint or the use of E-collars (cats and dogs).

5. Human and animal patients may exhibit allergic reactions to local anesthetics, usually in the form of a skin rash or hives. Anaphylaxis is also occasionally seen. Local anesthetics should not be used in patients in which an allergic reaction to these drugs has been previously observed.

6. Systemic toxicity may occur, particularly if a local anesthetic is inadvertently given intravenously without the use of a tourniquet. Systemic toxicity may be seen even if the drug is placed in the subcutaneous tissues, if a large amount of local anesthetic is injected. The most common signs of systemic toxicity originate in the central nervous system. The first sign of systemic toxicity is usually sedation, followed by nausea, restlessness, muscle twitching, hyperexcitability, seizures, respiratory depression, and, eventually, coma. Treatment of central nervous system signs may include intravenous or intrarectal diazepam (0.2 to 0.4 mg/kg) and administration of oxygen. Cardiovascular effects may also be observed, because of the direct effect of local anesthetics on the heart. Intravenous injection of lidocaine may inhibit the conduction of electrical impulses within the heart muscle and decrease the force of cardiac contractions. This is undesirable when local anesthesia is performed but makes this drug useful in the treatment of some types of ventricular arrhythmias. Bupivacaine is more cardiotoxic than lidocaine. The dose of lidocaine given subcutaneously to dogs, cows, and horses should not exceed 10 mg/kg and in cats should not exceed 4 mg/kg to avoid systemic toxicity. The smallest possible dose should be used. If the drug is given intravenously, the dose of lidocaine should not exceed 4 mg/kg in dogs, 2 mg/kg in large animals, and 0.5 mg/kg in cats. The dose of bupivacaine given subcutaneously should not exceed 2 mg/kg in dogs and 1 mg/kg in cats. For the average (4-kg) cat, the maximum dose of 2% (20 mg/mL) lidocaine is 0.8 mL (16 mg) if given subcutaneously and 0.1 mL (2 mg) if given intravenously. For 0.5% (5 mg/mL) bupivacaine, the maximum subcutaneous dose for a 4-kg cat is 4 mg (0.8 mL). Bupivacaine should not be given by intravenous injection. Dilution of the calculated dose of lidocaine or bupivacaine with sterile saline is helpful in small patients because it increases the volume and decreases the concentration of the solution to be injected.

7. Epidural or spinal injection may rarely traumatize the spinal cord or cauda equina, particularly if the animal is struggling during placement of the needle. Inflammation and fibrosis have been reported after epidural infiltration of local anesthetics containing preservatives. In addition, myelitis (spinal cord inflammation) and meningitis (inflammation of the pia mater, arachnoid, or dura mater) may occur if asepsis is not maintained.

8. If local anesthetics are permitted to infiltrate into the cranial portion of the spinal cord, serious toxicity and even death may occur. If the local anesthetic reaches the midthoracic vertebrae, innervation of the intercostal muscles may be blocked, interfering with normal respiration. If local anesthetic diffuses as far forward as the cervical spinal cord, the phrenic nerve may be affected. This nerve innervates the diaphragm, and loss of function may result in respiratory paralysis. When epidural anesthesia is performed, care should be taken to keep the patient's head elevated to avoid gravitational flow of the anesthetic into the anterior spinal canal around the thoracic and cervical spinal cord. The anesthetist should be prepared to intubate and artificially ventilate the lungs of any patient undergoing epidural anesthesia, because this may be necessary if intercostal and phrenic nerve function is impaired.

9. Diffusion of local anesthetic into the cervical and thoracic spinal cord may also affect sympathetic nerves supplying the heart and blood vessels, resulting in a sympathetic blockade with symptoms of bradycardia, decreased cardiac output, and hypotension. If blood pressure measurement is unavailable, careful monitoring of the capillary refill time, heart rate, and pulse strength will alert the anesthetist to a fall in blood pressure. Treatment consists of intravenous fluid administration at a rate of 20 mL/kg over a 15- to 20-minute period.

## ASSISTED AND CONTROLLED VENTILATION

The anesthetist may be called on to assist or control patient ventilation during any period of general anesthesia. In **assisted ventilation,** the anesthetist ensures that an increased volume of air or, more commonly, oxygen and anesthetic gases is delivered to the patient, although the patient initiates each inspiration. In **controlled ventilation,** the anesthetist delivers all of the air that is required by the patient, and the patient does not make spontaneous respiratory efforts. The anesthetist controls the respiratory rate and the volume and pressure of gas that the animal breathes.

Any procedure by which the anesthetist assists or controls the delivery of oxygen and anesthetic gas to the patient's lungs may be termed **positive pressure ventilation** (PPV). Whether achieved by bagging the patient (applying pressure to the reservoir bag with the pop-off valve fully or partially closed) or by using a mechanical ventilator, PPV is intended to ensure that the animal receives adequate oxygen and is able to exhale adequate amounts of carbon dioxide. This is a concern in veterinary anesthesia because the patient's own ventilation efforts may be inadequate to achieve these objectives.

## Ventilation in the Awake Animal

To understand the use of PPV in anesthesia, it is necessary to review the mechanics of normal breathing and the reasons why they may be ineffective in the anesthetized animal. Ventilation is the physical movement of air (and anesthetic gases in an anesthetized patient) into and out of the lungs and upper respiratory passageways. Ventilation has two parts: an active phase (inhalation) and a passive phase (exhalation). Inhalation is initiated by the respiratory center in the brain and is normally triggered by an increased level of carbon dioxide in the arterial blood ($Pa_{CO_2}$). As $Pa_{CO_2}$ rises above a threshold level (approximately 40 mm Hg), the respiratory center initiates the active inspiratory phase by stimulating the intercostal muscles and diaphragm to move, expanding the thorax. This creates a negative pressure (partial vacuum) within the chest, which causes the lungs to expand. As the lungs expand, air moves through the breathing passages and into the alveoli. When the lungs reach an adequate volume, nerve impulses feed back to the respiratory center, signaling the brain to stop the active phase of respiration. The intercostal muscles and diaphragm then relax, and exhalation takes place as the lungs deflate. Exhalation is passive, which means that no active muscle movement occurs (with the exception of exhalation during vigorous exercise, which has an active component). During exhalation, the carbon dioxide level in the blood begins to rise again, and after a short pause the respiratory center responds by initiating another inspiration.

Normally, exhalation lasts approximately twice as long as inspiration. For example, in an animal breathing 20 times per minute, each inspiration will last approximately 1 second and each exhalation will last approximately 2 seconds.

The amount of air that passes into or out of the lungs in a single breath is the **tidal volume** ($V_T$). Animals that are breathing deeply have a relatively large $V_T$, whereas animals that have shallow breathing or that are panting have a relatively small $V_T$. Normal $V_T$ in the awake animal is 10 to 15 mL/kg.

The respiratory rate or frequency is the number of breaths that occur in 1 minute. The **respiratory minute volume** is the total amount of air that moves into and out of the lungs in 1 minute. This value can be found by multiplying the average $V_T$ by the respiratory rate.

## Ventilation in the Anesthetized Animal

Ventilation in the anesthetized animal differs significantly from normal ventilation just described. These differences include the following:
- Tranquilizers and general anesthetics may decrease the responsiveness of the respiratory center in the brain to carbon dioxide. This means that inspiration does not occur as often in the anesthetized animal as in the healthy awake animal, despite the fact that the carbon dioxide level may be significantly elevated. This explains the observation that a respiratory rate of 8 to 20 breaths per minute is normal in cats and dogs under inhalation anesthesia, whereas the same animal would be expected to have a respiratory rate of 15 to 30 breaths per minute when awake.
- Tranquilizers and general anesthetics relax the intercostal muscles and diaphragm, causing them to expand less than they normally do during the inspiratory phase. Because the chest does not expand fully, the $V_T$ is reduced. The anesthetist may become aware of the reduced $V_T$ by noting that the reservoir bag does not collapse significantly during the inhalation phase (i.e., the volume of gas inhaled is relatively small). Because $V_T$ and respiratory rate are decreased, respiratory minute volume is also decreased.

As the amount of air entering and leaving the lungs in the anesthetized animal may be considerably reduced compared with the healthy awake animal, the anesthetist must be aware of the following potential problems:
- *Hypercarbia.* $Pa_{CO_2}$ may rise in the anesthetized patient, because carbon dioxide produced by the body is not eliminated as rapidly as in the awake animal. As the blood carbon dioxide level rises, carbon dioxide combines with water molecules in the bloodstream to form bicarbonate ions ($HCO_3^-$) and hydrogen ions ($H^+$). The accumulation of hydrogen ions causes the pH of circulating blood to fall, leading to respiratory acidosis. Blood pH in the healthy awake animal is 7.38 to 7.42, whereas in the anesthetized animal, blood pH may be as low as 7.20.
- *Hypoxemia.* If the anesthetized animal is breathing room air, $Pa_{O_2}$ may fall below normal values as a result of the decreased respiratory minute volume. Less oxygen enters the lungs, and therefore less is available to be absorbed into the blood.
- **Atelectasis.** Because $V_T$ is reduced, the alveoli do not expand as fully as normal on inspiration. The alveoli in some sections of the lung, particularly those that are lower in the animal's body, may partially collapse (a condition called atelectasis).

Some patients are at increased risk for having or developing these problems. Predisposing factors for hypercarbia, hypoxemia, and atelectasis include the following:
- Prolonged anesthesia (more than 90 minutes).
- Obesity.

- Administration of neuromuscular blocking agents (see following section).
- Preexisting lung disease such as pneumonia.
- Recent head trauma.
- Surgical procedures involving the chest or diaphragm. These animals may have preexisting cardiovascular or pulmonary disease and are at significant risk for cardiovascular collapse or respiratory arrest if conventional anesthesia with unassisted ventilation is attempted.
- Species differences. Horses in particular are prone to the problems listed previously, regardless of physical status. Adult ruminants also tend to hypoventilate and become hypercarbic.

The anesthetist has several ways of compensating for these effects. The $Pa_{O_2}$ can be elevated to normal levels (and, in fact, often above normal levels) if the patient is supplied with adequate oxygen. This is easily achieved because animals connected to anesthetic machines normally receive close to 100% oxygen. The anesthetized patient connected to an anesthetic machine is unlikely to have a reduced $Pa_{O_2}$ unless a problem such as pulmonary edema or upper airway obstruction is present.

It is more difficult to prevent atelectasis or an increase in $Pa_{CO_2}$ and resulting respiratory acidosis. In each of these situations, it may be advisable to take active steps to assist or control patient ventilation.

## Types of Controlled Ventilation

The following are two ways to control patient ventilation in the anesthetized patient:

1. The patient's lungs are ventilated by the anesthetist using the anesthetic breathing system; this technique is referred to as **manual ventilation.** A common term that is also used to indicate manual ventilation is **bagging.** In this type of PPV, the lungs are filled with oxygen by the pressure of gas entering the airways as the anesthetist squeezes the reservoir bag with the pop-off valve fully or partially closed. Exhalation is passive and occurs when the positive pressure is discontinued and the pop-off valve is opened fully, allowing the lungs to empty. For most patients, periodic bagging (one or two breaths every 2 to 5 minutes) is adequate to expand the lungs and reduce atelectasis. However, some patients require bagging throughout the anesthetic period, which is referred to as **intermittent mandatory ventilation.**
2. The patient's lungs are ventilated by a ventilator; this technique is called **mechanical ventilation.** In this type of PPV, the lungs are filled with oxygen by the pressure of gas from a special apparatus called a *ventilator.* As with manual ventilation, exhalation is passive and occurs when the positive pressure is discontinued. Ventilators used in anesthesia are not usually used to periodically ventilate patients, but

are most commonly used to provide intermittent mandatory ventilation.

Whether the patient's lungs are to be ventilated by manual or mechanical means, the patient must first be intubated and connected to an anesthetic machine. Ventilating the patient's lungs through an ordinary anesthesia mask does not deliver adequate amounts of oxygen to the lungs and may cause the stomach to fill with air, increasing the risk of regurgitation.

### Manual Ventilation

Manual ventilation can be performed on a periodic basis (one or two breaths every 2 to 5 minutes) on any anesthetized patient. These periodic breaths, also called "sighs," help expand collapsed alveoli and reverse atelectasis. For the patient's lungs to be manually ventilated, the pop-off valve is closed and the reservoir bag is compressed until the lungs are inflated. When pressure on the reservoir bag is released, exhalation can occur. The anesthetist must use caution to ensure that the pressure used is not excessive: the patient's chest should rise only to the same extent as with normal awake respiration. When normal lungs are ventilated, the pressure manometer reading should not exceed 20 cm $H_2O$ in small animal patients and 40 cm $H_2O$ in large animal patients. The bag should be squeezed for 1 to 1.5 seconds. Excessive or prolonged pressure may damage lung tissue and impede venous return to the heart.

For some patients, respiratory depression is so severe that periodic bagging does not provide the necessary level of ventilation, placing increased demand on the anesthetist's time and attention. Animals with preexisting heart or lung disease or diaphragmatic hernias may go into respiratory arrest immediately after induction. Other patients continue to breathe under anesthesia, but their $V_T$ is small (shallow breaths) and/or the respiratory rate is less than 6 breaths/min. These patients require intermittent mandatory ventilation. Ventilation can be assisted starting immediately after intubation, at which point the anesthetist should use the reservoir bag to superimpose positive pressure on the animal's own spontaneous breathing efforts. For many patients it is adequate to give a few larger than normal breaths manually then to connect the patient to a ventilator or to initiate manual ventilation. The initial large $V_T$ depresses the animal's urge to breathe by lowering blood carbon dioxide levels. Once the patient is connected to a ventilator or is undergoing appropriate manual ventilation, the patient usually stops spontaneous breathing efforts within 1 minute. Initially, the assisted ventilation rate should be 8 to 20 respirations per minute, depending on patient size. If after 3 to 5 minutes the patient still makes spontaneous breathing efforts, it may be necessary to use a neuromuscular blocking agent, which paralyzes the muscles of respiration (see the following section).

Once control has been established, a ventilation rate of 6 to 12 breaths/min is usually adequate. A pressure of

15 to 20 cm $H_2O$ is recommended in small animals (30 to 40 cm $H_2O$ in large animals), unless the chest is open, in which case higher pressures may be required depending on the degree to which the lungs are packed off by the surgeon to better expose the surgical field. When the reservoir bag is squeezed, the inspiratory time should be 1 to 1.5 seconds. Expiratory time should be at least twice as long as inspiratory time. The pop-off valve must be closed when the reservoir bag is squeezed; however, it should be opened briefly every two to three breaths to allow gas to escape from the circuit. The anesthetist must allow the airway pressure to return to zero during expiration so that cardiopulmonary function can normalize (improving venous return of blood to the heart and increasing stroke volume).

When assisting or controlling ventilation, the anesthetist may find it difficult to evaluate the adequacy of the ventilation efforts. Pulse oximetry and end-tidal capnography are valuable aids (see Chapter 5). For example, if the pulse oximeter reading is 95% or less in a patient undergoing manual ventilation, the patient may need more frequent ventilation or ventilation at a greater pressure or volume.

When the surgical procedure is nearing completion, the anesthetist must transition the patient from the intermittent mandatory breaths given by the ventilator, to spontaneous breathing. This is known as "weaning" the animal off the ventilator and is accomplished by turning off the anesthetic (and nitrous oxide if it is being used) while continuing to ventilate the patient's lungs with oxygen. If a neuromuscular blocking agent has been used, it should be reversed, if necessary. The anesthetist should gradually reduce the rate of inspirations to approximately two to four per minute while observing the animal for evidence of spontaneous breathing. When this is seen, the patient's ventilation can then be assisted by squeezing a small amount of air from the reservoir bag with each inspiration. Eventually, the animal will regain the ability to maintain a normal rate and $V_T$, and ventilation assistance can be discontinued. This may take several minutes to reestablish, particularly in older, hypothermic, or debilitated patients and in patients in which ventilation has been controlled for a long time. Warming the patient or stimulating the patient by pinching the toe pads or gently rubbing the thorax and abdomen (small animal), or twisting an ear (large animal), may help the patient regain spontaneous respiratory movements.

## Mechanical Ventilation

Mechanical ventilation is similar to intermittent mandatory manual ventilation in many respects. In mechanical ventilation, however, the patient's breathing is controlled by a ventilator, rather than by hand compression of the reservoir bag. When a ventilator is connected to the breathing circuit, it functionally replaces the reservoir bag and becomes a part of the breathing circuit. The ventilator automatically compresses a bellows, which forces

oxygen and anesthetic gas into the patient's airways via an endotracheal tube.

Many types of ventilators can be used with a veterinary anesthesia machine, and they vary in the number and complexity of the controls (Figure 6-2). The basic design is a bellows inside a housing, which is attached to the reservoir bag port of a circle breathing system. The bellows is compressed at a specified rate and a specified volume by a driving gas. Most ventilators have a double gas circuit pattern, with one circuit providing oxygen and anesthetic for the patient, and the other circuit containing a separate gas (oxygen or air) to drive the bellows. Ventilators are available for either large animal or small animal use. In both cases the scavenger should be attached to the exhaust port of the ventilator.

Depending on the type of ventilator used, the anesthetist may choose to deliver gases on inspiration according to a pressure cycle, volume cycle, or time cycle. A pressure-cycled ventilator (such as the Bird Mark 7 Respirator) will supply air until the pressure reaches a preset level. A time-cycled ventilator (such as the Small Animal Ventilator by Drager) supplies air according to a set inspiratory time. A volume-cycled type (such as the Ohio Metomatic) delivers a preset $V_T$ regardless of the pressure required. In volume-cycled ventilators, the anesthetist must adjust the volume of gas to be delivered on inspiration (usually 10 to 15 mL/kg, less if respiration is to be assisted rather than controlled).

After connecting the ventilator to the breathing circuit, the anesthetist should closely observe the patient to ensure that the chest rises with each inspiration. Respiratory rate is usually 6 to 12 breaths/min. Duration of inspiration is set at 1 to 1.5 seconds, and duration of expiration should

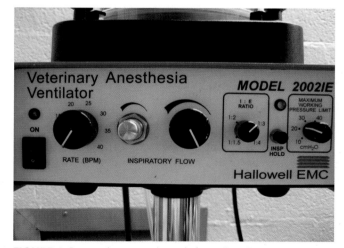

**FIGURE 6-2** Ventilator control panel of a Hallowell small animal anesthesia ventilator. From right to left, the controls are the on-off switch with indicator light; respiratory rate knob; inspiratory flow knobs (smaller silver knob for fine control, larger black knob for gross control); I:E ratio knob (controls ratio of inspiration to expiration); inspiratory hold button (allows the anesthetist to hold a breath on inflation); and the pressure limit knob (allows the anesthetist to set the maximum pressure within the breathing system on inspiration; an alarm will sound if this pressure is reached).

be 2 to 6 seconds with an inspiratory/expiratory ratio of 1:2 to 1:3. If a pressure-cycled ventilator is used, a pressure setting of 12 cm to 20 cm is normally selected. These settings may be varied to adapt to the special needs of selected patients. For example, a dog with gastric dilation–volvulus or a horse with colon torsion may need higher airway pressures to deliver a minimal effective $V_T$. Obese cats and dogs often require normal rates but higher airway pressures to overcome the thoracic effects of obesity.

Like manual ventilation, mechanical ventilation is particularly indicated for patients with compromised respiration. It is not normally necessary in healthy anesthetized patients, in which periodic manual bagging (once every 5 minutes) is usually sufficient. Mechanical ventilation is particularly helpful in animals undergoing a thoracotomy or other lengthy operation, in which manually providing intermittent mandatory ventilation would be difficult for the anesthetist.

### Technical Consideration for Intermittent Mandatory Ventilation of Anesthetized Patients

#### Rebreathing versus Non-rebreathing Systems

Intermittent mandatory manual ventilation can be performed using either a rebreathing or a non-rebreathing system. Non-rebreathing systems usually lack a manometer, and the anesthetist must use sight and touch to determine the optimal $V_T$.

### In-Circle versus Out-of-Circle Vaporizers

Patients connected to a circle system with an in-circle nonprecision vaporizer can be bagged every 5 minutes to assist ventilation. However, it is advisable to turn the vaporizer setting to zero before bagging the patient, to prevent sudden vaporization of large amounts of anesthetic as a result of the increased flow of carrier gas through the vaporizer. Mandatory controlled ventilation with an in-circle vaporizer is difficult and may be dangerous, unless the vaporizer is turned down or off or end-tidal anesthetic agent monitoring is available. Because of the increased gas flow associated with controlled ventilation and the lack of back pressure compensation in these vaporizers, the patient may receive excessive amounts of vaporized anesthetic.

In contrast, it is feasible to use mandatory manual or mechanical ventilation on patients connected to a circle system with an out-of-circle precision vaporizer. If the vaporizer is compensated for gas flow and back pressure, it is not necessary to turn the concentration setting to zero during controlled ventilation. However, if mandatory manual ventilation is used, it may be advisable to reduce the precision vaporizer setting, or the patient's level of anesthesia may become too deep because of increased delivery of anesthetic to the lungs. The anesthetist should closely monitor the patient and adjust the vaporizer setting according to the patient's anesthetic depth.

### Risks of Controlled Ventilation

Controlled ventilation, whether by manual ventilation with a reservoir bag or mechanical ventilation with a ventilator, has the potential to damage the animal's lungs if performed incorrectly.

- Excessive airway pressure may rupture alveoli, causing pneumothorax and/or pneumomediastinum.
- Cardiac output may be decreased if positive pressure is maintained throughout the respiratory cycle (during expiration and inspiration).
- If the ventilation rate is too high, excessive amounts of carbon dioxide may be exhaled, leading to respiratory alkalosis, which (if severe) can cause cerebral vasoconstriction and decreased cerebral blood flow.
- Controlled ventilation is generally more efficient at delivering anesthetic gas, even from a precision out-of-circle vaporizer. A ventilator will thus deliver more inhalant anesthetic to the patient, which may lead to exacerbation of side effects such as hypotension and increased central nervous system depression. Conversely, ventilators are often used in large animal patients as anesthetic delivery devices to maintain a smoother plane of anesthesia than sometimes occurs with spontaneous breathing.
- Mechanical ventilation is not intended to relieve the anesthetist of the necessity for patient monitoring. The anesthetist must closely monitor all animals in which ventilation is controlled or assisted to ensure that patient anesthetic depth and vital signs are maintained within acceptable limits.

## NEUROMUSCULAR BLOCKING AGENTS

Neuromuscular blocking agents (also called *muscle-paralyzing agents*) are often used in human anesthesia, but they have found only limited use in veterinary practice. Paralysis of the muscles of respiration is undesirable in conventional veterinary anesthesia; however, it is useful in the following situations:

- Patients that require mechanical ventilation. The use of neuromuscular blocking agents prevents spontaneous inspiratory efforts by the patient and allows more rapid and complete control of ventilation. This is particularly useful for thoracic or diaphragmatic surgery.
- Orthopedic surgery. Neuromuscular blocking agents provide excellent muscle relaxation, which is helpful in orthopedic procedures.
- Ophthalmic surgery. Neuromuscular blocking agents prevent movement of the eyeball and cause it to remain in a central rather than ventral position, which facilitates intraocular surgery.
- Cesarean sections. Neuromuscular blocking agents provide abdominal muscle relaxation and are not transferred across the placenta to the fetus.

- Neuromuscular blocking agents may be useful in facilitating difficult intubation (e.g., intubating animals with laryngospasm) because they allow rapid control of the airway without coughing or gagging.
- Occasionally, muscle-paralyzing agents are used in "balanced anesthesia" techniques. In balanced anesthesia, different drugs provide the three components of general anesthesia (unconsciousness, muscle relaxation, and analgesia). Instead of using a high dose of a single agent such as thiopental to induce general anesthesia, a balanced technique will include low doses of multiple agents (often an analgesic, a muscle-paralyzing agent, and an unconsciousness-inducing agent). The aim is to induce general anesthesia with a minimum of cardiovascular, respiratory, and other side effects.

Neuromuscular blocking agents should be administered only after the patient is unconscious and respiration has been controlled by means of intermittent mandatory manual or mechanical ventilation. These agents should be considered to be an adjunct to, rather than a replacement for, anesthesia with other agents. Use of neuromuscular blocking agents in a conscious animal is inhumane because these agents have no tranquilizing, analgesic, or anesthetic properties. The patient given only these drugs will be fully conscious and have normal sensitivity to pain, but will be unable to move or otherwise resist the surgeon's efforts. Control of respiration is also essential after the administration of these drugs because the respiratory muscles will be paralyzed, making it impossible for the patient to breathe on its own.

Neuromuscular blocking agents act by interrupting normal transmission of impulses from motor neurons to the muscle synapse. The site of action is the nerve-muscle junction, where acetylcholine is released by the neurons in proximity to the muscle end plate. There are two ways in which muscle-paralyzing agents may disrupt nervous transmission, and neuromuscular blocking agents are classified as depolarizing or nondepolarizing according to which of the two mechanisms applies.

Depolarizing agents, such as succinylcholine, cause a single surge of activity at the neuromuscular junction, which is followed by a period in which the muscle end plate is refractory to further stimulation. Animals given these agents may show spontaneous muscle twitching followed by paralysis. Succinylcholine has a fast onset (20 seconds) but a short duration of effect and is useful for rapid intubation. Potential adverse effects of succinylcholine include hyperkalemia and cardiac arrhythmias.

Nondepolarizing agents, such as gallamine, pancuronium, atracurium besylate, and cisatracurium, act by blocking the receptors at the end plates. As their classification suggests, they do not cause an initial surge of activity at the neuromuscular junction, and spontaneous muscle movements are not seen. Potential adverse effects of these agents include histamine release, hypotension or hypertension, tachycardia, and ventricular arrhythmias.

Concurrent use of inhalant anesthetics increases the potency of neuromuscular blocking agents. Animals that have undergone recent treatments with organophosphate insecticides also show an increased susceptibility to neuromuscular blocking agents. Other drugs, including corticosteroids, barbiturates, furosemide and other diuretics, anticancer drugs, epinephrine, tetracycline, and aminoglycoside antibiotics such as gentamicin, have been shown to affect the potency of neuromuscular blocking agents.

Muscle-paralyzing agents are normally given by slow intravenous injection. The dose required varies among patients and with the anesthetic protocol used. Most agents take effect within 2 minutes, and the duration of paralysis is approximately 10 to 30 minutes (although this varies considerably, depending on the agent used). If more prolonged paralysis is required, repeated doses can be given. Alternatively, some agents may be given by constant intravenous infusion.

Regardless of the agent used, only voluntary (skeletal) muscles are affected. These agents do not affect the involuntary muscles, including cardiac muscle and the smooth muscle of the intestine and bladder. Skeletal muscles are affected in a predictable order: facial and neck paralysis is seen first, followed by paralysis of the tail, limbs, and abdominal muscles. The intercostal muscles and diaphragm are affected last.

Anesthetic depth may be difficult to assess in animals that have been given muscle-paralyzing agents because of the inhibition or absence of normal reflex responses and the absence of jaw tone. Heart rate and blood pressure may give some indication of anesthetic depth. If salivation, tongue curling, or lacrimation is seen, the patient is likely not deeply anesthetized enough for surgery.

Animals given muscle-paralyzing agents cannot blink and are predisposed to corneal drying. An ophthalmic lubricant must be used. The anesthetist must also monitor the patient for hypothermia, which is a common side effect resulting from the decreased muscle tone seen in patients given these agents. Hypothermia can slow the metabolism of the agents and delay recovery from anesthesia.

Nondepolarizing agents should be reversed with an anticholinesterase agent, even if the effects appear to be wearing off. Reversal agents have no effect on depolarizing agents. The most commonly used reversal agents are edrophonium, neostigmine, and pyridostigmine. The patient should be maintained at a light anesthetic depth until the reversal agent has taken effect. After reversal of muscle-paralyzing agents, signs of returning muscle function include diaphragmatic movements, eye rotation, an active palpebral reflex, and increasing jaw tone. Sometimes the effect of the reversal agent wears off before the muscle-paralyzing agent is eliminated, in which case respiratory support may be required.

Reversal agents may have undesirable side effects such as bradycardia and increased bronchial and salivary secretions and should be given only after pretreatment with atropine or glycopyrrolate.

## KEY POINTS

1. Local anesthesia is the use of a chemical agent on sensory and motor neurons to produce a temporary loss of pain sensation and movement. Because of low patient toxicity, low cost, and minimal recovery time, local anesthesia may be preferred to general anesthesia in some patients. Disadvantages include lack of patient restraint, risk of overdose in smaller patients, and technical difficulties.

2. If sufficient quantity of local anesthetic reaches the sympathetic ganglia, sympathetic blockade may result. This causes flushing, increased skin temperature, and, occasionally, hypotension and bradycardia.

3. Local anesthetics have many topical uses, including application to the conjunctiva or the epithelium of the respiratory or urogenital tracts.

4. Local anesthetics may be injected in proximity to a peripheral nerve, blocking sensation from the tissues served by the nerve. Surgical preparation of the area is necessary before injection of a local anesthetic. Epinephrine is commonly added to the lidocaine to delay absorption of the local anesthetic agent from the site, but epinephrine must not be used at peripheral locations where blood supply may be compromised.

5. Epidural anesthesia is achieved by injecting local anesthetic in the epidural space, between the dura and the vertebrae. In dogs and cats, the injection is performed between the last lumbar vertebra and the sacrum. This technique is useful for surgical procedures in patients that are debilitated and in patients that require profound analgesia of the caudal abdomen, limbs, or pelvis.

6. Intravenous injection of local anesthetics may be useful for distal limb surgery, including amputation.

7. Local anesthetics may be harmful if injected into a nerve. They may also cause temporary paresthesia, which may result in self-mutilation.

8. Adverse systemic effects of local anesthesia include sedation, hyperexcitability, respiratory depression, and sympathetic blockade. Toxicity may be avoided by limiting the amount of lidocaine administered to the patient (a maximum of 10 mg/kg in dogs when given subcutaneously) and avoiding intravenous injection of bupivacaine.

9. Controlled or assisted ventilation may be used to deliver oxygen and anesthetic to the patient. Either a mechanical ventilator or manual bagging may be used. These procedures are particularly useful in patients with poor respiratory function. Controlled or assisted ventilation helps prevent the development of hypercarbia, respiratory acidosis, and pulmonary atelectasis.

10. Intermittent mandatory manual ventilation can be achieved by gently squeezing the reservoir bag at a rate of 8 to 12 breaths/min and a pressure of 15 to 20 cm $H_2O$. Inspiration time should be 1 to 1.5 seconds, and expiratory time should be at least 2 to 3 seconds. Manual ventilation is challenging and potentially dangerous to the patient if a nonprecision vaporizer is used.

11. Mechanical ventilators may be incorporated into either a rebreathing or a non-rebreathing system. Depending on the type of ventilator used, the anesthetist may control the pressure or volume of gas to be delivered, the respiratory rate, and the length of inspiration and expiration.

12. If controlled ventilation is used, the anesthetist must use caution to avoid excessive expansion of the alveoli, continuous positive pressure, and excessive ventilation rates.

13. Neuromuscular blocking agents may be useful in some anesthetic procedures to allow relaxation of voluntary muscles. They should never be used as the sole anesthetic agent.

14. Neuromuscular blocking agents may be depolarizing or nondepolarizing in their action. Nondepolarizing agents may be reversed by the administration of neostigmine or edrophonium.

15. Neuromuscular blocking agents may cause systemic effects such as hypothermia and respiratory failure. Mechanical or manual ventilation must be available when these agents are used.

16. Many drugs, including isoflurane, halothane, aminoglycoside antibiotics, organophosphates, and diuretics, may alter the potency of neuromuscular blocking agents.

## PROCEDURE 6-1 Performing Paravertebral Anesthesia in a Cow

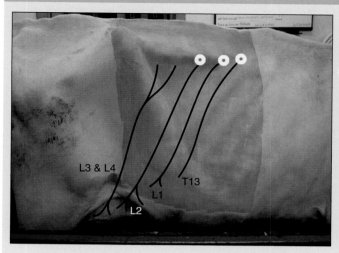

1. The sites for paravertebral anesthesia of spinal nerves T13 to L2 for flank laparotomy.

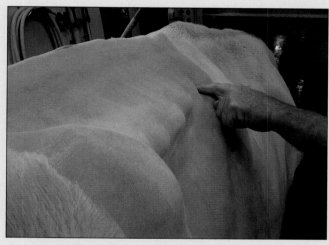

2. The space cranial to the transverse spinous process of L1 is palpated.

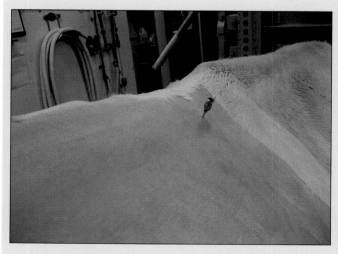

3. A short, large-gauge needle is inserted in the skin over the space, approximately 2.5 to 5 cm off the midline.

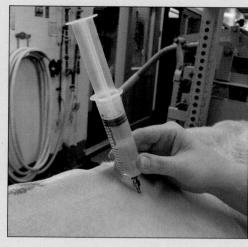

4. Two to 3 mL of lidocaine are injected into the subcutaneous tissues.

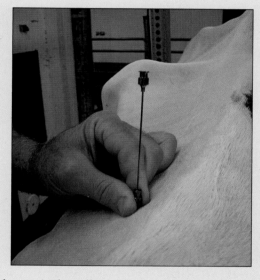

5. A long spinal needle is then passed through the anesthetized tissue, in this case inside the short needle.

*Continued*

## PROCEDURE 6-1    *Performing Paravertebral Anesthesia in a Cow—cont'd*

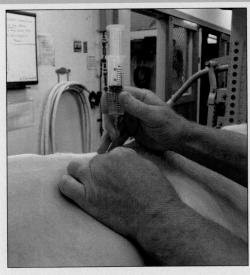

6. The remainder of the local anesthetic is deposited above and below the intertransverse fascia to anesthetize the dorsal and ventral branches of the spinal nerve.

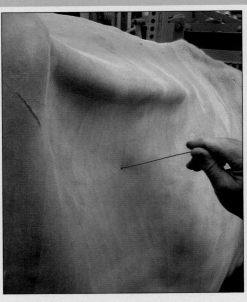

8. Skin sensitivity to a needle prick can be assessed before commencement of surgery.

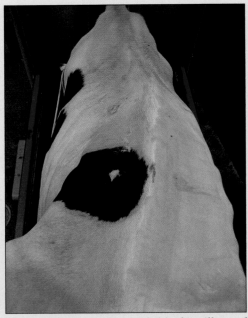

7. A correctly performed block will produce scoliosis toward the side of the block.

**PROCEDURE 6-2 Performing a Three-Point Nerve Block for Declawing a Cat**

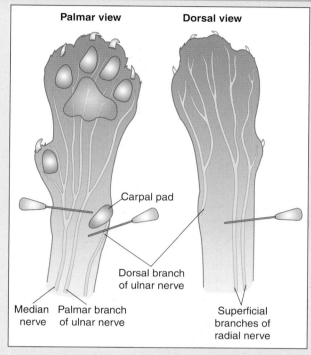

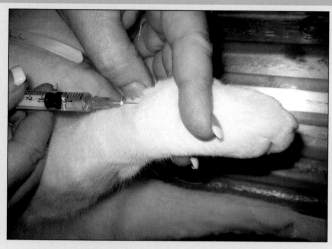

2. First 0.2 mL of 2% lidocaine is deposited dorsally proximal to the carpus to target the branches of the radial nerve.

1. Diagrammatic view of needle placement for three-point nerve block for right forelimb declaw in a cat.

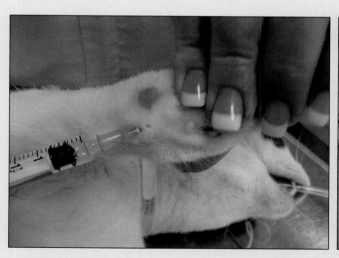

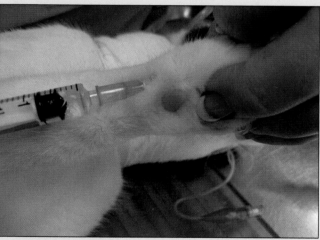

3. Then 0.1 mL of 2% lidocaine is deposited on either side of the superficial digital flexor to target the median nerve medially (left) and ulnar nerve laterally (right). Bupivacaine can be used in place of lidocaine, ensuring that a dose of 4 mg/kg is not exceeded.

# PROCEDURE 6-3 Performing an Epidural Injection in a Dog

## Steps

1. Gather the necessary equipment. This includes a short-beveled spinal needle with a stylet (18 to 22 gauge, 1.5 inches for small or thin dogs, and 2 to 3 inches for large or overweight dogs) and several sterile 3- or 5-ml syringes. If a catheter is to be placed, a thin-walled, 18-gauge, 3-inch needle is required.

2. Sedate (or anesthetize) the patient to achieve adequate restraint and place in sternal or lateral recumbency. The head is positioned higher than the spinal cord for at least the first 10 minutes of analgesia. This prevents forward migration of the drug into the region of the thoracic spinal cord, which could potentially affect the phrenic nerve (causing respiratory arrest) or cause a sympathetic blockade.

3. Identify the right and left cranial dorsal wings of the ilium, the spinous process of L7, and the sacral crest (Figures 1 and 2). Shave and prepare the area (approximately 10 cm × 10 cm) surrounding the injection site between L7 and the sacral crest. Wear surgical gloves for the procedure.

4. Palpate the lumbosacral space (between L7 and the sacrum), which is midway between the dorsal iliac wings (Figure 3). The lumbosacral space is the depression just caudal to the L7 process and immediately cranial to the sacral crest, which feels like a series of small bumps under the skin. Place the spinal needle in the area of greatest depression, perpendicular to the skin surface and exactly on the midline (Figure 4).The bevel should be directed cranially, and the stylet should be left in the needle to prevent introduction of skin into the epidural space. The needle is gently advanced perpendicular to the skin in the dog, passing through the skin, subcutaneous fat, supraspinous ligament, interspinous ligament, and ligamentum flavum (Figure 5). Resistance may be encountered, and a distinct pop often can be felt as the needle is advanced through the ligamentum flavum. Immediately after the ligamentum flavum is penetrated, the needle enters the epidural space. This usually occurs at a needle depth of 1 to 3 cm, depending on the size of the animal (Figure 6). Occasionally there is some difficulty in finding the intervertebral space, in which case the needle should be withdrawn, angled slightly caudally or cranially, and reinserted.

5. Remove the stylet and examine the needle hub for blood or cerebrospinal fluid (for 2 minutes). If cerebrospinal fluid is encountered, the needle is in the subarachnoid space. If this is the case, the procedure may be abandoned or the anesthetist may choose to administer 30% to 50% of the original dose, inducing spinal anesthesia (provided the agent used has minimal spinal toxicity). If blood is encountered, the needle has entered the venous sinus, and the procedure should be abandoned. If blood and cerebrospinal fluid are not observed, the needle should be aspirated to ensure that neither is present. To further check for proper needle placement, inject 1 to 2 mL of air; no resistance to air passage should be felt. For large dogs, it may be easier to remove the stylet as it enters the skin. The hub can be filled with saline, and as the needle penetrates the ligamentum flavum, the liquid will be drawn into the epidural space.

## Drug Selection for Epidural for Surgical Analgesia

If the epidural is performed for surgical analgesia and immobilization, lidocaine or bupivacaine is used. The dose of 2% lidocaine (without epinephrine) or 0.25% to 0.5% bupivacaine will vary with the extent of analgesia required. The anesthetist often will choose to produce anesthesia as far cranial as L2 (which is sufficient for most caudal abdominal procedures and all pelvic and rear limb procedures). The dose used in this case is 1 mL of 2% lidocaine for each 3.5 to 4.5 kg of body weight. The volume should be less than 0.25 mL/kg. Inject the calculated dose of lidocaine or bupivacaine over 1 minute. More rapid injection may cause pressure damage to the spinal cord and nerves or result in local anesthetic infiltrating too far forward along the spinal canal. Injection will be resistance-free if the needle is positioned correctly. If continuous epidural anesthesia is required, a polyethylene catheter may be advanced through the needle and the needle subsequently withdrawn, leaving the catheter in place. Advance the catheter only 1 cm into the epidural space.

Onset of analgesia is approximately 5 minutes after lidocaine injection or 20 minutes after bupivacaine injection (Figure 7).The block normally affects the most distal body parts (toes and tail) first. If a bilateral effect is desired, position the patient in dorsal recumbency for 20 minutes after the injection. If unilateral analgesia is required, place the patient in lateral recumbency with the desired side positioned ventrally, allowing for gravitation of the local anesthetic within the epidural space to the targeted side of the spinal canal.

It has been reported that 12% of correctly performed epidural blocks are ineffective, perhaps because of individual variations in anatomy. Effectiveness of the block may be determined through a test with a needle prick or may become evident during patient preparation or application of towel clamps.

Duration of analgesia is 4 to 6 hours for bupivacaine and 1.5 to 3 hours for lidocaine.

## Drug Selection for Epidural for Postoperative Pain Control

If the epidural is performed to provide postoperative analgesia, morphine or another opioid agent is used either alone or combined with a local anesthetic. The procedure used is the same as just described. It is advisable that single-use vials of preservative-free morphine be used. See Chapter 7 for more information on the use of morphine epidurals for pain control.

**PROCEDURE 6-3** **Performing an Epidural Injection in a Dog—cont'd**

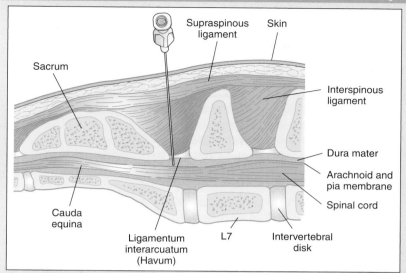

**FIGURE 1** Anatomy of the distal spinal canal, showing the placement of a needle for lumbosacral epidural analgesia.

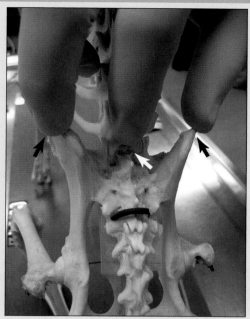

**FIGURE 2** Landmark palpation on a canine skeleton for lumbosacral epidural. *Black arrows,* the most dorsal points of the wings of the ilia. *White arrow,* the lumbosacral space.

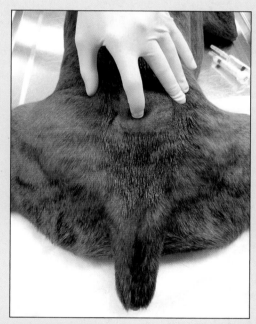

**FIGURE 3** Landmark palpation on a dog for lumbosacral epidural. The anesthetist places her thumb and middle finger on the most prominent points of the wings of the ilia. She places her index finger in the indentation at a midpoint between the thumb and middle finger, the lumbosacral junction.

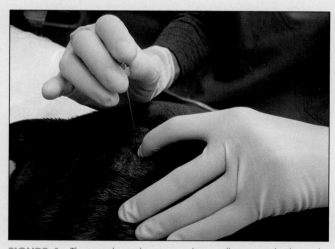

**FIGURE 4** The anesthetist then inserts the needle perpendicular to the spine.

*Continued*

## PROCEDURE 6-3    Performing an Epidural Injection in a Dog—cont'd

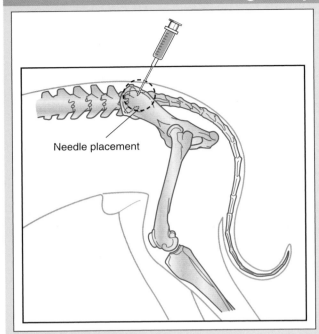

**FIGURE 5**    Needle placement for lumbosacral epidural in the dog.

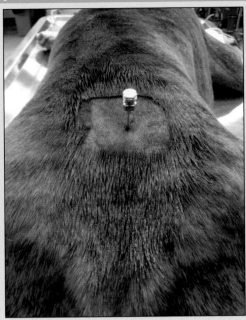

**FIGURE 6**    Spinal needle after the epidural space has been entered.

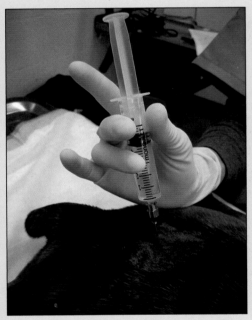

**FIGURE 7**    Injection of local anesthetic, opioid, or a combination of both is injected slowly. The anesthetist should feel no resistance to injection.

## PROCEDURE 6-4   Performing a Bier Block in a Dog Undergoing Toe Amputation

A 22-gauge, 1.5-inch catheter is placed in a vein in the distal part of the limb (because the valves of the veins prevent the backward flow of local anesthetic if the drug is injected too proximally). Once the catheter is in place, an elastic bandage is wrapped around the extremity, starting at the distal end and wrapping proximally to drive blood out of the veins (Figure 1). A tourniquet is applied just proximal to the area requiring anesthesia (e.g., immediately above the elbow if the foreleg is to be anesthetized). The tourniquet must be tight, or symptoms of local anesthetic toxicity may be evident after injection. The bandage is then removed and the drug injected into the vein via the catheter (Figure 2). The usual dose used is 2 to 3 mL of 1% lidocaine without epinephrine, not to exceed 2 mg/kg. Within 3 to 5 minutes, there is total desensitization of the limb distal to the tourniquet, allowing 25 to 30 minutes of analgesia. An additional advantage of this technique is the relatively blood-free surgery site that it affords after tourniquet application. As with other local anesthetic procedures, however, patient restraint may be a problem unless concurrent sedation or neuroleptanalgesia is provided. This technique can also be used in anesthetized patients.

Sensation returns to the affected area within a few minutes of release of the tourniquet. It is important to remove the tourniquet soon after the procedure has been completed. If the tourniquet is in place for more than 90 minutes, prolonged hypoxia of the tissues of the limb may result, leading to tissue damage and loss of function. In all patients, removal of the tourniquet should be gradual (i.e., over a 5-minute period) because this helps prevent an excessive concentration of local anesthetic from reaching the heart and brain.

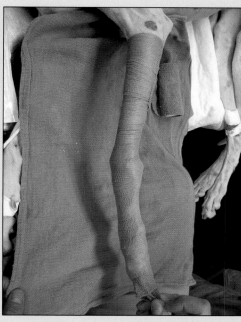

**FIGURE 1**   The leg is tightly wrapped using, in this case, Vetrap, or alternatively an Esmarch bandage, starting at and including the toes. A tourniquet is placed proximal to the bandage, and the bandage is then removed starting at the toes and moving proximally.

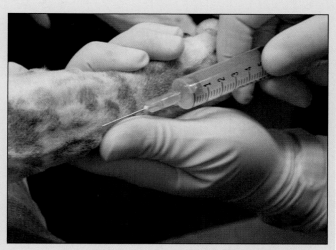

**FIGURE 2**   Local anesthetic is injected into a vein distal to the tourniquet. Very little blood should be present in the vein if the bandage and tourniquet have been applied correctly. The tourniquet should be removed after 60 minutes of intravenous regional anesthesia.

## REVIEW QUESTIONS

1. In the healthy awake animal, the main stimulus to breathe is the result of:
   a. Excess oxygen concentration in the blood
   b. Excess carbon dioxide concentration in the blood
   c. Insufficient oxygen in the blood
   d. Insufficient carbon dioxide in the blood

2. In the healthy awake animal, exhalation lasts at least __ times as long as inhalation.
   a. ½
   b. 2
   c. 3
   d. 4

3. The normal $V_T$ in an awake animal is __ mL/kg.
   a. 5 to 10
   b. 10 to 15
   c. 16 to 20
   d. 20 to 25

4. In the anesthetized animal that is breathing room air, the anesthetist may expect to see:
   a. An increase in the $Pa_{CO_2}$ and a decrease in the $Pa_{O_2}$
   b. A decrease in the $Pa_{CO_2}$ and an increase in the $Pa_{O_2}$
   c. A decrease in the $Pa_{CO_2}$ and a decrease in the $Pa_{O_2}$
   d. An increase in the $Pa_{CO_2}$ and an increase in the $Pa_{O_2}$

5. When used in a line block, a local anesthetic agent will have a direct effect on the:
   a. Peripheral nervous system
   b. Central nervous system
   c. Peripheral and central nervous systems
   d. Autonomic nervous system

6. Local anesthetics block transmission of nerve impulses from:
   a. Sensory neurons only
   b. Motor neurons only
   c. Sensory and motor neurons only
   d. Sensory, motor, and autonomic neurons

7. Local anesthetic agents work because:
   a. They mechanically block nerve impulse transmission
   b. They interfere with the movement of sodium ions
   c. They block all impulses at the spinal cord level
   d. They affect neurotransmission within the brain

8. When a local anesthetic is injected around a single major nerve, the procedure is referred to as a(n):
   a. Line block
   b. Epidural block
   c. Infiltration nerve block
   d. Intravenous anesthesia

9. Epinephrine may be mixed with a local anesthetic agent to prolong the effects of the drug.
   True                    False

10. When performing an epidural, one must be aware that the spinal cord in a cat may extend as far caudally as:
    a. T13
    b. L6
    c. L7
    d. S1
    e. The coccygeal vertebrae

11. The maximum subcutaneous dose of lidocaine for a dog is ___ mg/kg.
    a. 1
    b. 4
    c. 10
    d. 15

12. When performing intravenous regional anesthesia (Bier block), one should use lidocaine:
    a. With epinephrine
    b. Without epinephrine
    c. Either with or without epinephrine
    d. Lidocaine should not be used for this technique.

13. The term *atelectasis* refers to:
    a. Excess fluid in the respiratory system
    b. The absence of breathing
    c. Collapse of the alveoli
    d. Bronchial constriction

14. What is the most common acid-base abnormality in anesthetized patients?
    a. Respiratory alkalosis
    b. Metabolic alkalosis
    c. Respiratory acidosis
    d. Metabolic acidosis

15. When intermittent mandatory manual ventilation is applied to a patient that is connected to a circle system with a precision vaporizer, it is customary to:
    a. Increase the vaporizer setting
    b. Decrease the vaporizer setting
    c. Disconnect the patient from the circle system before starting manual ventilation
    d. The lungs of patients that are connected to a circle system should not be manually ventilated.

16. Which of the following can be used to monitor anesthetic depth in a patient that has been given a neuromuscular blocking agent?
    a. Heart rate
    b. Jaw tone
    c. Palpebral reflex
    d. Pedal reflex

17. A neuromuscular blocking agent not only will paralyze skeletal muscle, but also will give some analgesia.
    True                    False

18. When an animal is given a __ neuromuscular blocking drug, an initial surge of muscle activity may be seen before there is paralysis of the muscles.
    a. Depolarizing
    b. Nondepolarizing

19. The muscle type that is most affected by neuromuscular blocking agents is:
    a. Cardiac
    b. Smooth muscle
    c. Skeletal muscle
    d. All types are equally affected.

20. Both depolarizing and nondepolarizing drugs can be reversed.
    True                    False

For the following questions, more than one answer may be correct.
21. Problems that may result from excessive controlled ventilation may include:
    a. A decreased cardiac output
    b. Muscle twitching
    c. A state of respiratory alkalosis
    d. Ruptured alveoli

22. Local anesthetic agents such as lidocaine or proparacaine work well when applied:
    a. Topically on the epidermis
    b. Topically on mucous membranes
    c. Topically on the cornea
    d. Through injection

23. Factors that may interfere with the action of local anesthetic agents include:
    a. Fat
    b. Scar tissue
    c. Rapid heart rate
    d. Hemorrhage

24. Clinical signs of systemic toxicity from a local anesthetic agent may include:
    a. Sedation
    b. Convulsions
    c. Muscle twitching
    d. Respiratory depression

25. The effects that could result from an epidural anesthetic if the drug reached the thoracic and cervical spinal cord include:
    a. Sympathetic blockade
    b. Paralysis of intercostal muscles
    c. Paralysis of diaphragm
    d. Hypertension

## SELECTED READINGS

Anderson DE, Miesner MD: Field surgery of cattle, *Vet Clin North Am Food Anim Pract* 24(2):211-226, 2008.

Gaynor JS, Muir WW: *Handbook of veterinary pain management,* ed 2, Chapters 12, 15, 23, St Louis, 2009, Mosby.

Muir WW, Hubbell JAE: *Equine anesthesia,* ed 2, St Louis, 2009, Elsevier.

Tranquilli WJ, Grimm KA, Lamont LA: *Pain management for the small animal practitioner,* Jackson, 2000, Teton New Media.

Tranquilli WJ, Thurmon JC, Grimm KA: *Veterinary anesthesia and analgesia,* ed 4, Ames, Iowa, 2007, Blackwell.

# 7 Analgesia

## OUTLINE

Physiology of Pain, 207
Consequences of Untreated Pain, 208
Signs of Pain in Animals, 208
Pain Assessment Tools, 210
    *Assessing Response to Therapy, 210*
Perioperative Pain Management, 211
Pharmacologic Analgesic Therapy, 212

*Opioid Agents, 214*
*Nonsteroidal Antiinflammatory Drugs, 222*
*Other Analgesic Agents, 225*
*Multimodal Therapy, 226*
Home Analgesia, 227
Nursing Care, 227
Nonpharmacologic Therapies, 228

## LEARNING OBJECTIVES

*After completion of this chapter, the reader will be able to:*

- Define pain, nociception, physiologic pain, pathologic pain, neuropathic pain, idiopathic pain, visceral pain, somatic pain, preemptive analgesia, pain scale, and multimodal therapy.
- List the main steps of the pain pathway.
- List the benefits of multimodal analgesia.
- List the consequences of untreated pain.
- Explain how primary hyperalgesia (peripheral hypersensitivity) develops.
- Explain how secondary hyperalgesia (central hypersensitivity) develops.
- List common surgical and medical conditions that are considered to be painful.
- Describe how to recognize and assess pain-associated behaviors in animals.
- List the routes by which analgesic drugs are commonly administered.
- List the adverse effects of opioid drugs.
- Explain the mechanism of action of nonsteroidal antiinflammatory drugs.
- List the adverse effects of nonsteroidal antiinflammatory drugs.
- Describe the procedure for application of a fentanyl patch.
- Define multimodal therapy.
- List two examples of multimodal therapy.
- Describe nursing care that relieves discomfort in hospitalized patients.

## KEY TERMS

Algesia
Analgesia
Central nervous system hypersensitivity
Distress
Emergence delirium
Idiopathic
Locomotor
Mediators
Modulation
Morbidity
Mortality
Multimodal therapy
Neuropathic
Nociception
Pain
Pain scales
Pathologic pain
Perception
Perioperative analgesia
Physiologic pain
Pre-emptive analgesia
Primary hyperalgesia
Secondary hyperalgesia
Somatic pain
Transdermal patch
Transduction
Transmission
Visceral pain
Wasting
Windup

The veterinary team has the unique responsibility of assessing and treating animal **pain.** The role of the veterinary technician, either as anesthetist or patient caregiver, in the provision of **analgesia** cannot be overstated. The technician forms a vital part of the team through his or her understanding of pain physiology, pain-associated behaviors, pain assessment tools, analgesic drug pharmacology, and communication with the veterinarian-in-charge (VIC) regarding the welfare of patients. Pain assessment is currently considered to be an essential part of every patient evaluation, regardless of presenting complaint. Under the currently accepted standard of practice, provision of analgesia is mandatory for patients that are deemed to be in pain or that undergo painful procedures, including surgery for any reason. Clients expect, request, or sometimes even demand pain control for their pets. Consequently, failure to provide effective pain control not only results in patient discomfort but may evoke anger, could damage the doctor's reputation, or, in extreme circumstances, could result in disciplinary action by a Veterinary Medical Licensing Board.

Pain is a complex phenomenon that has been defined as an aversive sensory and emotional experience that elicits protective motor actions (such as a dog trying to bite when given an injection), results in learned avoidance (the same dog exhibits fear the next time it is taken to the vet for vaccine boosters), and may modify species-specific behavior traits, including social behavior. This experience is different for every individual animal, although within a given species some physiologic and behavioral responses will be similar (e.g., dogs in pain will often seek attention from their owners, whereas cats are more likely to hide). If left untreated, pain can negatively affect a patient's behavior, physiology, metabolism, and immune system, causing poor performance, weight loss, and increased susceptibility to infection.

## PHYSIOLOGY OF PAIN

Detection by the nervous system of the potential for or the actual occurrence of tissue injury is called **nociception.** This serves to protect the animal from painful or noxious stimuli. The protective sensation of pain that occurs when there is no or minimal tissue injury is referred to as **physiologic pain,** or "ouch" pain (e.g., the pain you would feel that would warn you if you touched something sharp,

hot, or chemically noxious). Pain that occurs after tissue injury is referred to as **pathologic pain** (e.g., the pain you would feel after a bone is broken). It is usually helpful to classify pathologic pain based on duration as either acute (hours) or chronic (days to years).

Pathologic pain is often classified based on the mechanism, origin, and severity of pain, as this may help determine treatment options. The mechanism of pain can be inflammation (e.g., after trauma or surgery), nerve injury **(neuropathic),** or cancer, or the pain can be **idiopathic** (of no identifiable cause). Pain can originate from organs, in which case it is **visceral pain** (e.g., pleuritis or colic), or from the musculoskeletal system, in which case it is **somatic pain.** Somatic pain can be divided into superficial (i.e., skin) and deep (i.e., joints, muscles, bones) pain. Some diseases or surgeries may result in more than one of these types of pain—for example, abdominal surgery has components of somatic pain (skin and abdominal wall incisions) and visceral pain (organ manipulation and surgery). Pain severity is often classified as none, mild, moderate, or severe, although more involved classifications exist (see the discussion of pain assessment tools later in this chapter).

Nociception, or the pain pathway, consists of four main steps (Figure 7-1). The first step is the transformation of noxious thermal, chemical, or mechanical stimuli into electrical signals called *action potentials* by peripheral A-delta and C nerve fibers, and is called **transduction.** These sensory impulses are then conducted to the spinal cord, a process known as **transmission.** In the spinal cord, where the A-delta and C fibers terminate, the

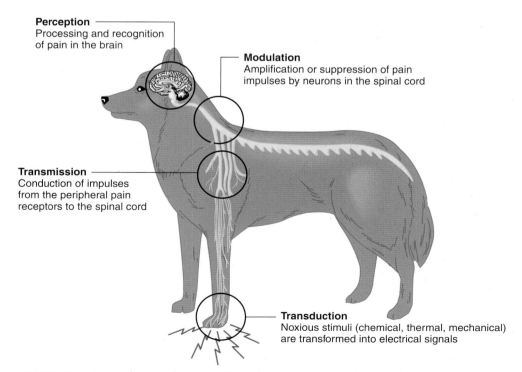

**Perception**
Processing and recognition
of pain in the brain

**Modulation**
Amplification or suppression of pain
impulses by neurons in the spinal cord

**Transmission**
Conduction of impulses
from the peripheral pain
receptors to the spinal cord

**Transduction**
Noxious stimuli (chemical, thermal, mechanical)
are transformed into electrical signals

**FIGURE 7-1** Pain pathway and receptors. Steps of the nociceptive (pain) pathway.

BOX 7-1   **Where Are Drugs Effective in the Nociceptive Pathway?**

- Transduction: Nonsteroidal antiinflammatory agents (NSAIDs), opioids, local anesthetics, corticosteroids
- Transmission: Local anesthetics, alpha$_2$-agonists
- Modulation: Local anesthetics, NSAIDs, opioids, alpha$_2$-agonists, ketamine, tricyclic antidepressants, anticonvulsants
- Perception: Opioids, sedatives, general anesthetics

impulses can be altered by other neurons, which either amplify or suppress them. The general term to cover both possibilities is **modulation.** The final step is **perception**, in which the impulses are transmitted to the brain, where they are processed and recognized. At each level of the pain pathway different receptors are involved in the nociceptive process, allowing the pain management team to choose drugs that target a specific receptor (e.g., nonsteroidal antiinflammatory drugs [NSAIDs], opioids, local anesthetics, or corticosteroids inhibit transduction) (Box 7-1). A goal of pain management, particularly severe pain, is to target two or more of these receptors. This pain management strategy is called **multimodal therapy** and is preferable to using a single analgesic because lower dosages can be used, which decreases adverse effects and improves safety.

> *TECHNICIAN NOTE* Using several analgesic drugs, each with a different mechanism of action, is called *multimodal therapy.* This results in lower doses, which increases safety.

## CONSEQUENCES OF UNTREATED PAIN

Pathologic pain that goes untreated has undesirable consequences for the patient.

- Pain produces a **catabolic state,** which may lead to **wasting.**
- Pain suppresses the immune response, predisposing to infection and increasing hospitalization time and cost.
- Pain promotes inflammation, which delays wound healing.
- Anesthetic risk is increased because higher doses of anesthetic drugs are required to maintain a stable plane of anesthesia.
- Pain causes patient suffering, which is also stressful for owners and caregivers.

Tissue damage results in constant stimulation of the nerves involved in the nociceptive process. This constant noxious stimulation of the central nervous system (CNS) can alter the function of neurons and receptors involved in the pain pathway. The ability of the CNS to change in this way can result in hypersensitivity in both acute and chronic pain. Neurons in the periphery (limbs, organs)

and central neurons (spinal cord) can be affected. Peripheral tissue trauma results in the release of substances called **mediators** from damaged cells and also attracts inflammatory cells, which also release mediators. These mediators combine to form what is called a "sensitizing soup" that lowers the threshold of the peripheral pain receptors, thus increasing their sensitivity. This peripheral hypersensitivity, referred to as **primary hyperalgesia,** manifests clinically as an area close to the site of tissue injury that, if stimulated with a normally non-noxious stimulus, is painful. Centrally, in the spinal cord, neurons that are stimulated by constant nociceptive input from the periphery become hyperexcitable and sensitive to low-intensity stimuli that would not normally elicit a pain response. This phenomenon is called **central nervous system hypersensitivity** and is also referred to as **"windup."** Clinically this may manifest as an area of hypersensitivity that is farther away from the initial injury, and is known as **secondary hyperalgesia.** A receptor that is activated in windup is the N-methyl-D-aspartate (NMDA) receptor. Drugs such as ketamine can block this receptor.

Pain also causes physiologic changes. Neuroendocrine changes that occur in response to pain include release of adrenocorticotropic hormone (ACTH); elevation in cortisol, norepinephrine, and epinephrine; and decrease in insulin. These changes result in a catabolic state, which, in addition to the fact that patients in pain may be reluctant or unable to eat, leads to wasting.

Sympathetic stimulation leads to vasoconstriction, increased myocardial work, and increased myocardial oxygen consumption, predisposing the patient to arrhythmias. Skeletal muscle blood flow tends to increase, whereas blood flow to the gastrointestinal and urinary tracts decreases.

The stress response caused by tissue injury (including surgery) is important for immediate survival but if left unchecked can lead to increased **morbidity** and **mortality.** An extreme form of stress, **distress,** occurs when stressors such as pain negatively affect the animal's physiology and behavior. An animal that is enduring pain is therefore suffering.

The quality of life of a patient in pain should be a concern of every veterinary professional and owner. Although not always easy to define, high quality of life requires that several basic needs be met. Representing these basic needs, the "five freedoms" can help those caring for animals assess quality of life (Box 7-2). As freedom from pain is a necessary element of a high quality of life, assessment of pain and provision of analgesia and comfort should be goals of treatment of veterinary patients.

## SIGNS OF PAIN IN ANIMALS

Animals cannot verbally express their pain. Pain recognition therefore relies on a sound understanding of normal animal physiology and behavior and stress-related or

## BOX 7-2 The Five Freedoms

- Freedom from hunger and thirst
- Freedom from discomfort
- Freedom from disease
- Freedom from injury
- Freedom from pain

## BOX 7-3 Pain-Related Physiologic Changes

**Cardiovascular**
Hypertension
Tachycardia, tachyarrhythmia
Peripheral vasoconstriction (pale mucosae)

**Respiratory**
Tachypnea
Shallow breathing (abdominal or thoracic guarding)
Exaggerated abdominal component
Panting (dogs)
Open-mouth breathing (cats)

**Ophthalmic**
Mydriasis

## BOX 7-4 Examples of Diseases and Surgeries Associated with Moderate to Severe Pain

**Painful Medical Conditions**
Arthritis
Cancer
Cystitis
Pancreatitis
Peritonitis
Pleuritis

**Painful Surgical Conditions**
Spinal surgery
Fracture repair
Total hip replacement
Joint surgery
Ear surgery
Dental extractions
Rhinotomy or sinus surgery
Trauma
Eye surgery
Thoracotomy
Gastric dilatation–volvulus, colon torsion
Pyometra

behavioral changes that may be indicative of painful conditions. A thorough, detailed history may also be helpful in assessing pain, because the owner is more likely to be aware of behaviors that may be masked during a visit to the hospital or when the veterinarian is at a farm or stable. An understanding of the degree of pain that is expected and associated with specific diseases and surgeries is also helpful.

There is no single physiologic parameter that is a specific indicator of pain. Common pain-related physiologic changes are presented in Box 7-3; however, note that there are other causes for each change. It is important to avoid projecting complex human emotions onto animals (anthropomorphizing); however, the pain pathways and therefore pain perceptions in animals and people have much in common. Therefore our personal experiences can help us determine whether a disease or procedure is likely to be painful or not.

Many disease processes and surgical procedures are associated with moderate to severe pain (see Box 7-4 for some examples). Pain management can be initiated for these types of patients when they are presented or before elective surgery. The administration of pain medication before pain occurs reduces the overall requirement for analgesics and the duration of analgesic administration postoperatively compared with waiting until after surgery to start analgesic therapy. Providing analgesia before tissue injury is called **preemptive analgesia.** Preemptive analgesia is most commonly achieved by adding an analgesic to the premedication before anesthetizing a patient for surgery. Preemptive analgesia also helps to prevent windup, which, through changes in the CNS from central sensitization, can lead to pain that lasts longer than anticipated and is more difficult to manage.

*TECHNICIAN NOTE* Administering analgesics before surgery decreases analgesic requirements and minimizes CNS sensitization. This is called *preemptive analgesia.*

Behavioral responses to pain vary depending on the species, age, breed, and temperament of the patient and the nature, duration, and severity of pain. Younger patients are less likely to tolerate pain and more likely to vocalize, whereas older animals may be more stoic and are more likely to become aggressive. Cattle are generally much more stoic than other species. Within a species certain breeds may have higher or lower pain thresholds (e.g., calm draught horses versus excitable thoroughbreds; large breed versus toy breed dogs; Labradors versus Siberian huskies and greyhounds). Individuals within a breed will also respond differently to pain. It is important to recognize that nonspecific behavioral indicators of pain may be present with painful as well as nonpainful conditions.

Assessment of pain-associated behavior is often best achieved by using a staged process. It may be useful to observe patient behavior when people are not present (e.g., via remote camera or one-way window), although this is more difficult to do in a busy hospital setting and requires special equipment or facilities. Many animals change their behavior when a human observer is watching the patient, when a person interacts verbally with a patient, and finally when the patient undergoes physical examination. A thorough assessment of pain-related behavior can therefore be time-consuming, although decreasing the time devoted to the assessment may result in subtle changes being overlooked. It is important to remember that animals may mask pain-related behavior in the presence of people, owing either to a protective response to avoid looking like prey or to socialization instincts. Different species often respond differently when they are in pain; cats tend to hide, dogs tend to seek attention from their owners, and herd or flock animals tend to separate from the other animals.

Changes in gait and level of activity such as lameness, limping, stiffness, and reluctance to move are all indicators of limb or joint pain. Development of exercise intolerance or a decrease in performance may also indicate the presence of limb pain. Arthritic dogs may not walk normally, whereas cats with arthritis show a reluctance to jump as high or as often as before. Horses will shift weight more frequently and point, rotate, or hang their limbs. Cows may arch their backs. A reluctance to lie down or a constant shifting of position is an indicator of thoracic or abdominal pain. Patients may stand, sit, or adopt a prayer position rather than lie down, eventually becoming exhausted. Pain may not consistently be present but can be elicited by an event such as palpation or manipulation of a joint or forced activity (e.g., a horse that is not lame at the walk but is when it is encouraged to trot).

Vocalization is frequently associated with pain. Dogs tend to whine, growl, whimper, and groan and may snarl or bite if manipulation is painful. Cats are more likely to groan, growl, or purr. They may also bite or hiss if palpation causes pain. Large animals do not vocalize as commonly; however, groaning and grunting are associated with pain in these species. Horses may bite or kick in response to pain or may try to flee. In small animals, particularly dogs, vocalization is common in the immediate postoperative period and may be caused by **emergence delirium** or pain. Emergence delirium can be differentiated from pain by the fact that it lasts for a short time and responds to sedation.

Facial expressions, appearance, and attitude may be altered in patients that are in pain. Common facial expressions encountered in dogs in pain include a glazed or fixed stare. Cats may squint and have a furrowed brow. Horses and cattle will have an altered head carriage and may also curl their lips. Cattle will grind their teeth. Animals in pain do not typically groom themselves and may appear unkempt. Hospitalized patients may sit staring at the back of the cage, or stand at the back of the stall. Such patients may be unaware of their surroundings and not interested in interacting, often appearing stuporous, or may be unwilling to move because of pain. Cats in pain will attempt to hide by moving as far from

view as possible, a form of escape behavior, and will often become unresponsive to people. Aggression is most commonly observed with severe acute pain that is elicited on palpation. (See Figure 7-2 for examples of pain-related behaviors.)

## PAIN ASSESSMENT TOOLS

Several pain assessment tools have been adapted from human medicine, evaluated, and used to quantify pain and response to therapy in animals. Most of these tools require evaluator training for consistently meaningful results to be obtained.

The pain assessment tools that have been developed for use in animals include verbal rating scales, simple descriptive scales, numeric rating scales, visual analogue scales, and comprehensive scales.

Verbal rating and simple descriptive scales (Figure 7-3) rate pain as absent, mild, moderate, or severe. They are quick and easy to use. These scales are not well suited to chronic or subtle changes, as they are not very detailed in their approach to assessing pain.

Numeric rating scales assign point values to various categories, such as physiologic parameters, **locomotor activity,** and behavior (Figure 7-4). Each category is subdivided with different descriptors, which are awarded different point scores. After the assessment the points are totaled, with a higher score indicating an animal in more pain. This type of scale can never include every possible pain-related behavior or measurable parameter, so the scales are usually simplified or designed for specific types of pain (e.g., a numeric rating scale for horses undergoing castration).

A visual analogue scale consists of a ruler where the left end of the line equates to no pain, and the right end of the line to the worst pain imaginable for the specific disease or surgical procedure (Figure 7-5). The assessor places a mark (usually an X) on the ruler corresponding to the level of pain the assessor feels the animal is experiencing.

Veterinary teaching hospitals often have their own pain assessment form that typically combines different types of pain assessment tools in order to assess pain and progression of signs in response to treatment (Figure 7-6).

Each type of assessment has its limitations. The least complex scales allow quicker assessment but are not as effective at detecting subtle changes. The common purpose of these tools is to help determine how much pain the animal is in and to assess response to treatment. **Pain scales** are more accurate when observers are trained and when the same observer performs all assessments on a given patient.

### Assessing Response to Therapy

Animals undergoing major surgery need to be assessed hourly or possibly more frequently in the first few hours of the postoperative period, whereas patients with diseases

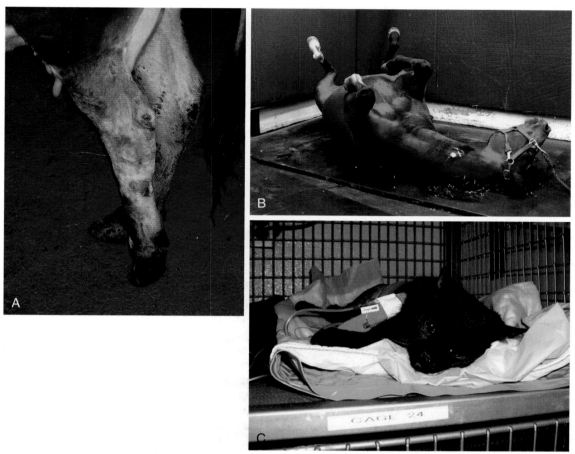

**FIGURE 7-2** Pain behaviors. **A,** Signs of locomotor pain in a cow. This cow had a chronic wound of the hock joint and was three-legged lame. **B,** Signs of abdominal pain in a horse. This horse with severely painful colic was violently thrashing in its stall and causing injury to itself. **C,** General signs of pain in a cat. This cat suffered multiple trauma (fractured femur and ruptured bladder) from being hit by a car. Note the laterally recumbent posture, the vacant stare with dilated pupils, and the lack of interest in the photographer. (**B** courtesy the OSU Equine Section.)

| No pain | |
|---|---|
| Mild pain | |
| Moderate pain | |
| Severe pain | |

**FIGURE 7-3** Simple descriptive scale. The observer makes an overall assessment of the animal's pain, and places an X in the box next to the descriptor.

associated with chronic pain such as arthritis require less frequent evaluation (monthly or at a longer interval). Effective analgesic treatment causes pain-associated behaviors to gradually recede. Hospitalized patients rest and sleep more easily and assume normal body positions and postures when asleep and awake. Appetite returns to normal, and appearance will improve as grooming behaviors also return to normal. When awake, animals will be more likely to interact with caregivers rather than ignore them or try to escape. Performance animals will return to form. Figure 7-7 shows examples of patients that seem comfortable after surgery.

Pain assessment scores will decrease if analgesic therapy is effective, although it is almost impossible to remove all pain that an animal experiences. Thus the aim is a reduction in the pain score and a more comfortable patient rather than the production of a pain-free patient.

> **TECHNICIAN NOTE** It is often not necessary to spend a lot of time trying to determine if a patient is in pain. Treat for pain and then observe the response to therapy.

## PERIOPERATIVE PAIN MANAGEMENT

Preemptive analgesia and multimodal therapy are key to providing successful **perioperative analgesia.** Multiple receptors and mechanisms have been identified that are

**Pain score 0-10. Choose one descriptor from each category**

| Interaction | Awake, willingly interacts, asleep | 0 | ☐ |
|---|---|---|---|
| | Awake, responds if encouraged | 1 | ☐ |
| | Awake, reluctant, unwilling | 2 | ☐ |
| Appearance | Asleep, calm | 0 | ☐ |
| | Agitated, vocalizing, looks at injury | 1 | ☐ |
| | Severely agitated, vocalizing, thrashing | 2 | ☐ |
| Posture | Normal, moves easily, asleep | 0 | ☐ |
| | Frequent position changes, guarded gait | 1 | ☐ |
| | Unwilling to lay down, abnormal gait | 2 | ☐ |
| Cardiovascular | HR and/or BP <10% elevated | 0 | ☐ |
| | HR and/or BP 10-20% elevated | 1 | ☐ |
| | HR and/or BP >20% elevated | 2 | ☐ |
| Respiration pattern | Normal | 0 | ☐ |
| | Guarded, mild abdominal | 1 | ☐ |
| | Marked abdominal | 2 | ☐ |

**FIGURE 7-4**   Numeric pain scale for use in small animal patients. The observer assigns a score for each category. Observations are performed before the animal is physically touched (e.g., to take a pulse rate). The overall score is used as a guide as to when to treat—for example, the veterinarian in charge may request that analgesics be administered if the pain score is ≥4—or as an assessment of response to treatment (i.e., a score that decreases after therapy).

**No Pain**                                   **Worst Possible Pain**

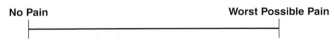

**FIGURE 7-5**   Visual analogue scale. The assessor places a mark (usually an X or a small vertical line) on the ruler corresponding to the level of pain the assessor feels the animal is experiencing.

responsible for pain and the development of windup. An analgesic plan for moderate to severe pain should make use of several drugs, each having a different mechanism of action. The benefits of multimodal analgesic therapy are that each individual drug dose is reduced, overall anesthetic drug requirement is reduced, and therefore the risk of toxicity and adverse effects is decreased.

Management of perioperative pain begins in the preoperative period. Premedication (see Chapter 3) offers an opportunity to administer analgesia before surgery (i.e., preemptively). Animals that are in pain before surgery will be in pain after surgery and should be treated for the anticipated severity of postoperative pain. Analgesics can be administered as part of the anesthetic premedication if they also provide or enhance sedation (opioids, alpha$_2$-adrenoceptor agonists, ketamine). Another

commonly used modality to provide preemptive analgesia in small animals is the application of a transdermal fentanyl patch at least 6 to 12 hours in advance of anticipated pain. NSAIDs are typically administered preoperatively in large animal patients and can be administered to small animal patients preoperatively when intravenous (IV) formulations are available and approved for this use.

## PHARMACOLOGIC ANALGESIC THERAPY

Pain control in the surgical patient should be available at every stage of hospitalization and treatment: during the preanesthetic period, the surgical procedure itself, the immediate postoperative period, the remainder of the hospital stay, and, if necessary, after the patient's return home.

The choice of analgesic is governed by the severity and type of pain and the animal's general condition. The veterinarian also selects the route of delivery, which may include injection (subcutaneous [SC], intramuscular [IM], IV, intraarticular, epidural, local infiltration), oral administration, or transdermal patch.

THE OHIO STATE UNIVERSITY VETERINARY TEACHING HOSPITAL
**PAIN MANAGEMENT PLAN**

"Pain assessment is considered part of every patient evaluation, regardless of presenting complaint."

PATIENT ID CARD

Date: _____ Department: _____

| Pulse rate: | Temperature: °C / °F | |
|---|---|---|
| Respiratory rate: | Weight: lbs / kg | Attitude: |

**Is pain present upon admission? Y ☐ N ☐**   Pain on palpation only? Y ☐ N ☐   Cause of pain:

**Signs of pain** (describe):   **Descriptors** (Please Circle):

| Behavior: | Normal ☐ | Depressed ☐ | Excited ☐ | Agitated ☐ | Guarding ☐ | Aggressive ☐ | Restless | Not grooming |
|---|---|---|---|---|---|---|---|---|
| Vocalization: | None ☐ | Occasional ☐ | Continuous ☐ | Other ☐ | | | Agitated | Obtunded |
| Posture: | Normal ☐ | Frozen ☐ | Rigid ☐ | Hunched ☐ | Recumbent ☐ | Reluctant to move ☐ | Trembling | Inappetant |
| Gait: | Sound ☐ | Lame weight bearing ☐ | | Lame non-weight bearing ☐ | | Non-ambulatory ☐ | Nervous | Biting or Licking area |

Other signs of pain:   Previous Analgesic History:

**Classification of pain:**   **Anatomical location of pain** (circle):

Acute ☐
Acute recurrent ☐
Chronic (>weeks) ☐
Chronic progressive ☐

Superficial ☐
Deep ☐
Visceral ☐

Inflammatory ☐
Neuropathic ☐
Both ☐

Primary hyperalgesia ☐
Secondary hyperalgesia ☐
Central algesia ☐

Ventral   Dorsal   Left   Comments:

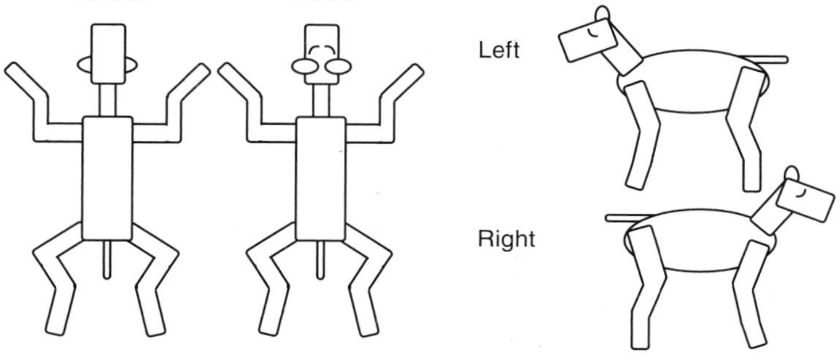

Right

**VISUAL ANALOGUE SCALE**

**No Pain**   **Worst Possible Pain**

| Event | Time(HH:MM): | Date: | Comments: |
|---|---|---|---|
| 1 | | | |
| 2 | | | |

**PAIN THERAPY**
(pharmacologic and alternative)

| | Date | Dose/Route | Efficacy/Duration | Comments |
|---|---|---|---|---|
| Current | | | | |
| Prescribed | | | | |
| | | | | |

**VISUAL ANALOGUE SCALE**

**No Analgesia**   **Complete Analgesia**

Clinician: _____   Release date: _____

**FIGURE 7-6**   The Ohio State pain assessment form. Note that there is a visual analogue scale to assess level of pain as well as degree of analgesia after therapy. Complex pain assessment forms or scales are useful for evaluating pain that is subtle, chronic, or difficult to treat. The main drawback of this type of pain assessment tool is that it is time-consuming.

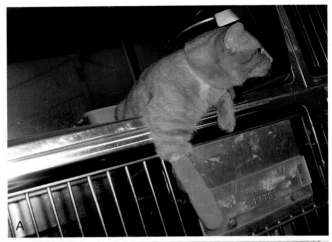

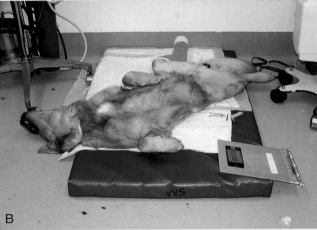

**FIGURE 7-7** Signs of comfort after surgery. **A,** One day after surgery for a forelimb wound this cat was playful and interactive. Analgesia consisted of oral buprenorphine and oral meloxicam. **B,** One hour after a tibial plateau leveling osteotomy, this golden retriever was sleeping on its back and seemed very comfortable. Analgesia consisted of a preoperative morphine epidural and postoperative intravenous carprofen.

Pharmacologic analgesia can be achieved through a variety of agents, including opioids, NSAIDs, alpha$_2$-agonists, ketamine, and local anesthetics.

## Opioid Agents

Opioids provide analgesia through their action on opioid receptors in both the spinal cord and brain, as well as in some peripheral tissues, such as the synovial membranes of joints. Opioid agonist drugs acting centrally inhibit perception in the brain and central sensitization in the spinal cord.

Doses, routes, and adverse effects of opioids used for postoperative analgesia are given in Table 7-1.

As outlined in Chapter 3, opioids have many uses in veterinary anesthesia, including the following:

- Opioids are commonly included in injectable premedications, often in combination with a tranquilizer such as acepromazine or dexmedetomidine.

When used preemptively, they diminish windup. The analgesic effect of these preanesthetic mixtures is generally gone by 2 to 4 hours after administration, however, and is usually inadequate to prevent or control even moderate pain after surgery.

- At higher doses, opioids can be used in combination with tranquilizers to induce a state of potent sedation (neuroleptanalgesia) that offers considerable analgesia throughout the surgical period and for some time after surgery. (See the discussions of neuroleptanalgesia in Chapter 3 and standing chemical restraint in Chapter 9.)
- Opioids can be used on their own or in combination with other agents (e.g., alpha$_2$-agonists, NSAIDs, and local anesthetics) to provide postoperative pain control (see later).

Individual opioids vary in their potency, duration, and adverse effects. Mu opioid receptor agonists (morphine, fentanyl, hydromorphone, oxymorphone, methadone, and meperidine) are generally considered to produce the most potent analgesic effects but are equally likely to induce unwanted adverse effects. They are used for moderate to severe pain. Partial mu agonists (buprenorphine, nalbuphine) and agonist-antagonists (nalbuphine, butorphanol) are less potent analgesics, and the degree of sedation is also less pronounced, as are adverse effects on the cardiovascular and respiratory systems. Because of their weaker analgesic effect, these agents should be reserved for use as preanesthetics and for treatment of mild to moderate pain.

In addition to their analgesic properties, many opioids cause some degree of sedation and relieve anxiety. If used as sole agents and at high doses, some may induce excitement in patients that are awake, particularly cats and horses.

Common gastrointestinal effects are characterized by an initial increase in gastrointestinal activity, including nausea and vomiting in cats and dogs, and defecation. This is followed by a relative slowdown of the gastrointestinal tract with the development of ileus, colic in horses, and constipation.

Opioids are metabolized in the liver. Animals with liver disease may have impaired drug metabolism, and these agents should be given at reduced doses.

## Opioid Agents Used for Moderate to Severe Pain

The potent opioid analgesics most commonly used in veterinary medicine are morphine, oxymorphone, hydromorphone, methadone, and fentanyl.

### Morphine

Morphine was the first opioid agent used in human and veterinary medicine and is still extensively used in veterinary practice as a preanesthetic and an analgesic. It is a pure agonist with affinity for both mu and kappa opioid receptors (see Chapter 3). Morphine can be used

## TABLE 7-1   Analgesics

| Drug | Species* | Route | Dose (mg/kg unless otherwise stated) | Notes |
|---|---|---|---|---|
| **OPIOIDS** | | | | |
| Morphine | Cat | IV (slow), IM, SC | 0.2-0.5 | Potential for excitement |
| | | CRI | 0.1-0.2 mg/kg/hr | |
| | | Epidural | 0.1 | Use preservative-free drug |
| | Dog | IV (slow), IM, SC | 0.5-1 | |
| | | CRI | 0.1-0.3 mg/kg/hr | |
| | | Epidural | 0.1 | Use preservative-free drug |
| | | PO | 2-5 | Give bid |
| | Horse | IV, IM, epidural | 0.05-0.1 | Potential for excitement, increased locomotor activity (e.g., stall walking), and ileus |
| | Cattle | IV, IM | 0.1-0.5 | |
| | | Epidural | 0.1 | |
| Hydromorphone | Cat | IV, IM, SC | 0.05-0.1 | |
| | | CRI | 0.01-0.03 mg/kg/hr | |
| | Dog | IV, IM, SC | 0.05-0.2 | |
| | | CRI | 0.01-0.03 mg/kg/hr | |
| Oxymorphone | Cat | IV, IM, SC | 0.05-0.1 | |
| | Dog | IV, IM, SC | 0.05-0.4 | |
| | Horse | IV | 0.001-0.005 | Potential for excitement and increased locomotor activity |
| Methadone | Dog | IV, IM, SC | 1-1.5 | |
| | Horse | IV | 0.05-1 | Potential for excitement and increased locomotor activity |
| Meperidine | Cat | IM, SC | 3-5 | May cause histamine release with IV administration |
| | Dog | IM, SC | 3-5 | May cause histamine release with IV administration |
| | Horse | IV | 0.2-1 | Potential for excitement and increased locomotor activity |
| Fentanyl | Cat | IV | 0.001-0.003 (1-3 mcg/kg) | |
| | | CRI | 1-4 mcg/kg/hr | Higher infusion rate for intraoperative analgesia |
| | | Transdermal patch | 2-5 mcg/kg/hr | |
| | Dog | IV | 0.002-0.005 (2-5 mcg/kg) | |
| | | CRI | 2-10 mcg/kg/hr | Higher infusion rate for intraoperative analgesia |
| | | Transdermal patch | 2-4 mcg/kg/hr | |
| | Horse | IV | 0.001-0.01 (1-10 mcg/kg) | Potential for excitement and increased locomotor activity |
| | | Transdermal patch | 0.5-1 mcg/kg/hr | |
| Buprenorphine | Cat | IV, IM, SC | 0.005-0.2 | Can be used to antagonize mu agonists |
| | | Transmucosal | 0.01-0.02 | Drip into cheek pouch using 1-mL syringe |
| | Dog | IV, IM, SC | 0.005-0.2 | Can be used to antagonize mu agonists |
| | Horse | IV | 0.01-0.04 | Potential for ataxia |

*Continued*

## TABLE 7-1   Analgesics—cont'd

| Drug | Species* | Route | Dose (mg/kg unless otherwise stated) | Notes |
|---|---|---|---|---|
| Butorphanol | Cat | IV, IM, SC<br>CRI<br>PO | 0.1-0.4<br>0.1-0.2 mg/kg/hr<br>0.5-1 | Can be used to reverse mu agonists |
| | Dog | IV, IM, SC<br>CRI<br>PO | 0.1-0.4<br>0.1-0.5<br>0.5-2 | Can be used to reverse mu agonists |
| | Horse | IV | 0.01-0.04 | Potential for ataxia |
| | Cattle | IV | 0.05-0.1 | |
| Pentazocine | Horse | IV | 0.5-1 | Potential for excitement and increased locomotor activity |

### ALPHA$_2$-ADRENOCEPTOR AGONISTS

| Drug | Species* | Route | Dose (mg/kg unless otherwise stated) | Notes |
|---|---|---|---|---|
| Xylazine | Cat | IV<br>IM, SC | 0.1-0.3<br>0.2-0.5 | Likely to cause vomition |
| | Dog | IV<br>IM, SC | 0.1-0.2<br>0.2-0.5 | Likely to cause vomition |
| | Horse | IV<br>Epidural | 0.5-1<br>0.03-0.05 | May cause bradycardia, ataxia |
| | Cattle | Epidural | 0.05 | |
| Dexmedetomidine | Cat | IM, SC | 10-40 mcg/kg | |
| | Dog | IM, SC<br>CRI | 5-20 mcg/kg<br>0.5-1 mcg/kg/hr | May cause bradycardia |
| Detomidine | Horse | IV<br>Epidural | 0.01-0.02<br>0.03-0.06 | May cause bradycardia, ataxia<br>Sedation, ataxia |
| | Cattle | Epidural | 0.06 | |
| Romifidine | Horse | IV<br>Epidural | 0.04-0.08<br>0.08 | May cause bradycardia |

### NONSTEROIDAL ANTIINFLAMMATORY DRUGS

All NSAIDs have the ability to cause renal toxicity.
Cox-2 selective drugs have lower gastrointestinal toxicity than COX-1 selective drugs.

#### COX-1 Selective NSAIDs

| Drug | Species* | Route | Dose (mg/kg unless otherwise stated) | Notes |
|---|---|---|---|---|
| Aspirin | Cat | PO, every 2-3 days | 10<br>(½ baby aspirin for a 4- to 5-kg cat) | Increased bleeding times |
| | Dog | PO, bid | 10-25 | Increased bleeding times |
| Acetaminophen | Dog | PO, tid | 5-10 | Highly toxic to cats |
| Flunixin meglumine | Cat | IM once, SC once | 0.25 | |
| | Dog | IV sid for three doses<br>IM sid for three doses<br>SC sid for three doses | 0.25-1 | |
| | Horse | IV | 0.2-1.1 | |
| | Cattle | IV | 1 | |

**TABLE 7-1  Analgesics—cont'd**

| Drug | Species* | Route | Dose (mg/kg unless otherwise stated) | Notes |
|---|---|---|---|---|
| Ketoprofen | Cat | SC (once) | 2 | Increased bleeding times |
| | | PO (for 5 days) | 0.5-1 | Increased bleeding times |
| | Dog | IV, IM, SC | 2 | Increased bleeding times |
| | | PO (for 5 days) | 0.5-2 | Increased bleeding times |
| | Horse | IV | 1.1-2.2 | |
| | Cattle | IV | 2 | |
| Ketorolac | Cat | IM, one or two treatments, 12 hr apart | 0.25 | |
| | Dog | IV or IM, one to three treatments, 12 hr apart | 0.3 | |
| Phenylbutazone | Horse | IV | 2-4 | Possible GI ulceration |
| Piroxicam | Dog | PO, sid | 0.3 | Antineoplastic (bladder tumors) |
| COX-2 Selective NSAIDs | | | | |
| Carprofen | Cat | SC | 2 | GI toxicity possible with chronic use |
| | | PO | 1 | GI toxicity possible with chronic use |
| | Dog | IV, IM, SC | 2-4 | Rarely, liver toxicity |
| | | PO | | Rarely, liver toxicity |
| | Horse | IV | 0.5-1.1 | |
| Meloxicam | Cat | IV, SC, PO, sid for 4 days | 0.1 | |
| | | PO, every 3-4 days | 0.025 | |
| | Dog | IV, SC, PO, sid | 0.1-0.2 | |
| Etodolac | Dog | PO, sid | 10-15 | Difficult to determine dose accurately in small dogs |
| Deracoxib | Dog | PO, sid | 1-4 | |
| Tepoxalin | Dog | PO, sid | 10 | Also blocks lipoxygenase |
| Firocoxib | Dog | PO, sid | 5 | |
| OTHER ANALGESIC DRUGS | | | | |
| Ketamine | Dog | CRI | 10-20 mcg/kg/hr | NMDA antagonist |
| | Horse | CRI | 10-20 mcg/kg/hr | NMDA antagonist |
| Amantadine | Dog | PO, sid | 3-5 | NMDA antagonist |
| Dextromethorphan | Dog | PO, sid | 0.5-2.0 | NMDA antagonist |
| Amitriptyline | Dog | PO, sid or bid | 1-2 | Inhibition of neurotransmitter reuptake |
| Tramadol | Dog | PO, sid or bid | 2-10 | Inhibition of neurotransmitter reuptake, weak mu opioid activity |
| Gabapentin | Dog | PO, sid | 3-5 | Unknown mechanism; wean off slowly to avoid rebound seizures |

*COX*, Cyclooxygenase; *CRI*, constant rate infusion; *GI*, gastrointestinal; *IM*, intramuscular; *IV*, intravenous; *NSAID*, nonsteroidal antiinflammatory drug; *NMDA*, N-methyl-D-aspartate; *PO*, by mouth; *SC*, subcutaneous.
*Where a species is not listed, no data are available for that specific drug.

in cats, dogs, and horses; however, as the likelihood for excitement or dysphoria is higher in cats and horses, it may be prudent to use lower doses initially in these species. Restlessness is seen in some dogs and horses (which manifests as an increase in **locomotor** activity) shortly after morphine administration, especially in the absence of pain. In addition, there is conflicting evidence as to whether morphine is an effective analgesic in horses when given systemically. For this reason morphine is more commonly administered to horses in combination with other drugs or administered epidurally.

Morphine is an inexpensive and effective option for treatment of moderate to severe pain in most patients. It is effective in treating both visceral and somatic pain and can be given by several routes, including slow IV, IM, SC, intraarticular, and epidural routes and by spinal injection.

Morphine is also available in regular or sustained release tablets for oral use, although efficacy of oral morphine varies considerably among patients.

When morphine is given intravenously, it must not be injected too rapidly, particularly in dogs, as rapid injection may cause release of histamine (characterized by a fall in blood pressure, flushing, and pruritus). One technique for use in dogs is to draw up a loading dose of 0.1 to 0.5 mg/kg, which is given slowly intravenously (over 5 minutes) and repeated until the patient appears free of pain or adverse effects occur. Morphine can also be administered intravenously by constant rate infusion (CRI). With this technique, morphine contained in a syringe is slowly administered through an IV catheter by means of a syringe pump at a rate of 0.05 to 0.3 mg/kg/hr.

IM administration of morphine (and other opioids) results in a slightly longer duration of action than IV administration and avoids the risk of hypotension, although IM injection appears to be somewhat painful. SC injections cause less patient discomfort (although SC injections have a slightly slower onset of effect). Also, the incidence of excitement, dysphoria, and vomiting in cats is lower when morphine is given subcutaneously rather than intramuscularly.

Although morphine provides potent analgesia and sedation, it is associated with several undesirable adverse effects. In cats and dogs there is initial gastrointestinal stimulation characterized by vomiting, salivation, and defecation. The incidence of vomiting can be reduced by pretreatment with acepromazine (0.02 mg/kg IM, 15 to 20 minutes before the morphine is given). In horses morphine may cause ileus and colic. Morphine also has the potential to cause severe respiratory depression, although this is less common in animals than in human patients. Excitement (particularly in cats given doses greater than 0.1 mg/kg), bradycardia, panting, increased intraocular pressure, increased intracranial pressure, urinary retention, miosis (in dogs), mydriasis (in cats), hypothermia, and hyperthermia (cats) are also encountered in some patients after morphine administration. Fortunately, these adverse effects are seldom a significant problem in patients in pain that are treated with analgesic doses. Morphine also reduces cardiac afterload and is sometimes used in dogs with congestive heart failure, especially if sedation is desirable.

Morphine has a strong tendency to cause physical dependence (addiction) in humans. It is therefore classified as a Schedule II drug in the United States and is designated as a narcotic in Canada.

### Oxymorphone

Oxymorphone is a pure opioid agonist with a greater analgesic potency and sedative effect than morphine, fewer adverse effects, and a longer duration of analgesia (4 hours). Despite these advantages, use of oxymorphone in veterinary practice is somewhat limited by its high cost.

Oxymorphone has a lesser tendency to induce vomiting in cats and dogs than morphine does. Also, unlike morphine, it does not induce histamine release and therefore does not decrease blood pressure. For this reason, it is preferred to morphine in patients with trauma, which may be in shock, or at increased risk for developing hypotension.

Oxymorphone may cause respiratory depression in some animals, especially in animals under inhalation anesthesia. Paradoxically, it also induces panting in many dogs, which may make some procedures (such as thoracic radiography) difficult. Oxymorphone causes some animals to become hyperresponsive to sound, and affected animals are easily startled by sudden noises. Bradycardia is also a potential adverse effect of this drug that can be prevented by pretreatment with atropine or glycopyrrolate.

Oxymorphone can be administered by many routes, including the IV, IM, SC, and epidural routes. Oxymorphone may be given rapidly intravenously to dogs, but rapid IV administration may cause excitement in cats. A tranquilizer such as dexmedetomidine, acepromazine, or diazepam may be used concurrently to prevent excitement and supplement the sedative effect of oxymorphone. Oxymorphone mixed with sterile saline and administered by IV drip is a safe analgesic agent in very sick or debilitated animals. Oxymorphone can be mixed with acepromazine (at a dose of 0.05 to 0.1 mg of acepromazine per kilogram, not to exceed 3 mg, and 0.2 mg of oxymorphone per kilogram) and used to induce anesthesia. Oxymorphone and diazepam (IV, administered alternately with separate syringes) can also be used to induce anesthesia with less risk of hypotension or decreased cardiac contractility than oxymorphone-acepromazine.

Oxymorphone is used infrequently in large animal patients because of cost and lack of information about adverse effects and analgesic efficacy.

Oxymorphone is classified as a Schedule II drug in the United States and as a narcotic in Canada.

### Hydromorphone

Hydromorphone is an opioid agonist with slightly less potency than oxymorphone and with a similar duration of effect. Hydromorphone is much less expensive than oxymorphone. It can be given via the IV, IM, and SC routes to both cats and dogs at a dose of 0.05 to 0.2 mg/kg. Unlike morphine, it is not associated with histamine release and has less potential to cause excitement in cats. Otherwise, adverse effects are similar to those seen with morphine: respiratory depression, bradycardia, vomiting, panting, excessive sedation, and excitement (seen especially at doses greater than 0.2 mg/kg).

Like oxymorphone, hydromorphone can be used as a premedication (at 0.1 to 0.2 mg/kg IM, alone or in combination with a tranquilizer), as an analgesic (at 0.05 to 0.2 mg/kg IM or SC for dogs and cats, repeated every 4 to 6 hours), or as an induction agent for high-risk patients (0.05 to 0.1 mg of hydromorphone per kilogram by slow IV injection followed by 0.05 to 0.2 mg of diazepam per kilogram intravenously). It is also given by the epidural route (0.03 to 0.1 mg) and has a similar effect to morphine.

Hydromorphone is used infrequently in large animal patients because of lack of information about adverse effects and analgesic efficacy.

Hydromorphone is classified as a Schedule II drug in the United States and as a narcotic in Canada.

### Methadone

Another synthetic opioid, methadone has similar characteristics to oxymorphone and hydromorphone with the exception that it has the lowest likelihood of causing vomiting in cats and dogs. This drug is also an antagonist at the NMDA receptor (see later), which may make it a favorable choice for treating pain when central sensitization is present or is likely to develop.

### Fentanyl

Among the most potent analgesics known, fentanyl has a rapid onset and short duration of effect in small animals (onset approximately 2 minutes, duration of effect approximately 20 to 30 minutes after IV injection). It is most commonly administered by continuous IV drip or by means of a **transdermal patch** (see following section). In small animal patients, fentanyl and midazolam or diazepam drawn into separate syringes can be used as induction agents. When fentanyl is given intravenously, a loading dose of 1 to 5 mcg/kg is typically administered, followed by a CRI of up to 10 mcg/kg/hr. It can also be given by IM, SC, or epidural injection.

Fentanyl can induce profound sedation, bradycardia, and respiratory depression in human patients, and like oxymorphone it may cause panting or increased sensitivity to sound. Adverse effects of fentanyl are further discussed in the section on transdermal patches later in the chapter.

Fentanyl was formerly sold in combination with the tranquilizer droperidol, in the injectable neuroleptanalgesic Innovar-Vet; however, this combination is no longer commercially available. Fentanyl is sold in combination with the tranquilizer fluanisone (under the name Hypnorm) in some countries.

Fentanyl (including fentanyl patches) is a Schedule II drug in the United States and is classified as a narcotic in Canada.

### Meperidine or pethidine

A synthetic opioid, meperidine has been extensively used in veterinary medicine as an analgesic and preanesthetic agent. Although meperidine is classified as a pure opioid agonist, its analgesic properties are less potent than those of the other pure agonists, and it is by comparison short acting. Meperidine is usually administered by SC injection, because IM injection may be painful and rapid IV injection may cause severe hypotension, excitement, and seizure-like activity.

Meperidine has a wide safety margin and causes less respiratory depression and gastrointestinal stimulation than morphine. It decreases salivary and respiratory secretions, a property that may be helpful in preanesthesia. Like morphine, it may cause histamine release in some patients, and pretreatment with histamine blockers may be advisable before IV injection.

In the past, meperidine was commonly used alone as a postoperative analgesic at a dose rate of 2 to 5 mg/kg IM or SC. Unfortunately, its analgesic effect is weak and of short duration, particularly in cats. For this reason it is no longer considered to be suitable for postoperative analgesia in animals, and in recent years it has been superseded by other opioids, particularly agonist-antagonists, buprenorphine, and butorphanol.

Despite its weak analgesic properties in animals, meperidine is still a useful drug for preanesthetic mixtures in combination with atropine and low doses of acepromazine. When administered with a tranquilizer (usually diazepam or acepromazine), meperidine also provides effective neuroleptanalgesia in puppies. Meperidine is also used in conjunction with injectable NSAIDs such as ketoprofen because it confers analgesia during the 30 to 60 minutes before the NSAID takes effect.

Meperidine is rarely used to provide analgesia in large animal patients.

Meperidine is a Schedule II drug in the United States and is classified as a narcotic in Canada.

### Butorphanol

A synthetic opioid with agonist and antagonist properties, butorphanol was first used in veterinary medicine as a cough suppressant. Butorphanol is widely used as a preanesthetic or sedative (at a dose of 0.1 to 0.4 mg/kg SC or IM or in mixtures with dexmedetomidine or acepromazine) and is also an effective postoperative analgesic for mild to moderate visceral pain.

Butorphanol is a mixed agonist-antagonist agent that stimulates kappa receptors and antagonizes or blocks mu receptors (see Chapter 3). As such, it is not as effective as the pure agonists for treating severe pain, especially orthopedic pain. Butorphanol is, however, an effective and safe treatment for mild to moderate visceral pain, especially cranial abdominal pain, in both dogs and cats. It is also extensively used in horses and ruminants.

Butorphanol is available in several concentrations, including 0.5 mg/mL, 2 mg/mL, and 10 mg/mL. Injectable butorphanol may be given via the IV, IM, or SC route. It is potentially toxic to the spinal cord, which limits its use for epidural injection. Tablets are available for long-term administration (at a dose of 0.4 to 1 mg/kg tid) and may be dispensed for postoperative pain.

The duration of analgesia provided by butorphanol may be short (as little as 1 hour in dogs after IM or SC injection). To avoid frequent readministration, butorphanol can be given as a CRI (in IV fluids or by syringe pump) at a dose of 0.1 to 0.2 mg/kg/hr, after a loading dose of 0.2 to 0.4 mg/kg.

Butorphanol produces less sedation, dysphoria, and respiratory depression than most opioids. Although moderate doses of butorphanol may cause some respiratory depression, higher doses do not depress respiration further (a phenomenon known as the *ceiling effect*). Heart rate, blood pressure, and cardiac output may be decreased after the administration of butorphanol; however, the effect is less than that of morphine, and pretreatment with atropine is not usually required. Panting, vomiting, and histamine release are seldom seen with this drug.

Butorphanol can be used as an antagonist to partially reverse respiratory depression and sedation induced by mu agonist opioids such as morphine or fentanyl, although the anesthetist must be aware that it will also partially reverse the analgesic effect of these drugs. The dose used for reversal is 0.2 to 0.4 mg/kg, administered intravenously to effect in increments of 0.01 to 0.05 mg/kg every 3 to 5 minutes. The antagonistic effect of butorphanol is less predictable and less potent than that of naloxone and can be overridden by subsequent administration of high doses (two to three times the normal dose) of morphine.

Since 1997, butorphanol has been classified as a Schedule IV drug in the United States. In Canada it is classified as a controlled drug.

### Buprenorphine

Buprenorphine is a partial mu agonist. It stimulates mu receptors, producing some analgesia, but is less effective than morphine and other pure agonists.

Buprenorphine can be given by the IV, IM, or epidural route. It has a delayed onset of action (15 minutes intravenously and 40 minutes intramuscularly) but provides a longer duration of analgesia than other opioids (authorities suggest as little as 6 hours or as long as 12 hours after IM injection and 18 to 24 hours after epidural injection). The injectable formulation of buprenorphine can be administered orally to cats; the pH of the feline mucosa allows excellent absorption via this route. Like butorphanol, buprenorphine does not provide adequate analgesia for severe pain (such as orthopedic pain), but it is useful for mild to moderate pain. It is commonly used to provide analgesia for rodents and other species used in research, as well as postoperative analgesia for dogs and cats.

Like butorphanol, buprenorphine can be used to reverse the sedation and respiratory depression induced by mu agonist opioids while maintaining some analgesic effect. Its effectiveness as a reversal agent is not as dramatic as butorphanol's because of the delay in its onset of action.

Buprenorphine at high doses may induce respiratory depression, which is difficult to reverse with naloxone. Analeptic agents such as doxapram may be somewhat effective in correcting buprenorphine-induced respiratory depression. Intubation and assisted ventilation are necessary in some patients because there is a potential for carbon dioxide retention and increased intracranial pressure.

Although buprenorphine has little sedative effect on its own, it can prolong sleep times when given with other agents.

Buprenorphine is a Schedule III drug in the United States and is unavailable in Canada. It is relatively expensive and is sometimes provided in ampules that are inconveniently large for small animal patients. Buprenorphine can, however, be transferred to sterile vials for use on multiple patients.

### Nalbuphine

Nalbuphine is a kappa agonist and mu antagonist like butorphanol, but its antagonist properties are greater. It is currently the only injectable opioid agent for veterinary use that is not classified as a controlled drug in the United States. It is a weak analgesic and sedative and can be used as a reversal agent for opioid agonists. Bradycardia, respiratory depression, and sedation are uncommon with this agent.

## Use of Opioid Injections to Treat Postoperative Pain

Opioids can be administered by a variety of routes for prevention or treatment of postoperative pain. In many practices, opioids are given by IM or SC injection, preferably before the animal regains consciousness from anesthesia. Injections may be repeated as necessary to prolong the analgesic effect (see Table 7-1 for information on dose and duration).

From the standpoint of analgesia, one major disadvantage of opioid agents is their relatively short duration of effect when given via the SC or IM route. Morphine offers 2 to 3 hours of analgesia for severe pain and 4 to 6 hours for moderate or mild pain; hydromorphone, 2 to 4 hours; oxymorphone, 1.5 to 5 hours; meperidine, less than 1 hour; fentanyl, approximately 20 minutes; and butorphanol, 1 to 2 hours in dogs and up to 4 hours in cats. Repeat injections can be given but are expensive, require hospitalization, and create "peak-and-trough" blood levels instead of a constant, effective blood concentration.

A second disadvantage of opioid use is the potential for adverse effects such as respiratory depression, bradycardia, excitement (usually exhibited as apprehension, hypersalivation, and mydriasis), excessive sedation, panting, increased sensitivity to sound, urinary retention, and gastrointestinal effects. These adverse effects are seldom severe when analgesic dosages are used. However, it is probably advisable to avoid opioid use or to use with caution in high-risk patients such as those with hypotension, hepatic disease, preexisting respiratory difficulties, CNS disorders such as head injuries or increased intracranial pressure, or altered bowel motility.

Both disadvantages of opioids—their short duration and potential for adverse effects—may be partially overcome by giving these drugs by routes other than IM or SC injection. Alternative routes for opioid administration include

IV infusion, epidural injection, transdermal patches, and intraarticular administration. When used by these alternative routes, opioids may produce effective, economical, and long-acting analgesia with minimal adverse effects. However, use of opioids by these routes constitutes off-label use in many animal species, and informed consent should be obtained from the animal's owner.

## Intravenous Infusion of Opioids

Morphine, fentanyl, oxymorphone, hydromorphone, methadone, and butorphanol can be given intravenously by CRI. This is sometimes the only method of analgesic delivery that is effective in constant, unremitting pain. Animals are given an initial loading dose (e.g., 0.1 mg of morphine per kilogram intravenously every 3 to 5 minutes) until the desired effect is achieved. The same dose is then given over 4 hours through a constant flow of IV fluids. At its most elaborate, IV infusion consists of an automated infusion pump or syringe pump. Practices that lack this type of specialized equipment can deliver opioid analgesics continuously in IV fluids by adding an opioid directly to the bag of fluids or burette, making sure to rotate the bag several times for adequate mixing (see Table 7-1 for doses). Patients must be frequently monitored for signs of inadequate pain control (in which case the rate of administration should be increased) or excessive sedation, dysphoria, respiratory depression, bradycardia, panting, and other signs that indicate an overdose. If these signs are present, the rate of administration should be decreased. The duration of pain control (for morphine) is 30 minutes past the discontinuation of the IV fluids. If morphine is inadequate to control pain, lidocaine also can be added to the fluids and infused at 5 to 20 mcg/kg/min. For severe pain, morphine, lidocaine, and ketamine can be co-infused (see later).

## Intraarticular Use of Opioids

Opioids may be given by the intraarticular route, particularly after elbow or stifle surgery. In this technique, 0.1 to 0.3 mg/kg of morphine is diluted in a volume of saline equivalent to 1 mL/10 kg body weight and instilled into the joint with a sterile catheter immediately after closure of the joint capsule. The morphine can also be combined with a local anesthetic such as 0.5% bupivacaine (at a dose of 1 mL/4.5 kg). This technique provides 8 to 12 hours of postoperative analgesia.

## Epidural Use of Opioids

With the instillation of a small dose of an opioid or other analgesic into the epidural space at the lumbosacral junction, it is possible to achieve excellent analgesia of the hind limbs, abdomen, caudal thorax, pelvis, and tail. Currently, morphine is the drug most commonly used for epidural analgesia. Oxymorphone is more expensive, butorphanol is less effective and may have some spinal toxicity, and local anesthetics such as lidocaine may impair movement, urination, and defecation and may cause a sympathetic

blockade if the drug diffuses too far cranially. Occasionally, morphine and local anesthetics are used epidurally in combination. Morphine is also sometimes combined with an alpha₂-agonist for epidurals in large animal patients.

Morphine given by the epidural route offers more profound analgesia for a longer time than when given by IM or SC injection. The analgesia is not sufficient for a surgical procedure unless supplemented with general anesthesia; however, it is an excellent means of achieving postoperative pain relief. Epidural morphine has a direct, long-lasting effect on the pain receptors in the spinal cord, but it does not reach high concentrations in the bloodstream because of low fat solubility. Adverse effects such as sedation (dogs), excitement (cats), respiratory depression, and nausea are therefore rare.

To achieve preemptive analgesia for postoperative pain, epidural morphine should be given after induction but before the surgical procedure. Epidural morphine is significantly less effective when administered in the postoperative period. Preservative-free morphine is preferred, because the preservatives typically found in morphine preparations (formaldehyde and phenol) are potentially neurotoxic.

The technique for epidural morphine administration is similar to epidural administration of lidocaine (see Procedure 6-3). Normally the animal is anesthetized or deeply sedated and is positioned in sternal recumbency with the head slightly elevated and the hind limbs pulled forward to open the lumbosacral space. An epidural puncture is performed. Once it has been determined that the needle is in the epidural space, morphine is injected over 30 seconds. Currently, the recommended dose for epidural morphine is 0.1 mg/kg in dogs and 0.05 to 0.1 mg/kg in cats. Ideally, a single-dose vial of preservative-free morphine should be used, diluted with sterile saline to a volume of 0.3 mL/kg. The recommended maximum volume that can be injected is 0.45 mL/kg. Onset of analgesia is approximately 20 to 60 minutes after injection, and analgesia lasts 6 to 24 hours. If more prolonged analgesia is required, an epidural catheter can be used to instill morphine into the epidural space over a longer period (hours to days).

Although epidural analgesia is regarded as a safe procedure, it should not be undertaken in animals with septicemia, local infections in the lumbosacral space, bleeding disorders, spinal trauma, or neurologic disease of the spinal cord. It is relatively difficult to administer epidural anesthetics to obese animals. Epidural hematomas and abscesses may result from improper needle placement or unsterile technique. Urinary retention may occur in the first 24 hours after surgery, and the bladder should be monitored closely in all patients that have received epidural analgesics. Urinary catheterization may be necessary in some patients. Pruritus, delayed respiratory depression, sedation, vomiting, and nausea have been reported in human patients but are uncommon in dogs. These symptoms, if they occur, can be treated with naloxone hydrochloride (0.01 mg/kg IV). Animals that have received epidural morphine should be repositioned every 2 to 4 hours because normal sensation may be absent. Failure to reposition animals may result in pulmonary atelectasis or prolonged pressure on superficial nerves, leading to temporary or permanent loss of function.

## Transdermal Use of Opioids

Transdermal patches containing fentanyl are another convenient option for long-term opioid administration. Fentanyl patches have been used for several years in the treatment of severe pain in human patients. The analgesic effect of a fentanyl patch is thought to be comparable to that of IM oxymorphone, but the duration of analgesia is considerably longer.

A "patch" consists of a reservoir of fentanyl enclosed in plastic. The patch is applied to the clipped skin of the animal and is left in place for several days (Procedure 7-1, p. 230). Patches come in different sizes that deliver different amounts of fentanyl each hour. A 12.5-mcg/hr patch is useful in animals weighing less than 4 kg. The 25-mcg/hr patch is used in cats and in dogs that weight less than 7 kg. A 50-mcg/hr patch is used in dogs weighing 7 to 20 kg; a 75-mcg/hr patch is used in dogs weighing 20 to 30 kg; and dogs that weigh more than 30 kg receive a 100-mcg/hr patch. Large animal patients may require several patches for effective plasma levels of fentanyl to be reached. Patches should not be cut or trimmed because this will cause erratic drug release and possible human exposure. In patients showing signs of inadequate pain control 24 hours after patch application, a second patch or another analgesic agent can be added.

Because fentanyl is relatively slowly absorbed through the skin, there is a delay of 4 to 12 hours in cats and 12 to 24 hours in dogs before therapeutic blood levels are achieved. To achieve preemptive analgesia, apply the patch at least 6 hours before the start of anesthesia in cats and at least 12 hours before the start of surgery in dogs. If application of the patch is delayed until after surgery, it is necessary to provide the patient with another opioid (e.g., morphine, hydromorphone, or oxymorphone) or NSAID such as meloxicam, ketoprofen, or carprofen until the patch takes effect. Butorphanol or buprenorphine should not be used concurrently with a fentanyl patch because either may partially block the opioid receptors, reducing the analgesic effect. Procedure 7-1 demonstrates how to apply a patch.

Many types of patients benefit from a fentanyl patch, including postoperative patients (e.g., after onychectomy, orthopedic procedures, or abdominal surgery) and those that have trauma, burns, cancer, or painful abdominal conditions such as pancreatitis.

Recent studies have shown considerable variation among animals in the concentration of fentanyl absorbed from a transdermal patch. One study showed that a 50-mcg/hr patch in dogs delivered as little as 13.7 and as much as 49.8 mcg/hr. Patients should be observed for signs of breakthrough pain (which may indicate a low plasma fentanyl concentration) and supplemented with morphine, oxymorphone, hydromorphone, or an NSAID as required.

Excessively high plasma fentanyl concentrations may develop in some patients. If this occurs, the most common signs are ataxia and sedation in dogs and dysphoria and disorientation in cats. Affected cats appear fearful or excited, are hypersensitive to sound, and may have widely dilated pupils. Panting is also a problem in some animals. Treatment, if necessary, consists of removing the patch and/or giving a narcotic antagonist (e.g., naloxone or butorphanol).

There have been some reports of death caused by respiratory failure when human patients self-administered more than one patch at a time, but respiratory depression is apparently uncommon in veterinary patients with fentanyl patches. Respiratory depression may be seen in trauma patients, particularly animals with CNS signs. Other adverse effects reported in human patients include constipation, physical dependence, muscle rigidity, miosis, mood changes, bradycardia, and bronchoconstriction. Use of fentanyl patches is not recommended in human patients with respiratory disease, increased intracranial pressure, impaired consciousness, bradycardia, pulmonary disease, hepatic or renal dysfunction, or brain tumors; these recommendations may also hold true for animals. Some patients may exhibit a mild transient dermatitis at the patch site after removal, and delayed hair regrowth at the patch site is common.

Transdermal patches may release excessive amounts of fentanyl if they are heated, and fentanyl overdoses have been reported in human beings who lie under electric blankets while wearing a patch. It is therefore suggested that fentanyl patches be avoided in animals with fevers and that patch contact with hot water bottles and other external sources of heat be avoided.

There is some concern regarding the potential for abuse by adult people or ingestion of a patch by a child. For this reason, the manufacturer does not support the use of fentanyl patches in animals. Some veterinarians address this concern by using the patch only on hospitalized animals or by carefully selecting and educating owners before discharging an animal that is wearing a patch.

## Nonsteroidal Antiinflammatory Drugs

NSAIDs, also called *nonsteroidal antiinflammatory analgesics* or NSAAs, are a large group of agents that have been used for many years to control minor pain in human beings and animals. The NSAID group includes such common drugs as acetylsalicylic acid (aspirin) and acetaminophen, and newer agents such as carprofen, meloxicam, etodolac, ketoprofen, tolfenamic acid, firocoxib, and deracoxib. Dose and toxicity information for individual NSAID agents are summarized in Table 7-1.

Traditionally veterinarians have thought that NSAIDs are not potent enough to treat anything other than mild postoperative pain. However, newer and more powerful NSAIDs such as ketoprofen, meloxicam, and carprofen are increasingly used for postoperative analgesia after procedures as diverse as ovariohysterectomy and fracture repair. NSAIDs are also useful for treatment of dental pain, panosteitis, osteoarthritis, meningitis, mastitis, and other painful medical conditions because of their strong antiinflammatory action.

## Mechanism of Action

NSAIDs have several beneficial effects on animal patients, including the following:

- All NSAIDs appear to be effective analgesics for somatic (musculoskeletal) pain. Some NSAIDs such as aspirin have little efficacy against visceral (organ-related) pain, whereas others such as ketoprofen and carprofen are potent analgesics with both somatic and visceral activity. All NSAIDs require approximately 30 to 60 minutes to achieve full analgesic effect, regardless of the route of administration.
- Many NSAIDs have potent antiinflammatory properties. This, combined with their analgesic effect, is the basis for the widespread use of drugs such as aspirin and carprofen in the treatment of osteoarthritis, panosteitis, hypertrophic osteodystrophy, and muscular pain.
- Some NSAIDs are antipyretic (reduce fevers).

The clinical effects of NSAIDs stem chiefly from their inhibition of prostaglandin synthesis. Prostaglandins (often abbreviated PGs) are a group of extremely potent chemicals that are normally present in all body tissues and are involved in the mediation of pain and inflammation following tissue injury. Prostaglandins are also responsible for a variety of homeostatic ("housekeeping") processes, including maintenance of normal gastrointestinal, reproductive, renal, and ophthalmologic function. Most NSAIDs prevent pain and inflammation by inactivating the enzyme cyclooxygenase (COX), which catalyzes one of the steps in the production of prostaglandins. There are two important COX isoenzymes that vary in importance from tissue to tissue. COX-1 is normally present (or constitutive) in most tissues, whereas COX-2 is constitutive in some, such as the kidney, reproductive organs, and eyes. COX-2 is inducible (i.e., not normally present, but is produced under certain circumstances), particularly during tissue damage and inflammation. Inhibition of both COX isoenzymes, but particularly COX-2, has been linked to analgesic effects. Most NSAIDs inhibit both COX-1 and COX-2, although the ratio of COX-1 to COX-2 inhibitory effects of individual NSAIDs vary considerably. Drugs that are COX-2 selective (carprofen, meloxicam, deracoxib) or specific (firocoxib) are less likely to interfere with intestinal barrier function and produce gastrointestinal ulceration; however, all NSAIDs have the potential to be nephrotoxic.

The relative effect of an NSAID on these enzymes will determine both the analgesic potency and the severity and type of adverse effects after the administration of that particular drug (see the separate section on adverse effects).

Although some NSAIDs are active against prostaglandins in peripheral tissues only, others (e.g., acetaminophen and ketorolac) exert their effects mainly on prostaglandin synthesis in brain tissue and are therefore said to be "central acting." Some agents (ketoprofen, meloxicam) appear to exert their effects both centrally and in the peripheral tissues.

As a group, NSAIDs are well absorbed orally, and many are available in tablet or liquid form. Recently, potent injectable NSAIDs have also become available. Injectable NSAIDs can be given at the end of surgery to provide 24 hours of pain relief. Some NSAIDs, for example, carprofen, can also be used before surgery in selected patients to achieve preemptive analgesia. If long-term analgesia is required, injections can be repeated in some cases, or tablets can be dispensed.

All NSAIDs are eliminated by metabolism and conjugation within the liver, followed by renal or biliary elimination. The NSAID group of drugs is unusual in that there is significant variation in duration of effect between species. For example, the plasma half-life of aspirin is 1 hour in the horse, 8 hours in the dog, and 38 hours in the cat. The prolonged half-life of aspirin in the cat is a result of the low levels of the enzyme glucuronyl transferase (one of the enzymes that metabolizes salicylate NSAIDs, such as aspirin) in that species. There is also significant variation among species in the toxicity of particular NSAIDs. For example, acetaminophen is extremely toxic in cats but is a useful agent in dogs. Similarly, ibuprofen is considered to be safe for use in humans but has significant toxicity in dogs and cats. Because of this variation, the safety of any NSAID in one species does not imply that it can be used with impunity in all species (see Table 7-1 for dosages and cautions for specific agents). In particular, it cannot be assumed that dosages and administration schedules that are appropriate for dogs can be safely used in cats.

NSAIDs have some advantages over opioids: they are not subject to the storage, handling, and record-keeping regulations that govern narcotics; they have little abuse potential; and they are effective when given orally. Unlike opioids, NSAIDs have a negligible effect on the cardiovascular and respiratory systems. NSAIDs also do not depress the CNS and therefore lack the sedative effect of opioids. When used in healthy young to middle-aged patients according to label directions, they provide effective and safe relief for mild to moderate pain. For some applications, their analgesic effect appears to be superior to that of butorphanol or meperidine.

## Adverse Effects

Unfortunately, NSAIDs as a group have significant potential for toxicity in small animal patients. Most people who work in veterinary hospitals are aware of the toxicity of acetaminophen in cats. A single 325-mg capsule may cause acute hepatotoxicosis within 4 hours of ingestion because of the formation of toxic metabolites within the liver. Many NSAIDs are safe for use in healthy animals but can have serious toxic effects in animals that are dehydrated or hypotensive.

Many of the adverse effects of NSAIDs are attributable to the fact that they reduce not only the production of the prostaglandins that mediate pain, inflammation, and fever, but also those that are beneficial. Pharmaceutical companies have attempted to formulate NSAIDs that will prevent the production of harmful prostaglandins while preserving the production of beneficial prostaglandins. This can be achieved if the NSAID inhibits the enzyme COX-2 (which is active in damaged or inflamed tissues and synthesizes the prostaglandins that cause pain) but does not affect COX-1 (which synthesizes the prostaglandins that help maintain normal physiologic functions such as protection of the gastric mucosa and modulation of blood flow to the kidney). In theory, it is possible to produce NSAIDs that have more than 1000-fold specificity for COX-2 over COX-1 and are therefore extremely safe for use in terms of their gastrointestinal adverse effects. However, the drugs currently available do not have this degree of specificity, and the COX-2 isoenzyme is important for normal function in some organs, such as the kidney and reproductive tract. Additionally confusing, an agent that has pronounced specificity for COX-2 in one species does not necessarily show the same specificity in another species.

One example of a beneficial prostaglandin that is adversely affected by many NSAIDs is prostacyclin, which is normally present within the stomach mucosa and helps reduce gastric acid secretion and promote mucous production. When prostacyclin levels are reduced by the administration of an NSAID, gastric acid secretion increases and mucous production decreases, which sometimes leads to the production of stomach ulcers. Up to 50% of dogs treated with aspirin have mild stomach ulceration within a few days of treatment, which may result in vomiting, gastrointestinal bleeding, and inappetence, but more often is not clinically apparent. Occasionally, animals with gastrointestinal ulceration resulting from NSAID use may undergo a sudden episode of life-threatening hemorrhage. In dogs, ulcerogenic potential appears to be high for ketoprofen, naproxen, ibuprofen, flunixin, piroxicam, and meclofenamic acid, and use of these agents for prolonged periods (over 5 days) is associated with a high incidence of adverse effects. Meloxicam, carprofen, and etodolac have less ulcerogenic activity in dogs and are preferred for long-term use, as in dogs with osteoarthritis.

In an effort to avoid gastrointestinal problems in human beings and animals receiving NSAIDs, pharmaceutical companies have prepared enteric-coated or buffered formulations. Enteric coating does not appear to reliably reduce the toxicity of these drugs; however, buffered formulations may have reduced toxicity. It is also helpful to administer oral NSAIDs with a meal to dilute the drug that is present in the stomach. In susceptible patients, it may be advisable to use gastrointestinal protectants such as sucralfate suspension (at a dose of 0.25 to 0.5 g by mouth [PO] tid in cats, 0.5 to 1 g PO tid in dogs) in conjunction with an NSAID to prevent or treat gastrointestinal effects. Sucralfate forms a proteinaceous complex that adheres to damaged gastric mucosa, preventing further injury. Sucralfate should be administered on an empty stomach at the same time as the NSAID. Another helpful gastrointestinal protectant is the synthetic prostaglandin misoprostol, which is given orally at a dose of 2 to 4 mg/kg tid. Histamine-2 ($H_2$)–receptor antagonists such as famotidine or ranitidine are also helpful in treatment of stomach ulcers but should not be given at the same time as sucralfate, which requires an acid environment to work.

Another potential adverse effect of NSAIDs is renal toxicity. A beneficial prostaglandin, $PGE_2$, normally maintains adequate blood flow within the kidney. In anesthetized animals and other animals that are prone to hypotension (such as trauma patients), $PGE_2$ plays a vital role in maintaining renal blood flow. By blocking synthesis of $PGE_2$, NSAIDs have the potential to decrease renal blood flow in these patients, leading to renal hypoxia. Dogs are apparently very susceptible to development of renal failure when blood pressure decreases, and there are several reports of acute renal failure after the administration of NSAIDs during anesthesia. To avoid the risk of renal damage in anesthetized patients, the use of NSAIDs should be postponed until after anesthesia, and preemptive or intraoperative use is not advised unless the patient is receiving intraoperative IV fluids and arterial blood pressure monitoring is available. Fortunately, NSAID-induced renal insufficiency is usually reversible (in young, healthy patients) with the administration of IV fluids. It is much more difficult to reverse in geriatric patients with preexisting renal failure. It is a prudent practice to screen geriatric patients for renal disease before anesthesia (by determining values for blood urea nitrogen, creatinine, and/or urine specific gravity) and to avoid NSAIDs in patients with decreased renal function.

Another potential adverse effect of NSAIDs is impaired platelet aggregation, which can lead to prolonged bleeding times. This effect may be beneficial in some circumstances (e.g., by lowering the risk of stroke in human patients who regularly take aspirin). However, there is a potential for increased bleeding in patients that are given NSAIDs before or during surgery. As with the potential for renal toxicity, this concern can be minimized by postponing the use of NSAID agents until after surgery has been completed. If preemptive use of an NSAID is indicated, carprofen can be used (in the dog), because it has been shown to have less renal toxicity and platelet-inhibiting effect than some other NSAID agents.

Liver damage appears to be associated with the use of NSAID agents in some patients. Carprofen has been extensively studied in this regard, and although the incidence of liver disease is small, this is a recognized adverse effect of this drug. Hepatocellular toxicosis appears to be most common in Labrador retrievers and may be evident as soon as 2 weeks after initiation of treatment. Monitoring bile acid levels appears to be a sensitive method of detecting early signs of toxicity.

NSAIDs may antagonize the action of several drugs commonly prescribed for cardiac disease and hypertension, including angiotensin-converting enzyme (ACE) inhibitors, and some diuretics.

As with most drugs, there is great variation among individual patients in the potency, duration, and adverse effects produced by NSAIDs. When used for postoperative pain control, NSAIDs are safe to use in well-hydrated young to middle-aged animals with normal renal and hemostatic function. NSAIDs should be used with care or avoided entirely in dehydrated patients and in animals with coagulopathies or liver or kidney dysfunction. Because of the potential for gastrointestinal ulceration, these agents should be avoided in patients with gastrointestinal disorders and in patients that are receiving corticosteroids (which also contribute to ulcer formation). Animals that have low blood pressure, congestive heart failure, or hemostatic disorders such as thrombocytopenia are generally high-risk candidates for NSAID therapy. Patients with trauma should not receive NSAIDs unless they are in stable condition with no indication of hemorrhage, they are receiving IV fluids, and no surgery is anticipated in the next 48 hours. For some patients (e.g., geriatric patients and patients with renal disease) NSAIDs should be used only in conjunction with IV fluids and blood pressure monitoring. Opioids appear to be a safer therapeutic option in these patients.

## Other Analgesic Agents

Opioids and NSAIDs are the mainstays of postoperative pain control; however, other agents may be useful in some circumstances. These include local anesthetics, alpha$_2$-adrenergic agonists, and ketamine.

### Local Anesthetics

Local anesthetic agents have long been used to allow surgical procedures to be performed in conscious animals, but their use in preventing or treating postoperative pain is relatively recent. The presence of local anesthetic blocks sodium channels, which prevents transduction and transmission of noxious stimuli into nerve impulses peripherally (local blocks) as well as centrally (if administered by epidural). Local anesthetic can be sprayed or injected at the site of an injury or a surgical site or infiltrated around nerves supplying the affected area. They can also be used to desensitize an entire region, as with epidural administration or IV infusion. Local anesthetics have many advantages, including complete anesthesia of the affected area, low toxicity (when given at the

appropriate dose), and rapid onset of action. Unfortunately, the duration of action is relatively short, and the danger of CNS and cardiac toxicity limits repeated use. The use of local anesthetics for pain control is discussed in detail in Chapter 6.

### Alpha$_2$-Adrenoceptor Agonists

Although alpha$_2$-adrenoceptor agonists such as xylazine and dexmedetomidine provide good analgesia by activating alpha$_2$-adrenergic receptors both centrally and in the periphery, their use for pain control in small animals is limited by three factors: (1) the short duration of their analgesic effect (in the case of xylazine, 30 to 60 minutes, and for dexmedetomidine, 30 to 90 minutes); (2) the profound sedative effect of these agents; and (3) the potential for serious adverse effects (respiratory depression, vomiting, bradycardia, heart block, and hypotension, which may be exacerbated by opioids). It is difficult to determine the quality or duration of analgesia in some patients because the sedative effect of these drugs remains even after the analgesic effect has worn off. In dogs and cats, these agents should be used only for young to middle-aged, healthy patients. However, when used in low doses (e.g., xylazine at 0.1 mg/kg IV, IM, SC; and dexmedetomidine at 0.001 to 0.005 mg/kg IV, IM, SC), these agents appear to potentiate the effect of opioids and may contribute to the quality of analgesia in the postoperative period. Butorphanol and dexmedetomidine in combination appear to provide effective analgesia and sedation for minor clinical procedures.

Recently, alpha$_2$-adrenoceptor agonists have been shown to produce significant analgesia when administered by the epidural route (alone or in combination with opioids and other agents). Dexmedetomidine (0.005 mg/kg) can be added to morphine to prolong the duration of epidural analgesia.

The analgesic effect of xylazine is antagonized by yohimbine, and the analgesic effect of dexmedetomidine is antagonized by atipamezole.

Alpha$_2$-adrenoceptor agonists (xylazine, detomidine, romifidine) are commonly administered to horses to provide sedation, muscle relaxation, and analgesia. The degree of sedation provided is typically less than seen in small animals, and horses typically remain standing although they may become ataxic. Analgesia is adequate for moderately to severely painful diseases or procedures. Cardiovascular adverse effects such as bradyarrhythmias (including second-degree atrioventricular block), initial hypertension, and ultimately hypotension are commonly seen. Heavy sedation should be induced cautiously in horses with preexisting upper airway stridor, as relaxation of the upper airway and pharyngeal muscles, along with congestion of the nares and nasal passages, may lead to respiratory obstruction in these patients. Alpha$_2$-adrenoceptor agonists cause decreased gut motility, which may lead to gas distension and colic postoperatively. Alpha$_2$-adrenoceptor antagonists (yohimbine, atipamezole) can be used to reverse these unwanted effects; however, analgesia and sedation will also be reversed. Use of these agents may even result in excitement.

## Ketamine

Ketamine is a dissociative injectable anesthetic (see Chapter 3) that has become popular as an adjunct to more potent analgesics (opioids, local anesthetics, alpha$_2$-agonists) because it blocks the NMDA receptors in the CNS at the level of the spinal cord. Antagonism of the NMDA receptors is important in preventing central sensitization, or windup. The dose of ketamine needed to antagonize these receptors is much lower than that required to induce anesthesia. Ketamine can be administered as IV boluses (0.5 mg/kg) or as a CRI (10 to 15 mcg/kg/hr). Ketamine alone does not typically provide sufficient analgesia; therefore it is most commonly administered in conjunction with other drugs. A commonly used approach to provide intraoperative analgesia for painful orthopedic surgery in healthy dogs is to co-infuse morphine, lidocaine, and ketamine, or MLK (see Table 7-1 and Procedure 7-2, p. 231).

Ketamine should be avoided or used with extreme caution in patients with hypertrophic cardiomyopathy or in cats with compromised renal function. Adverse effects of ketamine are dose related and rarely seen at analgesic dosages but may include tachycardia, increased blood pressure, increased intraocular and intracranial pressure, seizures and postoperative delirium, and salivation.

Orally administered NMDA antagonists include amantadine and dextromethorphan.

## Corticosteroids

These drugs (e.g., prednisone, dexamethasone) have strong antiinflammatory properties, which, as with the NSAIDs, act by decreasing prostaglandin activity. They should not be used concurrently with NSAIDs, as both drug classes are ulcerogenic. Other long-term adverse effects include immunosuppression and development of hyperadrenocorticism.

## Tramadol

Tramadol is a nonopiate drug that is given orally and has activity at the mu receptor. It is useful as a postoperative alternative to opioids once a patient has resumed eating (usually 12 to 24 hours after surgery) and can be prescribed for continuation of analgesic therapy at home. An additional mechanism of tramadol is inhibition of norepinephrine and serotonin reuptake, which also promotes analgesia. Tramadol should not be administered with other norepinephrine and serotonin reuptake inhibitors (e.g., amitriptyline).

## Tranquilizers

Although acepromazine, diazepam, and other tranquilizers are not considered to be analgesics, they may potentiate the effect of opioids in some patients. Possible explanations for this include the fact that pain appears to be intensified in anxious patients, and drugs that cause CNS depression also alter pain perception by the brain. Animals that have received adequate analgesia but are restless may become calmer after administration of acepromazine (0.01 to 0.05 mg/kg SC, IM, or IV) or diazepam (0.2 mg/kg IV). Tranquilizers are also useful in cats and horses that show excitement after opioid administration. Because tranquilizers have no analgesic effect, they should not be used as a substitute for opioids or other analgesic agents. Acepromazine should be used with caution in patients with blood loss, dehydration, or low blood pressure.

## Multimodal Therapy

Because there are several mechanisms by which pain is produced, it is often helpful to use more than one type of analgesic to relieve pain. Multimodal therapy (also known as *combination* or *balanced analgesia*) may be more successful than treatment with any single agent, because pain perception is affected at several points along the pain pathway and different mechanisms are targeted. For example, it has been shown in human patients that the use of piroxicam (an NSAID) and buprenorphine (an opioid) together provides analgesia that is superior to that with use of either agent alone. The concurrent use of NSAIDs with opioids may allow a 20% to 50% reduction in the opioid dose.

One familiar example of combination therapy is a mixture of acetaminophen and codeine, which is an effective oral treatment for moderate to severe pain in the dog. When given orally at a dose rate of 10 mg of acetaminophen per kilogram and 0.5 to 1 mg of codeine per kilogram every 6 to 12 hours, the combination is safe in healthy dogs for up to 5 days. If necessary, the codeine can be supplemented up to 4 mg/kg. Constipation and sedation are common adverse effects of this drug combination, and the diet should be supplemented with a fiber source such as bran or psyllium. Acetaminophen-codeine should never be given to cats and should also be avoided in dogs with hepatic disease.

Opioids and NSAIDs may be given to a patient simultaneously or at different times. For example, a fentanyl patch may be applied to a cat and a dose of meloxicam given at the same time to provide analgesia during the lag time when the patch has not yet taken effect. Alternatively, a dog undergoing an orthopedic operation can be premedicated with morphine (0.2 to 0.3 mg/kg IM) followed by administration of an injectable NSAID (such as meloxicam or carprofen) at the end of operation and followed up with an NSAID given orally for 3 days. This type of "balanced analgesia" allows the use of relatively modest doses of analgesics with a low risk of adverse effects, yet achieves effective pain relief in many patients.

Co-infusion of MLK is another type of combination therapy that is easily administered in IV fluids during surgery. Benefits include multimodal analgesia provided by three different mechanisms of action, and decreased inhalant anesthetic requirement. Problems encountered with MLK include delayed recovery from anesthesia and decreased accuracy of administration, especially with smaller patients. Delayed recovery can be avoided by decreasing the infusion rate until the patient is awake. Use of infusion pumps or burettes increases accuracy of delivery to smaller patients.

See Protocols 7-1 to 7-5 for examples of multimodal perioperative analgesia therapies.

## HOME ANALGESIA

There are several options for pain relief in dogs and cats discharged from the hospital. Fentanyl patches can be used sequentially for a period of up to several months in patients with chronic pain (e.g., cancer). Meloxicam, carprofen, etodolac, and other NSAIDs are commonly prescribed for long-term therapy of osteoarthritis and other chronic painful conditions. Oral morphine is available as a sustained-release tablet that is effective when given to dogs or cats twice daily, beginning with a low dose and gradually increasing the dose as needed. Tylenol with codeine (dogs only) and butorphanol are also available in tablet form and are suitable for treatment of mild to moderate chronic pain. Tramadol is also commonly prescribed for patients to take at home.

## NURSING CARE

Patient discomfort can also be reduced through conscientious nursing care, including keeping the animal and its cage or stall clean and dry, affording ample opportunity for defecation and urination (including bladder expression or catheterization if necessary), providing comfortable bedding and quiet surroundings, and gently reassuring the patient. The patient should be positioned so that it does not lie on a surgery site or traumatized area. Some patients benefit from being turned every 2 to 3 hours. Anxious patients may benefit from having a blanket or toy from home with them. Unconscious animals may require the application of ophthalmic ointment to prevent corneal

---

**PROTOCOL 7-1** | **Example of a Multimodal Pain Management Protocol for a Cat Undergoing Ovariohysterectomy (Spay) or Castration**

**Preemptive Analgesia**
- IM buprenorphine and a tranquilizer (premedication)

**Postoperative Analgesia**
- Buprenorphine orally every 6 to 8 hours for the first 12 to 24 hours
- Send home with buprenorphine and NSAIDs for 2 to 3 days; reassess if the cat seems to be in pain

*IM,* Intramuscular; *NSAID,* nonsteroidal antiinflammatory drug.

---

**PROTOCOL 7-2** | **Example of a Multimodal Pain Management Protocol for a Cat Undergoing Onychectomy (Declaw)**

**Preemptive Analgesia**
- IM buprenorphine and a tranquilizer (premedication), with or without ketamine (premedication or total injectable anesthesia)
- Three-point block with local anesthetic

**Postoperative Analgesia**
- Buprenorphine orally every 6 to 8 hours for the first 12 to 24 hours
- Send home with buprenorphine and NSAIDs for 2 to 3 days; reassess if the cat seems to be in pain

*IM,* Intramuscular; *NSAID,* nonsteroidal antiinflammatory drug.

---

**PROTOCOL 7-3** | **Example of a Multimodal Pain Management Protocol for a Dog Undergoing Ovariohysterectomy (Spay) or Castration**

**Preemptive Analgesia**
- IM morphine and a tranquilizer (premedication)

**Postoperative Analgesia**
- Injectable NSAID after anesthesia
- Tramadol orally every 8 to 12 hours for the first 12 to 24 hours
- Send home with tramadol and NSAIDs for 2 to 3 days; reassess if the dog seems to be in pain

*IM,* Intramuscular; *NSAID,* nonsteroidal antiinflammatory drug.

**PROTOCOL 7-4** | **Example of a Multimodal Pain Management Protocol for a Dog Undergoing Surgery to Repair a Fractured Humerus**

**Preemptive Analgesia**
- NSAID SC before surgery unless contraindicated
- IM morphine and a tranquilizer (premedication)

**Intraoperative Analgesia**
- Morphine, lidocaine, ketamine infusion

**Postoperative Analgesia**
- IM morphine every 4 to 6 hours for the first 12 to 24 hours
- Start oral NSAID therapy once the patient is alert enough to eat
- Send the dog home with NSAIDs and tramadol for 3 to 5 days; reassess earlier if the dog seems to be in pain

*IM,* Intramuscular; *NSAID,* nonsteroidal antiinflammatory drug; *SC,* subcutaneously.

**PROTOCOL 7-5** | **Example of a Multimodal Pain Management Protocol for a Horse Undergoing Bilateral Stifle Arthroscopy**

**Preemptive Analgesia**
- NSAID IV before surgery unless contraindicated
- Alpha$_2$-agonist and butorphanol as premedication

**Intraoperative Analgesia**
- Lidocaine infusion

**Postoperative Analgesia**
- Butorphanol as needed
- Oral NSAID therapy, which can be continued at home, reassessing if the horse seems to be in pain

*IV,* Intravenously; *NSAID,* nonsteroidal antiinflammatory drug.

drying. Treatments and monitoring should be scheduled so that the patient is not disturbed unnecessarily.

## NONPHARMACOLOGIC THERAPIES

Acupuncture and transcutaneous electric nerve stimulation may effectively treat pain by stimulating the release of endogenous opioids (endorphins). Other nonpharmacologic methods of pain control that may be effective in some situations include massage therapy, application of cold (for acute injuries) or heat (for chronic injuries), physiotherapy, laser therapy, magnetic therapy, and homeopathic or herbal remedies such as Bach flower remedies. Generally these methodologies are used in conjunction with and as an adjunct to pharmacologic therapy. The effectiveness of some of these therapies has not been demonstrated in controlled studies.

## KEY POINTS

1. The veterinary technician forms a vital part of the veterinary care-giving team. Through an understanding of pain physiology, pain-associated behaviors, pain assessment tools, analgesic drug pharmacology, and communication skills, the technician contributes significantly to the comfort and welfare of patients.

2. Pain assessment is an essential part of every patient evaluation, regardless of presenting complaint.

3. Pain is a complex, individual experience that has been defined as an aversive sensory and emotional experience that elicits protective motor actions, results in learned avoidance, and may modify species-specific behavior traits, including social behavior.

4. Untreated pain can negatively affect a patient's behavior, physiology, metabolism, and immune system, causing poor performance, weight loss, delayed wound healing, increased susceptibility to infection, and patient suffering.

5. Physiologic pain occurs in response to a noxious stimulus where there is no or minimal tissue injury, and is a protective mechanism.

6. Pathologic pain occurs after a noxious stimulus that results in tissue injury, and can be classified based on origin, duration, and severity.

7. The pain pathway consists of the following four components: transduction, transmission, modulation, and perception.

8. Peripheral hypersensitivity or primary hyperalgesia is caused by the presence of inflammation.

9. Central hypersensitivity or secondary hyperalgesia ("windup") is caused by changes to neurons in the spinal cord.

10. The practice of administering analgesics before surgery to decrease analgesic requirements and minimize central nervous system sensitization is called *preemptive analgesia.*

11. The practice of administering several analgesic drugs that work via different receptor mechanisms is called *multimodal analgesia.*

12. Pain assessment tools can be used to assess pain and response to analgesic therapy.

13. Opioid analgesics such as morphine, oxymorphone, hydromorphone, methadone, and fentanyl are opioid receptor agonists and are the most effective drugs for treating acute pain.

14. Potential side effects of the mu-agonist opioids are sedation, respiratory depression, vomition, defecation, gastrointestinal ileus, pruritus, excitement, hyperthermia, and dysphoria.

15. The partial agonist opioid buprenorphine has a long duration of action but may not provide sufficient analgesia for severe acute pain. It has been shown to provide good analgesia in rodents.

16. Agonist-antagonist opioid drugs such as butorphanol have a short duration of action and are not as effective at treating severe pain, but have fewer side effects and are used extensively in large animals.

17. Nonsteroidal antiinflammatory drugs decrease inflammation by inhibiting prostaglandin synthesis and are commonly used to provide analgesia postoperatively and in patients with less severe or inflammatory pain.

18. The side effects of NSAIDs include liver and renal toxicity, increased bleeding times, and gastrointestinal ulceration.

19. Local anesthetics provide analgesia via their sodium channel blocking activity and can be administered locally, epidurally, or, in the case of lidocaine, as a constant rate infusion.

20. Alpha$_2$-adrenoceptor agonists are effective analgesics; however, because of their side effects in small animals and ruminants, they are more commonly used for this purpose in horses.

21. Ketamine antagonizes NMDA receptors in the spinal cord, preventing central sensitization.

22. Corticosteroids have potent antiinflammatory activity and, because they act by the same mechanism as NSAIDs, should not be used concurrently with drugs of that class.

23. Tramadol is a nonopiate drug with activity at the mu receptor and is given orally, commonly as part of an analgesic plan for the patient at home.

24. Providing appropriate nursing care to the hospitalized animal is an important part of ensuring that a patient is comfortable when its pain is being treated.

25. Nonpharmacologic therapies, such as acupuncture, may effectively treat pain by stimulating the release of endorphins.

## PROCEDURE 7-1 Applying a Fentanyl Patch

1. Various locations can be used for patch application, including the lateral thorax, dorsal neck (commonly used in small animals), or upper part of the limb (commonly used in horses). Any location that is hard for the animal to reach with its mouth or limb will work. Once applied, the patch should not contact sources of external heat.

2. The skin is clipped, taking care not to nick the skin (which may result in the fentanyl being absorbed too rapidly). If soiled, the skin can be cleansed with water (only) and dried thoroughly.

3. The patch is removed from its protective backing and handled by the edges only. The adhesive side of the patch is held onto the skin for 1 to 2 minutes with hand pressure.

4. The patch should be handled by its edges, or gloves should be worn to avoid contact with the patch membrane.

5. The patch is applied to the shaved skin and held in place for 1 to 2 minutes. If the patch does not adhere to the skin, a Tegaderm patch or light dressing can be placed over the fentanyl patch. Skin staples can also be used to secure the patch if it is placed while the animal is anesthetized, taking care not to puncture the drug chamber (Figure 1). Tissue adhesive should not be used to attach the patch to the patient because it alters the absorption of the fentanyl. If necessary, the patch may be covered with bandage material to prevent removal by the patient (particularly dogs*).

6. The patch remains in place for several days, during which time the fentanyl is gradually absorbed. Blood levels remain at therapeutic levels for approximately 5 days in cats and 3 days in dogs, although there is considerable variation in duration and effectiveness among patients.

7. At the end of this time the patch should be peeled off and disposed as medical waste. If the patient has been discharged in the interim, it is advisable that the patient return to the clinic for patch removal and assessment.

8. If a longer duration of analgesia is required, a new patch can be applied at a separate, clipped site.

9. Fentanyl patches can be used in other species, following similar directions as for dogs. Figure 2 shows a fentanyl patch applied to a horse's forelimb.

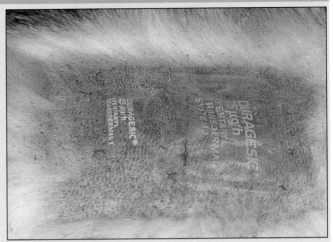

**FIGURE 1**  Fentanyl patch applied to the skin of a dog and secured using skin staples. Care should be taken not to place the staples through the drug reservoir chamber.

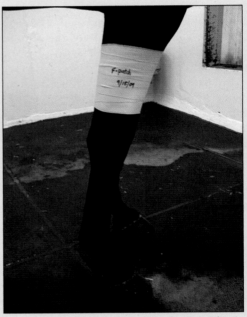

**FIGURE 2**  Fentanyl patch secured to the forelimb of a horse with Elastikon bandage. Note the writing on the bandage, which communicates to the caregivers that a patch is underneath, and when it was applied.

*Accidental ingestion of the patch produces no signs in dogs or cats if the patch reaches the stomach or intestines intact, because any fentanyl absorbed is metabolized rapidly by the liver. However, overdose may occur after oral absorption (e.g., if a patch is chewed and punctured).

## PROCEDURE 7-2 Procedure for Adding Morphine, Lidocaine, Ketamine to IV Fluids to Provide Analgesia for Dogs during Surgery

1. Add the following amounts of drugs to a 500-ml bag of crystalloid fluids:
   - 1.6 mL of morphine 15 mg/mL (24 mg morphine)
   - 15 mL of lidocaine 20 mg/mL (300 mg lidocaine)
   - 0.6 mL of ketamine 100 mg/mL (60 mg ketamine)
2. Remember to mark the bag of fluids using an appropriate additive label.
3. Administer the fluids at 5 mL/kg/hr during surgery.* The infusion rates will be:
   - Morphine 0.24 mg/kg/hr
   - Lidocaine 3 mg/kg/hr
   - Ketamine 0.6 mg/kg/hr
4. Important points to remember when administering the combination:
   - The combination should not be used to administer fluid boluses.
   - Lidocaine takes several hours to reach an effective concentration; therefore 2 mg/kg IV should be administered at the start of the anesthetic period or given before IV induction.
   - The effects of the combination will usually last for 1 hour after termination of the infusion, sometimes delaying recovery. Turning the infusion off before postoperative radiographs or bandage application will decrease time spent in recovery.
   - Particular care should be taken when administering this combination to small dogs; use of a smaller bag of fluids, a Buretrol, or an infusion pump is recommended.

*If fluids are being delivered at 10 mL/kg/hr, then the amount of drugs added should be halved.

## REVIEW QUESTIONS

1. *Idiopathic pain* is defined as:
   a. Pain that is caused by cancer
   b. Pain that is of unknown cause
   c. Pain that is caused by inflammation
   d. Pain that is caused by injury to nerves

2. *Pathologic pain* is defined as:
   a. Pain that is caused by cancer
   b. Pain that is of unknown cause
   c. Pain that is caused by tissue injury
   d. Pain that is not associated with tissue injury

3. An ovariohysterectomy, which involves surgically incising the skin and abdominal wall and excising the uterus and ovaries, has the following components of pain:
   a. Somatic pain only
   b. Visceral pain only
   c. Both somatic and visceral pain
   d. Neither somatic nor visceral pain

4. The process by which thermal, mechanical, or chemical noxious stimuli are converted into electrical signals called *action potentials* is:
   a. Perception
   b. Modulation
   c. Transduction
   d. Transmission

5. In the spinal cord, pain impulses can be altered by neurons that either suppress or amplify nerve impulses. This process is known as:
   a. Perception
   b. Modulation
   c. Transduction
   d. Transmission

6. Where in the pain pathway does secondary sensitization or "windup" occur?
   a. Brain
   b. Spinal cord
   c. Visceral pain receptors
   d. Peripheral pain receptors

7. Which of the following statements regarding multimodal analgesic therapy is true?
   a. The dose of each drug is decreased when several drugs are used.
   b. Multiple pain receptor mechanisms are targeted by one drug.
   c. One pain receptor mechanism is targeted by several drugs.
   d. Side effects are increased by using several drugs.

8. Which of the following anesthetic plans includes multimodal analgesic therapy?
   a. Dexmedetomidine, sevoflurane
   b. Acepromazine, ketamine, isoflurane
   c. Acepromazine, morphine, isoflurane
   d. Dexmedetomidine, morphine, ketamine

9. Which one of the following analgesic plans targets three different pain receptor mechanisms?
   a. Morphine IM, fentanyl CRI, lidocaine nerve block
   b. Morphine IM, fentanyl CRI, bupivacaine nerve block
   c. Morphine IM, ketamine CRI, lidocaine nerve block
   d. Ketamine CRI, lidocaine and bupivacaine nerve block

10. Treating pain does not improve wound healing.
    True          False

11. Administering analgesics before tissue injury is known as:
    a. Premedication
    b. Local analgesia
    c. Multimodal analgesia
    d. Preemptive analgesia

12. Which of the following is *not* a potential side effect of opioid administration in cats and dogs?
    a. Vomiting
    b. Dysphoria
    c. Renal failure
    d. Respiratory depression

13. What is the mechanism of action of nonsteroidal antiinflammatory drugs?
    a. They block sodium channels.
    b. They are alpha$_2$-receptor agonists.
    c. They inhibit prostaglandin synthesis.
    d. They are mu-opioid receptor agonists.

14. Which of the following is *not* a potential side effect of NSAID administration?
    a. Liver damage
    b. Kidney damage
    c. Gastrointestinal ulcers
    d. Respiratory depression

15. A pain scale can be used to assess pain as well as response to analgesic therapy.
    True          False

## SELECTED READINGS

Gaynor JS, Muir WW III: *Handbook of veterinary pain management*, St Louis, 2009, Mosby.

Lerche P, Muir WW III: Peri-operative pain management in horses. In Muir WW III, Hubbell JAE, editors: *Equine Anesthesia*, ed 2, St Louis, 2008, Mosby.

Perkowski SZ, Wetmore LA: The science and art of analgesia. In Gleed RD, Ludders JW, editors: *Recent advances in veterinary anesthesia and analgesia: companion Animals*, Ithaca, 2006, International Veterinary Information Service, (www.ivis.org), Document No. A1405.1006.

Shaffran N, Grubb T: Pain management. In Bassert JM, McCurnin DM, editors: *Clinical textbook for veterinary technicians*, ed 7, St Louis, 2010, Elsevier.

# Canine and Feline Anesthesia

8

## KEY TERMS

Anatomic dead space
Anesthetic induction
Anesthetic maintenance
Anesthetic protocol
Anesthetic recovery
Central nervous system
   (CNS) vital centers
Hypostatic congestion
Laryngospasm
Mechanical dead space
Pneumomediastinum
Pneumothorax
Stridor
Titration
Total intravenous
   anesthesia

## OUTLINE

Patient Preparation, 234
Selecting a Protocol, 235
Summary of a General Anesthetic
   Procedure, 236
   *Anesthetic Induction with an*
      *Intramuscular Agent or Combination,*
      *236*
   *Anesthetic Induction with an Intravenous*
      *Injection of an Ultra–Short-Acting*
      *Agent to Effect, 237*
   *Total Intravenous Anesthesia by*
      *Intravenous Boluses of an Ultra–Short-*
      *Acting Agent, 237*
   *Total Intravenous Anesthesia by Constant*
      *Rate Infusion, 237*
   *Induction and Maintenance with an*
      *Inhalant Agent, 237*
   *Intravenous Induction and*
      *Maintenance with an Inhalant Agent,*
      *239*
Equipment Preparation, 239
Premedication or Sedation, 240
Anesthetic Induction, 240
   *Intravenous Induction, 242*
   *Inhalation Agents, 242*
   *Mask Induction, 243*
   *Chamber Induction, 243*
   *Intramuscular Induction, 244*
   *Oral Administration, 244*

Endotracheal Intubation, 245
   *Equipment for Endotracheal Intubation, 245*
   *Selecting an Endotracheal Tube, 246*
   *Preparing the Tube, 247*
   *Intubation Procedure, 247*
   *Checking for Proper Placement, 248*
   *Securing the Tube, 248*
   *Cuff Inflation, 248*
   *Laryngospasm, 249*
   *Complications of Intubation, 250*
Maintenance of Anesthesia, 251
   *Maintenance with an Inhalant Agent, 251*
   *Maintenance with Repeat Boluses of*
      *Propofol or Another Ultra–Short-Acting*
      *Agent, 252*
   *Maintenance with a Constant Rate Infusion,*
      *252*
   *Maintenance with Injectable and Inhalant*
      *Agents, 252*
   *Maintenance with an Intramuscular*
      *Injection, 252*
Patient Positioning, Comfort, and Safety, 252
Anesthetic Recovery, 253
   *Anesthetist's Role in the Recovery Period, 253*
   *Signs of Recovery, 254*
   *Monitoring, 255*
   *Oxygen Therapy, 255*
   *Extubation, 255*
Postanesthetic Period, 256

## LEARNING OBJECTIVES

*After completion of this chapter, the reader will be able to:*
- Describe anesthetic techniques commonly used in small animal practices.
- List strategies used to minimize adverse effects when selecting an anesthetic protocol.
- Describe how different methods of anesthetic induction and maintenance influence the dynamics of an anesthetic event.
- Prepare a small animal patient, anesthetic equipment, and anesthetic agents and adjuncts for general anesthesia.
- Describe induction of general anesthesia by intravenous (IV) injection of an ultra–short-acting agent, by mask or chamber induction, or by intramuscular (IM) injection.
- Explain cautions and risks associated with each method of anesthetic induction, and strategies to maximize patient safety.
- List reasons for, advantages of, and potential complications of endotracheal intubation.
- Explain how to do each of the following: (1) select and prepare an endotracheal tube (ETT) for placement; (2) place an ETT in a dog or cat; (3) check for proper placement; (4) inflate the cuff; (5) minimize laryngospasm; and (6) extubate a patient during anesthetic recovery.
- Describe maintenance of general anesthesia by administration of an inhalant agent, injection of repeat IV boluses of an ultra–short-acting agent, or constant rate infusion (CRI).

- List principles of providing for patient positioning, comfort, and safety during anesthetic maintenance.
- List factors that affect patient recovery from anesthesia, the signs of recovery, appropriate monitoring during recovery, and oxygen therapy during recovery.
- Describe general nursing care during the postanesthetic period.

Small animal* patients are restrained and anesthetized by means of a variety of techniques including general anesthesia, sedation, neuroleptanalgesia, and local and regional anesthesia. Of these options, general anesthesia is most commonly used for several reasons. The immobilization and unconsciousness associated with general anesthesia enable most procedures to be performed more quickly and safely than is possible with alternative techniques. General anesthetics also produce analgesia during the period of unconsciousness and, if used along with an analgesic as a part of a balanced protocol, during the preoperative and postoperative periods as well. In addition, general anesthetic procedures can be performed with readily available resources and at a reasonable cost. In dogs and cats general anesthesia is induced and maintained using balanced protocols, exclusive use of inhalants, intramuscular (IM) protocols, and total intravenous (IV) techniques.

Mild to heavy sedation and neuroleptanalgesia are also frequently used to facilitate diagnostic and therapeutic procedures in small animals that are frightened, aggressive, or in pain. Box 8-1 lists some of the procedures commonly performed with patients under sedation or neuroleptanalgesia. Box 8-2 shows American College of Veterinary Anesthesiologists (ACVA) monitoring guidelines for sedated patients.

Although less frequently employed than general anesthesia, sedation, or neuroleptanalgesia, local and regional techniques are used along with general anesthesia in small animals to provide additional analgesia for dental, abdominal, orthopedic, and occasionally other procedures. Neuromuscular blockers are rarely used in general practice but are sometimes used to provide muscle relaxation for ocular and orthopedic procedures in veterinary schools and referral practices.

## PATIENT PREPARATION

The veterinary technician in any busy small animal practice routinely has a constant stream of demands placed on him or her from the time of arrival to the end of the day.

---

*Veterinary practices that provide health care services for dogs and cats are traditionally referred to as *small animal* or *companion animal practices,* although many other species, traditionally referred to as *exotic animals,* may also be served by these clinics. The term *exotic animal* includes mammals referred to as *pocket pets* or *small exotic mammals* (rabbits, ferrets, Guinea pigs, hamsters, gerbils, rats, and mice), birds, reptiles, amphibians, and fish. Although any of these species rightfully can be classified as small animals, in this chapter the term *small animal* will be used specifically in reference to dogs and cats.

---

| BOX 8-1 | **Examples of Procedures Commonly Performed under Sedation or Neuroleptanalgesia** |
|---|---|

- Radiographic studies
- Ultrasonographic studies
- Transtracheal washes
- Otic examination, flushing, and treatment
- Blood draws
- Wound treatment
- Bandage and splint application
- Toenail trims
- Grooming
- Orogastric intubation

---

| BOX 8-2 | **American College of Veterinary Anesthesiologists Monitoring Guidelines for Sedation without General Anesthesia** |
|---|---|

The objective of the American College of Veterinary Anesthesiologists (ACVA) monitoring guidelines for sedated patients is "to ensure adequate oxygenation and hemodynamic stability in the obtunded patient." To accomplish this, the ACVA makes the following recommendations:

"Intermittent monitoring of basic respiratory and cardiovascular parameters in the heavily sedated animal should be routine. Supplemental oxygen, an endotracheal tube, and materials for IV catheterization should always be readily available. Particular attention should be paid to brachycephalic breeds that are particularly at risk for airway obstruction under heavy sedation."

In order to function effectively in this environment, the technician must manage time efficiently so that the most pressing patient needs are met first. After essential tasks have been managed, often little time is left for less critical needs such as patient preparation. The technician must resist the temptation to limit or eliminate this important step, however, because incomplete patient preparation often results in complications ranging from mild to life-threatening, especially in anesthetized animals that are not young and healthy. Any time saved by abbreviating patient preparation is often offset managing problems that could have been prevented had it been given due attention. The reader is referred to Chapter 2 for a detailed discussion of the essentials of patient preparation. Procedure 8-1, p. 258, shows a summary of the steps required to prepare a small animal patient for general anesthesia.

## BOX 8-3 Dosage Calculations for Injectable Drugs

With the exception of a constant rate infusion (CRI), the volume of most injectable agents to be administered is calculated using the following standard formula:

$$\text{Volume (mL)} = \frac{\text{Patient body weight (kg or lb)} \times \text{Prescribed dose (mg or mcg/kg or lb body wt)}}{\text{Drug concentration (mg or mcg/mL)}}$$

The prescribed dose is the amount of the agent prescribed by the doctor in milligrams or micrograms per unit of body weight. The drug concentration is found on the drug vial label and is most often expressed in milligrams or micrograms per milliliter. For prevention of errors when this calculation is performed, all units must be the same. (All patient body weight units must be converted to either kilograms or pounds, and the prescribed dose and drug concentration units must be converted to either milligrams *or* micrograms.)

**Example**

How much propofol should you draw up to induce a 20-lb mixed-breed dog for a dental cleaning? The prescribed dose is 5 mg/kg body weight, and the drug concentration is 10 mg/mL.

$$\text{Patient body weight (kg)} = 20 \text{ lb} \times \frac{1 \text{ kg}}{2.2 \text{ lb}} = 9.1 \text{ kg}$$

$$\text{Volume (mL)} = \frac{9.1 \text{ kg} \times 5 \text{ mg/kg}}{10 \text{ mg/mL}} = 4.55 \text{ mL}$$

---

*TECHNICIAN NOTE* Incomplete patient preparation often results in complications ranging from mild to life-threatening, especially when anesthetic procedures are performed in animals that are not young and healthy. Any time saved by abbreviating patient preparation is often offset managing problems that could have been prevented.

### SELECTING A PROTOCOL

An **anesthetic protocol** is a list of the anesthetics and adjuncts prescribed for a particular patient, including dosages, routes, and order of administration. The veterinarian-in-charge (VIC) commonly selects anesthetic protocols, although he or she may authorize the experienced technician to suggest a protocol, which then must be approved before administration. A suitable protocol takes into account the minimum patient database, the patient's physical status class, and the procedure to be performed. Specific drug choices are also influenced by training, clinical experience, and personal preference and therefore vary widely from doctor to doctor.

*TECHNICIAN NOTE* Double-check all injectable drug doses before administration, and ensure that the concentration of an agent drawn into a syringe is the same as that used for drug calculations.

When the protocol is known, drug doses, oxygen flow rates, and fluid administration rates must be calculated and checked *carefully* by the veterinary technician to ensure that the correct drugs and amounts are prepared. Box 8-3 shows the steps required to calculate the doses of

most injectable drugs. Ill, geriatric, pediatric, or otherwise compromised patients (physical status class P3 to P5) require use of modified protocols based on the patient's primary condition. (See Chapter 12 for recommendations regarding class P3 to P5 small animal patients.) Management of these cases can be quite challenging and requires customization of the anesthetic protocol by the VIC.

*TECHNICIAN NOTE* Always label all syringes containing injectable agents with the name of the patient, the name of the drug, and the drug concentration if more than one concentration is available.

As discussed in the chapter on monitoring, anesthesia affects **central nervous system (CNS) vital centers**. Every anesthetized patient is at risk for potentially serious adverse effects such as hypotension, hypoventilation, hypoxemia, and hypothermia because of the actions of anesthetics and adjuncts on these centers. When choosing the protocol and preparing the agents, the anesthetist can use a number of strategies to minimize these adverse effects, as follows:

- Unless the procedure must be performed immediately for the patient's well-being, correct significant physiologic abnormalities such as dehydration, hypotension, and anemia before anesthesia.
- Base the anesthetic protocol on results of the minimum database. Do not use a single, standard protocol for all patients.
- Use a balanced protocol consisting of multiple agents. This approach reduces the required dose of any one agent, thus minimizing the adverse effects of all agents.

- Double-check all injectable drug doses before administration, and ensure that the concentration of an agent drawn into a syringe is the same as that used for the drug calculations.
- Label all syringes containing injectable anesthetic agents with the name of the patient, the name of the drug, and the drug concentration if more than one concentration is available.
- Administer no more than the minimum dose of drug needed to achieve the desired level of anesthesia.
- Unless told otherwise, administer all IV agents "to effect."

## SUMMARY OF A GENERAL ANESTHETIC PROCEDURE

In order to give anesthetic agents safely, it is important to have a clear understanding of the dynamics of an anesthetic procedure. The word *dynamics* refers to the changes in the patient's level of consciousness over time, including when, how extensively, and how quickly these changes occur. Armed with this understanding, the anesthetist is able to administer agents effectively, rapidly detect adverse reactions, and quickly recognize and respond to patient needs. An anesthetist without this knowledge is unable to make sound decisions, differentiate normal from abnormal responses, or react rapidly enough to protect the patient.

The protocol is the primary determinant of these dynamics. The agent used and the route of administration affect how quickly the patient becomes unconscious and awakens and the amount of control the anesthetist has over anesthetic depth. For instance, when given intramuscularly, most drugs begin to act, reach peak effect, and "wear off" relatively slowly and they afford the anesthetist very little control over anesthetic depth. In contrast, the commonly used inhalant agents act, reach peak effect, and are eliminated relatively quickly and they give the anesthetist excellent control. The dynamics for each of the commonly used protocols are summarized in the following sections.

### Anesthetic Induction with an Intramuscular Agent or Combination

When anesthetics are administered by IM injection, anesthetic depth gradually increases after injection (typically over 5 to 20 minutes) and, after peak effect, gradually decreases as the agent is metabolized (typically over 30 to 60 minutes or longer). Once the injection has been given, the anesthetist has little control over changes in depth or the peak effect. If the depth is inadequate, the anesthetist can give additional anesthetic, but if depth is excessive, the anesthetist can only monitor and support the patient until the agent is metabolized and the patient recovers naturally. The only exception to this is when using opioids, benzodiazepines, and alpha$_2$-agonists. In these cases the anesthetist can decrease anesthetic depth rapidly by administering the corresponding antagonist (reversal agent) (Figure 8-1).

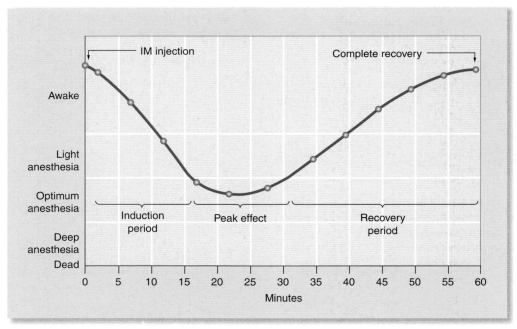

**FIGURE 8-1**   Induction with an intramuscular (IM) agent or combination. When this route is used, anesthetic induction is gradual, with peak effect about 15 to 20 minutes after a single IM injection. Recovery is even more gradual as the agent is metabolized or redistributed.

## Anesthetic Induction with an Intravenous Injection of an Ultra–Short-Acting Agent to Effect

**Anesthetic induction** with an intravenous injection of an ultra–short-acting agent to effect is a technique used for short procedures that require less than 10 minutes of anesthesia, such as removal of a Steinman bone pin, examination of the pharynx and larynx, or changing of a bandage. Propofol, methohexital, thiopental sodium, or etomidate may be used this way. When anesthesia is induced by IV injection, anesthetic depth typically increases rapidly over 15 seconds to a few minutes after the initial injection, then decreases gradually over 10 to 20 minutes. When using this technique, the anesthetist controls the peak effect and can increase anesthetic depth rapidly by giving additional boluses of the drug. However, as with IM anesthesia, there is little control over duration, and anesthetic depth cannot be decreased (Figure 8-2).

## Total Intravenous Anesthesia by Intravenous Boluses of an Ultra–Short-Acting Agent

With **total intravenous anesthesia** (TIVA) by IV boluses of an ultra–short-acting agent, anesthesia is induced as previously described and then is maintained by giving additional boluses every 3 to 5 minutes as needed to maintain surgical anesthesia. This technique is acceptable for noninvasive procedures of short to moderate length but is somewhat cumbersome for major surgeries because it is somewhat challenging to keep the patient at an optimum anesthetic depth even with constant monitoring. Propofol is the agent most commonly used to provide TIVA, although methohexital and etomidate are alternatives. With this technique the anesthetist can increase the depth rapidly by giving incremental boluses, but—as with IM administration—if the patient is deeply anesthetized, the anesthetist can only support the patient and wait until the agent is metabolized and the anesthetic depth naturally decreases (Figure 8-3).

## Total Intravenous Anesthesia by Constant Rate Infusion

TIVA by constant rate infusion (CRI) is similar to TIVA by bolus injections, except that anesthesia is maintained by infusing small amounts of anesthetic constantly with a syringe pump. Although similar in effect to maintenance with bolus injections, this technique moderates and slows down changes in depth by avoiding sudden infusion of a large amount of drug. Instead, only the amount needed to maintain anesthesia is infused on a continuous basis for the duration of the procedure (Figure 8-4).

## Induction and Maintenance with an Inhalant Agent

The use of an inhalation agent for induction and maintenance differs from injection techniques in several respects. Anesthetic induction with the commonly used inhalant agents is usually faster than IM induction but

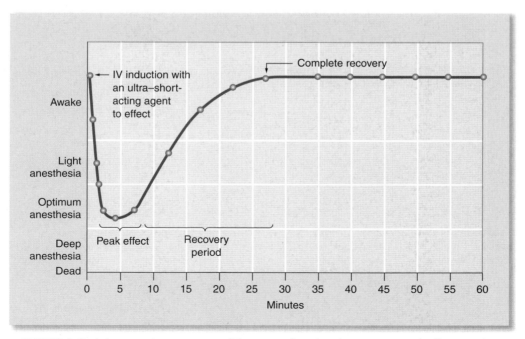

**FIGURE 8-2** Induction with an intravenous (IV) injection of an ultra–short-acting agent to effect. Anesthetic induction is very rapid, peak effect is short, and recovery is gradual but relatively rapid as the agent is metabolized or redistributed.

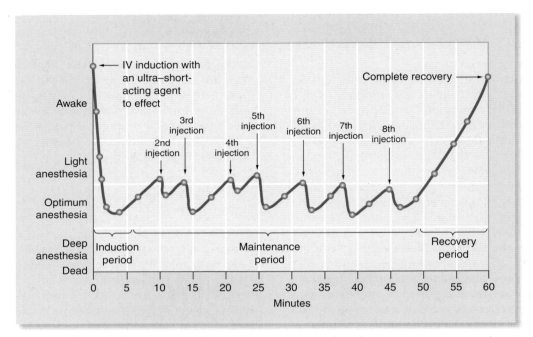

**FIGURE 8-3**   Total intravenous anesthesia (TIVA) by IV boluses of an ultra–short-acting agent. Anesthetic induction is very rapid, peak effect is short, and surgical anesthesia is maintained with administration of repeat boluses every 3 to 5 minutes to effect. As with a single injection, recovery is gradual after the final bolus but relatively rapid as the agent is metabolized or redistributed.

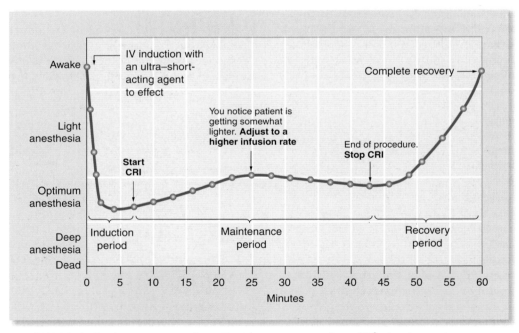

**FIGURE 8-4**   Total intravenous anesthesia (TIVA) by constant rate infusion (CRI). Anesthetic induction is very rapid, peak effect is short, and surgical anesthesia is maintained with a CRI. The rate of infusion is adjusted based on assessment of the anesthetic depth. After discontinuation of the CRI, recovery is gradual, but relatively rapid as the agent is metabolized or redistributed.

slower than IV induction (about 5 to 8 minutes with isoflurane or sevoflurane). Also, the anesthetist has excellent control over depth and can either increase or decrease depth relatively rapidly by changing the vaporizer dial setting. With inhalant agents, however, there is a delay between the time the dial setting is changed and the time it takes for patient anesthetic depth to change, because it takes at least several minutes for the new concentration to fill the breathing circuit, reach the patient's lungs, and equilibrate with the blood and CNS.

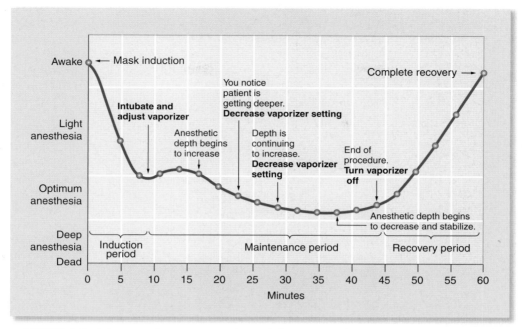

**FIGURE 8-5** Induction and maintenance with an inhalant agent. Induction is relatively rapid, but gradual. Anesthesia is maintained by continued administration of the inhalant agent. The percent administered is adjusted based on assessment of the anesthetic depth. After discontinuation of the agent, recovery is gradual, but relatively rapid as the agent is exhaled. Note that there is a delay after any change in the vaporizer setting. This is typical of inhalant anesthesia because of the time required for the concentration of the agent in the breathing circuit to reach the dialed concentration.

*TECHNICIAN NOTE* With inhalant agents there is a delay between when the dial setting is changed and when the patient depth changes. For this reason, vaporizer setting adjustments must be anticipated as much as possible through close monitoring.

The time required for anesthetic depth to change is influenced by a number of factors including the patient's respiratory drive, the agent used, the carrier gas flow rate, the type of breathing circuit, and the volume of the breathing circuit. For this reason, vaporizer setting adjustments must be anticipated as much as possible through close monitoring. In general, if a patient's anesthetic depth is significantly light or deep, larger dial changes are warranted, whereas if the patient is slightly too lightly or deeply anesthetized, more subtle changes are needed. The anesthetist will develop a "feel" for the exact amount to change the dial setting in any given circumstance through experience (Figure 8-5).

## Intravenous Induction and Maintenance with an Inhalant Agent

Intravenous induction and maintenance with an inhalant agent is the most commonly used method of inducing and maintaining general anesthesia in small animal patients. It has dynamic elements of both IV and inhalant administration, as illustrated in Figure 8-6, including rapid induction, good control over both increases and decreases in anesthetic depth, and a relatively rapid recovery. The sequence of events associated with this technique is summarized in Procedure 8-2, p. 258.

*TECHNICIAN NOTE* With inhalant agents, if a patient is significantly lightly or deeply anesthetized, larger dial changes are warranted, whereas if the patient's anesthetic depth is slightly too light or deep, more subtle changes are needed.

## EQUIPMENT PREPARATION

During a typical anesthetic induction, many events occur in rapid succession. Anesthetic agents are administered; the patient becomes unconscious and recumbent; the endotracheal tube is placed, secured, cuffed, and attached to the machine; the anesthetic vaporizer is turned on; the patient is positioned and monitored; and adjustments are made as needed, all within the first few minutes. Because these events follow one another so rapidly, the technician does not have the luxury of leaving the patient to locate equipment. For this reason, all equipment must be carefully gathered, checked, and organized before commencement of the procedure.

Unless IM or total IV techniques are used, most small animal patients are anesthetized by means of a small animal anesthesia machine configured as a semiclosed

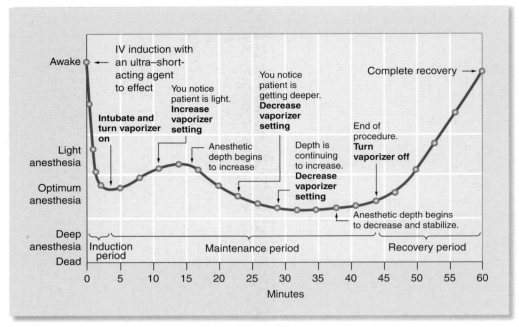

**FIGURE 8-6**  Intravenous (IV) induction and maintenance with an inhalant agent. This method has features of induction with an IV injection of an ultra–short-acting agent to effect and induction and maintenance with an inhalant agent. Anesthetic induction is very rapid, and the dynamics of maintenance are identical to those shown in Figure 8-5.

rebreathing system. Patients weighing less than 2.5 to 3 kg require a non-rebreathing circuit. Equipment required to intubate the patient, give injections, and administer fluids is also required—as is, especially if surgery will be performed, equipment designed to prevent hypothermia. A crash cart containing emergency equipment and drugs should also always be available.

> **TECHNICIAN NOTE**  Most small animal patients weighing more than 2.5 to 3 kg are anesthetized by means of a small animal anesthesia machine configured as a semiclosed rebreathing system. Patients weighing less than 2.5 to 3 kg require a non-rebreathing circuit.

## PREMEDICATION OR SEDATION

*Premedication* refers to the administration of anesthetic agents and adjuncts to calm and prepare the patient for anesthetic induction. Preanesthetic medications are chosen specifically to produce a set of desired effects such as sedation, cholinergic blockade, analgesia, and muscle relaxation. Tranquilizers, alpha$_2$-agonists, opioids, dissociatives, and anticholinergics are commonly used as preanesthetic medications and are most often given intramuscularly. See Protocols 8-1 and 8-2 for preanesthetic and sedative protocols in dogs and cats.

After IM injection of preanesthetic medications, the patient should be placed in a location that is quiet, but also one that permits close observation until the agent takes effect (for many drugs given intramuscularly, about

15 to 20 minutes). If the patient is excited or stimulated during this time, the beneficial effects of the drugs may be diminished. Especially if the patient is heavily sedated, observation every few minutes is paramount to permit prompt intervention in the event that the patient experiences complications. Once the patient is adequately sedated, anesthetic induction should immediately follow, or, as an alternative, these protocols can be used alone to provide sedation for diagnostic and therapeutic procedures.

> **TECHNICIAN NOTE**  After IM injection of preanesthetic medications, the patient should be placed in a location that is quiet, but also one that permits close observation until the agent takes effect (for many drugs given intramuscularly, about 15 to 20 minutes).

## ANESTHETIC INDUCTION

Anesthetic induction is the process by which an animal loses consciousness and enters surgical anesthesia. The goal of anesthetic induction is to take the patient from consciousness to stage III anesthesia smoothly and rapidly, so that an endotracheal tube can be placed. During any induction the patient passes through the excitement stage and therefore may show signs of uncoordination or struggling, followed by progressive relaxation and unconsciousness. Excitement and struggling during induction hamper restraint, increase the risk of unadvertent perivascular drug injection, and predispose the patient to traumatic injury, vomiting, cardiac arrhythmias, and other

**PROTOCOL 8-1** | **Premedication and Sedative Protocols for Physical Status Class (PSC) P1 and P2 Dogs**

**Protocols for Premedication or Light-Moderate Sedation**

1. **IM acepromazine:** Acepromazine 0.05 to 0.1 mg/kg IM with a maximum dose of 3 mg *(Not for use in old or debilitated patients, or in sensitive breeds.)*
2. **IM dexmedetomidine (microdose):** Dexmedetomidine 0.0015 to 0.003 mg/kg IM *(Equivalent to 1.5 to 3 mcg/kg.)*
3. **IM midazolam-butorphanol:** Midazolam 0.2 mg/kg and butorphanol 0.2 mg/kg IM *(Can add glycopyrrolate 0.01 mg/kg or atropine 0.04 mg/kg to this mixture. Halve the doses for IV administration. Can use hydromorphone 0.1 mg/kg in place of butorphanol.)*
4. **IM/IV hydromorphone:** Hydromorphone 0.05 to 0.1 mg/kg IM or IV

**Protocols for Premedication or Moderate-Deep Sedation (for Minor Procedures such as Radiography or Grooming)**

1. **IM or IV "BAG":** Butorphanol 0.2 mg/kg, acepromazine 0.05 mg/kg, and glycopyrrolate 0.005 mg/kg mixed in one syringe and given intramuscularly or intravenously *(As an alternative, mix 1 mL acepromazine, 4 mL butorphanol [10 mg/mL], and 5 mL glycopyrrolate, and give this mixture at a volume of 0.5 mL/10 to 20 lb of body weight.)*
2. **IM or IV "Super BAG":** Buprenorphine 0.01 mg/kg, acepromazine 0.05 mg/kg, and glycopyrrolate 0.005 mg/kg mixed in one syringe and given via IM or IV route
3. **IM dexmedetomidine-butorphanol:** Dexmedetomidine 0.005 to 0.01 mg/kg and butorphanol 0.2 to 0.4 mg/kg IM *(Can use hydromorphone 0.1 mg/kg in place of butorphanol.)*
4. **IM dexmedetomidine-ketamine:** Dexmedetomidine 0.015 mg/kg and ketamine 3 mg/kg IM *(Halve the doses for IV administration. Do not reverse the dexmedetomidine until at least 40 minutes later.)*
5. **IM or IV Telazol:** Telazol 4 mg/kg IM or IV to effect (for aggressive patients). This combination may cause light general anesthesia.

**PROTOCOL 8-2** | **Premedication and Sedative Protocols for PSC P1 and P2 Cats**

**Protocols for Premedication or Light-Moderate Sedation**

1. **IM acepromazine:** Acepromazine 0.05 to 0.1 mg/kg IM up to a maximum dose of 1 mg
2. **IM or IV "BAG":** *(Same dose as for the dog.)*
3. **IM dexmedetomidine:** Dexmedetomidine 0.005 to 0.02 mg/kg IM
4. **IM/IV hydromorphone:** Hydromorphone 0.05 to 0.1 mg/kg IM or IV

**Protocols for Premedication or Moderate-Deep Sedation (for Minor Procedures Such as Radiography or Grooming)**

1. **IM acepromazine-hydromorphone:** Acepromazine 0.2 mg/kg and hydromorphone 0.05 to 0.1 mg/kg IM
2. **IM dexmedetomidine-ketamine:** Dexmedetomidine 0.005 to 0.025 mg/kg and ketamine 5 mg/kg IM
3. **IM dexmedetomidine-butorphanol:** Dexmedetomidine 0.005 to 0.01 mg/kg and butorphanol 0.2 mg/kg IM *(Can use hydromorphone 0.1 mg/kg in place of butorphanol.)*
4. **IM "kitty magic" (ketamine-butorphanol-dexmedetomidine):** Ketamine 2.2 mg/kg, butorphanol 0.22 mg/kg, and dexmedetomidine 0.011 mg/kg mixed in the same syringe. This equates to 0.1 mL of each drug for an average sized (4.5 kg) cat.
5. **IM ketamine:** Ketamine 10 to 20 mg/kg IM *(Causes immobilization with muscle rigidity)*
6. **IM or IV Telazol:** Telazol 4 mg/kg IM or IV to effect *(For aggressive patients)*
7. **IM ketamine-acepromazine:** Ketamine 10 to 20 mg/kg and acepromazine 0.02 to 0.1 mg/kg IM

adverse effects, and so should be minimized through administration of preanesthetic medications.

> **TECHNICIAN NOTE** During anesthetic induction the patient should be sufficiently anesthetized to permit intubation, but anesthesia should generally be kept light until the tube is placed.

During induction, the patient should be sufficiently anesthetized to permit intubation, but anesthesia should generally be kept light until the tube is placed. At this point the anesthetic depth can be adjusted as needed.

Induction is most commonly accomplished by IV administration of injectable agents or by administration of inhalant agents via a mask or chamber. IM administration of drugs is a third method, which, although less common in general practice, is frequently used in animal shelters to induce and maintain anesthesia in patients undergoing routine procedures such as spays and castrations. Of these techniques, IV induction has the advantage of producing unconsciousness within seconds to a few minutes at most. Therefore most animals that undergo induction by this method pass through the excitement stage quickly, allowing rapid control of the airway. In contrast, mask or chamber induction typically

---

**PROTOCOL 8-3** | **Intravenous Induction Protocols for PSC P1 and P2 Dogs and Cats**

1. **IV ketamine/diazepam:** Ketamine 5.5 mg/kg IV and diazepam 0.28 mg/kg IV mixed in the same syringe. *(Equivalent to 1 mL of the mixture per 20 lb of body weight.)* An equivalent volume of midazolam can be substituted for diazepam. Butorphanol 0.1 to 0.2 mg/kg or hydromorphone 0.1 mg/kg can be given IV before induction, in a separate syringe, for additional analgesia.
2. **IV propofol:** Propofol 6 to 8 mg/kg IV to effect if not premedicated or 2 to 4 mg/kg IV after premedication
3. **IV diazepam/hydromorphone (This protocol is intended for older or depressed patients):** Diazepam 0.2 mg/kg (maximum dose of 5 mg) IV alternating with hydromorphone 0.1 mg/kg IV. *Use separate syringes.* Administer boluses of each agent alternately until the patient can be intubated. May need more to allow intubation.
   *(Midazolam may be substituted for diazepam at the same dose; fentanyl at 2 mcg/kg may be substituted for hydromorphone.)*
4. **IV thiopental sodium ± lidocaine:** Thiopental sodium 4 to 8 mg/kg IV to effect after premedication or 10 to 15 mg/kg IV if not premedicated *(Administration without premedication is not recommended.)*
   Lidocaine can be given to dogs at 2 to 4 mg/kg IV before the thiopental. This combination decreases cardiovascular depression and protects against arrhythmias.
5. **IV etomidate:** Etomidate 1 to 3 mg/kg IV to effect
6. **IV methohexital:** Methohexital 5 mg/kg IV to effect after premedication or 11 mg/kg IV if not premedicated *(administration without premedication is not recommended).*

**Additional Intravenous Induction Protocol for Use Only in PSC P1 and P2 Cats**

IV "kitty magic" (ketamine/butorphanol/dexmedetomidine): Ketamine 1.1 to 2.2 mg/kg, butorphanol 0.11 to 0.22 mg/kg, and dexmedetomidine 0.005 to 0.011 mg/kg IV mixed in the same syringe. This equates to 0.05 to 0.1 mL of each drug for an average sized (4.5-kg) cat.

---

takes at least 5 to 10 minutes, increasing the likelihood of undesirable effects. Induction after IM injection typically takes about 10 to 20 minutes but results in smooth, gradual CNS depression with little apparent excitement. What follows is a description of specific techniques used to induce anesthesia.

### Intravenous Induction

Agents commonly used to induce general anesthesia in dogs and cats by IV injection include (1) a mixture of equal volumes of ketamine and diazepam or midazolam, (2) propofol, (3) neuroleptanalgesics, (4) thiopental sodium, (5) etomidate, and (6) various other combinations containing dissociatives, tranquilizers, and opioids. Protocol 8-3 shows IV induction protocols in dogs and cats.

To induce general anesthesia by the IV route, a volume of the agent to be administered is calculated based on a prescribed dose and drawn into a syringe. The agent is then injected directly into the vein, or into a winged-infusion set or indwelling catheter *to effect* until the patient can be intubated or until the patient is at an adequate plane of anesthesia for completion of the planned procedure.

The term "to effect" means that only the amount of injectable anesthetic necessary to produce unconsciousness is given, rather than administering the entire dose calculated on a milligram per kilogram basis. This technique is necessary because the amount of drug needed to induce or maintain anesthesia cannot be accurately predicted for a given patient, and most anesthetic agents have narrow therapeutic indices.

For example, the amount of thiopental sodium required to induce anesthesia in a quiet, older dog may be one quarter to one half of the dose required for an active, young dog of equivalent body weight. Similarly, a cat with

a urinary obstruction may be deeply anesthetized after receiving a very small dose of ketamine, whereas a healthy cat may require several times more to reach an equivalent depth. The drugs used for premedication also affect the dose of general anesthetic required. For example, a patient that has not received any premedications may require two or three times as much as a patient that has been premedicated with a neuroleptanalgesic combination to reach a comparable plane of anesthesia.

For these reasons, IV drugs are given as a series of bolus injections and discontinued when the desired depth is reached—a process known as **titration.** A competent anesthetist monitors the patient closely and alters the amount of anesthetic given to suit the patient's requirements, rather than relying solely on a calculated dose. (See Procedure 8-3, p. 259, for IV induction techniques in dogs and cats.)

After induction with the commonly used IV injectable agents, the duration of anesthesia varies but is usually no more than 10 to 20 minutes. If more than 20 minutes is required, anesthesia is maintained with inhalation anesthetics or administration of propofol, methohexital, or etomidate by repeat boluses or CRI. This is not recommended with other injectable agents such as thiopental sodium, because if such drugs are given this way, large amounts of anesthetic will accumulate in the body and prolong recovery.

### Inhalation Agents

Inhalation agents commonly used to induce general anesthesia in dogs and cats include isoflurane and sevoflurane. These agents are administered by means of a facemask or anesthetic chamber. Protocol 8-4 shows inhalant induction protocols in dogs and cats.

---

**PROTOCOL 8-4** | **Inhalant Induction Protocols for PSC P1 and P2 Dogs and Cats**

1. **Isoflurane:** Administer isoflurane at 3% to 5% by mask or chamber.
2. **Sevoflurane:** Administer sevoflurane at 4% to 6% by mask or chamber.
*(Patients should receive rates in the lower end of these ranges if preanesthetic medications have been administered.)*

---

## Mask Induction

Mask induction involves administration of an inhalant anesthetic such as isoflurane or sevoflurane via a facemask. This method of induction is feasible only with use of inhalation anesthetics with a low blood-gas solubility coefficient, such as isoflurane or sevoflurane, because the rapid induction time associated with these agents results in passage through stage II anesthesia quickly enough to minimize excitement. In contrast, mask induction is difficult and, in some cases, not possible with agents with a higher solubility coefficient because of the prolonged length of time required to reach stage III anesthesia. For some patients in critical condition, induction by mask may be safer than induction with injectable agents because the anesthetist can decrease anesthetic depth or discontinue the agent by adjusting the vaporizer setting if problems arise.

> **TECHNICIAN NOTE** Successful mask induction requires skillful restraint (enough to prevent operator and patient injury, but not so much as to restrict chest excursions or the airway). Mucous membrane color and refill time as well as ocular indicators of anesthetic depth are not easily observed, although monitoring requirements are no different with this method of induction.

Mask induction is challenging for several reasons. Many patients struggle, necessitating skillful restraint (enough to prevent operator and patient injury, but not so much as to restrict chest excursions or the airway). The fear associated with passage through stage I and the excitement associated with passage through stage II cause release of epinephrine and other catecholamines, which can predispose the patient to cardiac arrhythmias, hypotension, and other adverse effects. Also, mucous membrane color and refill time as well as ocular indicators of anesthetic depth are not as easily observed because the mask partially obscures the eyes and muzzle, although monitoring requirements are no different with this method of induction.

The mask should be carefully fitted before commencement of mask induction. There should be a reasonably tight seal between the muzzle and the rubber gasket without constriction of the tissues or discomfort. The mask should be long enough to accommodate the full length of the muzzle (so that the nares do not press against the end of the mask when the muzzle is fully inserted), but not too long. Be aware that relatively higher oxygen flow rates are required than when an endotracheal tube is used. The technique for mask induction is described and illustrated in Procedure 8-4, p. 259.

There are several cautions associated with mask induction with which the anesthetist must be aware:
- Mask induction may result in significant exposure of personnel to waste anesthetic gas, because no matter how well the mask is fitted, some leakage is inevitable. Therefore adequate room ventilation is necessary to prevent excess inhalation of waste gas (see Chapter 13).
- If the animal resists mask induction, struggling may cause the release of epinephrine, which predisposes the patient to potentially fatal cardiac arrhythmias and hypotension. To avoid this, induce anesthesia in only calm or sedated patients by mask.
- Because of the longer induction time compared with IV administration, mask induction is not appropriate for patients with poor respiratory function (e.g., upper airway disease or obstruction, difficult breathing because of brachycephalic conformation, diaphragmatic hernia, pleural effusion, or pulmonary edema), unfasted patients, or patients at risk for vomiting during induction. These patients must be intubated immediately to prevent serious adverse effects and permit rapid control of the airway and ventilatory support.
- The anesthetist must ensure that the airway is kept open at all times during mask induction. The mask must not occlude the patient's nostrils, as might happen with a cat or brachycephalic patient if the mask is too small or tight. The anesthetist must not compress the airway or chest during restraint.

Although a mask can be used to maintain anesthesia, the anesthetist is not able to protect the airway, prevent aspiration, provide ventilatory support, or observe respirations as readily as when a tube is present. For these reasons, most anesthetists intubate the patient immediately after induction.

## Chamber Induction

Chamber induction involves placing the patient in a closed chamber infused with anesthetic gas. This technique is feasible only for patients small enough to fit comfortably into a chamber (typically weighing less than 5 to 7 kg) and is therefore primarily used for small patients that are aggressive or difficult to handle.

> **TECHNICIAN NOTE** During chamber induction, it is impossible to accurately assess most monitoring parameters. Thus, the anesthetist must be vigilant and prepared to act quickly if the patient shows signs of compromise.

Most chambers are small clear boxes that resemble a 5-gallon aquarium (see Figure 4-6). The chamber should be examined before induction. A tight-fitting lid and two ports (one for entry of fresh gas and another for exit of excess gas) are required. Although there is more than one way to supply oxygen and anesthetic gases to a chamber, a common way is to remove the Y-piece from the corrugated breathing tubes of a semiclosed rebreathing system and attach the inspiratory tube to one chamber port and the expiratory tube to the other port. Place the patient in the chamber, close the lid, and proceed, following the instructions summarized in Procedure 8-5, p. 260, and illustrated in Figure 4-6.

Anesthetic chambers allow the induction of anesthesia in even the most uncooperative animal but are associated with complications from stress, trauma, vomiting, airway blockage, and other issues:

- Because it is impossible to accurately assess most monitoring parameters while the patient is inside a chamber, the anesthetist must be vigilant and prepared to act quickly if the patient shows signs of compromise.
- As with mask induction, there is some risk of regurgitation or vomiting, especially in the nonfasted patient. Because the airway is unprotected, aspiration of stomach contents may occur.
- There is considerable risk of exposure of hospital personnel to waste anesthetic gas, particularly when removing the patient from the chamber. The chamber must be equipped with a scavenger, and ideally the anesthetic gas should be evacuated before the chamber is opened so that waste gas exposure can be avoided. This is often not possible in a clinical setting, however, because of the need to remove the patient quickly.
- As with induction by mask, epinephrine release will predispose the patient to cardiac arrhythmias and hypotension.
- As with mask induction, chamber induction is not appropriate for patients in which rapid control of the airway is required.

## Intramuscular Induction

Agents commonly used to induce general anesthesia in dogs and cats by IM injection include neuroleptanalgesic combinations and a variety of combinations of tranquilizers, dissociatives, and opioids. IM induction is useful for animals in which IV injections are difficult, such as ferrets and very young puppies and kittens. IM induction using restraint equipment such as a squeeze cage or rabies pole is necessary to induce anesthesia in extremely aggressive domestic animals. IM induction is also standard in animals that are difficult to approach or impossible to handle or in which IV or mask induction not feasible (e.g., wild animals and captive animals in zoos). In these animals, dissociative-tranquilizer mixtures, neuroleptanalgesics,

or opioids (particularly etorphine and carfentanil) are usually administered by means of a blowpipe or tranquilizing gun.

Induction by IM injection differs from IV induction in several important respects.

- IM injections cannot be titrated or given "to effect." Usually the entire calculated dose is given at once.
- In general, the dose for IM injection is about twice the corresponding IV dose.
- Drugs administered by the IM route require more time to reach a high enough concentration in the brain to induce anesthesia. IM induction is therefore characterized by a relatively slow onset of anesthesia compared with IV induction (typically 10 to 20 minutes). Occasionally, if drugs are deposited in a fascial plane between muscles, or in subcutaneous (SC) tissue, slow or incomplete absorption may result in an even longer induction or a blunted effect.
- After peak effect, if the patient's depth of anesthesia is still inadequate, additional drug must be given or an inhalant agent must be administered with a mask until the patient can be intubated. (Remember that some drugs such as propofol, thiopental sodium, and etomidate *must not* be given intramuscularly.)
- IM induction is characterized by a lengthy recovery period because the animal requires considerable time to metabolize the relatively large dose of drug given by this route.

The differences between IM and IV administration are illustrated by the use of ketamine in cats. When ketamine is given intravenously at a dose of 5 mg/kg, induction of anesthesia occurs in less than 1 minute. Alternatively, the drug can be given intramuscularly at a dose of 15 mg/kg, inducing anesthesia in 5 to 10 minutes. Recovery from IV ketamine administration usually begins in 10 to 15 minutes, and healthy animals often appear fully recovered within 1 to 2 hours. In contrast, complete recovery from IM ketamine administration may require several hours.

## Oral Administration

Oral administration of certain anesthetics (most notably ketamine) is occasionally used in circumstances in which injection is dangerous or difficult, such as induction of anesthesia in feral cats. With an open-ended tom-cat urethral catheter and syringe, the drug is forcefully squirted into the animal's mouth from a distance when the patient opens its mouth to hiss or vocalize. When this route is used, care must be taken to avoid pulmonary aspiration or contact with the eyes. Alternatively, the agent can be mixed with a small amount of palatable food. Because ketamine is not labeled for oral use, administration by this route constitutes extra-label use.

Other routes of administration for injectable agents include the SC, rectal, and intraperitoneal routes. For dogs and cats, these routes are too slow or impractical for routine use.

## ENDOTRACHEAL INTUBATION

After induction of general anesthesia, an endotracheal tube is usually placed in the patient's airway. This tube conducts air or anesthetic gases directly from the oral cavity to the trachea, bypassing the nasal passages and pharynx (Figure 8-7). Placement of an endotracheal tube is especially beneficial for maintaining anesthesia with inhalant anesthetics, but also offers several key advantages even when anesthesia is maintained with injectable protocols.

- When properly maintained, an endotracheal tube helps to maintain an open airway, decreasing the likelihood of airway obstruction caused by patient position, collapse of pharyngeal tissues, foreign material, or any other cause. Because of the importance of maintaining a patent airway, it is customary to leave the tube in place throughout anesthesia and into the recovery period, until the animal regains the swallowing reflex.
- Intubation allows more efficient delivery of anesthetic gas to the animal than does a mask. Because gas flow rates can be lowered, intubation results in reduced exposure of hospital personnel to waste anesthetic gas and increased economy.
- Use of an endotracheal tube with an inflated cuff reduces the risk of aspiration of vomitus, blood, saliva, or other material that may be present in the oral cavity or breathing passages. This material may accumulate during any procedure; however, the risk of aspiration is particularly high during oral surgery or dentistry and in patients that have not been fasted.
- An endotracheal tube of the correct diameter and length will improve efficiency of gas exchange by reducing the amount of **anatomic dead space.** Anatomic dead space is composed of the portions of the breathing passages that contain air but in which no gas exchange can occur (i.e., the mouth, nasal passages, pharynx, trachea, and bronchi). With the anatomic dead space minimized, the endotracheal

tube ensures that a larger proportion of the gas delivered to the patient reaches the exchange surface in the alveoli.

- The anesthetist can support ventilation in intubated patients by manual or mechanical means. *Manual ventilation* refers to forced delivery of oxygen and anesthetic gases by squeezing the reservoir bag of the anesthetic machine. *Mechanical ventilation* refers to use of a mechanical ventilator to achieve the same result. Manual and mechanical ventilation are discussed in detail in Chapter 6. Because of the respiratory depression associated with anesthesia, periodic manual or mechanical ventilation is necessary in most anesthetized patients to ensure adequate gas exchange. Intermittent mandatory manual or mechanical ventilation is required in patients that have been given neuromuscular blocking agents or in which the thoracic cavity is open.
- Endotracheal intubation followed by manual or mechanical ventilation is also essential for patients in respiratory or cardiac arrest. For this reason it is advisable to have a laryngoscope and an endotracheal tube of correct size readily available for all anesthetized patients, even if endotracheal intubation is not planned.

### Equipment for Endotracheal Intubation

The following equipment is required to perform endotracheal intubation (Figure 8-8):
- Appropriately sized endotracheal tubes (at least three of slightly different diameters)
- A 2-foot length of IV tubing or rolled gauze to secure the tube
- A gauze sponge to grasp the tongue
- A 12-mL syringe to inflate the cuff
- A good examination light

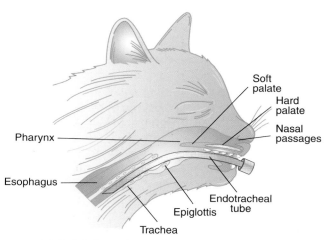

FIGURE 8-7 Intubation of the cat, showing anatomy.

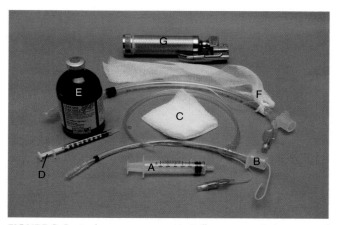

FIGURE 8-8 Intubation equipment. *A*, Cuffing syringe; *B*, 4-mm internal diameter (ID), polyvinyl chloride (PVC) endotracheal tube (ETT) with stylette and intravenous (IV) tubing tie; *C*, 3 × 3 gauze sponge; *D*, 1-mL syringe containing 0.1 mL of injectable lidocaine; *E*, 2% lidocaine injectable solution; *F*, 8-mm ID PVC ETT with gauze tie; *G*, laryngoscope (optional).

- A stylette if using a narrow-diameter tube (this is most important for cats) or any other tube that requires additional support
- Lidocaine injectable solution or lidocaine gel to control **laryngospasm** (in cats only)
- A laryngoscope with an appropriately sized blade if desired

> **TECHNICIAN NOTE** When preparing for endotracheal intubation, select at least three tubes of slightly different diameters so that you are prepared if your first choice does not fit. Ideally the endotracheal tube should extend from the tip of the nose to the thoracic inlet.

## Selecting an Endotracheal Tube

Endotracheal tubes are available in a wide variety of diameters and lengths. The tube must be of a diameter that is small enough to allow placement without causing trauma to the trachea, but large enough to produce a seal when the cuff is inflated. It must be of sufficient length to reach the thoracic inlet when fully inserted, but must not be so long as to reach the main stem bronchi or to extend beyond the end of the muzzle when inserted the correct distance.

At least three tubes of slightly different diameters should be selected so that you are prepared if your first choice does not fit. The size required by any given patient is influenced by patient species, conformation, and breed. For instance, cats require smaller-diameter tubes than dogs of comparable body weight. Most brachycephalic breeds require a tube several sizes smaller than mesocephalic or dolichocephalic breeds. An obese patient will require a smaller tube, and an emaciated patient will require a larger tube than a patient of normal conformation that weighs the same.

In view of these variances, the following guidelines can be used to estimate the proper size based on patient body weight. Most cats require a 3- to 4.5-mm tube. A dog weighing 20 kg will require a 9.5- to 10-mm tube. Increase or decrease the size approximately 1 mm for each 5 kg of body weight under or over 20 kg. For example, prepare a 7.5- to 8-mm tube for a 10-kg patient, and a 10.5- to 11-mm tube for a 25-kg patient. This guideline applies to canine patients weighing about 10 to 40 kg. (See Table 8-1 for size recommendations.)

Next determine if the tube is the appropriate length. The endotracheal tube should ideally extend from the tip of the nose to the thoracic inlet. If it is too short, it may not be long enough to reach the trachea at all. If the tube is too long, one of two problems may occur. If inserted too far, the beveled end may advance into only one main stem bronchus, thus supplying only one lung with oxygen and anesthetic. If inserted only to the thoracic inlet, the portion of the tube extending from the mouth will increase **mechanical dead space** (Figure 8-9). Either situation predisposes the patient to hypoventilation and hypoxemia. If a tube of the appropriate length is unavailable, the machine end of the tube can be trimmed, with care being taken to avoid cutting into the cuff inflation apparatus. Endotracheal tubes are further discussed in Chapter 4.

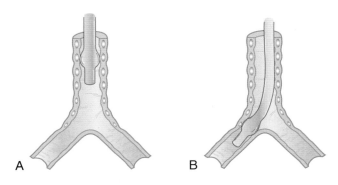

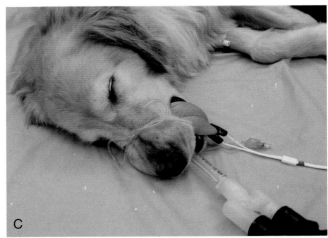

**FIGURE 8-9** **A,** Endotracheal tube placed the correct distance in the trachea. **B,** Endotracheal tube advanced too far into the trachea. **C,** Endotracheal tube extending beyond the nasal planum, which increases mechanical dead space.

| TABLE 8-1 | **Recommended Endotracheal Tube Sizes** |
|---|---|
| Species and Body Weight (kg) | Tube Size (Internal Diameter [mm]) |
| Cat | |
| 1 | 2.5-3 |
| 2-4 | 3.5-4 |
| 5 or greater | 4.5-5 |
| Dog | |
| 2 | 5 |
| 4 | 5.5-6 |
| 7 | 6.5-7 |
| 10 | 7.5-8 |
| 15 | 8.5-9 |
| 20 | 9.5-10 |
| 25 | 10.5-11 |
| 30 | 11.5-12 |
| 40 | 13-14 |

## Preparing the Tube

Before an endotracheal tube is used, it must be checked for integrity. It should be clean, sanitized, and free of blockages, holes, deterioration, or other damage. The connector must be securely attached, and the cuff must inflate and hold pressure after the syringe is detached from the valve. A soft or narrow tube may require use of a stylette, which does *not* extend beyond the end of the tube, to stiffen it during placement. The tube should be lubricated with a small amount of sterile water-soluble lubricant or with the patient's saliva immediately before placement.

## Intubation Procedure

Successful endotracheal tube placement requires knowledge of the anatomy of the pharynx and larynx including the glottis, epiglottis, vocal folds, and soft palate. (See Figure 8-10 for a review of the anatomy.) Careful restraint, positioning, and lighting are necessary to maximize visibility of the larynx. Very subtle differences in these factors can make the difference between success and failure. This is especially true in cats. If you cannot easily see the larynx, insist that your assistant alter the patient position, the way the head is held, or the lighting until you can. A failure to do this frequently results in delay, frustration, and failure to successfully intubate the patient. A little time spent optimizing these factors is well worth the effort.

Endotracheal intubation is performed essentially the same way in both dogs and cats, although it is typically more challenging in cats owing to the smaller size of the larynx, decreased visibility, and the predisposition to laryngospasm typical of feline patients.

> **TECHNICIAN NOTE** Readiness for endotracheal intubation is characterized by unconsciousness, a lack of voluntary movement, an absent pedal reflex, sufficient muscle relaxation to allow the mouth to be held open, and no swallowing when the tongue is grasped.

First prepare the necessary equipment, and prepare the patient for anesthetic induction. Induce anesthesia by IV injection, mask, or chamber until the patient is in a state of readiness for intubation. This requires administration of anesthetic, combined with careful monitoring, until the patient passes through stage II. Readiness for intubation is characterized by unconsciousness, a lack of voluntary movement, an absent pedal reflex, sufficient muscle relaxation to allow the mouth to be held open, and no swallowing when the tongue is grasped. As soon as the patient reaches this point, proceed with intubation as described in Procedure 8-6, p. 260.

In most cases intubation must be performed rapidly and efficiently, because the window for successful intubation is short (typically 1 to 2 minutes with injectable protocols and often less than a minute with inhalation protocols). Immediately after intubation, place the patient in lateral recumbency, secure and cuff the tube, turn on

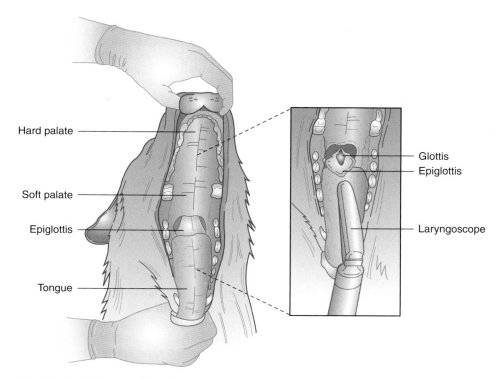

Hard palate

Soft palate

Epiglottis

Tongue

Glottis
Epiglottis

Laryngoscope

**FIGURE 8-10** Anatomy of the pharynx. When the epiglottis is depressed, the glottis is exposed. The endotracheal tube is then advanced through the glottis.

the oxygen, attach the breathing circuit, turn on the anesthetic vaporizer, and immediately start monitoring.

With typical protocols (assuming the patient has not been overdosed), many patients are in a light plane of stage III anesthesia after intubation, although the stage and plane vary case to case. If the patient is in a light plane (as characterized by one or two forceful exhalations immediately after placement, strong jaw tone, present palpebral reflex, and in some cases spontaneous movement, swallowing, or chewing), use high oxygen flow, and keep the inhalant anesthetic agent on induction level (3% to 5% isoflurane or 4% to 6% sevoflurane), until the patient begins to enter a deeper plane. Then immediately decrease the vaporizer setting to a safe level while continuing to monitor. Adjustments are then made in response to monitoring parameters. As soon as the patient's condition is stable, attach any mechanical monitoring devices and prepare the patient for the procedure. Details of the intubation procedure are given and illustrated in Procedure 8-6, p.

### Checking for Proper Placement

The entrance to the esophagus lies just dorsal to the entrance to the trachea, and although difficult to see, easily accommodates the endotracheal tube. Inadvertent misplacement in the esophagus is common and sometimes not detected, because air may appear to move in and out of the tube and reservoir bag even if the tube is not in the trachea. This will result in an inability to keep the patient anesthetized, and possible airway blockage and hypoxemia. The following techniques may be used to confirm proper placement in the trachea:

- Revisualize the larynx, and confirm that the tube is in the correct location.
- Watch for expansion and contraction of the reservoir bag as the animal breathes.
- Feel for air movement from the tube connector as the patient exhales or when light, quick pressure is applied to the chest wall.
- Watch for fogging of the tube with condensation during exhalation.
- Check that the motion of the unidirectional valves coincides with breathing. The inhalation valve should open as the patient inhales, and the exhalation valve should open when the patient exhales.
- Palpate the neck. The trachea is the only naturally firm structure in the neck. If the tube is inside the trachea, only the trachea will be palpable. If the tube is in the esophagus, both the tube and trachea may be palpable. It is not always easy to feel the tube, however, so mastery of this technique requires practice.
- The ability of the patient to vocalize (growl, whine, or cry) indicates a misplaced tube. This is because vocalization requires the vocal cords to vibrate together, which is impossible if the tube is properly placed.

- Many patients, especially if in a light plane of anesthesia, will cough or exhale forcefully during intubation. This is indicative of proper placement, although not all patients exhibit this sign, especially if anesthesia is deep.
- Connecting a capnograph to the endotracheal tube will reveal an appropriate waveform and level of end-tidal $CO_2$ if the animal is correctly intubated.

### Securing the Tube

The tube is secured in place with a 2-foot-long piece of rolled gauze or IV tubing. Tie the gauze around the tube near the connector using a surgeon's knot, or IV tubing around the tube using a Lark's head knot. Do not place the tie around the small tube supplying the pilot balloon. Be sure that the tie is secure enough that it does not slide up or down the tube, but not so tight that it compresses the tube. Then tie the loose ends over the nose for dolichocephalic dogs or behind the head for cats and brachycephalic dogs. When properly secured, the tube should not move in or out when manipulated (Figure 8-11).

### Cuff Inflation

Immediately after successful intubation, the cuff of the endotracheal tube must be gently inflated until a seal is formed between the trachea and the cuff. "Cuffing" prevents leakage of anesthetic gases and inhalation of room air, which will result in a variety of complications including contamination of the surgery suite with waste gases and difficulty keeping the patient anesthetized. To inflate the cuff, first extend the patient's head to straighten the airway. Attach an air-filled 12-mL syringe to the valve port. Have an assistant close the pop-off valve and gently compress the reservoir bag, watching the pressure manometer. Listen for gas leakage around the tube, which may sound like a soft hiss or gurgling. Slowly inflate the cuff until the leaking just ceases at a pressure of 20 cm $H_2O$ but resumes at higher pressures. Avoid overinflation of the cuff, which can result in a variety of mild to serious complications. Inflation should be checked again after 15 or 30 minutes of anesthesia, because tracheal diameter may increase as a result of muscle relaxation, or a slow, undetected leak in the cuff or pilot line may cause the cuff to deflate.

Sometimes the anesthetist may see or hear recommendations that suggest use of a specific volume of air to inflate the cuff. These recommendations are not valid and in fact are potentially dangerous, because the volume necessary to seal the cuff depends on the relationship among the external diameter of the tube, the internal diameter of the trachea, and the size and type of the cuff and is thus somewhat different for every patient and anesthetic procedure.

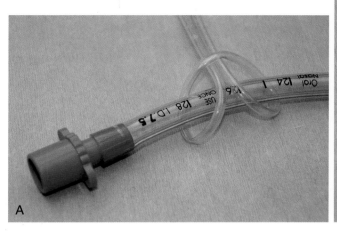
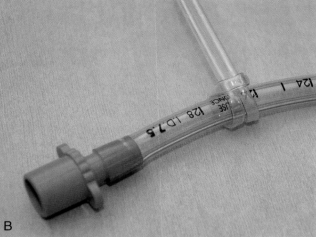
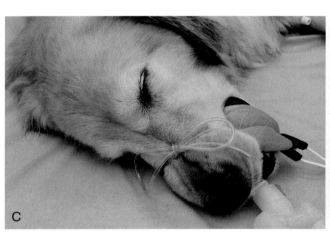
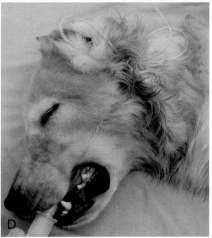

**FIGURE 8-11** **A,** Endotracheal tube (ETT) with intravenous (IV) tubing tie showing lark's head knot. **B,** ETT with lark's head knot pulled tight to prevent the tube from slipping. **C,** ETT IV tubing tie firmly secured around the nose of a dolichocephalic animal to prevent movement. **D,** ETT IV tubing tie secured around the back of the head. Used for cats, brachycephalic dogs, and possibly for patients undergoing dental cleanings.

*TECHNICIAN NOTE* Slowly inflate the cuff until the leaking just ceases at a pressure of 20 cm $H_2O$ but resumes at higher pressures. Inflation should be checked again after 15 or 30 minutes of anesthesia, because tracheal diameter may increase as a result of muscle relaxation, or a slow, undetected leak in the cuff or pilot line may cause the cuff to deflate.

*TECHNICIAN NOTE* Particular care should be used when intubating cats, which have a narrow glottis that is easily traumatized. Irritation of the larynx during intubation causes laryngospasm, which can occlude the airway if severe.

## Laryngospasm

Laryngospasm is a reflex closure of the glottis in response to contact with any object or substance. This reflex will cause the glottis to forcibly close during intubation. This complication is most commonly encountered in cats, swine, and small ruminants, especially when in a light plane of anesthesia. It is extremely difficult to place a tube in a patient experiencing laryngospasm because the glottis closes as soon as it is touched with the tube and cannot be forced open without damaging the larynx.

Laryngospasm is frustrating, makes successful intubation difficult, and in extreme cases causes hypoxemia and cyanosis. If the patient becomes cyanotic, immediately release the tongue and administer oxygen by mask. In most cases the cyanosis will quickly resolve. Laryngospasm can be prevented by using one or more of the following strategies.

- Apply no more than 0.1 mL of 2% injectable lidocaine directly to the glottis before placement. Aerosolize it with a 25- to 26-gauge needle, or apply 2 to 4 drops on the arytenoid cartilages with a tomcat catheter attached to a 1-mL syringe. Wait 30 to 60 seconds for the lidocaine to take effect before attempting intubation. As an alternative, a small amount of lidocaine gel can be gently applied with a sterile cotton swab.

- Be sure the patient is adequately anesthetized before attempting to intubate the patient, because increased anesthetic depth decreases the incidence and severity of laryngospasm.

- Prepare carefully, wait for the glottis to open before attempting placement, and try to get the tube in the first time. Repeat attempts worsen laryngospasm.

- *Do not force the tube!* This can lead to severe and potentially life-threatening complications including tracheal rupture, **pneumothorax,** and **pneumomediastinum.**

## Complications of Intubation

A number of hazards are associated with endotracheal intubation (Box 8-4). Most are associated with tracheal irritation, trauma, or failure to protect the airway. Although the larynx and trachea of mammals are relatively resilient structures, excessive force will result in damage, perforation, rupture, or irritation of the delicate mucosa. An endotracheal tube must therefore be chosen, maintained, placed, and monitored with care.

- Intubation may stimulate the vagus nerve and cause an increase in parasympathetic tone, particularly in brachycephalic dogs. This in turn may cause bradycardia, hypotension, and cardiac arrhythmias. Occasionally, cardiac arrest may occur, particularly in an animal with preexisting cardiovascular disease. Anticholinergics given in the preanesthetic period help to prevent parasympathetic stimulation.

- Some animals are difficult to intubate. Brachycephalic dogs, for example, have a large amount of redundant tissue within the oral cavity that falls over the back of the pharynx when the animal's mouth is opened, obscuring the glottis. To compound this challenge, these animals must be intubated quickly after induction to prevent airway collapse, so the anesthetist must use all means to facilitate intubation. A laryngoscope is helpful in these patients to increase visibility of the oropharynx, to gently retract the redundant tissue away from the glottis, and to avoid airway trauma during intubation.

- Overzealous efforts to intubate may damage the larynx, pharynx, or soft palate. Particular care should be used when intubating cats, which have a narrow glottis that is easily traumatized. Irritation of the larynx during intubation causes laryngospasm, which can occlude the airway if severe.

- Overinflation of the cuff may cause pressure necrosis of the tracheal mucosa. Cats are particularly sensitive to pressure necrosis from endotracheal tubes, and it is sometimes recommended that uncuffed tubes or tubes with low-pressure cuffs be used with this species. Some anesthetists suggest that if tubes

---

### BOX 8-4 Complications of Endotracheal Intubation

**Cuff Not Inflated or Underinflated**
- Inability to create a seal between the cuff and trachea
- Difficulty or inability to keep the patient anesthetized
- Aspiration of stomach contents
- Aspiration of foreign material and fluid during dental cleaning
- Pollution of the work space with anesthetic gas

**Tube Diameter Too Small**
- Inability to create a seal between the cuff and trachea, leading to the same complications listed earlier
- Small tubes are more likely to block with mucus
- Increased resistance to breathing with increased respiratory effort

**Cuff Overinflated or Tube Diameter Too Large**
- Necrosis of the tracheal mucosa
- Possibility of tracheal rupture in extreme situations

**Tube Too Long**
- If placed past the thoracic inlet, intubation of only one main stem bronchus, leading to hypoxemia and difficulty in keeping the patient anesthetized
- If extending beyond the mouth, increased mechanical dead space leading to hypoventilation and hypoxemia

**Tube Too Short**
- Inability to intubate the patient successfully
- Changes in patient position may dislodge the tube from glottis

**Overzealous Intubation**
- Tracheal irritation leading to tracheitis and postoperative cough
- Trauma or tracheal rupture resulting in pneumomediastinum and/or pneumothorax

**Tube Kinked or Obstructed**
- Dyspnea and hypoxemia
- Asphyxia and cardiac arrest if not corrected

**Tube Not Removed before Return to Consciousness**
- Damage to the tube from chewing
- Blockage of the airway
- In extreme situations, a severed portion of the tube can be aspirated or swallowed

**Tube Not Cleaned and Disinfected**
- Transmission of infectious agents leading to tracheitis, bronchitis, or pneumonia
- Blockage of the tube with dried mucus or other foreign material

From Bassert JM, McCurnin DM: *McCurnin's clinical textbook for veterinary technicians,* ed 7, St Louis, 2010, Elsevier.

with high-pressure cuffs are used, the cuff should be inflated for no longer than 30 minutes before being deflated and moved slightly to a new location in the trachea. Others suggest that more risk to the patient, through accidental extubation, inadvertent esophageal intubation, or damage to the tracheal mucosa, is caused by moving the tube.

- Endotracheal tubes may become obstructed by saliva, mucus, blood, or foreign material such as gauze. This material may also occlude the patient end of the tube after use, making this a hazard for the next patient if the tube is not cleaned properly. Obstruction may also occur if the tube is kinked or twisted or if the end is occluded against the wall of the trachea. If the endotracheal tube is obstructed for any of these reasons, the patient will not receive oxygen, resulting in hypoxemia.
- Intubated animals require careful monitoring during recovery to ensure that the tube is removed when the animal begins to swallow. If the patient regains consciousness with the tube in place, the patient may chew the tube. In fact, patients can chew the tube in half and aspirate the distal portion into the airway. The presence of such a tracheal foreign body is dangerous, requires bronchoscopy to remove, and is difficult to explain to the owner.
- Although endotracheal tubes used in human patients are routinely discarded after a single use, tubes used in veterinary patients are commonly reused. Tubes must therefore be thoroughly disinfected between patients to prevent the spread of infectious diseases such as infectious tracheobronchitis ("kennel cough"). Keep in mind that red rubber tubes soaked in a disinfectant solution for too long or in a solution that is too concentrated will become impregnated with the disinfectant. When next used, the disinfectant may irritate the tracheal mucosa. This can result in coughing after anesthesia or may even cause the tracheal mucosa to slough.
- Despite all precautions, some intubated patients will develop minor irritation of the trachea and larynx. Animal owners should be warned that it is common for animals to cough for 1 to 2 days after anesthesia if an endotracheal tube is used.

Because of the problems associated with the use of endotracheal tubes and for reasons of convenience, not all animals undergo endotracheal intubation during anesthesia. If an endotracheal tube is not used, the inhalation agent is delivered by mask throughout the procedure. Animals lightly anesthetized with IM or IV agents for the performance of short procedures may not require the use of an endotracheal tube if the animal maintains the ability to swallow throughout the anesthesia and can breathe adequately. There should be no sounds indicating airway obstruction (such as fluid sounds in the airway), and the chest wall should move normally. With these exceptions, intubation is recommended for safety reasons if inhalation anesthetics are used or if a lengthy procedure is performed with the patient under injectable anesthesia.

## MAINTENANCE OF ANESTHESIA

After anesthetic induction and endotracheal intubation, patients that are in a light plane of anesthesia must be brought into surgical anesthesia. When the patient reaches the desired anesthetic depth, general anesthesia is maintained with injectable anesthetics, inhalant anesthetics, or a combination thereof. General anesthesia is most commonly maintained with inhalant agents delivered via an anesthetic machine. Less frequently, anesthesia is maintained with IV boluses every 3 to 5 minutes or a CRI of an ultra–short-acting agent such as propofol, or with IM protocols. See Protocol 8-5 for maintenance protocols in dogs and cats, and Procedure 8-7, p. 262, for details regarding **anesthetic maintenance**.

### Maintenance with an Inhalant Agent

To maintain general anesthesia with an inhalant agent, periodic changes in the vaporizer dial setting must be made based on information derived from physical and machine generated monitoring parameters. Frequent and effective monitoring is paramount, so that subtle changes in anesthetic depth are detected in time to make adjustments before the anesthetic depth becomes seriously too light or deep, thus risking that the patient will move or become aware or will be endangered.

In general, if the anesthetic depth is slightly too light or deep, small dial changes are necessary (about 0.5% to 1% increments with isoflurane and sevoflurane). In contrast, if anesthetic depth is significantly light or deep, large dial changes are necessary. For instance, if the patient's anesthetic depth is significantly light (patient exhibits spontaneous movement, swallowing, active reflexes, strong muscle tone), settings of 3% to 5% isoflurane or 4% to 6% sevoflurane and a high oxygen flow rate are generally necessary to bring the patient back into surgical anesthesia. If the patient's anesthetic depth is significantly too deep (e.g., absent reflexes; flaccid jaw tone; central, dilated pupils), then the vaporizer should be turned off, the oxygen flow increased, and the patient monitored

## PROTOCOL 8-5 | Maintenance Protocols for PSC P1 and P2 Dogs and Cats

1. **Isoflurane:** Administer isoflurane at 1.5% to 2.5%.
2. **Sevoflurane:** Administer sevoflurane at 2.5% to 4%.
3. **IV propofol:** Propofol by repeat boluses to effect every 3 to 5 minutes, or 0.2 to 0.4 mg/kg/minute by constant rate infusion.
4. **Desflurane:** Administer desflurane at 8% to 12%.

| **PROTOCOL 8-6** | **IM Anesthetic Protocols for PSC P1 and P2 Cats** |

1. **IM dexmedetomidine/ketamine/butorphanol:** Dexmedetomidine 0.03 mg/kg with ketamine 5 mg/kg and butorphanol 0.2 mg/kg IM for elective surgeries.
2. **IM "TKX" (Telazol/ketamine/xylazine):** Add 4 mL of ketamine and 1 mL 10% (LA) xylazine to 1 vial of Telazol powder. Give at a dose of 0.015 mL/kg IM. Must dose accurately!
3. **IM "TTDex" (Telazol/butorphanol/dexmedetomidine):** Add 2.5 mL butorphanol (10 mg/mL) and 2.5 mL dexmedetomidine to 1 vial of Telazol powder. Give at a rate of 0.015 mL/kg IM for castration and 0.02 mL/kg IM for ovariohysterectomy.

carefully until signs of decreased depth are evident. Be aware that these are only general guidelines, and each case must be handled differently as the circumstances warrant.

## Maintenance with Repeat Boluses of Propofol or Another Ultra–Short-Acting Agent

As when maintaining anesthesia with an inhalant agent, frequent and effective monitoring is necessary so that the anesthetist has an accurate assessment of the patient's condition and anesthetic depth. Every 3 to 5 minutes, additional boluses are administered to effect, often in volumes of approximately $\frac{1}{10}$ to $\frac{1}{4}$ of that required for induction, as needed to maintain depth at an optimal plane. If the anesthetist is distracted during this process, there is a danger that the patient will unexpectedly awake in the midst of a procedure, endangering itself and hospital staff.

## Maintenance with a Constant Rate Infusion

Before induction and intubation, a calculated volume of anesthetic is drawn into a syringe large enough to accommodate the anticipated amount needed to maintain surgical anesthesia for the duration of the procedure. The syringe is placed in a syringe pump that has been programmed with an infusion rate based on a calculated dose, and attached to a winged infusion set, which in turn is placed in the injection port of an IV administration set. After induction, the pump is started, causing the agent to be delivered at a constant rate. Based on results of monitoring parameters, subtle changes are made in the infusion rate as needed to maintain surgical anesthesia. This method of administration is most suited to propofol, which does not accumulate in body fat stores, because it is rapidly metabolized. Although etomidate or methohexital can also be used to maintain anesthesia, these agents are rarely used for this purpose in small animal practice.

## Maintenance with Injectable and Inhalant Agents

As an alternative, inhalant and injectable agents can be used in combination to maintain anesthesia. For example, if a patient in which anesthesia is maintained with an inhalant agent shows a response to a painful surgical stimulus or wakes prematurely, small doses of an opioid or other appropriate injectable agent can be given intravenously to rapidly deepen the anesthetic plane.

## Maintenance with an Intramuscular Injection

Finally, anesthesia can be induced and maintained with a single IM injection. IM protocols generally produce general anesthesia of relatively short duration (only long enough to perform routine procedures such as spays and castrations). This technique is most commonly used in shelter medicine for elective surgeries in cats. Only tranquilizers, alpha$_2$-agonists, opioids, dissociatives, and anticholinergics can be given intramuscularly. In contrast, propofol, etomidate, and barbiturates should be given only by the IV route. Protocol 8-6 describes IM anesthetic protocols in cats.

## PATIENT POSITIONING, COMFORT, AND SAFETY

During anesthetic induction and maintenance, a number of considerations must be observed to ensure that the patient is not harmed.

- During induction the animal should be supported as it loses consciousness. Particular care should be taken to be sure that the animal does not strike its head on the table during induction or transfer to surgery.
- After IV induction, as soon as the patient is intubated, remove the needle and syringe to avoid accidental overdose in the event that the syringe plunger is accidentally pushed while the patient is being moved.
- Immediately after intubation, lay the patient in lateral recumbency, then secure and cuff the tube.
- Before preparing the patient for surgery, the anesthetist must ensure that the patient's endotracheal tube is correctly placed (i.e., in the trachea) and that the cuff is functional and inflated. Once the surgical preparation begins, it is difficult to position the animal to allow reintubation without compromising aseptic technique.
- Check the endotracheal tube for kinks or bends. An open airway must be maintained at all times (Figure 8-12).

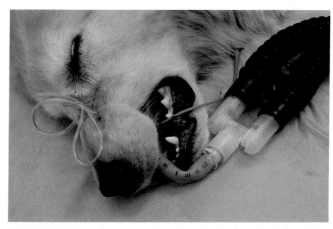

**FIGURE 8-12** In this patient the endotracheal tube is kinked, and the airway is blocked because of the position of the breathing tubes in relation to the position of the patient.

- Any time an intubated patient is turned over, the endotracheal tube should be temporarily disconnected from the anesthetic circuit. Rolling or twisting the animal while it is still connected to the circuit may cause the endotracheal tube to twist and collapse, resulting in an airway obstruction, or may cause the distal end of the tube to traumatize or lacerate the trachea.
- The hoses of the anesthetic machine should be supported so that there is no drag on the endotracheal tube. This could result in tracheal trauma or displacement of the tube.
- The position of the hoses and endotracheal tube should be checked during patient transfer and after repositioning. Hyperflexion of the neck should be avoided because it may lead to endotracheal tube obstruction.
- The reservoir bag should be placed so that it is clearly visible at all times.
- When positioning the animal on the surgery table, the anesthetist should ensure that the animal assumes as normal a posture as possible. In particular, hyperextension or hyperflexion of the limbs should be avoided because either may result in permanent neurologic injury.
- Heavy drapes or instruments must not compress the chest of small patients, because this may interfere with respiration.
- Do not overtighten leg restraint ropes, or circulation may be compromised.
- Place the patient on a heat-retaining surface such as a warm-water circulating blanket. Do *not* use an electric heating pad, which can burn the patient!
- If one lung is diseased, place the normal side up whenever possible, to maximize oxygen exchange.
- Tilting the surgery table so that the patient's head is down gives the surgeon easier access to some abdominal organs, particularly the uterus and ovaries. However, the anesthetist should be aware that

more than a 15-degree elevation of the caudal aspect of the body may cause the abdominal organs to compress the diaphragm, which may compromise heart and lung function. Head-down tilted positions should be avoided entirely in animals with breathing difficulties, especially those with diaphragmatic hernia.
- Artificial tear solution or other corneal lubricant should be instilled into the eyes of an anesthetized patient every hour, unless the patient is undergoing ocular surgery. This is particularly important if an anticholinergic is used. General anesthesia decreases tear secretion for a period of up to 24 hours after anesthesia, and some dogs may need periodic application of a corneal lubricant for up to 36 hours after anesthesia. Cats maintain some tear production throughout anesthesia; however, lubrication is advisable if an anticholinergic or ketamine is given.

> *TECHNICIAN NOTE* Artificial tear solution or other corneal lubricant should be instilled into the eyes of an anesthetized patient every hour. General anesthesia decreases tear secretion for a period of up to 24 hours after anesthesia, and some dogs may need periodic application of a corneal lubricant for up to 36 hours after anesthesia.

## ANESTHETIC RECOVERY

The **anesthetic recovery** period may be defined as the period between the time the anesthetic is discontinued and the time the animal is able to stand and walk without assistance. The length of the recovery period depends on many factors, including the following:
- The length of the anesthetic period. As a general rule, the longer the patient is under anesthesia, the longer the expected recovery.
- The condition of the patient. Lengthy recoveries are seen in animals that have almost any debilitating disease (particularly liver and kidney disease).
- The type of anesthetic given and the route of administration. Lengthy recoveries are more common if an injectable agent is given intramuscularly rather than intravenously.
- The patient's temperature. Hypothermic patients are slow to metabolize and excrete anesthetic drugs.
- The breed of the patient. Certain canine breeds (e.g., greyhounds, salukis, Afghan hounds, whippets, and Russian wolfhounds) are slow to recover from certain anesthetic agents, especially barbiturates.

### Anesthetist's Role in the Recovery Period

The anesthetist's duty toward the patient does not end until the patient is awake and sternal. On completion of the procedure, the patient should be transferred to a recovery area where it can be monitored. A crash cart,

---

**PROTOCOL 8-7** | **Reversal Agent Protocols for Dogs**

1. **Yohimbine:** To reverse the effects of xylazine, administer yohimbine slowly intravenously at a 10:1 agonist-antagonist ratio (1 mg of xylazine per kilogram is reversed with 0.1 mg of yohimbine per kilogram).
2. **Atipamezole:** Administer intramuscularly according to the following dosage guidelines. Give intravenously only for emergency resuscitation.
   a. To reverse the effects of dexmedetomidine, administer atipamezole intramuscularly at a 1:10 agonist-antagonist ratio (0.01 mg of dexmedetomidine per kilogram is reversed with 0.1 mg of atipamezole per kilogram). Equal volumes of the two drugs should be administered.
   b. To reverse the effects of medetomidine, administer atipamezole intramuscularly at a 1:5 agonist-antagonist ratio (0.01 mg of medetomidine per kilogram is reversed with 0.05 mg of atipamezole per kilogram). Equal volumes of the two drugs should be administered.
3. **Naloxone:** To reverse the effects of opioids, administer naloxone at a dose of 0.002 to 0.02 mg/kg IM or by slow IV injection. If renarcotization occurs, additional doses may be needed.

---

**PROTOCOL 8-8** | **Reversal Agent Protocols for Cats**

1. **Yohimbine:** To reverse the effects of xylazine, administer yohimbine slowly intravenously at a 2:1 ratio in cats (1 mg of xylazine per kilogram is reversed with 0.5 mg of yohimbine per kilogram).
2. **Atipamezole:** Administer intramuscularly according to the following dosage guidelines. Because of marked side effects, atipamezole should not be given intravenously except when necessary for emergency resuscitation.
   a. To reverse the effects of dexmedetomidine, administer atipamezole intramuscularly at a 1:5 agonist-antagonist ratio in cats (0.01 mg of dexmedetomidine per kilogram is reversed with 0.05 mg of atipamezole per kilogram).
   b. To reverse the effects of medetomidine, administer atipamezole intramuscularly at a 1:2.5 agonist-antagonist ratio in cats (0.01 mg of medetomidine per kilogram is reversed with 0.025 mg of atipamezole per kilogram).
3. **Naloxone:** To reverse the effects of opioids, administer naloxone at a dose of 0.002 to 0.02 mg/kg IM or by slow IV injection. If renarcotization occurs, additional doses may be needed.

---

monitoring equipment, and oxygen should be readily available. The anesthetist must remain vigilant during recovery because this is often one of the most dangerous periods even for animals that have had no problems during induction or maintenance.

During anesthetic recovery, the anesthetist must fulfill each of the following responsibilities:
- Discontinue administration of all anesthetic agents.
- Monitor the patient on a continual basis.
- Administer oxygen as necessary.
- Administer reversal agents (see Protocol 8-7 for reversal agent protocols in dogs and Protocol 8-8 for reversal agent protocols in cats).
- Maintain a patent airway, and extubate the patient at the appropriate time.
- Provide general nursing care (reassure the patient, provide patient hygiene, warm the patient, and prevent self-injury).
- Provide adequate analgesia, and administer other medications as requested by the veterinarian.

Procedure 8-8, p. 262, shows the sequence of events during the recovery period.

> **TECHNICIAN NOTE**  During recovery the patient must be watched continuously at close range. This is often one of the most dangerous periods even for animals that have had no problems during induction or maintenance.

## Signs of Recovery

An animal recovering from general anesthesia gradually progresses back through the anesthetic stages and planes. As the animal moves from deep to moderate to light anesthesia, vital signs and reflexes change in predictable ways. The heart rate, respiratory rate, and respiratory volume increase. After assuming a ventromedial position, the eyeballs move back to a central position. Reflex responses return, and muscle tone strengthens. The animal may shiver, swallow, chew, or attempt to lick. Shortly after swallowing reflexes return, the animal will normally show signs of consciousness, including voluntary movement of the head or limbs and possibly vocalization.

While passing through stage II, some patients may exhibit a variety of alarming signs including head-bobbing, delirium, hyperventilation, head-thrashing, and rapid limb paddling, especially if not premedicated. Occasionally a patient may attempt to stand and fall or may appear blind and bump into the sides of the cage. Some patients (particularly those recovering from ketamine anesthesia) may chew at their paws or claw their faces. Animals showing these signs of a "rough" or "stormy" recovery usually return to normal within a short time, but steps must be taken to prevent self-trauma or disruption of the surgical wound. Administration of preanesthetic medications before the procedure often prevents or moderates these signs, but additional tranquilization or administration of analgesics during the postoperative period may be necessary in these patients.

## Monitoring

During recovery, the patient must be watched continuously at close range because a recovering animal may develop hypoxemia, cardiac arrhythmias, or other complications yet show no signs that are evident to the casual observer. Evaluation from across the room is not acceptable because problems such as vomiting, chewing the tube, and airway occlusion occur with some regularity and must be managed without delay to prevent serious consequences. These problems are discussed in detail in Chapter 12.

To minimize these risks, the patient should be positioned in the cage so that mucous membranes and respirations can be observed. Vital signs should be evaluated at least every 5 minutes. Abnormal vital signs or a delayed return to consciousness may indicate a variety of serious conditions that must be treated promptly by the veterinarian, such as shock, hemorrhage, hypoglycemia, or hypothermia. See Box 8-5 for ACVA monitoring guidelines for the recovery period.

## Oxygen Therapy

As soon as the anesthetic depth decreases sufficiently, most recovering patients begin to shiver. Shivering is a protective response to hypothermia that raises the body temperature. During shivering, contracting muscle tissue converts oxygen and chemical fuel into heat. Consequently, muscle contractions associated with shivering increase oxygen consumption. Oxygen administration during recovery is necessary to meet these needs and to compensate for residual respiratory depression until anesthetic depth decreases.

> **TECHNICIAN NOTE** Recovering patients often consume more oxygen as a result of shivering. Oxygen administration during recovery is necessary to meet these needs.

Oxygen should be administered via the endotracheal tube at a rate of 50 to 100 mL/kg/min (0.5 to 1 L/10 kg body weight up to a maximum of 5 L/min) for 5 minutes after discontinuation of the anesthetic or until the animal swallows. This route of administration allows waste anesthetic gases to be scavenged and gives the anesthetist the ability to bag the patient during recovery to help reinflate collapsed alveoli.

If the patient is at a light depth and must be extubated, oxygen can be administered by mask. Some patients do not tolerate a mask without becoming agitated, however, and may require an alternative means of oxygen delivery.

---

**BOX 8-5** | **American College of Veterinary Anesthesiologists Monitoring Guidelines for the Recovery Period**

The objective of the American College of Veterinary Anesthesiologists (ACVA) monitoring guidelines for recovery is "to ensure a safe and comfortable recovery from anesthesia." To accomplish this, the ACVA makes the following recommendations: "Monitoring in recovery should include at the minimum evaluation of pulse rate and quality, mucous membrane color, respiratory pattern, signs of pain, and temperature."

---

The following options are alternatives to the use of a mask during the postoperative period.

- An oxygen source such as the Y-piece or the fresh gas inlet of a non-rebreathing system can be placed near the nasal openings.
- An Elizabethan collar can be placed around the patient's neck, with an oxygen line secured to the inside of the collar. The front of the collar is covered with cellophane, with a small ventilation hole. A flow rate of 1 L/min provides 30% to 40% oxygen.
- Oxygen can be delivered via a nasal catheter. A lubricated soft red rubber catheter (5 to 10 French depending on the size of the patient) is introduced into the ventral nasal meatus. Intranasal proparacaine or 2% lidocaine can be used to desensitize the nasal tissues to allow insertion. The catheter is advanced to the level of the carnassial teeth and attached to the dorsum of the nose with tissue glue (cyanoacrylate). A flow rate of 100 to 150 mL/kg provides 30% to 50% oxygen. Alternatively, nasal prongs used in human hospitals may be used. They can be secured to the patient with tissue glue or staples.
- The patient can be placed in an oxygen cage.

Note that a patient that is intubated and breathing oxygen from an anesthetic machine receives close to 100% oxygen. This is beneficial for the relatively short duration of most procedures, but prolonged inhalation of high levels of oxygen (e.g., greater than 50% oxygen for more than 24 hours) can be toxic.

## Extubation

To prepare the patient for extubation, deflate the cuff by drawing out all the air until the pilot balloon is empty. Untie the tube so that it can be rapidly removed. At all times during recovery, keep the neck in a natural but extended position to protect the airway. Some anesthetists prefer to deflate the cuff and untie the gauze before signs of arousal are seen so that the tube can be quickly removed when swallowing occurs.

As soon as the patient shows signs of imminent arousal, the endotracheal tube must be removed using a slow, steady motion. In dogs, return of the swallowing reflex is the most appropriate time to remove the tube because this reflex will help protect the animal from pulmonary aspiration if vomiting occurs during recovery. Animals that show voluntary limb, head, or chewing movements are close to consciousness, however, and should be extubated even if swallowing has not been observed. These patients typically swallow on removal of the endotracheal tube.

A notable exception to this general rule is brachycephalic dogs. In these patients, many anesthetists prefer to delay extubation until the patient is able to lift its head unassisted, as early extubation may lead to respiratory distress from upper airway obstruction. In these patients it is wise to prepare by having a laryngoscope, an endotracheal tube (the same size as or one size smaller than used during the procedure), and the appropriate dose of an ultra–short-acting IV induction agent such as propofol nearby in case reintubation is necessary.

If a recovering patient shows signs of respiratory distress after extubation, the anesthetist must determine whether this is because of pulmonary disease (in which case oxygen therapy may be needed) or upper airway obstruction. One helpful clue is that upper airway obstruction is often associated with **stridor** (noisy respirations), especially on inspiration. If obstruction is present, the anesthetist should reposition the patient and gently pull the tongue forward. If the obstruction persists, it may be necessary to reinduce and reintubate the patient.

In cats the endotracheal tube may be removed when signs of impending arousal are observed. These include swallowing, an active palpebral reflex, and voluntary limb, tail, or head movements. Delaying extubation is not advisable in cats because it may predispose the patient to laryngospasm.

> **TECHNICIAN NOTE**  After dental cleaning, oral surgery, or any other procedure in which blood or other fluids are present in the oral cavity, the cuff should be left partially inflated during removal to sweep out the fluid and prevent it from entering the airways.

After dental cleaning, oral surgery, or any other procedure in which blood or other fluids are present in the oral cavity, the cuff should be left partially inflated during removal to sweep out the fluid, and prevent it from entering the airways. After extubation, all animals should be placed in lateral or sternal recumbency with the neck extended. This position helps maintain a patent airway. Occasionally, fluid or mucus may accumulate in the pharynx or trachea and must be removed by suction. The anesthetist should do this before the patient is fully awake to avoid being bitten.

## POSTANESTHETIC PERIOD

In the postanesthetic period, patients require general nursing care to ease recovery, ensure their safety, and prepare them for return to the hospital ward. The anesthetist should be sensitive to the fact that the animal has no means of understanding the events that have produced the disorientation, fear, and discomfort that often accompanies the return to consciousness. Quiet, calm handling, reassurance, and attention to the patient's comfort level are therefore essential.

The anesthetist can take several steps to minimize patient discomfort during recovery. All ties restraining the animal to the surgery table should be removed before the animal regains consciousness. The anesthetist should ensure that all accessory procedures, such as bandaging, chest tube placement, and urinary catheterization, have been completed and that all monitoring equipment probes, cuffs, and electrocardiographic electrodes have been removed. The anesthetist should also be gentle when moving a recovering patient, so as not to increase discomfort and pain.

The IV catheter should be left in place until the endotracheal tube has been removed and it is clear that the patient is recovering normally. This provides venous access in the event that the patient's current condition or an unexpected complication necessitates administration of IV drugs or fluids.

Patient recovery may be hastened by gentle stimulation in the form of talking softly to the patient, patting or rubbing the chest, turning the patient, or gently moving the endotracheal tube. These actions stimulate breathing and increase the flow of information to the reticular activating system (RAS) of the brain—the area responsible for maintaining consciousness in the awake animal. A lack of stimulation of the RAS may cause drowsiness in the conscious animal. It is therefore speculated that stimulation of this area may help the animal to awaken.

> **TECHNICIAN NOTE**  A recovering patient should also be turned every 10 to 15 minutes to prevent pooling of blood in the dependent lung and tissues—a condition called *hypostatic congestion*.

A recovering patient should also be turned every 10 to 15 minutes to prevent pooling of blood in the dependent lung and tissues—a condition called **hypostatic congestion.** When the intubated patient is turned from one side to another, the breathing circuit must be briefly detached from the endotracheal tube, and the head and neck should be turned as a single unit to minimize the risk of tracheal damage by the tube. Although not proven, there may be a risk of causing the stomach to twist if a patient is turned by moving the limbs over the body from one side to the other. For this reason, some professionals recommend turning a patient by sliding the limbs under the body instead, especially if the patient is a member of a breed prone to gastric dilatation–volvulus.

Never leave a recovering patient in an open cage or on a table unattended, because once spontaneous movement returns, a recovering patient may fall and be injured. Food and water should not be left in the cage during recovery because it is possible for a recovering animal to drown in a water bowl or suffocate in a food bowl. Some patients may be able to drink soon after standing; however, most have little appetite for food for several hours after recovery anyway. Vomiting during the recovery period is not uncommon, but provided the patient is conscious, this is seldom dangerous.

Nursing care of hypothermic patients should include the provision of heat. This can be accomplished by a variety of means including warm air or water blankets, heat lamps, warm water bottles, and incubators. Never use electric heating pads, which have a significant potential to burn a recovering patient. Box 8-6 lists recommended heat sources. Recovering patients are unable to voluntarily move away from a heat source if excessive; therefore the anesthetist must prevent burns by ensuring that the heat source never exceeds 42° C (approximately 107.6° F). Gradual rewarming is preferred to rapid rewarming because the latter may cause dilation of cutaneous vessels, leading to hypotension.

Analgesics should be administered as requested by the veterinarian, preferably before the onset of pain (see Chapter 7). If analgesia is adequate, the patient should be able to sleep comfortably and should demonstrate minimal signs of discomfort. A change in the dose or frequency of administration or use of a different or additional agent may be necessary if postoperative pain is not well controlled.

> **BOX 8-6 Acceptable Heat Sources for Recovering Patients***
>
> - Provide ample bedding.
> - Place warm towels over the patient.
> - Place warm water bottles wrapped in towels on either side of the patient, taking care not to restrict respiratory movements, especially in small patients.
> - Place an infrared heat lamp approximately 1 m (3 feet) from the patient.
> - Wrap the patient in a warm air blanket.
> - Use a hair dryer on low heat.
> - Heat bags containing rice or oats in a microwave, and place them next to the patient.
> - Place the patient on a circulating warm water blanket.
> - Place the patient in an incubator designed for human babies.
>
> *Note that heat sources should never exceed 42° C (107.6° F).

After recovery the anesthetist must provide ongoing care and prepare the patient for release or continued hospitalization. Most small animal patients should be given nothing by mouth for the first hour or two and no food for at least several hours. On discharge, the client should be instructed to reintroduce water gradually after arriving home and to feed a small meal after several hours. Exceptions to these guidelines include very small and neonatal patients, which require reintroduction of water and food more rapidly.

## KEY POINTS

1. Small animal patients are restrained and anesthetized with a variety of techniques, but general anesthesia is most commonly selected for many procedures. In many practices intravenous (IV) or mask induction followed by maintenance with an inhalant agent is most commonly employed.
2. When a protocol is being selected, great care must be used in calculating drug dosages, oxygen flow rates, and fluid administration rates, and in drawing up and administering anesthetic agents and adjuncts.
3. To safely and effectively anesthetize a patient, the anesthetist must have a clear understanding of the expected sequence of events and dynamics associated with each anesthetic technique.
4. Equipment must be carefully prepared before anesthetic induction, because once induction commences, the anesthetist has little to no time to gather missing equipment.
5. The goal of anesthetic induction is to take the patient from consciousness to stage III anesthesia smoothly and rapidly. This requires finesse, watchfulness, and an ability to make decisions rapidly and act quickly based on patient monitoring parameters.
6. IV induction agents are most often given "to effect" by using a process called *titration*. When inducing anesthesia by IV injection, in general the entire calculated dose should not be administered at once.
7. Mask and chamber inductions involve risks of which the anesthetist must be aware to prevent serious complications. Vigilant patient monitoring is required when these methods are used.
8. There are many advantages to endotracheal intubation, which justify this technique even in patients anesthetized only with injectable drugs.
9. Successful and safe endotracheal intubation requires careful preparation, excellent technique, and watchfulness for potential complications.
10. The anesthetic period can be divided into preanesthesia, induction, maintenance, and recovery. Traditionally, anesthetic depth has been described in terms of stages and planes of anesthesia, with stage III, plane 2, being suitable for most surgical procedures.
11. Patient positioning, comfort, and safety must be considered during anesthetic maintenance to avoid problems such as traumatic injury, accidental overdose, airway blockage, hypoxemia, circulatory compromise, burns, hypostatic congestion, and corneal drying.

12. The length of the recovery period depends on many factors, including the anesthetic protocol and the patient's condition. Return to consciousness is accompanied by increasing heart and respiratory rates, increased reflex responses, and voluntary movement.

13. During the recovery period, the anesthetist must continue to monitor the patient's vital signs, particularly temperature, as anesthetic complications commonly occur during this period. It is often helpful to administer oxygen for several minutes after the anesthetic has been discontinued.

14. In dogs extubation should occur when the swallowing reflex returns. In cats extubation should occur when the patient shows signs of impending arousal, such as voluntary movements, swallowing, or active reflexes.

15. Other duties during recovery include stimulation of the patient, administration of oxygen, postoperative analgesia, and general nursing care.

16. Anesthetic safety is improved through the use of preanesthetic agents, use of the minimum effective dosages, selection of a protocol well suited to the patient, and close monitoring of the patient.

---

## PROCEDURE 8-1   Preparation of the Dog and Cat for Anesthesia

1. Assess, prepare, and weigh the patient. (See Chapter 2 for a discussion of patient assessment, preparation, and stabilization.)
2. Determine the protocol (anesthetic agents, doses, and routes and sequence of administration).
3. Calculate the volume of each agent to give (preanesthetic, induction, maintenance, and analgesic agents) and fluid administration rates.
4. Calculate the oxygen flow rates (see Chapter 4, p. 126).
5. Prepare equipment required to administer drugs (scales, syringes, needles, agents, reversal agents, emergency cart, controlled substance log).
6. Prepare fluid administration equipment (clippers, antiseptic scrub, catheters, tape, heparinized saline, catheter cap, administration and extension set, fluids).
7. Prepare equipment for endotracheal intubation (see Figure 8-8, p. 245).
8. Prepare monitoring equipment, including anesthesia record, stethoscope, monitors, and probes (see Chapter 5).
9. Assemble and test the anesthetic machine.

---

## PROCEDURE 8-2   Sequence of Events for Induction of General Anesthesia with an IV Agent and Maintenance with an Inhalant Agent in a Small Animal Patient

1. Administer premedications intramuscularly approximately 15 to 20 minutes, or intravenously approximately 5 to 10 minutes, before anesthetic induction.
2. Place an intravenous catheter, attach a fluid administration set, and begin fluid administration.
3. Administer the induction agent.
4. Check the patient's readiness for intubation.
5. Place and secure the endotracheal tube.
6. Check the patient's vital signs.
7. Turn on the oxygen, and connect the endotracheal tube to the breathing circuit.
8. Inflate the endotracheal tube cuff.
9. Turn the vaporizer on to the appropriate setting.
10. Determine the patient's anesthetic depth, and commence regular monitoring.
11. Position and secure the patient for the procedure, giving attention to padding, maintenance of an open airway, unrestricted blood flow, and unrestricted chest excursions.
12. Attach monitoring devices.
13. Continue to monitor and adjust the anesthetic and oxygen levels as needed until completion of the procedure.

## PROCEDURE 8-3  IV Induction in a Dog or Cat

Although each IV agent or combination is given somewhat differently, all intravenously administered general anesthetics should be given "to effect" so that the patient receives only the minimum amount necessary to induce anesthesia.

### Giving an IV Anesthetic "to Effect"

Give an initial bolus of ¼ to ½ the calculated dose. Immediately after giving the initial bolus, check the heart rate and respiratory rate to be sure the patient is stable and is breathing (while keeping in mind that a brief period of apnea is a common adverse effect of some intravenous anesthetics). As soon as the patient relaxes, remove muzzles and other restraint devices. Continue monitoring and give additional boluses as necessary until the patient has passed through stage II. When signs of readiness for intubation are present, intubate the patient and take the steps necessary to bring the patient into surgical anesthesia.

During this process, there must be interplay between administration of the drug and patient monitoring. Give the initial dose; then rapidly check the vital signs, pedal reflex, palpebral reflex, and jaw tone; give more if needed; check again; and so on, until the patient is in a plane of anesthesia sufficient to permit intubation. After the initial dose, subsequent doses should generally be about ⅕ to ⅒ the calculated dose.

- **Propofol:** Give propofol slowly at a rate of ¼ to ½ the calculated dose every 30 seconds to effect. A more rapid injection rate may be helpful in uncooperative patients but is more likely to induce apnea. If the injection is too slow, excitement may be seen.
- **Ketamine-diazepam** and other **ketamine-tranquilizer mixtures:** Give slowly to effect over 60 to 120 seconds.

Slow injection minimizes the adverse effects of these combinations, which may take as long as 2 minutes to reach peak effect. Therefore an overly rapid injection rate may result in overdose. If a bolus injection technique is preferred, ⅓ to ½ the calculated dose can be given over 15 to 30 seconds, with further increments every 30 to 60 seconds until the desired depth is reached.

- **Thiopental sodium:** Give thiopental via an indwelling catheter to reduce the risk of perivascular injection. Alternatively, a skilled anesthetist may use a needle and syringe, using extreme care to stay within the vein. In healthy patients give ½ the calculated dose over 10 to 15 seconds, then to effect. If intubation is not possible after 45 seconds, a second dose (approximately ¼ the calculated dose) may be given. Continue until the desired depth is reached. This technique allows rapid induction of stage III anesthesia with minimal stage II excitement. Old, ill, and debilitated patients may need much less and require that the drug be given much more cautiously and slowly.
- **Neuroleptanalgesic combinations** (e.g., hydromorphone and diazepam): Give an IV bolus of diazepam, followed by a bolus of hydromorphone. Some patients may require an additional bolus of each drug to allow intubation and occasionally may require a third bolus.
- **Etomidate:** Give rapidly to effect after premedication with a tranquilizer, or concurrently with IV diazepam or midazolam (use a separate syringe if diazepam is chosen). Some anesthetists recommend administering it via the port of a fluid administration set with the fluids running to reduce adverse effects.

## PROCEDURE 8-4  Mask Induction in a Dog or Cat

1. Use either a malleable black rubber mask or a clear plastic mask with a rubber diaphragm for mask induction. The mask should fit tightly on the animal's face to reduce leakage of waste gas and should not be any larger than necessary in order to minimize dead space.
2. Connect the mask to the Y-piece of a rebreathing circuit or the endotracheal tube connector of a non-rebreathing circuit, and hold it in place over the animal's muzzle (Figure 1).
3. Give 100% oxygen for 2 to 3 minutes to allow the patient to adjust to the mask and to increase the amount of oxygen in the blood. The oxygen flow rate should be set at 30 times the patient's tidal volume (1 to 3 L/min for patients weighing less than or equal to 10 kg and 3 to 5 L/min for patients weighing more than 10 kg) because higher flow rates help speed induction.
4. Set the anesthetic vaporizer to deliver 0.5% isoflurane or 1% sevoflurane. Sevoflurane is less pungent than isoflurane and better accepted.
5a. Gradually increase the concentration of anesthetic by small increments (0.5% every 30 seconds for isoflurane and 1% every 30 seconds for sevoflurane) until an anesthetic concentration of 3% to 5% for isoflurane or 4% to 6% for sevoflurane is reached. This is higher than maintenance level but allows a rapid uptake of the anesthetic and a faster induction. The slow increase helps reduce struggling, prevents cardiac arrhythmias, and allows the animal to become accustomed to the smell of the anesthetic. This method is often well accepted by cats and small dogs, although some struggling may be seen after 2 to 3 minutes when isoflurane is given, corresponding to stage II excitement. Most patients reach stage III, plane 1, in about 5 to 10 minutes, depending on the agent used.
5b. Other anesthetists suggest increasing the vaporizer setting to the induction level immediately, especially if the patient is difficult to handle, to minimize the time spent in stage II. If the patient struggles, the anesthetist must observe the patient closely for cyanosis, hypotension, or other problems and be ready to act quickly if the patient becomes compromised.

*Continued*

## PROCEDURE 8-4    Mask Induction in a Dog or Cat—cont'd

6. As soon as the patient is laterally recumbent, assess readiness for intubation and adjust the anesthetic level as appropriate, then place an endotracheal tube. From this point on the patient is managed much the same as for intravenous induction.

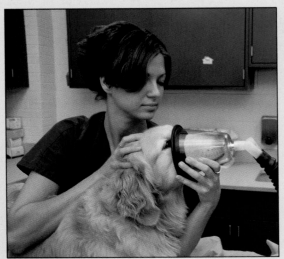

**FIGURE 1**    Mask induction. Note the good fit of the mask around the muzzle to minimize leakage.

## PROCEDURE 8-5    Chamber Induction in a Dog or Cat

1. Place the conscious animal inside an anesthetic chamber. The chamber should be large enough for the patient to lie down with its neck extended. If the patient can be handled, an ophthalmic lubricant should be applied before the patient is placed in the induction chamber.
2. Remove the Y-piece of a rebreathing circuit, and attach one corrugated hose to each port.
3. Deliver a mixture of oxygen at 5 L/minute, and isoflurane at 3% to 5% or sevoflurane at 4% to 6%.
4. During passage through stages I and II, patients typically exhibit fear and agitation. The patient may attempt to escape or vocalize. Gradually, with the onset of anesthesia, the patient will become increasingly depressed and immobile.
5. As soon as the patient can no longer stand, rock the chamber gently to assess the patient's status. Initially the patient will respond by righting itself until anesthesia is of sufficient depth to prevent purposeful movement. When the patient is immobile enough to allow it to be safely handled, remove it from the chamber, place a mask, and proceed as with mask induction.

## PROCEDURE 8-6    Intubation Procedure for a Dog or Cat

1. Place the patient in sternal recumbency.*
2. Have an assistant grasp the maxilla behind the canine teeth, extend the neck, and raise the head so that the head and neck are in a straight line. Be sure the lips and whiskers are pulled dorsally and out of the line of sight. The neck should be propped upright and not allowed to sag. The assistant should not push on the ventral aspect of the neck or head because this may obscure the view, making intubation difficult.
3. Grasp the tongue with a gauze sponge, and open the mouth fully by firmly pulling the tongue out and down. A mouth gag can be used to hold the mouth open.
4. Adjust the light so that the larynx is well illuminated.
5. If necessary, use the tube or laryngoscope to gently displace the epiglottis ventrally, or the soft palate dorsally, until the glottis can be visualized† (Figure 1).
6. Gently insert the tube past the vocal folds using a rotating motion. If the tube is too large to pass easily, change the tube for one of smaller diameter, but *never force the tube!*
7. After the tube has been placed, gently transfer the patient into lateral recumbency.

## PROCEDURE 8-6   Intubation Procedure for a Dog or Cat—cont'd

8. Check the tube to ensure that it is in the trachea. Then check that it is inserted to an appropriate distance and is oriented to match the natural curve of the trachea.

9. Secure the tube in place with a length of rolled gauze or used IV tubing.

10. Position the tongue so that it hangs loosely from the mouth and is not compressed by the tie.

11. Turn on the oxygen flow meter(s).

12. Connect the ET tube connector to the breathing circuit.

13. Inflate the cuff, and check for leaks.

14. Turn on the anesthetic vaporizer, and select the appropriate setting.

15. Commence regular monitoring.

16. Ensure a patent airway by checking the position of the patient and tube. The neck and tube should assume a gentle natural curve.

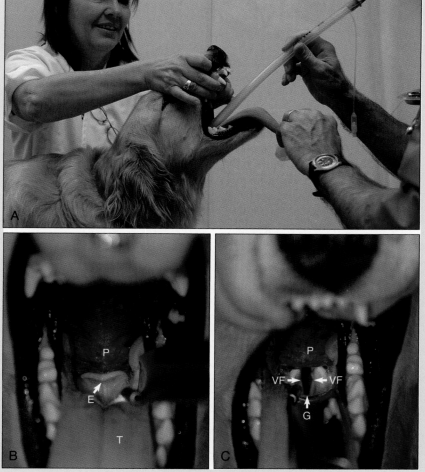

**FIGURE 1   A,** Proper position for endotracheal intubation in a small animal. **B,** The anatomy of the pharynx and larynx: *E,* epiglottis, which in this view is covering the glottis; *P,* palate; *T,* tongue. **C,** In this view the epiglottis has been displaced ventrally with a laryngoscope. The glottis *(G)* is visible as the dark, oval opening between the vocal folds *(VF),* which move apart when the patient inhales and relax as the patient exhales.

*Some anesthetists prefer to position the patient in dorsal recumbency. If this position is used, a laryngoscope held with the handle up is used to displace the epiglottis against the base of the tongue.

†Some anesthetists prefer to intubate dogs blindly (by feel). The patient is placed in lateral recumbency, and the tube is passed along the roof of the mouth, over the epiglottis, and into the trachea. If this technique is used, care must be taken to prevent trauma to the delicate tissues of the pharynx and larynx.

## PROCEDURE 8-7    Anesthetic Maintenance in a Dog or Cat

General anesthesia is maintained with inhalant or injectable agents. As with anesthetic induction, there are subtleties in the way each agent is handled to ensure that the patient is at an optimum anesthetic depth and is safe. The administration of these agents is summarized here.

### Maintenance with an Inhalant Agent

- Choose the initial dial setting based on the anesthetic depth following intubation.
- Make periodic changes in the vaporizer dial setting based on monitoring parameters.
- If the anesthetic depth is slightly too light or deep, make small dial changes of approximately 0.5% to 1% increments with isoflurane or sevoflurane.
- If the patient's anesthetic depth is significantly light (e.g., patient exhibits spontaneous movement, swallowing, active reflexes, strong muscle tone), increase the oxygen flow to 50 to 100 mL/kg body weight per minute, and set isoflurane at 3% to 5% or sevoflurane at 4% to 6% (induction levels).
- If anesthetic depth is significantly too deep (e.g., absent reflexes; flaccid jaw tone; central, dilated pupils), then increase the oxygen flow to 50 to 100 mL/kg body weight per minute; turn off the vaporizer, and monitor the patient carefully until signs of decreased depth are evident. As soon as depth starts to decrease and the patient is safe, resume the anesthetic.

### Maintenance with Repeat Boluses of Propofol or Another Ultra–Short-Acting Agent

- Monitor the patient every few minutes.
- Administer additional boluses as needed to effect, typically every 3 to 5 minutes.
- The necessary volume for each bolus varies but is often approximately 1/10 to 1/4 of that required for induction.

- Maintain the patient at an optimal plane and avoid overdose.

### Maintenance with a CRI of Propofol

- Place an IV catheter, attach an administration set, and begin IV fluid administration.
- Calculate the volume of anesthetic needed to last the anticipated length of the procedure.
- Draw this volume into a syringe.
- Place the syringe in a syringe pump and program in the infusion rate in milliliters or microliters per minute, or in milliliters or microliters per hour (the manual will indicate accepted units).
- Attach the syringe to the port of a winged infusion set primed with anesthetic to be administered.
- Place the needle of the winged infusion set into the injection port of an IV administration set near the catheter.
- After induction and intubation, start the syringe pump at the calculated rate.
- Based on results of monitoring parameters, make subtle changes in the infusion rate as needed to maintain the patient in surgical anesthesia.

### Induction and Maintenance with an IM Injection

- Calculate the volume to be administered.
- Administer the agent via the IM route.
- Place the patient in a quiet area for 15 to 20 minutes, where it can be monitored.
- After peak effect, check the anesthetic depth and start the procedure if depth is adequate.
- If the anesthetic depth is inadequate, give additional drug intramuscularly or intravenously or administer an inhalant agent by mask.

## PROCEDURE 8-8    Recovery from General Anesthesia in a Dog or Cat

1. Prepare the patient for recovery, including removal of drapes, any other equipment used for the procedure, and monitoring equipment.
2. Prepare a cage without food, water, a litter pan, or anything else that has the potential to cause patient injury during the recovery period.
3. Discontinue the anesthetic, but continue administering oxygen at a rate of 50 to 100 mL/kg/min up to a maximum of 5 L/min for 5 minutes or until the patient is extubated (which ever comes first).
4. Transfer the patient to the recovery area or cage, paying attention to positioning so that an open airway is maintained, and continue monitoring.
5. Deflate the cuff, untie the endotracheal tube, and extubate the patient at the appropriate time. Ensure that the airway is open and the patient is breathing without difficulty.
6. Calm, reassure, and warm the patient. Turn the patient every 10 to 15 minutes. Take precautions to prevent self-trauma or injury.
7. As soon as it is clear that the patient is recovering normally, ask the VIC if continued IV access is needed for ongoing care. When and if ordered by the VIC, stop fluid administration and remove the IV catheter.
8. Prepare the patient for continued hospitalization or discharge by applying bandages, administering medications, and performing any other procedures ordered by the doctor.
9. When the patient is able to remain in sternal recumbency unsupported, return the patient to the cage (if not already done) and close the cage door securely.

# REVIEW QUESTIONS

1. Consider the following scenario: You are performing a procedure on a canine patient that you feel is at an appropriate anesthetic depth. Which of the following settings would be most appropriate if using sevoflurane in this patient?
   a. 2%
   b. 2 L/minute
   c. 3.5%
   d. 4 mL/minute
   e. 6%

2. Which of the following statements about how to induce anesthesia in a young healthy patient using an IV agent such as thiopental or propofol is least accurate?
   a. If, after giving the initial amount, the patient is not adequately anesthetized to allow intubation, give the rest of the calculated dose.
   b. Draw up the calculated dose, give about ¼ to ½ first, and give the rest to effect.
   c. You must be sure the drug gets in the vein.
   d. Old, sick, or debilitated patients often require less.

3. Which of the following statements regarding IV induction agents is least accurate?
   a. Ketamine-diazepam takes slightly longer to act and lasts somewhat longer than propofol.
   b. When using propofol, give about 25% to 50% of the calculated dose every 30 seconds to effect.
   c. Significantly lower doses of thiopental sodium must be used in sick, old, or debilitated patients.
   d. Thiopental sodium is generally given intravenously but can be given intramuscularly in uncooperative patients.

4. Which of the following barbiturates can be used to maintain anesthesia without prolonging recovery?
   a. Pentobarbital
   b. Methohexital
   c. Thiopental sodium
   d. Phenobarbital

5. Which of the following statements about thiopental sodium is least accurate?
   a. It is likely to cause tissue necrosis if injected outside of the vein.
   b. Due to the patient's age and condition, you may have to give less of the drug.
   c. It commonly induces seizures during recovery.
   d. It is more likely than propofol to depress respirations in neonates.
   e. It is more likely than propofol to cause cardiac arrhythmias such as bigeminy and PVCs.

6. Which of the following statements concerning endotracheal intubation is false?
   a. Choosing a tube that is too short may cause increased mechanical dead space.
   b. Choosing a tube that is too small may result in increased resistance to breathing.
   c. Choosing a tube that is too long may result in hypoxemia.
   d. Failure to cuff the tube may result in aspiration of foreign material.

7. Which of the following is an indicator that the endotracheal tube has been placed in the esophagus instead of the trachea?
   a. The patient coughs when the tube is placed.
   b. The unidirectional valves don't move.
   c. The pressure manometer indicates 0 to 2 cm $H_2O$ while the patient is spontaneously breathing.
   d. Only one firm structure in the neck is palpated.

8. The term atelectasis refers to:
   a. Increased fluid in the alveoli
   b. Hyperinflation of the alveoli
   c. A decrease in the perfusion of blood around the alveoli
   d. Collapsed alveoli

9. After an anesthetic procedure, when is it best to extubate a dog?
   a. Right after you turn off the vaporizer
   b. About 10 minutes after turning off the vaporizer
   c. When the animal begins to swallow
   d. Any time that is convenient

10. Hypostatic congestion may be present at the end of the anesthetic protocol. This term refers to the:
    a. Accumulation of mucus in the trachea
    b. Pooling of blood in the dependent lung
    c. Leakage of fluid into the chest
    d. Pooling of ingesta in one area of the gastrointestinal tract

11. Which of the following protocols would result in the fastest induction time and the best control over anesthetic depth?
    a. IM induction and maintenance
    b. IV induction with an ultra–short-acting agent, and maintenance with bolus injections of the same
    c. Inhalant induction and maintenance
    d. IV induction with an ultra–short-acting agent, and maintenance with an inhalant

12. Mask inductions in small animal patients are:
    a. Easier for the anesthetist than IV inductions
    b. Less likely to cause cardiac arrhythmias and hypotension than IV inductions
    c. An excellent technique for brachycephalic breeds
    d. Possible only with use of inhalant agents with a low solubility coefficient

13. Which of the following techniques are used most often in most general small animal practices?
    a. General anesthesia and sedation
    b. Sedatives and local techniques
    c. Neuromuscular blockade and neuroleptanalgesia
    d. Local and general anesthesia

14. An 18-kg adult dog of normal conformation would likely require a _____ endotracheal tube.
    a. 7- to 7.5-mm
    b. 8- to 8.5-mm
    c. 9- to 9.5-mm
    d. 10- to 10.5-mm

The following questions may have more than one correct answer. Select all that apply.

15. An endotracheal tube is used to:
    a. Decrease dead space
    b. Maintain a patent airway
    c. Protect the patient from aspiration of vomitus
    d. Allow the anesthetist to ventilate the patient

16. Problems associated with endotracheal intubation include:
    a. Decreased dead space
    b. Pressure necrosis of the tracheal mucosa
    c. Intubation of a bronchus
    d. Spread of infectious disease

17. During anesthetic maintenance:
    a. The patient should be supported as it loses consciousness
    b. The patient should be placed on an electric heating pad to prevent hypothermia
    c. If a patient has one diseased lung, it should be positioned with the diseased side down
    d. The anesthetist should avoid any more than a 15-degree elevation of the rear quarters

18. The length of the anesthetic recovery period may be influenced by:
    a. Body temperature
    b. Patient condition
    c. The length of time the patient was under
    d. The breed of the patient

19. Which of the following is/are not a normal sign(s) of recovery?
    a. Head-bobbing
    b. Mydriasis
    c. Seizures
    d. Rapid limb paddling

20. Which of the following actions is appropriate during anesthetic recovery?
    a. Administer oxygen at a high flow rate for 5 minutes after discontinuation of the anesthetic or until extubation.
    b. Leave the cage door open so you can monitor the patient from across the room.
    c. Turn the patient about every 10 to 15 minutes.
    d. Use warming methods to increase the body temperature.

## SELECTED READINGS

Bednarski RM: Dogs and cats. In Thurmon JC, Tranquilli WJ, Benson GJ, editors: *Essentials of small animal anesthesia and analgesia*, Baltimore, 1999, Lippincott Williams & Wilkins, pp 367-381.

Bednarski RM: Dogs and Cats. In Tranquilli WJ, Thurmon JC, Grimm KA, editors: *Lumb and Jones' veterinary anesthesia and analgesia*, ed 4, Ames, Iowa, 2007, Blackwell, pp 705-715.

DiBartola S: *Fluid, electrolyte, and acid-base disorders*, ed 3, St Louis, 2006, Elsevier.

Kaiser-Klinger S: Balanced anesthesia in small animals, *Vet Tech* 28(11):711-718, 2007.

Lerche P, Muir WW, Grub TL: Mask induction of anesthesia with isoflurane or sevoflurane in premedicated cats, *J Small Anim Pract* 43(1):12-15, 2002.

Love L, Egger C: Balanced anesthesia protocols for cats and dogs, *compendiumvet.com*, June 2008.

Lucero R: Brachycephalic breeds and anesthesia, *Vet Tech* 27(5): 302-310, 2006.

Macintire D, Drobatz K, Haskins S, Saxon W: *Manual of small animal emergency and critical care medicine*, Philadelphia, 2005, Lippincott Williams & Wilkins, pp 38-54.

Muir WW, Hubbell JA, Bednarski RM: *Handbook of veterinary anesthesia*, ed 4, St Louis, 2007, Elsevier, pp 361-388.

Norkus C: Balancing Act—Combining inhalant anesthetics and injectable drugs, *Vet Tech* 27(12):770-779, 2006.

Ortel S: Constant-rate infusions, *Vet Tech* 27(1):47-50, 2006.

Plumb, Donald C: *Plumb's veterinary drug handbook*, ed 6, Ames, 2008, Blackwell.

Roach W, Krahwinkel DJ: Obstructive lesions and traumatic injuries of the canine and feline tracheas, *Compendium*. 31(2): 86-93, 2009.

# Equine Anesthesia

# 9

## OUTLINE

Patient Preparation, 267
Selecting a Protocol, 267
Summary of a General Anesthetic
 Procedure, 267
Equipment Preparation, 267
Premedication or Sedation, 268
 *Standing Chemical Restraint, 268*
Anesthetic Induction, 269
 *Intravenous Induction, 269*
 *Inhalation Induction via Nasotracheal*
 *Tube, 272*
Endotracheal Intubation, 272
 *Equipment for Endotracheal Intubation, 272*
 *Selecting an Endotracheal Tube, 272*
 *Preparing the Tube, 272*
 *Intubation Procedure, 272*
 *Complications of Intubation, 273*

Maintenance of Anesthesia, 273
 *Maintenance with an Inhalant Agent, 273*
 *Maintenance with Intravenous Agents*
 *(Total Intravenous Anesthesia), 275*
 *Maintenance with Injectable and*
 *Inhalant Agents, 275*
Patient Positioning, Comfort, and Safety, 275
Anesthetic Recovery, 275
 *Preparation for Recovery, 276*
 *Monitoring during Recovery, 276*
 *Signs of Recovery, 277*
 *Extubation, 277*
 *Standing after Regaining Consciousness, 277*
Postanesthetic Period, 278

## KEY TERMS

Atelectasis
Demand valve
Epistaxis
Field anesthesia
Hypotension
Hypoventilation
Hypoxemia
Insufflation
Myopathy
Neuropathy
Positive inotrope
Standing chemical
 restraint
Total intravenous
 anesthesia
Ventilation-perfusion
 mismatch

## LEARNING OBJECTIVES

*After completion of this chapter, the reader will be able to:*
- Describe anesthetic techniques commonly used in equine practice.
- Explain the special anesthetic challenges resulting from patient temperament, large body size, and equine anatomy and physiology.
- List the causes of nasal congestion, atelectasis, neuropathy, and myopathy, and describe strategies to prevent these anesthetic complications.
- Describe the differences between anesthetic protocols and procedures used for field anesthesia and anesthesia in a clinic.
- Explain the indications for, the advantages of, and risks associated with standing chemical restraint.
- Describe anesthetic induction by intravenous injection and by inhalation via a nasotracheal tube.
- Prepare an equine patient, anesthetic equipment, and anesthetic agents and adjuncts for general anesthesia.
- Explain cautions and risks associated with each method of anesthetic induction, and strategies to maximize patient safety.
- Explain how to do each of the following: (1) select and prepare an endotracheal tube (ETT) for placement; (2) place an ETT in a horse; (3) check for proper placement; (4) inflate the cuff; (5) extubate a patient during anesthetic recovery.
- Describe maintenance of general anesthesia with an inhalant agent and with intravenous agents.
- List principles of providing appropriate patient positioning, comfort, and safety during anesthetic maintenance.
- Explain the significance of hypoventilation, hypoxemia, and hypotension in equine patients, as well as describe prevention and management strategies of these anesthetic complications.
- List factors that affect patient recovery from anesthesia, the signs of recovery, appropriate monitoring during recovery, and oxygen therapy during recovery.
- Describe general nursing care during the postanesthetic period.

The basic principles of anesthesia discussed in Chapter 8 apply to equine anesthesia. Horses present unique challenges to the anesthetist because of their temperament, size, anatomy, and physiology. The anesthetist should be aware of these concerns before anesthetizing equine patients.

Different breeds of horse, and even individuals within the same breed, can have varying temperaments ranging from calm and stoic to excitable and nervous. Also, because horses are "flight" animals (animals that tend to run away from stressful situations), even a normally calm, stoic horse can become excited in an unfamiliar environment such as a veterinary hospital. An excited horse may behave unpredictably and can cause injury to itself and veterinary personnel. A complete discussion of handling the equine patient is beyond the scope of this chapter; however, it is important to have a good understanding of how to catch, handle, and physically restrain a horse in order to minimize risk to the horse, the anesthetist, and other personnel. An aspect of equine behavior that differs from that of other species is that horses have an instinctive desire to stand shortly after awakening from anesthesia, a behavior that makes any equine anesthetic recovery relatively high risk. Ideally both induction and recovery from anesthesia should occur in a calm, quiet environment, with subdued lighting if possible.

The average adult horse weighs 350 to 500 kg, and some larger breed horses may weigh as much as 1000 kg. This necessitates having specialized equipment such as induction and recovery stalls, hoists, and special large animal surgery tables and anesthetic machines in addition to small animal machines and equipment, which are used for patients weighing less that 150 kg (foals, miniature horses). The equine anesthetist must be familiar with the operation of all related equipment in addition to anesthetic machines and monitors.

Anatomic concerns involve the respiratory, gastrointestinal, and musculoskeletal systems. Horses are obligate nasal breathers; thus anything that causes nasal obstruction, such as congestion (which develops when the head is below the withers during general anesthesia) or a horse pressing its nostrils against the recovery stall wall, can quickly lead to respiratory compromise and death without intervention. The large, heavy gastrointestinal tract places pressure on the lungs when horses are placed in dorsal or lateral recumbency, causing **atelectasis** (collapsed alveoli). Atelectatic lung tissue is not available for gas exchange; thus horses are prone to hypoxemia under anesthesia. Many anesthetic drugs affect the gastrointestinal tract (anticholinergics, opioids, alpha$_2$-agonists), which must be taken into consideration when protocols are selected, as horses are susceptible to developing colic. Some superficial nerves (e.g., facial nerve, radial nerve) can become damaged (**neuropathy**) if intraoperative padding is not appropriate or if the halter is inadvertently left on during anesthesia. Muscle blood flow must be maintained during anesthesia in order to prevent **myopathy**, which manifests in recovery as muscle hardness, pain, and weakness and is commonly referred to using the lay term "tying up." Insufficient padding can also lead to myopathy.

Because of these challenges, it is preferable, if the horse's temperament and the surgical approach allow, to perform procedures on lightly or heavily sedated horses. Heavy sedation is often referred to as **standing chemical restraint,** and these terms are used interchangeably. Many diagnostic and surgical procedures can be performed with the patient under standing chemical restraint with the addition of local anesthetic nerve blocks (Box 9-1). Horses that are not cooperative after sedation and horses undergoing more complex procedures (e.g., abdominal surgery, arthroscopy) do, however, require general anesthesia. General anesthesia is frequently carried out at farms or stables and is referred to as **field anesthesia.** As the name implies, field anesthesia occurs away from the veterinary hospital in a relatively clean stall or paddock and is appropriate for short procedures (20 to 45 minutes). Procedures that will last longer than 60 minutes, those that are complex, and those involving compromised patients should be performed at a veterinary clinic where inhalant anesthetics and oxygen can be administered using an anesthetic machine and where anesthetic monitoring is available. As with small animal anesthesia, neuromuscular blockers are rarely used in general practice but are sometimes used to provide muscle relaxation for ocular and orthopedic procedures in veterinary schools and referral practices.

---

**BOX 9-1    Examples of Procedures Commonly Performed under Sedation or Standing Chemical Restraint**

**Sedation**
- Radiographic studies
- Ultrasonographic studies
- Endoscopy
- Teeth floating
- Minor wound suturing
- Hoof trimming and shoeing
- Nasogastric intubation
- Venipuncture for catheter placement

**Standing Chemical Restraint in Conjunction with Local Nerve Blocks or Epidural Anesthesia**
- Eye and eyelid surgery
- Sinus and dental surgery
- Castration
- Major wound evaluation and repair
- Mass removals
- Rectovaginal fistula repair
- Laparoscopy
- Ovariectomy

## PATIENT PREPARATION

The reader is referred to Chapters 2 and 8 for a detailed discussion of the essentials of patient preparation before anesthesia. See Procedure 9-1, p. 279, for additional tasks pertinent to preparation of the equine patient undergoing general anesthesia. In addition, the anesthetist should be familiar with operation of additional equipment such as surgical tables and hoists that will be used during the anesthetic episode.

## SELECTING A PROTOCOL

A suitable protocol takes into account the minimum patient database, the patient's physical status class, and the type and duration of the procedure to be performed. Location also plays a role; field anesthesia is most commonly performed under **total intravenous anesthesia** (TIVA) whereas in a veterinary clinic the anesthetic protocol may be TIVA, or induction with an injectable drug followed by maintenance with an inhalant agent.

Regardless of the protocol, the correct drugs and amounts must be prepared. Box 8-2 shows the steps required to calculate the doses of most injectable drugs, and Box 9-2 shows an example of drug calculations for a horse. Ill, geriatric, pediatric, or otherwise compromised patients (physical status class P3 to P5) require use of modified protocols based on the patient's primary condition. Management of these cases can be quite challenging and requires customization of the anesthetic protocol by the veterinarian-in-charge (VIC).

## SUMMARY OF A GENERAL ANESTHETIC PROCEDURE

The dynamics for the commonly used protocols in equine anesthesia are similar to those for small animal (see Chapter 8), with the exception that induction with an intramuscular (IM) agent is not done in clinical practice, although it is used for capture of feral horses.

## EQUIPMENT PREPARATION

During a typical anesthetic induction, many events occur in rapid succession. Anesthetic agents are administered, the patient becomes unconscious and recumbent, and the endotracheal tube is placed, secured, and cuffed. The horse is then hoisted onto the surgery table, the halter is removed, and the endotracheal tube is connected to the anesthetic machine and the anesthetic gas level is adjusted, all within the first few minutes. Because these events follow one another so rapidly, the technician does not have the luxury of leaving the patient to locate equipment. For this reason, all equipment must be carefully gathered, checked, and organized before commencement of the procedure.

Equine patients weighing more than 150 kg are usually placed on a large animal anesthetic machine (Figure 9-1). Most large animal anesthetic machines incorporate a ventilator (Figure 9-1, *D*). Both the circle system and the ventilator of the machine should be checked before use. Smaller horses, ponies, and foals weighing less than 150 kg

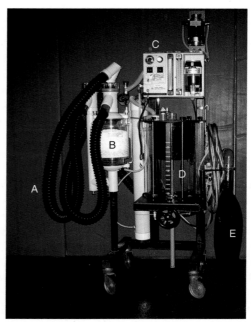

**FIGURE 9-1** Large animal anesthetic machine (Drager). *A,* Large animal breathing tubes and Y-piece. *B,* $CO_2$ absorber canister. *C,* Ventilator control panel, flow meters, and vaporizers. *D,* Ventilator bellows and housing. *E,* 35-L reservoir bag.

---

**BOX 9-2    Example of Dosage Calculations for Injectable Drugs**

How much ketamine and diazepam should you draw up to induce anesthesia in a 1200-lb quarter horse for arthroscopy? The prescribed dose of ketamine is 2.2 mg/kg, and the drug concentration is 100 mg/mL. The prescribed dose of diazepam is 0.05 mg/kg, and the drug concentration is 5 mg/mL.

$$\text{Patient body weight (kg)} = \frac{1200\ \text{lb} \times 1\ \text{kg}}{2.2\ \text{lb}} = 545\ \text{kg}$$

$$\text{Volume of ketamine (mL)} = \frac{545\ \text{kg} \times 2.2\ \text{mg/kg}}{100\ \text{mg/mL}} = 12\ \text{mL}$$

$$\text{Volume of diazepam (mL)} = \frac{545\ \text{kg} \times 0.05\ \text{mg/kg}}{5\ \text{mg/mL}} = 5.45\ \text{mL}$$

## PROTOCOL 9-1 — Premedication or Sedative Protocols for Physical Status Classification P1 and P2 Horses

### Protocols for Mild-Moderate Sedation (for Minor Procedures Such as Wound Debridement or Radiography)

1. **Acepromazine:** 0.03 to 0.05 mg/kg IV or IM *(Not for use in debilitated patients or in breeding stallions)*
2. **Xylazine:** 0.1 to 0.3 mg/kg IV
3. **Detomidine:** 0.005 to 0.01 mg/kg IV
4. **Romifidine:** 0.03 to 0.05 mg/kg IV
5. **Butorphanol:** 0.02 to 0.05 mg/kg can be combined in the same syringe with any one of the sedatives listed above and given intravenously for additional sedation

### Protocols for Premedication or Moderate-Deep Sedation

1. **Xylazine:** 1.1 mg/kg IV
2. **Detomidine:** 0.01 to 0.02 mg/kg IV
3. **Romifidine:** 0.05 to 0.1 mg/kg IV
4. **Butorphanol:** 0.05 to 0.2 mg/kg IV can be added to any of the alpha$_2$-agonists listed above to provide neuroleptanalgesia
5. **Morphine:** 0.05 to 0.1 mg/kg IV can be added to any of the alpha$_2$-agonists listed above to provide neuroleptanalgesia

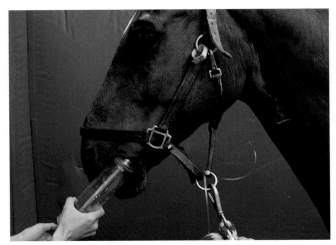

**FIGURE 9-2** Preparing a horse for general anesthesia. Flushing a horse's mouth with water using a large dosing syringe. The nozzle of the syringe is inserted between the horse's cheek and teeth. This is done on both sides of the mouth to flush out feed material.

can be placed on a small animal anesthetic machine. Hypothermia is uncommon in anesthetized adult horses; however, methods such as forced air warming and warm water circulating blankets can be used in smaller horses and foals. A crash cart containing emergency equipment and drugs should also always be available.

## PREMEDICATION OR SEDATION

*Premedication* refers to the administration of anesthetic agents and adjuncts to calm and prepare the patient for anesthetic induction. Preanesthetic medications are chosen specifically to produce a set of desired effects such as sedation, analgesia, and muscle relaxation. Tranquilizers, alpha$_2$-agonists, and opioids are commonly used as preanesthetic medications and are given via the IM or intravenous (IV) route. Anticholinergic drugs are not used to premedicate horses because they reduce gastrointestinal motility, which may result in colic. This class of drugs is therefore reserved for treatment of arrhythmias and for cardiopulmonary resuscitation (CPR) in this species.

The preanesthetic procedure in horses differs slightly from that used for small animals. After appropriate patient assessment, the first step is placement of an IV catheter (4 to 6 inch, 14 to 16 gauge), almost always in one of the jugular veins. Some horses object to venipuncture and must be sedated first. Such horses may be premedicated at this time (Protocol 9-1). Alternatively, a low dose of

xylazine (0.2 to 0.5 mg/kg IV) may be sufficient to achieve catheter placement. Once the horse is cooperative, a small bleb of local anesthetic is administered over the proposed site of catheterization to desensitize the skin.

After catheterization, the horse's mouth should be washed out with a large syringe (Figure 9-2) to flush out any feed material. This prevents aspiration of the material during intubation or in recovery. Feet should be cleaned before sedation, and then shoes should be removed or wrapped. Just before or immediately after premedication, the horse is positioned in an induction area or placed adjacent to a tilt table. Some breeds generally require higher doses of sedatives than others—for example, Arabians and thoroughbreds, particularly those in training—whereas draught horses typically require lower doses. See Protocol 9-1 for preanesthetic and sedative protocols in horses.

### Standing Chemical Restraint

Standing chemical restraint is essentially a continuation or extension of sedation. The patient is prepared as if it were having surgery, with placement of an IV catheter and extension set. The patient is usually secured in stocks for the procedure (Figure 9-3). If the level of sedation required for the procedure is inadequate, additional drugs are given intravenously. See Protocol 9-2 for standing chemical restraint protocols in horses. The dynamics of standing chemical restraint differ because general anesthesia is not the goal; the horse remains standing. The horse's level of consciousness may change from light to heavy sedation, which can be gauged based on the horse's level of interest in the environment, head position, and stance. On rare occasions general anesthesia may be required after or during standing restraint. If a horse becomes oversedated or becomes excited and falls

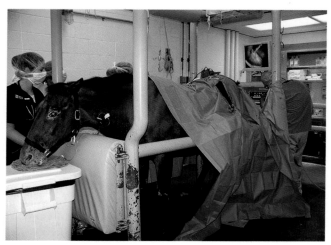

**FIGURE 9-3** Standing chemical restraint. Sedated horse standing in the stocks before preparation for procedure. An assistant should always be present to control the head of the horse.

## PROTOCOL 9-2 | Protocols for Standing Chemical Restraint

These protocols are used for major procedures such as laparoscopy; rectovaginal fistula repair; and sinus, eye, or dental surgery. Note that local anesthetic blocks or opioid epidurals may be required to facilitate these procedures.

1. **Xylazine + butorphanol IV**: Xylazine 0.5 to 1.1 mg/kg + butorphanol 0.05 to 0.1 mg/kg *(provides 20 to 30 minutes of chemical restraint).* Extend sedation with xylazine 0.025 to 0.5 mg/kg + butorphanol 0.025 to 0.05 mg/kg as needed.
2. **Detomidine + morphine IV**: Detomidine 0.02 mg/kg IV + morphine 0.1 mg/kg *(provides approximately 60 minutes of sedation).* Administer detomidine 0.01 mg/kg to extend sedation. *(Morphine has a longer duration of action than detomidine and thus does not need to be readministered).*

in the stocks, or if the veterinarian cannot perform the procedure because of inadequate sedation or surgical access, the anesthetist should be prepared to anesthetize the horse under instructions from the VIC. If the procedure lasts for a considerable period of time, the horse may develop nasal congestion, which could lead to respiratory obstruction. To avoid this, the head should be held up in a neutral position. If the horse is placed in stocks, cross-ties can be used for this purpose.

Signs of appropriate sedation before anesthetic induction or for standing restraint include lowering of the head and neck, drooping of the lower lip, a reluctance to move, a wide-based stance, and a lack of interest in the surrounding activity. Some horses remain sensitive to sudden loud noises and movements. This can be diminished by ensuring the work area of the induction stall is quiet, by covering the horse's eyes, or by placing cotton in the horse's ears. Moving a horse into position behind

a squeeze gate or into stocks may cause brief excitement or loss of sedation. Waiting for a few minutes will usually allow the horse to settle down. It may also be necessary to give additional sedative drug if the horse is not adequately sedated. It is also possible that external stimuli in an environment unfamiliar to the horse may result in the excitement, even if the horse initially appeared to be adequately sedated with acepromazine or an alpha$_2$-agonist. If this occurs, the horse should be given time to calm down (decrease external stimuli, refrain from trying to move the horse into the induction area) before proceeding. Again, additional sedation may also be required. Once the patient is adequately sedated, anesthetic induction should immediately follow, or, as an alternative, these protocols can be used alone to provide sedation for diagnostic and therapeutic procedures.

**TECHNICIAN NOTE** Remember that a horse can easily become aroused or excited after sedation with an alpha$_2$-agonist or acepromazine. Covering the horse's eyes with a towel or placing cotton in the horse's ears will decrease visual and auditory stimuli, which may enhance sedation.

## ANESTHETIC INDUCTION

Anesthetic induction is the process by which an animal loses consciousness and enters surgical anesthesia. In addition to the goals set out for induction in Chapter 8, an additional goal for equine anesthetic induction is to render the horse unconscious as quickly as possible so that its transition from standing to lateral recumbency occurs with minimal risk of injury to the horse or personnel. In healthy horses induction drugs are therefore given as rapid bolus injections, rather than "to effect." Induction is most commonly accomplished by IV administration of injectable agents, typically ketamine alone or in combination with other agents. Inhalant induction is reserved for foals that can be nasotracheally intubated while still awake; foals that will tolerate this are typically compromised and will require careful anesthetic management. What follows is a description of specific techniques used to induce anesthesia. (See Protocol 9-3 for IV induction protocols in horses, and Procedure 9-2, p. 279, for the sequence of events.)

**TECHNICIAN NOTE** One of the main goals of anesthetic induction is to render the horse unconscious as quickly as possible so that its transition from standing to lateral recumbency occurs with minimal risk of injury to the horse or personnel.

### Intravenous Induction

Unless it occurs in the field, induction typically occurs in a special induction stall that has padded walls and often a padded floor. Induction may be done "free fall" or behind

| **PROTOCOL 9-3** | **IV Induction Protocols for PSC P1 and P2 Horses** |
|---|---|

1. **Ketamine IV:** Ketamine 2.2 mg/kg
2. **Ketamine-diazepam IV:** Ketamine 2.2 mg/kg IV and diazepam 0.05 to 0.1 mg/kg IV mixed in the same syringe administered as a rapid bolus (*An equivalent volume of midazolam can be substituted for diazepam.*)
3. **Guaifenesin IV + ketamine IV:** Guaifenesin 25 to 50 mg/kg is administered under pressure to effect (horse becomes ataxic and "buckles" at the carpus joints), followed by ketamine 2.2 mg/kg bolus IV.

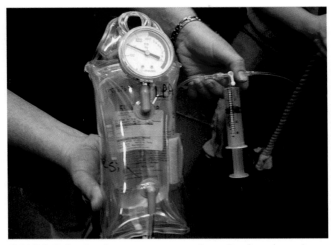

**FIGURE 9-5** Guaifenesin in a pressure bag. Guaifenesin is administered as a rapid infusion using a pressure bag. Note that the induction drug (in this case ketamine) is attached to the three-way stopcock so that once the desired level of muscle relaxation has been reached, anesthesia can be induced.

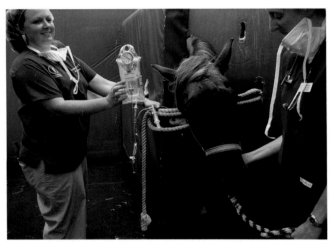

**FIGURE 9-4** Equine anesthetic induction gate. Premedicated horse restrained behind a gate before induction. The purpose of the rope (which is looped through a ring in the wall of the induction stall) is to prevent the horse from moving forward during induction and potentially injuring itself or personnel. One person controls the rope, and an assistant should always be present to control the head of the horse.

a gate that restrains the horse (Figure 9-4). Sometimes the induction stall is also used for recovery. In comparison to small animals, in which IV induction is given to effect, the goal of induction in horses is to rapidly take the horse from standing (sedated) to lateral recumbency (unconscious) so as to minimize excitement, which can lead to the horse's injuring itself or personnel. All drugs are therefore given as a bolus, with the exception of the muscle relaxant guaifenesin, which is administered rapidly intravenously to effect by placing it in a pressure bag (Figure 9-5). Once the horse shows signs of ataxia, typically knuckling of the forelimbs at the carpi and/or fetlocks, the induction agent is given as a bolus.

Once anesthesia has been induced, the vital signs should be briefly checked. The horse is then intubated.

In some practices the floor of the induction stall forms part of the surgery table, but in many the horse must be hoisted onto a table (Figure 9-6). It is important to understand how the hoist functions so that the horse can be transported safely and any problems can be resolved rapidly.

It is important to ensure that muscles and prominent nerves are protected when a horse is placed on a surgical table or surface. The anesthetist should make sure that muscle groups are well supported and do not rest on hard surfaces to prevent myopathy ("tying up") and that the facial and radial nerves are protected. Horses in lateral recumbency should have the forelimb closest to the table pulled forward if possible to decrease the pressure placed on it by the chest and opposite limb, and the hindlimbs should be separated by padding so that they are in a neutral position (Figure 9-7).

> **TECHNICIAN NOTE** It is important to ensure that the horse's muscles and prominent nerves are protected when it is placed on a surgical table or surface. The anesthetist should make sure that muscle groups are well supported and do not rest on hard surfaces during anesthesia, in order to prevent myopathies and neuropathies.

Agents commonly used to induce general anesthesia in horses by IV injection include (1) ketamine as a bolus injection, (2) a mixture of either ketamine and diazepam or midazolam as a bolus injection, and (3) guaifenesin infused under pressure to effect followed by ketamine as a bolus injection.

After induction with the commonly used IV injectable agents, the duration of anesthesia varies but is usually no more than 10 to 20 minutes. If a period longer than 20 minutes is required, anesthesia is maintained with inhalation anesthetics or administration of repeat boluses or a constant rate infusion (CRI) of ketamine. Occasionally horses will be too lightly anesthetized to intubate or place on the hoist after the induction dose. If this is the case, a bolus dose of ketamine at 0.4 mg/kg (one fifth of the induction dose) or thiopental at 0.5 mg/kg is given intravenously. See Procedure 9-3, p. 279, for IV induction in horses.

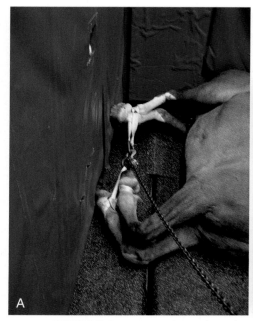
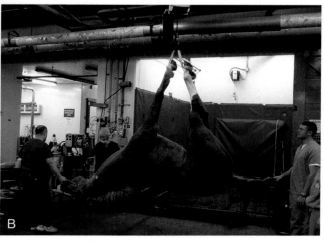

**FIGURE 9-6** Hoisting a horse after induction. **A,** Hobbles are placed distal to the fetlock joints of the front and hindlimbs and attached to the hook of a hoist. **B,** The horse is then hoisted so that a large animal surgery table can be positioned underneath it. The hoist can then be used to facilitate correct positioning on the table. The anesthetist controls and supports the head while an assistant controls the tail.

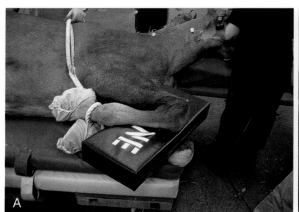
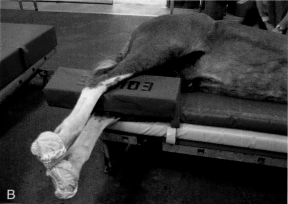
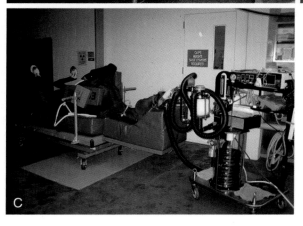

**FIGURE 9-7** Correct padding of a horse on a surgery table. **A,** In lateral recumbency the dependent forelimb is pulled forward before both forelimbs are secured with a rope. **B,** In lateral recumbency a pad is placed between the hindlimbs so they remain in a neutral position. **C,** In dorsal recumbency the horse's front limbs are tied and supported with pads. The hindlimbs are not tied and are left in a neutral, flexed position whenever possible. Note the thick foam pad used to support the horse; this prevents muscles of the rump and back from coming into contact with hard surfaces, which could lead to development of myopathy.

## Inhalation Induction via Nasotracheal Tube

This technique is limited to use in young foals, particularly those that are sick or those that will tolerate nasotracheal intubation. The anatomy of the horse's nasal passages and nasopharynx is such that an endotracheal tube passed from the nostril into the ventral nasal meatus will emerge in the nasopharynx in a position that favors entry into the larynx. Once the nasotracheal tube has been placed and the cuff inflated, the tube is connected to the breathing system of a small animal machine. Oxygen and inhalant are then administered. (See Protocol 9-4 for inhalant induction protocols in foals and Procedure 9-4, p. 280, for the technique.)

This technique has the same risks as mask induction in small animals (see Chapter 8). The placement of the nasotracheal tube has the advantage of having few, if any, leaks compared with mask induction; thus induction should be faster and can occur at lower vaporizer settings, and causes far less environmental pollution.

Foals that require general anesthesia and are amenable to nasotracheal intubation without sedation are often compromised. Care should be taken during inhalant induction in these patients because anesthesia may become deep relatively quickly compared with anesthesia in their healthy counterparts.

## ENDOTRACHEAL INTUBATION

After induction of general anesthesia, an endotracheal tube is usually placed. The advantages of intubation are discussed in Chapter 4, p. 97 and Chapter 8, p. 245.

## Equipment for Endotracheal Intubation

The following equipment is required to perform endotracheal intubation (Figure 9-8):
- Appropriately sized endotracheal tubes (at least two of slightly different diameters)
- A mouth gag to hold the jaws apart
- A 60-mL syringe to inflate the cuff
- Gauze sponge to grasp the tongue (if preferred)

## Selecting an Endotracheal Tube

The general principles for selecting an endotracheal tube are discussed in Chapter 8. Adult horses typically require a 22-mm, 26-mm, or 30-mm diameter cuffed tube. Because of head and neck length in horses, endobronchial intubation is rarely of concern. Typically two tube sizes are selected for intubation—the anticipated size and one size smaller. Foals require smaller tubes, but rarely smaller than 10 mm in diameter. Longer tubes of smaller diameter may be required for successful nasotracheal intubation in foals.

Endotracheal tubes are further discussed in Chapter 4.

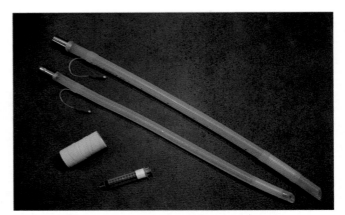

**FIGURE 9-8** Equipment for intubation of the horse. Appropriately sized endotracheal tubes, a mouth gag ("homemade" from polyvinyl chloride [PVC] pipe in this case), and a 60-mL syringe for inflating the cuff.

## Preparing the Tube

Before an endotracheal tube is used, it must be checked for integrity. It should be clean, sanitized, and free of blockages, holes, deterioration, or other damage. The connector must be securely attached, and the cuff must inflate and hold pressure after the syringe is detached from the valve. The tube may be lubricated with a small amount of sterile water-soluble lubricant, although this is not essential in most horses.

| PROTOCOL 9-4 | Inhalant Induction Protocols for PSC P1 and P2 Foals |
|---|---|

1. **Isoflurane:** Administer isoflurane at 4% to 5% by nasotracheal tube.*
2. **Sevoflurane:** Administer sevoflurane at 5% to 8% by nasotracheal tube.*

*Lower percentages should be used in sick foals.

## Intubation Procedure

Intubation in the horse is performed blindly. This means that the anesthetist does not directly visualize the larynx but instead passes the tube more by feel. The oral and oropharyngeal anatomy of the horse make blind intubation relatively easy. Unlike in other species, it is uncommon for the tube to pass into the esophagus.

The horse's head is extended, the tongue is gently pulled to the side of the mouth, and a mouth gag or speculum is placed. Mouth gags can be proprietary, or homemade from polyvinyl chloride (PVC) piping. The endotracheal tube is then passed through the mouth gag, over the base of the tongue, and into the larynx. If the anesthetist meets resistance at the level of the laryngopharynx, he or she should withdraw the tube 1 to 2 inches, rotate it 90 degrees, and advance it again (Figure 9-9 and Procedure 9-5, p. 280).

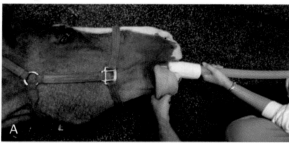
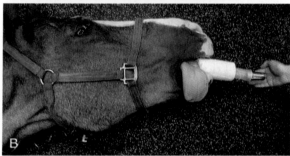

**FIGURE 9-9** Intubation of the horse. **A,** The anesthetist advances the endotracheal tube blindly through a speculum in the mouth into the larynx with the head extended. **B,** The anesthetist feels for movement of air when the horse breathes out to confirm correct placement of the tube in the trachea.

Advancement of the tube without resistance indicates successful placement in the trachea. Intubation is confirmed by feeling air move when the horse exhales, or when an assistant pushes on the thoracic wall. The endotracheal tube in horses is either tied to the mouth speculum or taped to the horse's muzzle. In the event that a tube will not pass into the larynx, changing the angle of the head slightly, changing the angle of the tube slightly, or trying with a smaller tube usually results in success. If there is any resistance, it is important not to force the tube, as this may damage the larynx.

> **TECHNICIAN NOTE** Orotracheal intubation in the horse is performed with the head and neck of the horse extended using a blind technique.

The cuff is inflated as for small animal intubation (see Chapter 8). Often it is partially inflated before hoisting, then, once the patient is connected to the anesthetic machine, the cuff is checked for proper inflation in the same way as for a small animal patient.

Nasotracheal intubation may be preferred over orotracheal intubation in horses undergoing some surgeries of the head and neck (e.g., sinus surgery, dental surgery). Nasotracheal intubation is performed by passing a well-lubricated tube, one size smaller than will likely pass orotracheally, into the ventral nasal meatus with the head in the same position as for orotracheal intubation.

The tube should be passed very gently in order to avoid damaging the nasal mucosa and turbinates and causing **epistaxis** (nosebleed).

## Complications of Intubation

Complications are similar to those in small animal anesthesia. Additional concerns include the following:

- Epistaxis may occur as a result of nasal intubation.
- Animals with abnormal anatomy (miniature horses, horses with diseases of the oral and nasal cavity, horses with laryngeal paralysis) may be difficult or impossible to intubate. These patients may require endoscopy-assisted intubation, in which an endoscope is passed through the tube and into the larynx, then the tube is threaded off the endoscope. In some cases placement of an endotracheal tube through a tracheostomy incision may be indicated.

Because healthy horses do not regurgitate under anesthesia, when horses are undergoing intraoral surgery, and for reasons of convenience, not all horses undergo endotracheal intubation during anesthesia. This is particularly true of field anesthesia. When oxygen is available, it is recommended that anesthetized horses be intubated and allowed to breathe oxygen.

## MAINTENANCE OF ANESTHESIA

After anesthetic induction and endotracheal intubation, patients that are in a light plane of anesthesia must be brought into surgical anesthesia. When the patient reaches the desired anesthetic depth, general anesthesia is maintained with injectable anesthetics (using TIVA), inhalant anesthetics delivered via an anesthetic machine, or a combination thereof. See Protocol 9-5 for maintenance protocols in horses.

### Maintenance with an Inhalant Agent

Maintenance of anesthesia with an inhalant agent is similar to that in a small animal patient, with the exception that sudden unexpected movement can occur without any change in signs of depth. Because of the large breathing circuit volume and patient size, response to changes in inhalant anesthetic and oxygen flow rates occur too slowly to return the patient to surgical anesthesia simply by altering machine settings. A syringe of thiopental or ketamine is typically drawn up before anesthesia and either attached to a three-way stopcock in the fluid administration line or kept close to the IV port for this purpose. Approximately one fifth of the IV induction dose is administered to the horse to return it to surgical anesthesia, which corresponds to 0.4 mg of ketamine per kilogram intravenously or 0.5 mg of thiopental per kilogram intravenously. See Procedure 9-6, p. 281.

## PROTOCOL 9-5   Maintenance Protocols for PSC P1 and P2 Horses

1. **Isoflurane:** Administer isoflurane at 1.5% to 2.5%.
2. **Sevoflurane:** Administer sevoflurane at 2.5% to 4%.
3. **Desflurane:** Administer desflurane at 8% to 12%.
4. **"Triple drip" CRI:** Administer at 1.5 mL/kg/hr (see Procedure 9-8 for details).
5. **Xylazine + ketamine IV:** Xylazine 0.25 mg/kg IV + ketamine 0.5 mg/kg IV. This is repeated each time the horse's anesthetic depth becomes light.

Compared with other species, horses are more likely to develop hypoxemia, hypoventilation, and hypotension during maintenance of anesthesia, particularly when inhalant agents are used.

In order to monitor blood pressure more accurately and to obtain arterial blood gas values, it is recommended that horses anesthetized with inhalant anesthetics for procedures lasting longer than 1 hour have an arterial catheter placed in a peripheral artery (facial, transverse facial, dorsal pedal) (Figure 9-10). Blood gas samples should be taken every 30 to 60 minutes, or more frequently if the situation warrants.

> **TECHNICIAN NOTE** Hypotension, hypoventilation, and hypoxemia are common complications in horses anesthetized with inhalant agents.

**Hypoventilation** is so common in anesthetized horses, particularly those placed in dorsal recumbency, that a ventilator is often used to maintain normal ventilation. See Chapter 6 for a discussion of mechanical ventilation.

**Hypotension** (mean arterial blood pressure <70 mm Hg) has been shown to contribute to myopathy, so treatment with drugs is frequently indicated if increased IV fluid rate, decreased anesthetic depth, and surgical stimulation do not increase blood pressure. The most common drug used to support blood pressure is the

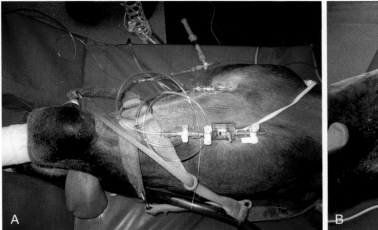
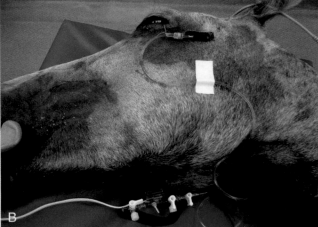
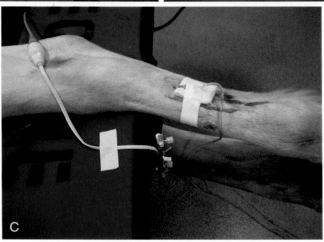

**FIGURE 9-10**   Direct blood pressure monitoring in the anesthetized horse. **A,** Catheter placed in the facial artery. **B,** Catheter placed in the transverse facial artery. **C,** Catheter placed in the dorsal metatarsal artery.

**positive inotrope** dobutamine (commonly administered via a syringe pump). Dobutamine and many other positive inotropes may cause arrhythmias, so it is important to monitor the electrocardiogram (ECG) closely when an infusion is being administered. See Procedure 9-7, p. 281, for preparation and administration of dobutamine.

> **TECHNICIAN NOTE** Dobutamine, a positive inotrope, is commonly used to treat hypotension in horses. Positive inotropes may cause arrhythmias, so the ECG should be closely monitored during infusion of dobutamine.

**Hypoxemia,** usually defined as a $PaO_2$ lower than 80 mm Hg, can occur in any horse, regardless of the physical status class. It is more common in horses that are obese, are pregnant, have torsed intestines, or are placed in dorsal recumbency. Hypoxemia has several possible causes, including hypoventilation, **ventilation-perfusion mismatch,** lung disease, and low cardiac output. Wherever possible the cause should be investigated and corrected.

### Maintenance with Intravenous Agents (Total Intravenous Anesthesia)

IV maintenance of anesthesia in horses is generally reserved for shorter procedures (less than 1 hour) in healthy patients, and for procedures done away from a veterinary clinic ("field anesthesia"). TIVA is generally characterized by higher blood pressure, less respiratory depression, and more active palpebral reflexes than inhalant anesthesia. When used for procedures lasting less than 1 hour, TIVA is associated with recoveries of good quality.

Anesthesia can be extended by administering additional doses of an alpha$_2$-agonist and ketamine. Typically half the amount of each drug used to sedate and induce anesthesia in the horse is administered intravenously to prolong anesthesia. The mainstay of TIVA in horses is, however, a combination commonly referred to as "triple drip." As its name suggests, this is a combination of three drugs: guaifenesin, ketamine, and xylazine (or any other alpha$_2$-agonist). Ketamine and xylazine are added to the guaifenesin and infused together to maintain anesthesia (see Procedure 9-8, p. 281, for preparation and administration of "triple drip").

> **TECHNICIAN NOTE** Maintenance of anesthesia in the field and for procedures of less than 1 hour in duration is typically accomplished using TIVA. The most common drug combination used for TIVA is a co-infusion of guaifenesin, ketamine, and xylazine, known as "triple drip."

### Maintenance with Injectable and Inhalant Agents

As an alternative, inhalant and injectable agents can be used in combination to maintain anesthesia. In equine anesthesia triple drip can be infused at a very slow rate (with a 10-gtt/mL administration set, 1 drop every 5 to 10 seconds is delivered to an adult horse), which will allow some reduction in the amount of inhalant required as well as providing muscle relaxation and analgesia. Lidocaine or detomidine infusions are also commonly administered to decrease inhalant requirements in horses and to produce analgesia.

## PATIENT POSITIONING, COMFORT, AND SAFETY

During anesthetic induction and maintenance, a number of considerations must be observed to ensure that the patient is not harmed. Many of the same principles of small animal anesthesia apply to equine anesthesia (see Chapter 8). Additional concerns are as follows:

- Take care to physically control the head to protect the eyes during gate inductions; horses will tend to fall against the wall or the gate, which leaves their eyes vulnerable to corneal scrapes.
- When hoisting horses, ensure that hobbles are correctly applied so that the horse cannot fall from the hoist or be injured by hobble placement.
- Correct positioning and padding on the surgery table are paramount to prevent neuropathies and myopathies.

## ANESTHETIC RECOVERY

Horses have a psychologic need to stand up shortly after awakening from anesthesia, and it is this that makes recovery particularly dangerous. Some steps can be taken to minimize injury to the horse and anesthetist, but there is a high incidence of complications from anesthetic recovery in horses, and clients should be informed of the risks. In veterinary clinics and hospitals, specific padded areas or rooms are dedicated as recovery stalls. In some clinics the induction stall is also used for recovery. Depending on the facilities and personnel available, horses may be left to recover unassisted after extubation, or may have ropes attached to the halter and tail with which personnel can assist the horse as it attempts to stand (Figure 9-11). Under field conditions the anesthetist typically restrains the horse by kneeling on its neck until the anesthetist believes the horse is ready to make a successful attempt to stand (see later for signs of recovery) (Figure 9-12). Personnel then typically hold the head and tail until the horse is able to stand unassisted.

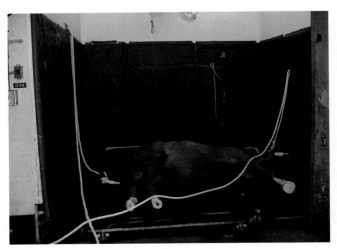

**FIGURE 9-11**   Rope placement for assisted recovery in a horse. One rope is attached to the halter, and the other is attached to the tail.

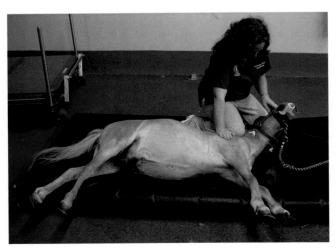

**FIGURE 9-12**   Anesthetist restraining a horse. The anesthetist can restrain a horse by kneeling on the horse's neck and lifting the muzzle slightly off the ground. Once the horse is awake enough to "lift" the anesthetist off its neck, the anesthetist may leave the recovery area and allow the horse to make an attempt to stand. This technique is useful in any size horse—in this case, a miniature horse.

## Preparation for Recovery

Replace the halter. Place a nasopharyngeal tube before movement if nasal congestion or edema is present (Figure 9-13). On completion of the procedure, turn off the inhalant and transfer the horse to a padded recovery stall, where it can be extubated and monitored. Horses are often placed on thick foam or air mattresses, although a padded floor may also give enough support. If possible, and particularly if the horse was hypoxemic during anesthesia, provide oxygen support using a **demand valve** (Figure 9-14) or **insufflation** (5 to 10 L/min nasally or through the endotracheal tube) until the horse is extubated or anesthesia is too light for the horse to tolerate an insufflation hose. A demand valve provides oxygen at a very high flow rate (160 to 280 L/min).

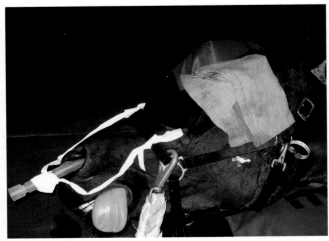

**FIGURE 9-13**   Nasopharyngeal tube placed for recovery. Through use of the same technique as for nasotracheal tube placement, a nasopharyngeal tube can be placed for recovery and secured to the halter. The tube is gently removed after the horse stands.

An assisted breath can be given as follows: remove the endotracheal tube connector from the tube; connect the demand valve to the endotracheal tube of the intubated horse; and manually depress the button while observing the chest wall (oxygen should flow into the patient's lungs and expand the chest). Once an adequate chest expansion is observed, release the button and disconnect the demand valve from the endotracheal tube to allow complete exhalation. Insufflation is the passive provision of oxygen: a tube that is able to fit inside the endotracheal tube, nasopharyngeal tube, or nostril is advanced to at least the level of the oropharynx; oxygen flow is set at 10 L/min.

> **TECHNICIAN NOTE**   If nasal congestion is present after anesthesia, a nasopharyngeal tube should be placed for recovery.

If the recovery is to be assisted by ropes, a head rope should be attached to the halter and another rope tied to the tail (see Figure 9-11). See Procedure 9-9, p. 281, for the sequence of events for preparing a horse for recovery.

## Monitoring during Recovery

During recovery it is ideal to watch the horse on a continual basis so that it can be assisted or sedated if necessary. While the horse is lying quietly the anesthetist should watch respirations to make sure the horse is breathing normally, take the pulse (facial artery) every 5 to 10 minutes, and assess the eye for depth of anesthesia. The anesthetist stays close to the head of the horse in order to monitor the pulse, to be ready for extubation, and to control the horse if it attempts to stand too soon.

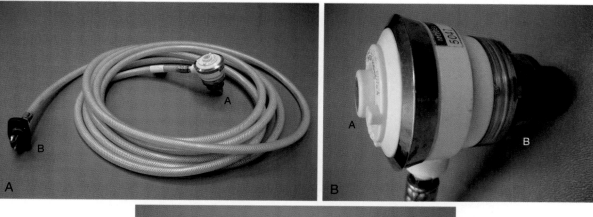

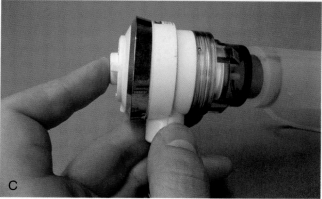

**FIGURE 9-14** Oxygen demand valve. **A,** An oxygen demand valve showing *A,* the demand valve and *B,* the quick-release connector, which is inserted into the hospital oxygen supply hose. **B,** Close up view of the demand valve showing *A,* manual button and *B,* connector for endotracheal tube. **C,** Demand valve connected to endotracheal tube (it is usually easier to remove the endotracheal tube connector when the demand valve is used).

## Signs of Recovery

As the patient recovers, it will progress back through the stages and planes of anesthesia. Many horses develop nystagmus during recovery, and rapid nystagmus accompanied by 'paddling' of the limbs generally means that a horse will try to get up too soon and will have a 'rough' recovery. In this event it may be prudent to sedate the horse with 0.1 to 0.2 mg of xylazine per kilogram intravenously and/or 0.01 to 0.03 mg of acepromazine per kilogram intravenously. Generally, maintaining control of the head by sitting on the neck or holding the head up off the floor will provide some control over the horse. However, once the horse is strong enough to lift an anesthetist off its neck, the anesthetist should retreat to a safe distance to observe the remainder of recovery. Other signs that a horse is recovering and may be close to extubation are chewing, swallowing, and purposeful ear, limb, or tail movement.

## Extubation

To prepare the patient for extubation, deflate the cuff by drawing out all the air until the pilot balloon is empty. Both before and after removal, keep the neck in a natural but extended position to protect the airway. Remove the endotracheal tube gently when the swallowing reflex returns, using a slow, steady motion. You may also remove it when signs of imminent arousal are present such as voluntary movement of the limbs or head, movement of the tongue, or chewing. Check to make sure the horse can breathe without obstruction. Horses can breathe only through their noses and will become distressed and compromised if they are unable to. If a nasopharyngeal tube has not been placed and the nasal passages are or become obstructed, one must be placed immediately. In the event that a nasopharyngeal tube does not alleviate the obstruction, a tracheostomy must be performed by the veterinarian, so materials for performing one must be close to the recovery stall at all times.

## Standing after Regaining Consciousness

The ideal recovery to standing is one in which the horse, after it is extubated, rolls smoothly from lateral to sternal recumbency. After lying in sternal recumbency for several minutes, the horse ideally makes a coordinated, strong attempt to stand and is successful on its first try.

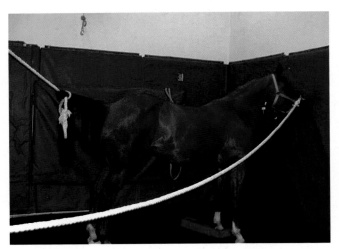

**FIGURE 9-15** Assisted anesthetic recovery using ropes with a horse. The head and tail rope are used to guide the horse as it attempts to stand. After the horse has made a successful attempt to stand, it may be necessary to leave the ropes on for several minutes as the horse continues to recover.

Head and tail ropes are used to assist the horse each time it attempts to stand (Figure 9-15). Unfortunately many horses, particularly those anesthetized for several hours with inhalant anesthesia, do not have ideal recoveries. With experience the anesthetist will learn when it is appropriate to provide additional sedation, analgesia, or physical assistance in the recovery stall to minimize injury to the horse. There is always the possibility that a horse may experience a catastrophic event during recovery, such as a fractured long bone (femur, tibia, humerus, radius). In such an event the VIC should assist the anesthetist in immediately reanesthetizing the horse to assess the situation.

## POSTANESTHETIC PERIOD

Once the horse is standing and able to walk steadily, it can be returned to its stall. This can be assessed by walking the horse in a circle inside the recovery stall. Once back in its own stall, the horse should be muzzled for 1 to 3 hours but should have free access to water. The horse should also be observed for any signs of neuropathy (e.g., facial nerve paralysis—drooping eyelid and lip on the affected side; radial nerve paralysis—inability to fully extend affected forelimb), myopathy (hard, swollen muscles, stiff and painful gait), or colic (rolling, kicking at the abdomen) in the postanesthetic period.

## KEY POINTS

1. Horses present unique challenges to the anesthetist because of their size, physiology, and temperament. Horses also seem to have a psychologic need to stand after anesthesia, making recovery from anesthesia challenging and potentially dangerous to horse and anesthetist.
2. Horses are susceptible to hypoventilation, nasal congestion, atelectasis, and hypoxemia during general anesthesia.
3. Superficial nerves are susceptible to pressure injury leading to neuropathy, and muscles are prone to injury if blood flow to them is inadequate during anesthesia. Attention must be paid to positioning and padding on the surgery table and in recovery.
4. Standing chemical restraint may be used to perform many surgical and medical procedures in horses, instead of general anesthesia, which is fraught with risks to the patient. The head should be supported in a neutral position in a standing sedated horse in order to minimize nasal congestion.
5. A horse should always be appropriately sedated before induction of general anesthesia.
6. Induction of anesthesia is typically done by injecting a rapid bolus of injectable anesthetic intravenously. This provides a smooth transition from standing to lateral recumbency with minimal risk of injury to the horse and anesthetist.
7. Maintenance of anesthesia in the field and for short procedures (<1 hour in duration) is typically accomplished using total intravenous anesthesia (TIVA). The most common drug combination used for this is a co-infusion of guaifenesin, ketamine, and xylazine, known as "triple drip."
8. Foals that are easily restrained may be nasotracheally intubated after sedation. The nasotracheal tube can then be attached to an anesthetic machine, and anesthesia can be induced using an inhalant anesthetic.
9. Intubation in equine patients is a blind procedure that is facilitated by extending the horse's head and neck.
10. Common problems encountered during maintenance of anesthesia are hypoventilation, hypoxemia, and hypotension. These problems are more common when anesthesia is maintained with inhalant anesthetics and in horses positioned in dorsal recumbency.
11. Recovery is the most challenging part of equine anesthesia. Various strategies can be employed to minimize injury to the horse and personnel; however, it is possible for any horse to have a recovery that is not ideal.
12. After general anesthesia horses should be monitored for signs of neuropathy, myopathy, pain, and colic.

## PROCEDURE 9-1　Preparation for Anesthesia of the Horse

1. Assess, prepare, and weigh the patient. If a large animal scale is not available, the weight must be estimated, preferably with a weight tape. (See section on patient preparation for a discussion of patient assessment, preparation, and stabilization.)
2. Prepare equipment for and place intravenous (IV) catheter, which may require intramuscular (IM) sedation in some horses (local anesthetic, antiseptic scrub, catheters, tape, heparinized saline, suture material, catheter cap, and/or extension line with three-way stopcock).
3. Rinse the horse's mouth, clean the hooves, and remove or wrap shoes when appropriate.
4. Determine the protocol (anesthetic agents including doses and routes and sequence of administration).
5. Calculate the volume of each agent to give including fluid administration rates (preanesthetic, induction, maintenance and analgesic agents).
6. Review oxygen flow rates (see Chapter 4).
7. Prepare equipment required to administer drugs (syringes, needles, agents, reversal agents, emergency cart, controlled substance log).
8. Prepare fluid administration equipment (fluids, administration and extension set, syringe pump).
9. Prepare equipment for endotracheal intubation (see Chapter 4).
10. Prepare monitoring equipment including arterial catheterization materials, anesthesia record, monitors, and probes (see Chapter 5).
11. Assemble and test the anesthetic machine and ventilator.

## PROCEDURE 9-2　Sequence of Events for Induction with an IV Agent and Maintenance with an Inhalant Agent in a Horse

1. Administer premedications intramuscularly approximately 20 to 30 minutes before or intravenously approximately 5 to 10 minutes before anesthetic induction.
2. If the horse is adequately sedated, administer the induction agent; otherwise give additional sedation before induction.
3. Check the patient's readiness for intubation.
4. Place and secure the endotracheal tube.
5. Inflate the endotracheal tube cuff.
6. Check the patient's vital signs.
7. Hoist, position, and secure the patient for the procedure, paying attention to padding of the face and lower limbs if the horse is in lateral recumbency, maintenance of an open airway, unrestricted blood flow, and unrestricted chest excursions. If the patient is placed in lateral recumbency, the dependent forelimb should be extended forward as far as possible, and padding should be placed between the hindlimbs. The forelimbs are usually secured with a rope.
8. Remove the halter.
9. Turn on the oxygen, and attach the endotracheal tube to the breathing circuit.
10. Turn on the inhalant anesthetic to the appropriate level.
11. Determine the patient's anesthetic depth, and commence regular monitoring.
12. Attach intravenous fluid administration line, commence fluid administration at appropriate rate.
13. Attach noninvasive monitoring devices.
14. Place arterial catheter and connect to direct blood pressure monitor.
15. Continue to monitor and adjust the anesthetic and oxygen levels as needed until completion of the procedure.

## PROCEDURE 9-3　IV Induction in Horses

Induction of anesthesia in horses differs from that in small animals in that the goal is to achieve lateral recumbency without excitement or injury to the horse or personnel. In order to do this, the induction agent is given as a rapid IV bolus in PSC P1 and P2 horses. The only induction drug that is given "to effect" (see Procedure 8-3) is guaifenesin.

- **Ketamine-diazepam** and **ketamine-midazolam mixtures:** The anesthetist checks to make sure that the IV catheter is patent and still in the jugular vein, then the entire syringe of the calculated dose of drugs is rapidly injected into the catheter or extension set, then flushed using heparinized saline. Care must be taken to ensure all connections are secure prior to injecting to avoid administering partial doses, which could result in a partially induced and excited horse.
- **Guaifenesin** and **ketamine:** A bag of guaifenesin with an IV administration set attached is placed in a pressure sleeve, which is inflated up to 300 mm Hg pressure. The administration set is connected to the IV catheter or extension set. The anesthetist checks to make sure that the IV catheter is patent and still in the jugular vein, then the guaifenesin is administered under pressure to effect. Approximately 0.5 to 1 mL/kg will produce signs of ataxia (knuckling over at the carpus and fetlock), at which point ketamine is administered as a bolus.

## PROCEDURE 9-4    Inhalant Induction via Nasotracheal Intubation in Foals

1. In a tractable or sedated foal, place a nasotracheal tube by the following method: extend the head and neck, and pass a lubricated endotracheal tube through a nostril into the ventral meatus of the nasal cavity (Figure 1). Gently advance the tube into the nasopharynx. As the foal inhales, advance the tube into the larynx (Figure 2).
2. Connect the Y-piece of a rebreathing circuit to the endotracheal tube.
3. Give 100% oxygen for 2 to 3 minutes at 1 to 3 L/min.
4. Set the anesthetic vaporizer to deliver 0.5% isoflurane or 1% sevoflurane. Sevoflurane is less pungent than isoflurane and better accepted.

5. Gradually increase the concentration of anesthetic by small increments (0.5% every 30 seconds for isoflurane and 1% every 30 seconds for sevoflurane) until an anesthetic concentration of 4% to 5% is reached for isoflurane and 6% to 8% for sevoflurane. Use lower maximum concentrations in compromised or very young foals. If the foal struggles, the vaporizer concentration can be increased more rapidly.
6. Monitor the foal carefully for increasing depth of anesthesia, and turn the vaporizer to maintenance levels as soon as the patient is in a surgical plane of anesthesia (1.5% to 2% for isoflurane and 2.5% to 3.5% for sevoflurane).

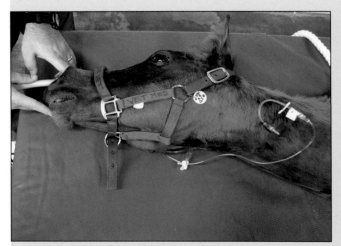

**FIGURE 1**   In an amenable or sedated foal, the anesthetist directs the tube into the ventral nasal meatus. It is helpful to use the finger of the hand not holding the tube to palpate the ventral meatus, as well as to direct the tube ventrally into it. As with orotracheal intubation, the head and neck should be extended.

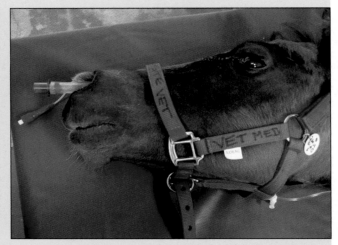

**FIGURE 2**   Once the tube has been placed in the ventral meatus it is gently advanced toward and into the larynx. The tube can then be connected to an anesthetic machine for inhalant induction.

## PROCEDURE 9-5    Intubation Procedure for Horses

Horses are generally intubated in lateral recumbency.*
1. Place a mouth speculum or gag between the incisors.
2. Grasp the tongue and pull it out of the mouth between the lips and the speculum.
3. Extend the head and neck: the person intubating can use a knee to press the head away, or the hand that grasps the tongue can push.
4. With care taken to keep the tube in the center of the oral cavity to avoid laceration of the cuff by the molars, the tube is gently advanced toward, then through, the larynx.
5. If the anesthetist encounters resistance at the level of the larynx, the tube is withdrawn 1 to 2 inches and rotated 90 degrees before he or she tries to advance it again.

6. Check to ensure that the tube is in the trachea by feeling air pass during exhalation or when an assistant presses down on the horse's chest.
7. A small volume of air may be placed in the cuff (20 to 60 mL) before the horse is hoisted.
8. After the horse has been positioned on the surgery table, connect the endotracheal tube to the anesthetic breathing system and allow the horse to breathe 100% oxygen.
9. Check the tube for leaks.
10. Turn on the anesthetic vaporizer, and adjust the appropriate level.
11. Commence regular monitoring.

*Horses can be intubated in sternal recumbency, although this requires that the horse be supported in this position. Sternal intubation is typically reserved for horses that have significant nasogastric reflux because of colic.

## PROCEDURE 9-6  Anesthetic Maintenance with Inhalant Anesthetic in Horses

General anesthesia maintained with inhalant is similar to the procedure described for small animals (see Procedure 8-7).

1. Choose the initial dial setting based on the anesthetic depth after intubation.
2. Set the oxygen flow rate to 8 to 10 L/min for an adult horse for 10 to 15 minutes to wash out the large amount of nitrogen that is present in a horse's lungs. Then turn the flow rate down to 3 to 5 L/min for the remainder of the procedure.
3. Make periodic changes in the vaporizer dial setting based on monitoring parameters.
4. If the anesthetic depth is slightly too light or deep, make small dial changes of approximately 0.5% to 1% increments with isoflurane and sevoflurane.
5. If the patient's anesthetic depth is significantly light (e.g., patient exhibits spontaneous movement, swallowing, active reflexes, strong muscle tone), administer a bolus of thiopental 0.5 mg/kg IV or ketamine 0.4 mg/kg IV. It may also be necessary to increase the oxygen flow to 8 to 10 L/min and set isoflurane at 4% to 5%, or sevoflurane at 5% to 8% (induction levels).

## PROCEDURE 9-7  How to Prepare and Administer Dobutamine Using a Syringe Pump

1. Draw 56 mL of 0.9% sodium chloride into a 60-mL syringe.
2. Draw 4 mL of dobutamine (15 mg/mL) into the syringe.
3. The concentration of dobutamine is now 1 mg/mL (1000 mcg/mL).
4. Place the syringe in a syringe pump and program in the infusion rate in milliliters or micrograms per minute, or in milliliters or micrograms per hour (the prompts displayed by the pump's menu will give accepted units).
5. Typical infusion rates for dobutamine in horses range from 0.5 to 5 mcg/kg/min, usually starting at the lower end. Administering 1 mcg/kg/min to a 500-kg horse results in an infusion rate of 30 mL/hr.
6. Attach the syringe to the port of a primed infusion set.
7. Place the needle of the winged infusion set into the injection port of an IV administration set near the catheter.

## PROCEDURE 9-8  How to Prepare and Administer "Triple Drip"*

1. Add 2.5 mL of xylazine (100 mg/mL) to 500 mL of 5% guaifenesin.
2. Add 5 mL of ketamine (100 mg/mL) to 500 mL of 5% guaifenesin.
3. Each milliliter of "triple drip" contains 0.5 mg xylazine, 1 mg ketamine, and 50 mg guaifenesin.
4. Administer via CRI at 1.5 mL/kg/hr, which equates to xylazine 0.75 mg/kg/hr, ketamine 1.5 mg/kg/hr, and guaifenesin 75 mg/kg/hr.
5. Temporarily increase infusion rate if patient's anesthetic depth becomes light (e.g., patient exhibits movement, rapid nystagmus, swallowing).

*Note that there are other ways to formulate "triple drip." Some practices substitute detomidine or romifidine for xylazine, and some will use different final concentrations of drugs. In the latter case, infusion rates will vary.

## PROCEDURE 9-9  Recovery from General Anesthesia in the Horse

1. Prepare the patient for recovery, including placement of a nasopharyngeal tube and removal of monitoring equipment. Ensure the recovery area has been prepared.
2. Discontinue the anesthetic, and transfer the horse to the recovery area, paying attention to positioning.
3. Extubate the patient at the appropriate time, and ensure the horse can breath through its nostrils without obstruction.
4. Assist the horse until it stands as directed by the veterinarian.
5. Prepare the patient for continued hospitalization or discharge by applying bandages, administering medications, and performing any other procedures ordered by the doctor.

## REVIEW QUESTIONS

1. Which of the following is true regarding use of standing chemical restraint for performing surgery on a horse?
   a. Horses must be endotracheally intubated for standing chemical restraint.
   b. Risk of myopathy or neuropathy is higher with standing chemical restraint.
   c. The head must be supported in a normal position to avoid nasal congestion.
   d. Hypoxemia is a common complication of standing chemical restraint.

2. If a horse becomes excited after it has been premedicated with xylazine intravenously before general anesthesia, the next step the anesthetist should take is to:
   a. Allow the horse time to calm down before proceeding
   b. Physically restrain the horse using ropes
   c. Induce anesthesia with acepromazine
   d. Induce anesthesia with ketamine

3. Appropriate positioning and padding of the horse on the surgery table is essential to prevent:
   a. Hypoxemia and hypotension
   b. Myopathies and neuropathies
   c. Hypoventilation and hypertension
   d. Regurgitation and aspiration

4. What is the main reason for including guaifenesin in an induction protocol in horses?
   a. Muscle relaxation
   b. Analgesia
   c. Sedation
   d. All of the above

5. An inhalant induction via nasotracheal tube placement is appropriate for which of the following patients?
   a. A 2-year-old Arabian stallion undergoing arthroscopy
   b. A 25-year-old thoroughbred mare undergoing sinus surgery
   c. A 3-week-old foal undergoing colic surgery
   d. A 6-month-old foal undergoing umbilical hernia repair

6. Which of the following statements best describes endotracheal intubation in the horse?
   a. Intubation is performed blindly with the head and neck extended.
   b. Intubation can be performed only with the patient in lateral recumbency.
   c. A laryngoscope is useful for visualization of the larynx.
   d. An endoscope is commonly used to facilitate intubation.

7. The most common complications during maintenance of anesthesia in horses with inhalant anesthetics are:
   a. Hypoxemia, hypertension, and bradycardia
   b. Hypoxemia, hypotension, and bradycardia
   c. Hypoxemia, hypertension, and hypoventilation
   d. Hypoxemia, hypotension, and hypoventilation

8. Which drug is used to treat hypotension in the anesthetized horse?
   a. Dextrose
   b. Digoxin
   c. Dobutamine
   d. Doxycycline

9. Of all phases of anesthesia, recovery poses the highest risk to the horse and is the phase over which the anesthetist has the least control.
   True                    False

10. A horse has recovered from anesthesia for arthroscopy and shows the following symptoms: hard, swollen gluteal muscles, stiff gait, and reluctance to walk. The most likely diagnosis is:
    a. Colic
    b. Myopathy
    c. Neuropathy
    d. Nephropathy

## SELECTED READINGS

Muir WW, Hubbell JAE: *Equine anesthesia*, ed 2, St Louis, 2009, Elsevier.

Robertson SA: Sedation and anesthesia of the foal, *Equine Vet Educ* 9:37–44, 1997.

Tranquilli WJ, Thurmon JC, Grimm KA: *Veterinary anesthesia and analgesia*, ed 4, Ames, Iowa, 2007, Blackwell.

# Ruminant and Swine Anesthesia

# 10

## KEY TERMS

Bolus
Eructate
Porcine stress
  syndrome
Regurgitus
Tilt tables
TKX
Total injectable
  anesthesia

## OUTLINE

**Ruminants,** 283
Patient Preparation, 284
Selecting a Protocol, 284
Summary of a General Anesthetic
    Procedure, 284
    *Equipment Preparation, 284*
    *Premedication or Sedation, 285*
    *Anesthetic Induction, 285*
    *Endotracheal Intubation, 286*
    *Maintenance of Anesthesia, 287*
    *Patient Positioning, Comfort,*
        *and Safety, 288*

*Anesthetic Recovery, 288*
*Postanesthetic Period, 289*
**Swine,** 289
Physical Examination, 289
Summary of a General Anesthetic
    Procedure, 289
    *Sedation, 289*
    *Anesthetic Induction, 290*
    *Intubation, 290*
    *Maintenance of Anesthesia, 290*
    *Monitoring, 292*
    *Recovery, 292*

## LEARNING OBJECTIVES

*After completion of this chapter, the reader will be able to:*
* Describe the main physiologic and anatomic differences that influence anesthetic management of ruminants and swine.
* Explain how to prepare a ruminant or porcine patient for anesthesia.
* Select an anesthetic protocol for an American Society of Anesthesiologists (ASA) PS1 or PS2 adult cow, small ruminant, and pig.
* Explain how to intubate an adult cow, a small ruminant or calf, and a pig.
* Explain the importance of positioning of ruminants under general anesthesia.
* Explain how to position a ruminant for recovery.
* Explain the anesthetic concerns and challenges regarding anesthetizing pigs.
* Describe the signs of porcine stress syndrome.

## RUMINANTS

The basic principles of anesthesia discussed in Chapter 8 apply to ruminant anesthesia. Ruminants do not pose quite the same challenge to the anesthetist as horses; however, an understanding of their unique digestive physiology is important because it affects the well-being of the patient under general anesthesia. In addition, ruminants are presented for general anesthesia less frequently than small animals or horses are, so it takes longer to gain anesthetic experience. There are several reasons for this. Because of their relatively calm nature, ruminants require general anesthesia for relatively few procedures. Many surgeries can be conducted using local or regional anesthetic techniques (see Chapter 6) in conjunction with physical restraint. Consideration must also be given to drug withdrawal times when dealing with animals that produce milk or meat for human consumption. Finally, administration of general anesthesia to production animals is often uneconomical.

Ruminant patients range in size from a few kilograms (lambs and kids) to over 1000 kg (adult bull). Thus, as with horses, specialized **tilt tables,** head gates, hoists, and transporters may be required to allow the veterinarian to perform surgery or procedures such as hoof-trimming safely without injury to the animal. Equipment suitable for anesthetizing small animal patients is commonly used for smaller patients (sheep, goats, calves). However if young cattle >150 kg and adult cattle are to undergo general anesthesia, the anesthetist must have access to a large animal anesthesia machine and be familiar with its operation as well as that of related equipment and monitors.

The main anesthetic concerns in ruminants result from their unique digestive anatomy and physiology. Ruminants constantly produce large volumes of saliva compared with other species, and this is generally not inhibited by general anesthesia. They are thus prone to aspiration if the airway is not protected. In addition, regurgitation of ruminal contents (known as **regurgitus**) can occur at any stage of general anesthesia and occur most commonly in light and deep planes. Fermentation in the rumen is only slightly decreased by general anesthesia; thus ruminants are predisposed to bloat, as they cannot **eructate** when they are unconscious.

As with small animal anesthesia, neuromuscular blockers are rarely used in general practice but are sometimes used to provide muscle relaxation for ocular and orthopedic procedures in veterinary schools and referral practices.

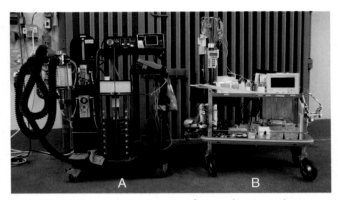

**FIGURE 10-1**   Anesthetic equipment for anesthetizing a large ruminant. *A,* Large animal anesthetic machine and ventilator. *B,* An anesthetic cart with drugs, syringes, endotracheal tubes, a mouth gag for adult cattle, and anesthetic monitor ready for anesthetizing a large ruminant.

## PATIENT PREPARATION

The reader is referred to Chapters 2 and 8 for a detailed discussion of the essentials of patient preparation before anesthesia. See Procedure 10-1, p. 294, for additional tasks pertinent to preparation of the ruminant patient undergoing general anesthesia. In addition, the anesthetist should be familiar with operation of additional equipment such as surgical tables, transporters, head gates, and hoists that will be used during the anesthetic episode.

It is key to ensure that ruminants have been adequately fasted before anesthesia. Fasting reduces the size of the rumen and also decreases microbial activity. This in turn decreases gas production during anesthesia. Normally ruminants eructate to expel the gas from the rumen; however, under anesthesia this does not happen, which can lead to bloating. A bloated rumen can put pressure on the diaphragm and large blood vessels (aorta, caudal vena cava) in the abdomen, resulting in respiratory as well as circulatory compromise. Once an anesthetized ruminant has developed severe bloat, it can be very difficult to treat and may lead to the death of the patient if it goes unnoticed or untreated. Bloat often goes unrecognized when a patient is small and covered by surgical drapes. Signs include development of a distended, tight abdomen, decreased blood pressure, increased heart rate, and decreased ventilation.

## SELECTING A PROTOCOL

A suitable protocol takes into account the minimum patient database, the patient's physical status class, and the type and duration of procedure to be performed. Regardless of the protocol, the correct drugs and amounts must be prepared. Ill, geriatric, pediatric, or otherwise compromised patients (physical status class P3 to P5) require use of modified protocols based on the patient's primary condition. Management of these cases can be quite challenging and requires customization of the anesthetic protocol by the veterinarian-in-charge (VIC).

## SUMMARY OF A GENERAL ANESTHETIC PROCEDURE

The dynamics for the commonly used protocols in ruminant anesthesia are very similar to those for small animals (see Chapter 8, p. 236), with the exception that induction with an intramuscular (IM) agent is not commonly done in clinical practice.

### Equipment Preparation

During a typical anesthetic induction, many events occur in rapid succession. Anesthetic agents are administered, the patient becomes unconscious and recumbent, and the endotracheal tube is placed, secured, and cuffed. The patient is then lifted or hoisted onto the surgery table, the endotracheal tube is connected to the anesthetic machine, and the anesthetic gas level is adjusted, all within the first few minutes. Because these events follow one another so rapidly, the technician does not have the luxury of leaving the patient to locate equipment (Figure 10-1). For this reason, all equipment must be carefully gathered, checked, and organized before commencement of the procedure.

Patients weighing more than 150 kg are usually placed on a large animal anesthetic machine (see Figure 9-1). Most large animal anesthetic machines incorporate a ventilator (see Figure 9-1, *D*). Both the circle system and the ventilator of the machine should be checked before use. Small ruminants and calves weighing less than 150 kg can be placed on a small animal anesthetic machine. Hypothermia is uncommon in anesthetized adult cattle; however, devices such as warm air blankets or warm water circulating blankets can be used to maintain body temperature in small ruminants and calves as for small animal patients.

Any specialized equipment required for restraining or positioning anesthetized ruminants, such as head gates, transporters, and tilt tables, should be checked. In addition to the items from the standard checklist, it is extremely helpful to have suction available for small ruminants to allow feed material, regurgitus, or saliva to be removed from the pharynx during intubation.

A crash cart containing emergency equipment and drugs should also always be available.

## Premedication or Sedation

Many ruminants are calm and tractable enough to allow intravenous (IV) catheterization and induction of anesthesia with minimal or no premedication and mild restraint. Adult cattle are typically restrained using the head gate of a transporter or chute, or against a tilt-table. Premedication is often reserved for patients that are aggressive, excited, or stressed. Despite the fact that many ruminants do not require sedation before anesthesia, premedication will still provide benefits such as decreased dose of induction and maintenance drugs, muscle relaxation, and analgesia.

> **TECHNICIAN NOTE** Ruminants are very sensitive to xylazine, requiring one tenth the dose that horses do.

Anticholinergic drugs are not used to premedicate ruminants because they do not reduce salivation but instead cause the saliva to become thick and ropy. These thicker strands of saliva are more easily aspirated. This class of drugs is therefore reserved for treatment of arrhythmias and for cardiopulmonary resuscitation (CPR) in this species. See Protocol 10-1 for sedative and premedication drugs and doses in ruminants.

> **TECHNICIAN NOTE** Anticholinergics should not be used for premedication of ruminants, because they do not decrease salivation but instead make it thick and ropy, increasing the risk of aspiration.

## Anesthetic Induction

Anesthetic induction is the process by which an animal loses consciousness and enters surgical anesthesia. Of the goals set out for induction in Chapter 8, it is particularly important to gain control of and protect the airway as quickly as possible in ruminants.

What follows is a description of specific techniques used to induce anesthesia. See Protocol 10-2 for IV induction protocols in ruminants, and Procedure 10-2, p. 290, for the sequence of events for induction with an IV agent and maintenance with an inhalant agent in a ruminant.

---

**PROTOCOL 10-1** | **Premedication and Sedative Protocols for Physical Status Classification (PSC) P1 and P2 Ruminants**

**Protocols for Mild-Moderate Sedation***
1. **Acepromazine:** 0.01 to 0.03 mg/kg IV (May increase regurgitation)
2. **Xylazine:** 0.01 to 0.05 mg/kg IV or IM (Unlikely to cause recumbency)
3. **Detomidine:** 0.005 to 0.02 mg/kg IV

**Protocols for Moderate-Heavy Sedation (for Minor Procedures Such as Radiography or Wound Assessment) or for Premedication†**
1. **Acepromazine:** 0.03 to 0.05 mg/kg IV
2. **Xylazine:** 0.05 to 0.1 mg/kg IV or 0.05 to 0.2 mg/kg IM (Likely to cause recumbency and potentially light anesthesia)
3. **Detomidine:** 0.01 to 0.03 mg/kg IV
4. **Midazolam + butorphanol:** Midazolam 0.1 mg/kg plus butorphanol 0.1 to 0.2 mg/kg IV (May produce ataxia, so recommended for small ruminants or restrained cattle)

*Many ruminants require no sedation for standing procedures performed with local anesthetic.
†Many ruminants do not require premedication before anesthesia.

---

**PROTOCOL 10-2** | **IV Induction Protocols for PSC P1 and P2 Ruminants**

1. **Ketamine + diazepam:** Ketamine 2.5 mg/kg IV and diazepam* 0.12 mg/kg IV mixed in the same syringe. (Dose is calculated as 1 mL of the mixture per 20 kg of body weight most commonly for small ruminants. Note the difference from the small animal dosage of 1 mL per 10 kg of body weight.)
2. **"Double drip":** Administered to effect (approximately 1 to 2 mL/kg) IV. ("Double drip" can be made by adding 500 mg of ketamine to a 500-mL bag of 5% guaifenesin. Each milliliter of 'double drip' therefore contains 1 mg of ketamine and 50 mg of guaifenesin.)
3. **Telazol:** 1 to 4 mg/kg IV (Lower dose after xylazine premedication.)
4. **Propofol:** 2 to 4 mg/kg IV (For small ruminants only; not economical for adult cattle.)

*An equivalent volume of midazolam can be used in place of diazepam.

## Intravenous Induction

Induction in large cattle may occur in a special induction stall that has padded walls and often a padded floor, in a transporter, or on a tilt table. Smaller ruminants can generally undergo induction next to the surgery table or, if small or severely compromised, while lying on the surgery table. Although ruminants do not typically become excited during induction of anesthesia, the goal with adult cattle is similar to that in horses: to rapidly produce

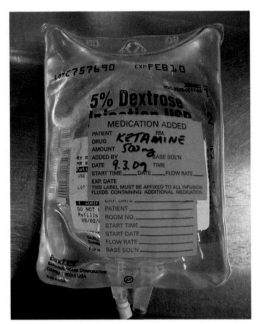

**FIGURE 10-2**   "Double drip." A 500-mL bag of 5% dextrose in water containing 5% guaifenesin, to which 5 mL of ketamine has been added. Final concentrations are therefore 1 mg of ketamine per milliliter and 50 mg of guaifenesin per milliliter.

unconsciousness and minimize injury of the patient or personnel. Drugs are thus given to the larger ruminants as a **bolus,** with the exception of "double drip" (see Protocol 10-2 and Figure 10-2), which is administered rapidly intravenously to effect. Smaller ruminants, particularly those that are compromised, can be given induction drugs to effect as for small animal patients.

Once the patient is unconscious, it should be kept in sternal recumbency for intubation whenever possible. It is important to be vigilant for regurgitation, which can occur at any point of the anesthetic procedure but occurs most frequently when anesthesia is light or too deep. If regurgitation occurs the head should immediately be positioned so that it is lower than the body to prevent aspiration.

Once anesthesia has been induced, the vital signs should be briefly checked before intubation. See Procedure 10-3, p. 295, for IV induction techniques in adult cattle.

## Endotracheal Intubation

After induction of general anesthesia, an endotracheal tube is usually placed in the patient's airway. The advantages of intubation are discussed in Chapter 4 on p. 98 and Chapter 8 on p. 245.

### Equipment for Endotracheal Intubation

The following equipment is required for endotracheal intubation:

- Appropriately sized endotracheal tubes (at least two of slightly different diameters)
- Stylette (small ruminants and calves only)
- A mouth gag to hold the jaws apart (adult cattle only)
- Laryngoscope (small ruminants and calves)
- Gauze sponge to grasp the tongue (if preferred)
- A syringe to inflate the cuff (10 mL for small ruminants and calves or 60 mL for adult cattle)

### Selecting an Endotracheal Tube

The general principles for selecting an endotracheal tube are discussed in Chapter 8. Adult cattle typically require a 22-mm–, 26-mm–, or 30-mm–diameter cuffed tube. Typically two tube sizes are selected for intubation—the anticipated size and one size smaller. Small ruminants and calves require smaller tubes.

Endotracheal tubes are further discussed in Chapter 4.

### Preparing the Tube

Before an endotracheal tube is used, it must be checked for integrity. It should be clean, sanitized, and free of blockages, holes, deterioration, or other damage. The connector must be securely attached, and the cuff must inflate and hold pressure after detaching the syringe from the valve. The tube may be lubricated with a small amount of sterile water-soluble lubricant, although this is not essential in adult cattle.

### Intubation Procedure

The procedure for intubation of small ruminants and calves differs from that for adult cattle.

#### Small Ruminants and Calves

Intubation in small ruminants and calves is accomplished as for small animal patients. The oral opening is small in these patients compared with the distance between the mouth and larynx, so visualization of the airway can be challenging. In addition, the caudal half of the tongue is thickened, which further obstructs the anesthetist's view. Attempting to pass the endotracheal tube alone typically completely obstructs the view, making successful placement extremely challenging, and more a matter of luck than skill. Thus using a stylette that protrudes beyond the end of the tube allows better visualization of the larynx.

With the head extended by an assistant, the anesthetist places a laryngoscope to visualize the larynx. It often helps to grasp the tongue with a gauze sponge and gently pull it forward. The anesthetist then passes the stylette into the airway, taking care not to cause injury to the larynx or trachea. The endotracheal tube can then be passed over the stylette and into the larynx (Figure 10-3).

The cuff is inflated as for small animal intubation (see Chapter 8).

#### Adult Cattle

Adult cattle are intubated manually using a blind technique (Procedure 10-4, p. 295). A speculum or mouth gag is placed, which prevents the cow from closing its mouth. This protects the anesthetist's arm and hand from being damaged if the cow should become lightly anesthetized

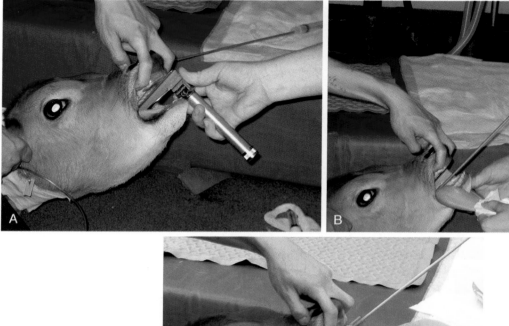

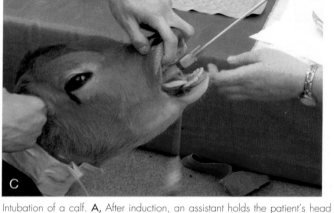

**FIGURE 10-3** Intubation of a calf. **A,** After induction, an assistant holds the patient's head in an extended position. The anesthetist places a laryngoscope and directly visualizes the larynx. The tongue of ruminants, particularly sheep and goats, has a raised area in the caudal portion that makes correct positioning of the laryngoscope more difficult than in small animals. **B,** A stylette, which is pre-placed within and extends beyond the endotracheal tube, is advanced until it is positioned 2 to 5 cm within the larynx. **C,** The tube is then advanced over the stylette into the trachea. The stylette can then be removed. This technique is also used for intubating sheep and goats.

enough to chew. The anesthetist then inserts the nondominant hand into the mouth up to the larynx, holding (and protecting) the endotracheal tube in this hand. The dominant hand holds the connector end of the tube and is used to advance the tube. Once the nondominant hand is at the level of the larynx, the anesthetist palpates the epiglottis, reflects it forward if necessary, and directs the end of the endotracheal tube into the trachea, advancing it into the larynx with the dominant hand. Extending the head and neck of the cow, although sometimes challenging because of the weight, is often helpful while the tube is being passed. On successful placement, the endotracheal cuff is inflated. The tube is then tied in place, either to the halter or around the muzzle as in a dog.

## Maintenance of Anesthesia

After anesthetic induction and endotracheal intubation, patients that are in a light plane of anesthesia must be brought into surgical anesthesia. When the patient reaches

| **PROTOCOL 10-3** | **Anesthetic Maintenance Protocols for PSC P1 and P2 Ruminants** |
|---|---|

1. **Isoflurane or sevoflurane:** Isoflurane 1.5% to 2.5% or sevoflurane 2.5% to 4%
2. **"Double drip:"** Can be used to maintain anesthesia at 1 to 2 mL/kg/hr IV

the desired anesthetic depth, general anesthesia is most commonly maintained with inhalant anesthetics but can also be maintained with total intravenous anesthesia (TIVA). See Protocol 10-3 for maintenance protocols in ruminants.

### Maintenance of Anesthesia with Inhalant

Maintenance of anesthesia in small ruminants and calves is similar to that in small animals (see Procedure 8-7). Maintenance of anesthesia in adult cattle is similar to that

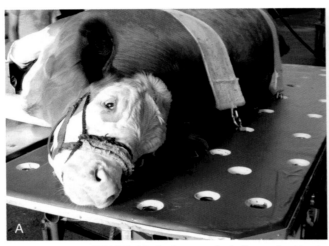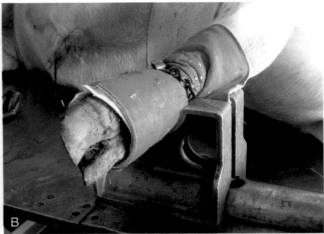

**FIGURE 10-4** Restraint of a bull on a tilt table. **A,** A bull appropriately restrained with two support bands on a tilt table that has a padded surface. The bull's halter is secured by passing a rope through one of the holes and tying it underneath the table. **B,** Appropriate padding of the bull's distal right forelimb, which is placed in a metal foot support.

in horses (see Procedure 9-6). Healthy ruminants typically have relatively few problems during the maintenance phase of anesthesia. Blood pressure is usually well maintained and is often much higher than that seen in small animal and equine patients. Ruminants do, however, tend to hypoventilate and are often observed to breathe rapidly and shallowly, somewhat like a panting dog. This type of breathing pattern may lead to hypercarbia, hypoxemia, and difficulty keeping the patient anesthetized because of inadequate delivery of inhalant anesthetic to the lungs. Patients that demonstrate this breathing pattern should be placed on a ventilator (see Chapter 6).

Most ruminants have accessible arteries in their ears, and these are often catheterized so that blood pressure can be monitored directly and blood samples can be taken for blood gas analysis, particularly for long surgeries or in compromised patients.

## Intravenous Maintenance of Anesthesia

IV maintenance of anesthesia in ruminants is generally reserved for shorter (less than 20 minutes) procedures in healthy patients, although if the patient is intubated the duration of anesthesia can be extended. "Double drip" is commonly used for this purpose.

## Patient Positioning, Comfort, and Safety

During anesthetic induction and maintenance, a number of considerations must be observed to ensure that the patient is not harmed. Many of the same principles of small animal anesthesia apply to ruminant anesthesia (see Chapter 8, p. 252). Additional concerns include the following:

- All ruminants should be positioned for surgery with the mouth lower than the pharynx to allow drainage of saliva and any regurgitated material from the mouth, preventing buildup in the pharynx, which could lead to aspiration in recovery.

- Ruminants, even large cattle, are not predisposed to developing myopathy or neuropathy as horses are; however, appropriate physical support and padding during anesthesia is prudent (Figure 10-4).

## Anesthetic Recovery

Unlike horses, ruminants are generally content to lie in sternal recumbency after anesthesia. The development of complications from anesthetic recovery is generally limited to the residual effects of bloat. Ruminants rarely develop nasal edema during anesthesia and usually do not require nasal intubation. See Procedure 10-5, p. 296, for information regarding anesthetic recovery.

## Preparation for Recovery

On completion of the procedure, turn off the inhalant and transfer the patient to a padded recovery stall where it can be extubated and monitored (large cattle) or to a quiet, clean area on the floor (small ruminant). Support or prop the patient in sternal recumbency with the mouth lower than the pharynx. This allows eructation as the patient regains consciousness, as well as drainage of saliva and/or regurgitus that may have accumulated during anesthesia (Figure 10-5).

## Monitoring during Recovery

The patient should be monitored for signs of excessive bloating (visually large abdomen that feels tight to the touch).

## Signs of Recovery

As the patient recovers, it will progress back through the stages and planes of anesthesia. Generally this is not as dramatic in ruminants as it is in horses, even if the patient did not receive a premedication.

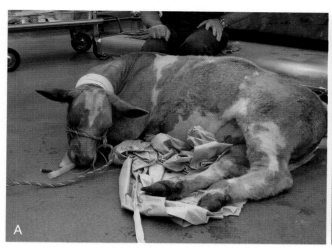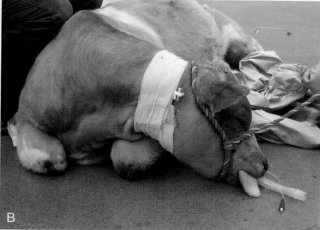

**FIGURE 10-5** Appropriate positioning of a ruminant for anesthetic recovery. **A,** This heifer recovering from anesthesia for umbilical hernia repair is placed in sternal recumbency and maintained in that position, in this case by an assistant, to allow for eructation. The head is positioned so that the pharynx is higher than the mouth, thus allowing for drainage of saliva and regurgitus. **B,** Folding the front limbs underneath the heifer makes it easier to keep her in sternal recumbency.

## Extubation

In contrast to other patients, the endotracheal tube cuff should be either kept inflated or only partially deflated in order to prevent aspiration of any material that may have become lodged in the pharynx during anesthesia. The anesthetist should wait for strong swallowing movements or coughing before extubation. Both before and after removal, keep the neck in a natural but extended position to protect the airway. Remove the endotracheal tube gently using a slow, steady motion. If there is difficulty removing the tube, remove some more air from the cuff and try again.

> TECHNICIAN NOTE Ruminants should be placed in sternal recumbency for recovery from anesthesia to allow the patient to eructate. The endotracheal tube should be only partially deflated to assist removal of saliva and regurgitus from the laryngopharynx on extubation.

## Postanesthetic Period

Once a ruminant is lying in sternal recumbency without support and is no longer in danger of bloating, it can be left unattended. Many ruminants will lie quietly after anesthesia, standing only some time after the anesthetic period, unless they are stimulated to rise. It is not necessary to withhold food or water from ruminants postoperatively unless specifically instructed to do so.

### SWINE

Pigs are challenging patients to restrain, sedate, and anesthetize because of unique characteristics in this species that make physical examination, sedation, IV catheterization,

and intubation much more difficult than in the species discussed so far.

> TECHNICIAN NOTE Pigs are challenging patients to restrain, sedate, and anesthetize because of unique characteristics in this species that make physical examination, sedation, IV catheterization, and intubation difficult.

## PHYSICAL EXAMINATION

In most swine, examination is impossible beyond general observation of the animal, assessment of respiratory rate and character, and observation of obvious problems such as nasal discharge. Restraint of conscious pigs typically results in them squealing in protest, making procedures such as thoracic auscultation impossible. The anesthetist must often rely on patient history to determine health status. Pigs also do not have readily accessible peripheral veins or arteries, making further investigation of cardiovascular status and obtaining blood samples very difficult to impossible without causing extreme stress to the animal and to the handler.

## SUMMARY OF A GENERAL ANESTHETIC PROCEDURE

### Sedation

Sedative drugs are most commonly administered by IM injection in pigs owing to the lack of easily accessible peripheral veins and the presence of a thick layer of subcutaneous fat, which makes IM administration of drugs difficult without the use of needles that are at least 1½ inches long. The most accessible site for IM

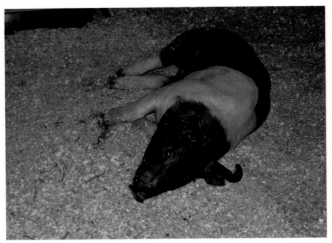

**FIGURE 10-6** Pig sedated with Telazol-ketamine-xylazine (TKX). This pig became laterally recumbent 15 minutes after IM injection of TKX (the blood on the side of the neck marks the site of IM injection).

**PROTOCOL 10-4** | **Premedication and Sedative Protocols for PSC P1 and P2 Swine**

**Protocols for Mild-Moderate Sedation**
1. **Acepromazine + butorphanol:** Acepromazine 0.04 to 0.09 mg/kg + butorphanol 0.05 to 0.1 mg/kg IM*
2. **Dexmedetomidine + butorphanol:** Dexmedetomidine 0.02 to 0.03 mg/kg + butorphanol 0.05 to 0.1 mg/kg IM*

**Protocols for Moderate-Heavy Sedation**
1. **Telazol-ketamine-xylazine (TKX):** TKX administered intramuscularly at 1 mL/50 kg to a maximum of 3 mL
2. **Dexmedetomidine + ketamine + butorphanol:** Dexmedetomidine 0.02 mg/kg + ketamine 5 mg/kg + butorphanol 0.2 mg/kg IM*
3. **Romifidine + ketamine + butorphanol:** Romifidine 0.12 mg/kg + ketamine 8 mg/kg + butorphanol 0.1 mg/kg IM*

*Combine the drugs in one syringe before IM administration.

injection is in the muscles of the neck caudal to the ear and at least 3 to 5 cm lateral to the dorsal midline (Figure 10-6).

Swine are generally considered to be the most resistant to sedative drugs of the domestic species, and many protocols for IM sedation, premedication, or **total injectable anesthesia** include a tranquilizer or sedative, an opioid, and a dissociative. Various combinations of drugs have been used to sedate swine (Protocol 10-4). Generally, drug combinations that include a dissociative produce more predictable and heavier sedation that, in some pigs, may produce anesthesia for short surgical and nonsurgical procedures. A combination that is widely used to produce heavy sedation to anesthesia is Telazol, ketamine, and xylazine, or **TKX** (Procedure 10-6, p. 296).

### Anesthetic Induction

Using a combination of drugs such as TKX will often induce anesthesia in pigs. The eyes of pigs are very small and sunken in and do not provide reliable information about depth of anesthesia. Readiness for intubation is often best assessed by seeing if the mouth can be opened without resistance. If after administration of TKX the patient is not quite deeply anesthetized enough to intubate, the anesthetist has two options. He or she can place an IV catheter in an aural vein (Figure 10-7) and administer small increments of an IV induction drug such as ketamine (i.e., 0.5- to 1.0-mg/kg boluses), or deepen anesthesia by administering an inhalant anesthetic via face mask (Figure 10-8).

### Intubation

Intubation of swine is particularly challenging because of poor visualization resulting from the limited opening of the mouth, the relatively narrow dental arcade, and the

anatomy of the larynx and proximal trachea. A ventral laryngeal diverticulum is present into which the tube can easily be misdirected, and the laryngotracheal junction is at an angle rather than being straight as is seen in other domestic species. Finally, the larynx in pigs is sensitive and may spasm when stimulated, making intubation even harder. The novice anesthetist should seek assistance from an experienced person when intubating a pig, as it is easy to damage the larynx by forcing the tube. There are several methods of intubating pigs. The pig may be placed in either sternal or dorsal recumbency. Similarly to small ruminants, a straight stylette is placed within the tube and extends beyond it. With a laryngoscope used to visualize the airway, the stylette is passed into the larynx, bypassing the diverticulum. The tube can then be gently threaded over the stylette into the trachea. Care must be taken with the stylette to avoid damage to the larynx and trachea (Figure 10-9). Alternatively, a stylette with a 20- to 30-degree curve in it is placed in the tube, ensuring that it does not extend beyond the end of the tube. The tube is inserted into the larynx with the convex surface against the palate. Once the tube is placed in the larynx, the tube and stylette are rotated 180 degrees and advanced into the trachea. Patience should be exercised, and if anesthesia becomes light during intubation, further attempts at intubation should be halted until IV or inhalant drugs are administered and an appropriate depth of anesthesia for intubation is achieved.

### Maintenance of Anesthesia

Anesthesia in most pigs can be maintained with inhalant anesthetic delivered using a small animal anesthetic machine and circle system. Maintenance of anesthesia is similar to that in small animal patients (see Chapter 8). In the case of very large pigs that can be intubated with

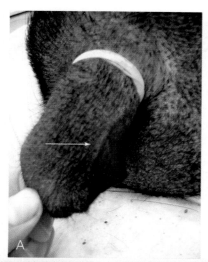

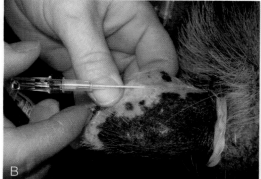

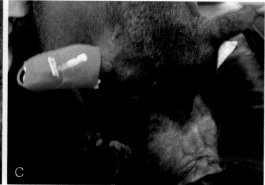

**FIGURE 10-7**   Placing a catheter in an aural vein of a pig. **A,** A rubber band placed around the base of the ear acts as a tourniquet, causing the marginal ear vein to distend *(white arrow).* **B,** Placement of an IV catheter in the vein. Note the blood flashback in the hub of the catheter. Because of the small size of ear veins in pigs, blood does not commonly flow out of the catheter after the stylette has been removed. After the catheter has been placed, the rubber band is removed. It is usually easier to cut the rubber band off, taking care not to cut the ear, than risk dislodging the catheter while moving the rubber band over the catheter and off the ear. **C,** If required, the catheter can be secured and wrapped to allow for administration of postoperative intravenous medication.

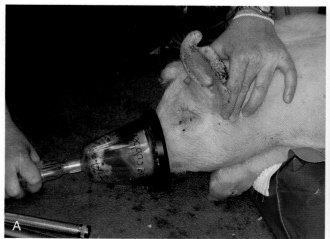

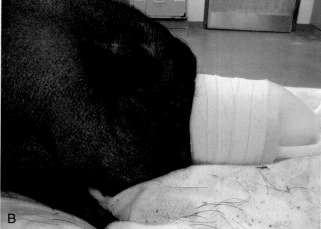

**FIGURE 10-8**   Administering an inhalant anesthetic via a face mask in a pig. **A,** Use of a small animal clear face mask in a small pig. **B,** Use of a homemade face mask in a large pig. In both cases it is important that the mask be tight fitting to avoid pollution of the work area and to ensure that the inhalant anesthetic is not diluted by room air, which will delay induction.

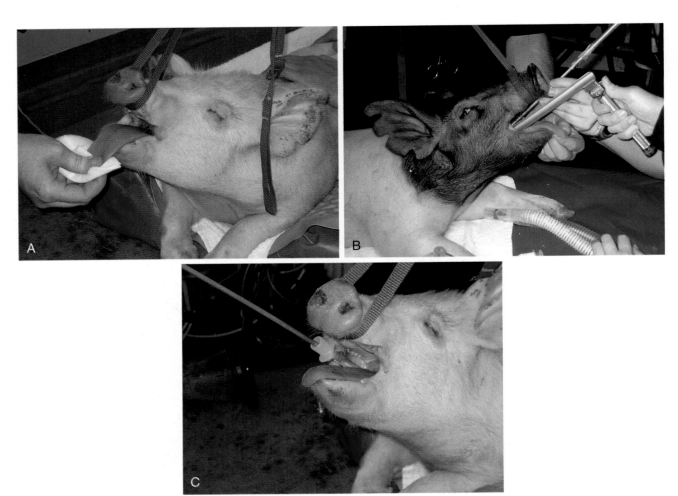

**FIGURE 10-9** Intubation of a pig. **A,** After anesthetic induction, the tongue is gently pulled forward and down while the upper jaw is pulled upward using a lead. **B,** With a laryngoscope used to aid visualization, a stylette placed through and beyond the end of an endotracheal tube is advanced into the larynx. **C,** The tube is advanced over the stylette into the larynx.

a size 16-mm endotracheal tube, a large animal machine can be used.

## Monitoring

Pigs can be challenging to monitor effectively, because they have few palpable peripheral arteries and their cone-shaped legs make the use of blood pressure cuffs, which are designed for the more cylindric arms of people, more difficult. In most pigs pulses can be palpated in the ear and on the medical aspect of the carpus. In smaller pigs the brachial artery may be palpable, a Doppler signal may be obtained from it, and oscillometric cuffs will often give pressure readings (Figure 10-10). A Doppler signal is also relatively easy to elicit from the tail artery, which runs in the ventral midline of the tail. Pulse oximeter transmission probes will usually work on the tongue but can also be placed on other areas such as the snout and ears of pink pigs (Figure 10-11).

The respiratory system can be monitored by observing the breathing bag and with capnometry as for other species.

## Porcine Stress Syndrome

**Porcine stress syndrome,** also known as *malignant hyperthermia,* has been associated with anesthesia, particularly inhalant anesthetics. This metabolic condition occurs in affected animals because of a mutation in one of the genes that controls calcium metabolism in the muscle. Signs include muscle rigidity, rapid rise in temperature, hypercapnia, hyperkalemia, and death. Treatment includes immediate termination of all anesthetic drugs, delivery of oxygen at high flow rates, and treatment with dantrolene.

## Recovery

The general principles applicable to extubation and recovery for small animals apply to pigs, including detection and treatment of hypothermia. Typically the IV catheter is removed before full awakening, although if a pig is to be hospitalized it may be prudent to secure the IV catheter for administration of IV medications (see Figure 10-7, *C*).

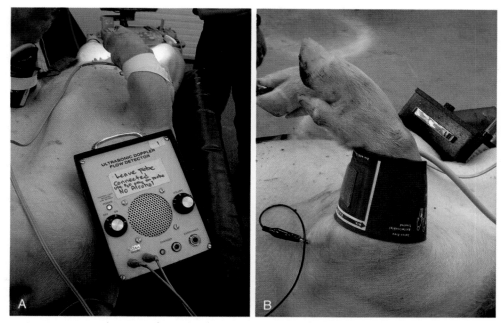

**FIGURE 10-10** Placement of Doppler probe and oscillometric blood pressure cuff on the forelimb of a small pig. **A,** Placement of the Doppler probe on the medial aspect of the carpus. **B,** Placement of an oscillometric blood pressure cuff on the forelimb.

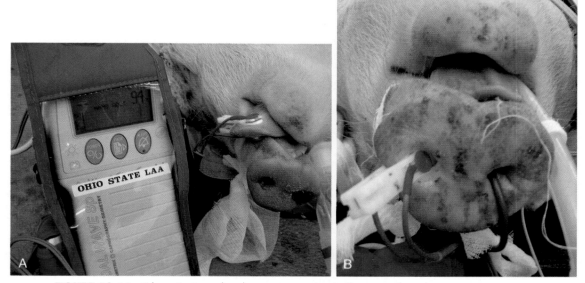

**FIGURE 10-11** Pulse oximetry probe placement on a pig. **A,** Placement of a pulse oximetry transmission probe on a pig's tongue. **B,** Placement of a pulse oximetry transmission probe on a pig's snout. Note the temperature probe entering the pig's right nostril.

## KEY POINTS

1. The main anesthetic concerns in ruminants arise from their unique digestive anatomy and physiology.

2. Ruminants are susceptible to bloat, regurgitation, and hypoventilation under general anesthesia.

3. Ruminants are generally very tractable, and surgery, particularly flank laparotomy, is often accomplished using local anesthesia with or without sedation.

4. Intubation is performed under direct visualization with a laryngoscope in small ruminants and calves, often with the use of a stylette.

5. Intubation of adult cattle is performed manually using a blind technique that involves direct palpation of the larynx.

6. During recovery from anesthesia ruminants should be placed in sternal recumbency to allow for eructation. The endotracheal tube should be left in place with the cuff partially inflated to minimize the risk of aspirating rumen contents or saliva.

7. Preoperative physical examination of swine is limited to observation.

8. The main anesthetic concerns in swine are inability to perform blood work, resistance to sedation, paucity of peripheral veins and arteries, and difficulty of intubation.

9. Pigs are resistant to sedation compared with other species. The combination of Telazol, ketamine, and xylazine (TKX) is commonly used to provide heavy sedation or total intravenous anesthesia (TIVA) in pigs.

10. After sedation or induction, the ear vein is usually accessible for catheterization in pigs.

11. Intubation of swine is challenging because of poor visualization of the larynx, and the potential for laryngospasm.

12. There are few palpable arteries in pigs, making monitoring difficult. Oscillometric blood pressure cuffs may not work well on the cone-shaped limbs of pigs.

---

### PROCEDURE 10-1    *Preparation for Anesthesia of a Ruminant*

1. Assess, prepare, and weigh the patient. (See section on patient preparation for a discussion of patient assessment, preparation, and stabilization.)

2. Prepare equipment for and place intravenous (IV) catheter, which may require restraint in a chute with a head gate for larger or aggressive cattle (clippers, local anesthetic, antiseptic scrub, catheters, tape, heparinized saline, suture material, catheter cap and/or extension line with three-way stopcock).

3. Determine the protocol (anesthetic agents including doses, routes, and sequence of administration).

4. Calculate the volume of each agent to give, including fluid administration rates (preanesthetic, induction, maintenance, and analgesic agents).

5. Review the oxygen flow rates (see Chapter 4, p. 127).

6. Prepare equipment required to administer drugs (syringes, needles, agents, reversal agents, emergency cart, controlled substance log).

7. Prepare fluid administration equipment (fluids, administration and extension set, syringe pump, tape, heparinized saline).

8. Prepare equipment for endotracheal intubation. Have suction equipment assembled and turned on for small ruminants. Remove jewelry and watch, and ensure fingernails are trimmed short for digital intubation of adult cattle (see Chapter 4).

9. Prepare monitoring equipment including arterial catheterization materials, anesthesia record, monitors, and probes (see Chapter 5).

10. Assemble and test the anesthetic machine and ventilator.

---

### PROCEDURE 10-2    *Sequence of Events for Induction with an IV Agent and Maintenance with an Inhalant Agent in a Ruminant*

1. Administer premedications approximately 20 to 30 minutes intramuscularly or 5 to 10 minutes intravenously before anesthetic induction if this is considered necessary.

2. Administer the induction agent.

3. Check the patient's readiness for intubation.

4. Place and secure the endotracheal tube.

5. Inflate the endotracheal tube cuff.

6. Check the patient's vital signs.

7. Hoist or lift (as appropriate), position, and secure the patient for the procedure. It is imperative that the pharynx be positioned higher than the head whenever possible.

8. Turn on the oxygen, and attach the endotracheal tube to the breathing circuit.

9. Turn on the inhalant anesthetic to the appropriate level.

10. Determine the patient's anesthetic depth, and commence regular monitoring.

11. Attach monitoring devices, including placement of an arterial catheter.

12. Continue to monitor and adjust the anesthetic and oxygen levels as needed until completion of the procedure.

## PROCEDURE 10-3 IV Induction in Adult Cattle

Induction of adult cattle is similar to horses in that the goal is to achieve lateral recumbency without excitement or injury to the patient or personnel. In order to do this, the induction agent is given as a rapid IV bolus in PS1 and PS2 cows. The only induction drug that is given "to effect" (see Procedure 8-3) is "double drip."

- **Ketamine-diazepam and ketamine-midazolam mixtures:** After a check to make sure that the IV catheter is patent and still in the jugular vein, the entire syringe of the calculated dose of drugs is rapidly injected into the catheter or extension set, then flushed using heparinized saline.

- **Double drip (guaifenesin 50 mg/mL and ketamine 1 mg/mL):** A bag of double drip with an IV administration set attached is placed in a pressure sleeve, which is inflated up to 300 mm Hg pressure. The administration set is connected to the IV catheter or extension set. After a check to make sure that the IV catheter is patent and still in the jugular vein, the double drip is then administered under pressure to effect. Approximately 1 to 2 mL/kg will produce signs of ataxia (swaying) followed by recumbency. If intubation is not possible, a further 1 to 2 mL/kg may be administered more slowly, or a bolus of ketamine 1 mg/kg IV may be given.

## PROCEDURE 10-4 Intubation Procedure for Adult Cattle

1. Ruminants are generally intubated in sternal recumbency.
2. Place a mouth speculum or gag.
3. Grasp the tongue and pull it forward.
4. Extend the head and neck (Figure 1).

5. Hold the tube at the patient end, and cover the cuff with the nondominant hand (Figure 2).
6. Holding the tube in this manner, extend the nondominant arm into the mouth and advance to the larynx. Use the dominant hand to assist with advancement of the machine end of the tube (Figure 3).
7. Palpate the epiglottis and laryngeal opening with one or two fingers of the nondominant hand.

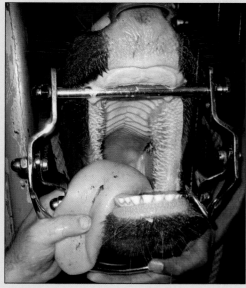

**FIGURE 1** A mouth gag is placed and the head extended by an assistant.

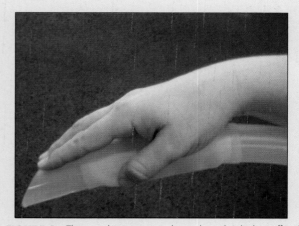

**FIGURE 2** The anesthetist protects the endotracheal tube cuff with the nondominant hand.

*Continued*

## PROCEDURE 10-4    Intubation Procedure for Adult Cattle—cont'd

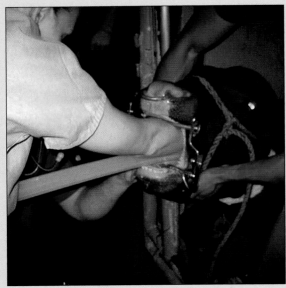

**FIGURE 3** Using the nondominant hand, the anesthetist palpates the larynx with the fingers and directs the endotracheal tube into the larynx, while advancing the tube with the dominant hand.

8. Pass the tube into the larynx, using the nondominant hand to push the end of the tube into the airway, and the dominant hand to advance the tube.
9. Check to ensure that the tube is in the trachea by feeling air pass during exhalation or when an assistant presses down on the patient's chest.
10. A small volume of air may be placed in the cuff (20 to 60 mL) before the cow is hoisted or positioned.
11. Secure the tube to the halter or to the muzzle.

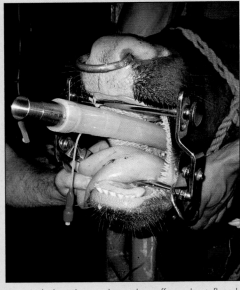

**FIGURE 4** With the tube in place, the cuff can be inflated and the mouth gag removed.

12. After the cow has been positioned on the surgery table, connect the endotracheal tube to the anesthetic breathing system and allow the patient to breathe 100% oxygen (Figure 4).
13. Check the tube for leaks.
14. Turn on the anesthetic vaporizer, and adjust to the appropriate level.
15. Commence regular monitoring.

## PROCEDURE 10-5    Recovery from General Anesthesia in Ruminants

1. Prepare the patient for recovery, including removal of monitoring equipment, and ensure that the recovery area has been prepared.
2. Discontinue the anesthetic, and transfer the patient to the recovery area.
3. Extubate the patient at the appropriate time with the cuff partially inflated. Place or prop the patient in sternal recumbency so that it can eructate.

4. Prepare the patient for continued hospitalization or discharge by applying bandages, administering medications, and performing any other procedures ordered by the veterinarian.

## PROCEDURE 10-6    How to Prepare and Administer TKX (Telazol, Ketamine, Xylazine) to Swine

1. Reconstitute a bottle of Telazol with 2.5 mL of ketamine 100 mg/mL and 2.5 mL of xylazine 100 mg/mL.
2. The final mixture of TKX contains the following drugs and concentrations:
   Tiletamine 50 mg/mL
   Zolazepam 50 mg/mL
   Ketamine 50 mg/mL
   Xylazine 50 mg/mL

3. Administer TKX at 1 mL/50 kg intramuscularly up to a maximum of 3 mL.

## REVIEW QUESTIONS

1. Comparing the sensitivity of cattle, horses, and swine to xylazine, which of the following is true?
   a. Cattle are more sensitive than horses, which are more sensitive than swine.
   b. Cattle are more sensitive than swine, which are more sensitive than horses.
   c. Horses are more sensitive than cattle, which are more sensitive than swine.
   d. Swine are more sensitive than cattle, which are more sensitive than horses.

2. An anticholinergic is an essential component of premedication in ruminants.
   True            False

3. "Double drip" contains which two drugs?
   a. Guaifenesin and dobutamine
   b. Guaifenesin and ketamine
   c. Xylazine and ketamine
   d. Acepromazine and ketamine

4. You plan to anesthetize a 1000-kg bull and maintain anesthesia using an inhalant technique. Which of the following statements regarding intubation is correct?
   a. The inhalant can be safely delivered via a face mask.
   b. You will need a laryngoscope to visualize the larynx.
   c. You will have to manually intubate the bull.
   d. All of the above

5. It is common for anesthetized ruminants to hypoventilate.
   True            False

6. Positioning the head of an anesthetized ruminant with the pharynx higher than the mouth helps to prevent:
   a. Hyperventilation
   b. Hypotension
   c. Aspiration
   d. Hypoxemia

7. Ruminants should be placed in sternal recumbency during recovery to allow them to:
   a. Eructate
   b. Regurgitate
   c. Salivate
   d. Hyperventilate

8. Intubation is made easier in pigs by:
   a. The presence of a laryngeal diverticulum
   b. The possibility of laryngospasm
   c. The use of a stylette
   d. The angle of the laryngotracheal junction

9. Which of the following statements regarding porcine anesthesia is true?
   a. Oscillometric blood pressure monitors work well in pigs.
   b. All pigs should have complete blood work before anesthesia.
   c. Pigs are very sensitive to alpha$_2$-agonists.
   d. Intravenous sedation is virtually impossible in healthy pigs.

10. Which of the following is *not* a sign of porcine stress syndrome?
    a. Hypothermia
    b. Hyperthermia
    c. Hyperkalemia
    d. Hypercapnia

## SELECTED READINGS

Greene SA: Protocols for anesthesia of cattle, *Vet Clin North Am Food Anim Pract* Vol. 19(Issue 3):679-693, November 2003.

Tranquilli WJ, Thurmon JC, Grimm KA: *Veterinary anesthesia and analgesia*, ed 4, Ames, Iowa, 2007, Blackwell.

# 11

# Rodent and Rabbit Anesthesia

*Paul Flecknell*

## OUTLINE

Patient Evaluation, 298
    *Handling and Restraint, 299*
    *Physical Examination of Small*
        *Mammals, 302*
    *Diagnostic Tests, 303*
Preanesthetic Patient Care, 303
    *Withholding Food before Anesthesia, 303*
    *Correction of Preexisting Problems, 304*
Preanesthetic Agents, 304
    *Anticholinergics, 304*
    *Phenothiazines, 304*
    *Benzodiazepines, 304*
    *Alpha$_2$-Adrenoreceptor Agonists, 305*
    *Opioids, 305*

General Anesthesia, 306
    *Induction Techniques and Agents, 306*
    *Intubation and Maintenance of*
        *Anesthesia, 309*
Postoperative Care, 312
Anesthetic Emergencies, 312
    *Respiratory Depression, 312*
    *Circulatory Failure, 312*
Postoperative Analgesia, 313
    *Pain Assessment in Small Mammals, 313*
    *Analgesic Agents, 314*
    *Chronic Pain, 315*
    *Administration of Analgesics, 315*

## KEY TERMS

Droperidol
Fluanisone
Intraosseous
Intraperitoneal
Laryngeal mask
Neuroleptanalgesia

## LEARNING OBJECTIVES

*After completion of this chapter, the reader will be able to:*
- Summarize the common problems that may arise when anesthetizing rodents and rabbits.
- List the preanesthetic and anesthetic agents suitable for use in these species.
- Describe the technique of endotracheal intubation in rabbits.
- Describe the problems that can arise when monitoring anesthesia in rodents and rabbits.
- State aspects of intraoperative care that are of particular importance when anesthetizing rodents and rabbits.
- Describe how to cope with common anesthetic emergencies in rodents and rabbits.
- Describe the most common problems associated with postanesthetic care of rodents and rabbits.
- List the analgesics that can be used in rodents and rabbits.

Anesthesia of small mammals (rabbits, guinea pigs, rats, mice, gerbils, and hamsters) is a specialized branch of veterinary anesthesia, but the general principles of good anesthetic practice provide basic guidance. The main difficulties encountered when anesthetizing these animals result from the following situations:
- Lack of familiarity with the species
- Lack of suitable equipment
- A failure to appreciate the poor health status of some patients
- The difficulties of providing supportive care

Once these problems are appreciated, anesthesia of small mammals and other exotic species should be as successful as anesthesia of dogs and cats.

## PATIENT EVALUATION

To anesthetize small mammals safely and effectively, it is important to perform a clinical examination and obtain a case history. Although the information required is similar to that needed for more familiar species, many of these small animals are owned by children, and accurate information may not always be obtainable. Even when an adult or older child is caring for the animal, it may be difficult to be certain that the animal is eating and drinking normally, because many of these species are fed ad lib.

| TABLE 11-1 | Biologic Data for Small Mammals | | | | | |
|---|---|---|---|---|---|---|
| | Gerbil | Guinea Pig | Hamster | Mouse | Rabbit | Rat |
| Adult body weight (g) | 85-150 | 700-1200 | 85-150 | 25-40 | 2000-6000 | 300-500 |
| Respiratory rate (breaths/min) | 90 | 50-140 | 80-135 | 80-200 | 40-60 | 70-115 |
| Heart rate (bpm) | 260-300 | 150-250 | 250-500 | 350-600 | 135-325 | 250-350 |
| Average adult blood volume (mL) (65-70 mL/kg) | 9 | 60 | 9 | 2.5 | 250 | 30 |
| PCV (%) | 41-52 | 37-48 | 36-55 | 36-49 | 36-48 | 38-50 |
| Blood glucose (mmol/L) | 3-7 | 4.5-6 | 3-8 | 3.5-9 | 4-8 | 3-8 |
| Total protein (g/dL) | 4.3-12.5 | 4.6-6.2 | 5.9-6.5 | 3.5-7.2 | 5.4-7.5 | 5.6-7.6 |
| BUN (mg/dL) | 17-27 | 9-32 | 10-25 | 12-28 | 17-23.5 | 6-23 |
| ALT (IU) | — | 25-59 | 12-36 | 74-232 | 35-38 | 17.5-30 |
| Life span (yr) | 3-5 | 4-8 | 1.5-2 | 2-2.5 | 5-10 | 2-3.5 |

*ALT*, Alanine aminotransferase; *BUN*, blood urea nitrogen; *IU*, international units; *PCV*, packed cell volume.

It should be recalled that the life span of these small mammals is considerably shorter than that of dogs and cats. Geriatric animals present a greater risk when anesthetized; a hamster, for example, will be nearing the end of its natural life when aged only 18 to 24 months. Some basic biologic data are given in Table 11-1.

> **TECHNICIAN NOTE** It is important that the techniques for restraining the different species of small mammals be understood so that injury to the patient and handler can be avoided.

For a physical examination to be performed, any animal must be safely and humanely handled and restrained. Handling is easier if small rodents are brought to the veterinary clinic in a small container, although they should not be left in a cardboard box for a prolonged period because they can easily gnaw through the container and escape. Rabbits can usually be transported in a small transport box, and cat-sized carriers are suitable. Because rabbits are a prey species and cats are one of their predators, it is not surprising that placing a rabbit in a transport box that has been previously used for cats can be extremely stressful; this should be avoided. Similarly, it is advisable for the technician to wash the hands and preferably wear a fresh gown or coat before examining and handling these species if he or she has previously been working with dogs and cats.

Before the animal is handled, it should be observed undisturbed so that its normal behavior and respiratory pattern and rate can be noted.

## Handling and Restraint
### Mouse

Mice are best picked up by the base of the tail and lifted clear of their transport box. They can then be allowed to rest on the operator's forearm and their external

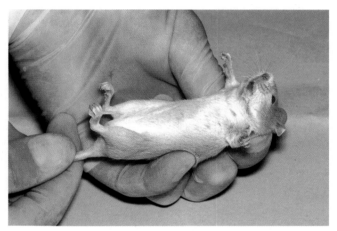

**FIGURE 11-1** Restraint of a mouse. Mice can be restrained by the skin overlying the shoulders, with the tail held between the operator's fingers.

appearance assessed. To restrain them for administration of injectable anesthetics or other drugs, allow mice to rest on a rough surface (e.g., a towel or the bars of their cage). They can then be grasped by the skin overlying the shoulders and lifted clear. The tail can be gripped between the operator's fingers as shown in Figure 11-1. Subcutaneous administration of medication is made into the skin overlying the shoulders and can be carried out single-handedly. An assistant should administer **intraperitoneal** and intramuscular injections while the operator restrains the animal as shown in Figures 11-2 and 11-3. Restraining the mouse by its scruff can interfere with respiration. This causes no problems in healthy animals, but care should be taken if the animal is showing signs of respiratory disease. Young mice can be extremely active and may jump out of their transport box as soon as the lid is removed; handling these agile young animals requires fast reactions.

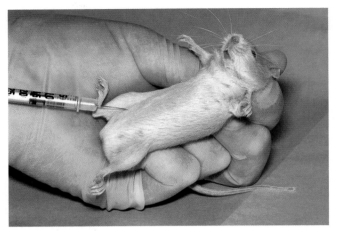

**FIGURE 11-2** Intraperitoneal injection in a mouse. Intraperitoneal injection in mice is made into one posterior quadrant of the abdomen, along the line of the hindlimb.

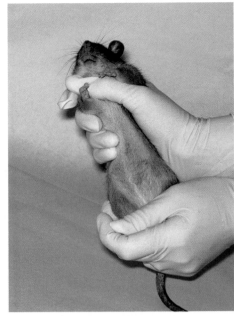

**FIGURE 11-4** Restraint of a rat. Note that the thumb is positioned below the mandible to prevent biting. The chest is held gently to avoid interfering with respiration.

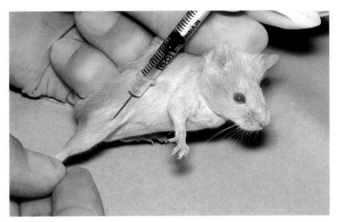

**FIGURE 11-3** Intramuscular injection in a mouse. Intramuscular injection in mice is made into the quadriceps muscle.

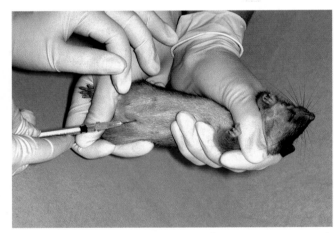

**FIGURE 11-5** Intraperitoneal injection in the rat. An assistant extends one hindlimb and injects into one posterior quadrant of the abdomen.

## Rat

Most pet rats are friendly and easy to handle. They should be picked up around the shoulders and lifted clear of the transport box. They can then be allowed to rest on the handler's forearm and be gently restrained by the tail or around the shoulders. If the animal resents handling (which it may if it is in pain—for example, if it has arthritis), it can be picked up by the base of the tail as mice are. It can then be placed on a rough surface and grasped around the shoulders. When holding a rat in this way, the operator can avoid being bitten by positioning the thumb under the mandible as shown in Figure 11-4. It is important not to grasp the animal's chest too firmly because this can interfere with respiratory movements, causing the animal to panic and struggle. Although subcutaneous injections can be given into the scruff while the animal is also being restrained, it is usually easier to obtain the assistance of a colleague. Intramuscular and intraperitoneal injections are given in the same way as in the mouse, but an assistant is needed for these procedures (Figures 11-5 and 11-6).

## Hamster

Hamsters vary considerably in their temperament, and care should be taken when handling them. This species is normally active at night and asleep during the day, and if necessary they should be gently awakened before being handled. Most animals can be cupped in the operator's hands, as shown in Figure 11-7, and an external examination carried out. If it is necessary to immobilize the animal, it should be covered by the operator's hand with the skin overlying the shoulders and back grasped firmly (Figure 11-8). It is important to grasp sufficient skin; otherwise, the animal can turn in the operator's grasp and may bite (Figure 11-9). An assistant can make intramuscular, intraperitoneal, or subcutaneous injections into the

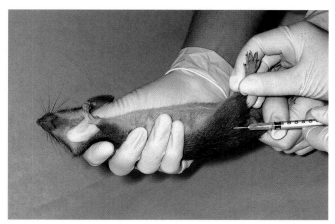

**FIGURE 11-6** Intramuscular injection in the rat. An assistant extends and immobilizes one hindleg and injects into the quadriceps muscle.

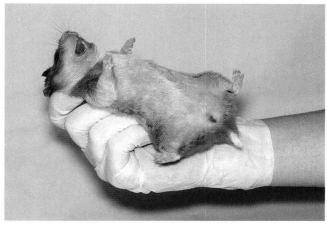

**FIGURE 11-8** Secure restraint of a hamster. For more secure restraint, the hamster should first be immobilized with the operator's hand and the skin overlying the back and shoulders grasped firmly.

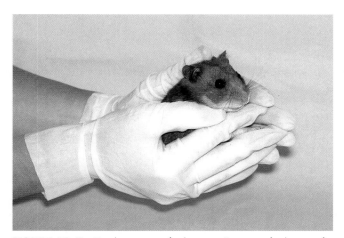

**FIGURE 11-7** Gentle restraint of a hamster. Restraint of a hamster for clinical examination by cupping in the operator's hands.

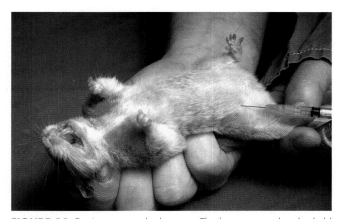

**FIGURE 11-9** Injection in the hamster. The hamster can then be held securely for injections to be carried out by an assistant.

same sites as in the rat and mouse. Hamsters should not be allowed to run unrestrained on the consulting room table because they appear to lack depth perception and may fall to the floor and injure themselves.

## Gerbil

Gerbils are very active and can easily escape from their transport container unless quickly immobilized. Preventing escape is best achieved by the operator covering the animal with a hand and grasping around the animal's shoulders with the thumb positioned under the mandible to prevent biting. With the animal immobilized in this way, an assistant can administer subcutaneous injections into the flank and intramuscular and intraperitoneal injections in the same site as for other small rodents. Gerbils can also be immobilized by grasping the base of the tail, but the skin of the tail is delicate and easily damaged.

## Guinea Pig

On initial examination a guinea pig may be completely immobile, but when attempts are made to restrain it, the animal can become very agitated and run around its

transport box at high speed. It should be immobilized by grasping it swiftly and firmly around the shoulders. It can then be lifted clear of the transport container, and the operator's other hand can be used to support its hindquarters (Figure 11-10). With the animal restrained in this way an assistant can administer subcutaneous injections into the flank and intramuscular and intraperitoneal injections into the same site as with other rodents. If drugs are to be given by the subcutaneous route, an alternative approach is placing the restrainer's hands on either side of the guinea pig's body to immobilize the animal on the examination table. An assistant can then inject into the skin overlying the shoulders.

## Rabbit

Rabbits vary considerably in body weight, ranging from dwarf breeds weighing as little as 400 g up to giant breeds that can weigh 10 kg. Most domestic rabbits weigh 2 to 5 kg and are relatively easy to restrain, but care must be taken because they are easily frightened. When attempting to escape, they may kick out with their back legs. This can injure the person attempting to handle them and

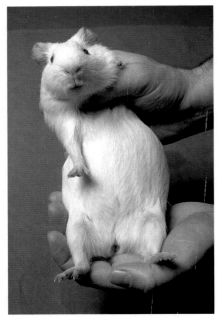

FIGURE 11-10    Restraint of a guinea pig. Guinea pigs should be grasped around the shoulders, with the hindquarters supported.

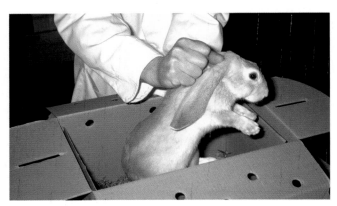

FIGURE 11-11    Lifting a rabbit. When a rabbit is lifted out of its transport box or cage, the skin overlying the shoulders should be grasped firmly and the abdomen supported. The operator's forearms are used to provide support to the animal's back.

may also result in serious injury to the rabbit (e.g., fracture of the lumbar vertebrae). It is therefore important to provide support to the animal's back at all times and never to leave the animal unrestrained on the consulting room table.

Rabbits should be grasped by the skin overlying the shoulders and lifted clear of the transport container. As the rabbit is lifted, the operator's other hand should be positioned under the animal's abdomen to support its body weight as shown in Figure 11-11. The rabbit can then be placed on the examination table. The animal should not be released until its feet are in firm contact with the table surface. It can then be restrained by gently holding the skin over the shoulders. Rabbits should never be picked up by the ears because these are delicate structures.

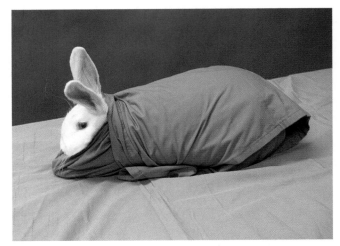

FIGURE 11-12    Restraint of a rabbit. Restraint of a rabbit by wrapping it in a surgical gown.

An assistant can make intramuscular injections into the quadriceps or into the lumbar muscles while the operator restrains the animal by placing hands and arms along either side of its body. Intravenous injection is most easily carried out into the marginal ear veins. The skin of the ears is sensitive, and animals will often jerk in response to venipuncture. To avoid a jerk and to prevent discomfort, the skin overlying the vein can be desensitized using a local anesthetic cream (e.g., EMLA, AstraZeneca). The cream is applied thickly over the vein and covered with a waterproof dressing (e.g., plastic food wrap) and a protective adhesive bandage. The cream is left in place for approximately 45 minutes and then removed and the ear wiped clean. This provides full skin thickness anesthesia for at least an hour. This technique is particularly useful for placing "over-the-needle" catheters. As an alternative to the ear veins, the cephalic veins on the forelegs can also be used, or the lateral saphenous veins on the hindleg. These vessels are fragile, and it is easy to produce a hematoma, even when venipuncture has been carried out successfully on the initial attempt.

If an assistant is unavailable, rabbits can be securely restrained by wrapping them in a towel, lab coat, or surgical gown, as shown in Figure 11-12. Provided it is wrapped securely, the animal will remain immobile, and it is usually possible to carry out venipuncture successfully with the marginal ear veins.

> TECHNICIAN NOTE    The patient should first be observed undisturbed in its transport box. Respiratory rate and character can be noted during observation.

## Physical Examination of Small Mammals

As mentioned earlier, the animal should first be observed undisturbed in its transport box if possible and can then be restrained as previously described for more detailed examination. The animal's respiratory rate and pattern can be assessed and its heart rate recorded either by palpating the heartbeat or by using a stethoscope. Although normal rates are given in Table 11-1, these will rarely be observed in patients because most will show a marked increase in heart and respiratory rates owing to the stress of examination. Rabbits, for example, frequently have respiratory rates in excess of 250 breaths/min during routine clinical examination. The type of examination that can be carried out is limited by the size of the animal being examined, but in rabbits it is possible to auscultate and percuss the chest as in cats.

In all species, the following are of particular importance:

- Discharges from the eyes and nose may indicate the presence of respiratory disease. Rats are commonly seen with a black or reddish brown discharge around their eyes or nose. This is a buildup of porphyrin secretions, which when wiped with a damp swab will appear bright red. This can lead owners to report that their animal has been bleeding from its eyes or nose. These secretions are a nonspecific response to stress or illnesses such as chronic respiratory disease.
- Labored or noisy respiration is also indicative of respiratory disease.
- Soiling of the perineum can indicate gastrointestinal disturbances.
- An unkempt or "starey" appearance of the coat is a general sign of ill health in small mammals.
- Loss of skin tone in response to dehydration is more difficult to detect in small mammals than in dogs and cats. If loss of elasticity is noted, it usually indicates that more than 10% of body weight has been lost as fluid. When small mammals are markedly dehydrated, the eyes become sunken. This is commonly seen in rabbits and small mammals that are anesthetized for treatment of dental disease. Because the disease may have been present for some time, the animal may have had a prolonged period of reduced food and water intake. It is essential that these animals receive supportive fluid therapy before anesthesia.
- Palpation of the regions overlying the back and pelvis is helpful in assessing body condition. If the prominences of the vertebrae and of the pelvis are easily palpable, it is likely that the animal has lost a considerable amount of body fat.
- It is difficult to examine the mucous membranes in small rodents, but in the rabbit both the gingiva and conjunctiva can be inspected easily. They should have a normal reddish coloration, and the capillary refill time should be under 1 second. As with dogs and cats, abnormal coloration of the mucous membranes may indicate underlying disease.

> **TECHNICIAN NOTE** Dehydration is more difficult to detect in small mammals than in dogs and cats. If loss of skin elasticity is noted, it usually indicates that more than 10% of body weight has been lost as fluid.

### Diagnostic Tests

Preanesthetic blood tests are rarely undertaken in small rodents but may be of value in some circumstances (e.g., in rabbits with suspected hepatic lipidosis). Urine samples are easily obtained from small rodents because these species frequently urinate when handled. Diabetes mellitus is relatively common in Chinese hamsters and is also seen occasionally in rabbits and guinea pigs. In these latter species it is frequently asymptomatic.

Radiography may be required before some surgical procedures. For example, radiography of the skull is helpful in assessing underlying dental problems before flushing the tear ducts to correct blockage. Radiography is also indicated before removal of suspected uterine adenocarcinoma in rabbits to identify secondary tumors in the lungs.

## PREANESTHETIC PATIENT CARE

> **TECHNICIAN NOTE** There is generally no reason to withhold food or water before anesthesia because small rodents and rabbits do not vomit, and this practice may lead to hypoglycemia. Food should be made available until 1 to 2 hours before anesthesia and immediately after recovery from anesthesia.

### Withholding Food before Anesthesia

Small rodents and rabbits do not vomit, and there is generally no reason to withhold food or water before anesthesia. Withholding food from small rodents for prolonged periods can be detrimental because it can predispose to hypoglycemia. Withholding food from rabbits and guinea pigs can also trigger digestive disturbances that can result in enterotoxemia, which can be fatal. One exception to the no-fasting rule is if the planned operation involves the stomach, in which case a 3- to 4-hour fasting period will reduce the volume of digesta.

Successful recovery from an operation and anesthesia in these species is critically dependent on reestablishing a normal feeding pattern. It is therefore strongly recommended that food be available up until 1 to 2 hours before anesthesia and provided again as soon as the animal has recovered. The anesthetist should be aware that many of these animals are nocturnal and will not feed during the day. Postoperative pain and discomfort can also decrease appetite in the period after the operation.

| TABLE 11-2 | Volumes of Fluid Administration for Adult Small Mammals* | | | | | |
|---|---|---|---|---|---|---|
| Route | Gerbil | Guinea Pig | Hamster | Mouse | Rabbit | Rat |
| Intraperitoneal | 2-3 mL | 20 mL | 3 mL | 2 mL | 50 mL | 5 mL |
| Subcutaneous | 1-2 mL | 10-20 mL | 3 mL | 1-2 mL | 30-50 mL | 5 mL |

*All fluids should be warmed to body temperature before administration.

## Correction of Preexisting Problems

If animals are in poor condition, every attempt should be made to commence supportive therapy before anesthesia. One common problem is dehydration. Unfortunately the small body size of these animals makes administration of fluids difficult. In rabbits the marginal ear veins and cephalic veins can be used, but in rodents the small size of the veins does not allow easy intravenous catheterization. One alternative is to administer fluids by the subcutaneous or intraperitoneal route, although subcutaneous administration is unlikely to be effective if dehydration is severe. The **intraosseous** route can also be used and can be a valuable means of providing prolonged fluid therapy in rabbits, guinea pigs, and rats.

Calculation of fluid volume and administration rates is done according to body weight. Small mammals require higher maintenance rates than dogs and cats (100 mL/kg every 24 hours). All of the commonly used fluids used in small animal practice can be administered to rodents and rabbits. Suggested volumes for administration are listed in Table 11-2.

## PREANESTHETIC AGENTS

> *TECHNICIAN NOTE*  Atropine is often relatively ineffective in rabbits because many animals have high levels of atropinase, an enzyme that inactivates atropine. Glycopyrrolate should be used instead.

Although the general principles governing the use of preanesthetic agents (see Chapter 3) apply in small mammals, these agents are less frequently used than in dogs and cats. This is primarily because of the methods of anesthesia that are used in small mammals. Because many anesthetic protocols include a combination of anesthetic agents to be given by subcutaneous, intraperitoneal, or intramuscular injection, there is often little advantage in giving a sedative agent before this. If anesthesia is to be induced with an anesthetic chamber, prior sedation is rarely needed except in rabbits. However, preanesthetic agents should be used in the following circumstances:
- Preanesthetics can be used to reduce salivation associated with some anesthetics (e.g., ketamine) and to reduce bronchial secretions, particularly in animals with preexisting respiratory disease. Atropine is frequently used for this purpose, but in rabbits it is often relatively ineffective, because many animals have high levels of atropinase. It is therefore advisable to use glycopyrrolate in rabbits.
- Opioid analgesics may be given 30 to 45 minutes before induction of anesthesia. This reduces the concentration of volatile anesthetic needed to maintain anesthesia and provides preemptive analgesia (see Chapter 7).
- Sedatives or tranquilizers should be given to rabbits before induction of anesthesia with volatile agents (see detailed discussion later in this section).

All of the agents that are commonly used for preanesthetic medication in dogs and cats can be used in small mammals. Their properties and side effects are very similar, but some vary in their actions. Suggested dose rates and effects are listed in Table 11-3.

### Anticholinergics

Both atropine and glycopyrrolate can be used in small mammals with the same indications as in dogs and cats. As mentioned earlier, glycopyrrolate is preferred to atropine for use in rabbits because the effect of atropine is less predictable in this species.

### Phenothiazines

Phenothiazines such as acepromazine can be used to sedate small mammals. When used in rodents, acepromazine will sedate the animal but will not immobilize it. In rabbits, acepromazine has excellent sedative effects and will often provide sufficient restraint for procedures such as radiography.

### Benzodiazepines

Both diazepam and midazolam have marked sedative effects in rodents and rabbits, unlike their effects in dogs and cats. They can be administered by intraperitoneal, intramuscular, or intravenous injection and are often used in combination with other agents to produce balanced anesthesia. The sedative properties, although pronounced, are not usually sufficient to immobilize an animal for a minor procedure such as radiography.

| TABLE 11-3 | Preanesthetic Agents for Use in Small Mammals | | |
|---|---|---|---|
| Drug | Species | Dose Rate | Effect |
| Acepromazine | Rat, guinea pig | 2.5 mg/kg IP or SC | Sedation, but still active |
| | Mouse, hamster, gerbil | 3-5 mg/kg IP or SC | |
| | Rabbit | 1 mg/kg SC or IM | Sedation, often immobilized |
| Acepromazine and butorphanol | Rabbit | 0.5 mg/kg + 1 mg/kg IM or SC | Sedation, often immobilized, some analgesia |
| Atropine | Mouse, hamster, gerbil, rat, guinea pig | 40 mg/kg SC or IM | Reduced bronchial and salivary secretions, inhibition of vagal responses, ineffective in many rabbits |
| Diazepam | Mouse, hamster, gerbil, guinea pig | 5 mg/kg IP | Sedation |
| | Rat | 2.5 mg/kg IP | |
| | Rabbit | 1-2 mg/kg IM | |
| Glycopyrrolate | Rabbit | 0.01 mg/kg IV or 0.1 mg/kg SC or IM | Reduced bronchial and salivary secretions, inhibition of vagal responses |
| Innovar Vet (fentanyl-droperidol) | Rabbit | 0.22 mL/kg IM | Sedation and analgesia, often sufficiently immobilized for minor surgical procedures |
| | Mouse | 0.5 mL/kg IM | |
| | Hamster | 1.5 mL/kg IM | |
| | Guinea pig | 0.4 mL/kg IM | |
| Hypnorm (fentanyl-fluanisone) | Mouse, hamster, gerbil, rat, guinea pig | 0.5 mL/kg SC or IP | Sedation and analgesia, often sufficiently immobilized for minor surgical procedures |
| | Rabbit | 0.3-0.5 mL/kg SC or IM | |
| Medetomidine | Mouse, hamster, rat | 30-100 mg/kg SC or IP | Sedation and some analgesia, immobilized at higher dose rates |
| | Rabbit | 100-500 mg SC or IP | |
| Midazolam | Mouse, hamster, gerbil, guinea pig | 5 mg/kg IP | Sedation |
| | Rat | 2.5 mg/kg IP | |
| | Rabbit | 1-2 mg/kg IM | |
| Xylazine | Mouse, hamster, rat | 5 mg/kg SC or IM | Sedation and some analgesia, immobilized at higher dose rates |
| | Rabbit | 2.5 mg/kg SC or IM | |

*IM*, Intramuscular; *IP*, intraperitoneal; *IV*, intravenous; *SC*, subcutaneous.

## Alpha$_2$-Adrenoreceptor Agonists

Xylazine, medetomidine, and dexmedetomidine can be used to produce sedation with some analgesia in small mammals. At higher dose rates the effects can be sufficient to immobilize some animals. This effect is most reliable in the rabbit, and medetomidine or dexmedetomidine can be used to provide sedation and restraint for radiography in this species. One side effect of medetomidine and dexmedetomidine, vomiting (which is often seen in dogs and cats), does not occur in small mammals because these animals do not vomit. The other side effects of these agents, such as hyperglycemia, diuresis, and respiratory and cardiovascular system depression, do occur. A major advantage of these sedatives is that their action can be reversed by administration of specific antagonists. Both yohimbine and atipamezole have been used for this purpose in small mammals. Atipamezole is preferable because it has fewer side effects. It can be given through the subcutaneous, intraperitoneal, intramuscular, and intravenous routes. Absorption after subcutaneous injection is rapid; the drug generally acts within 5 to 10 minutes. Dose rates of 0.5 to 1.0 mg/kg are required, depending on the dose of medetomidine that has been administered.

## Opioids

The use of opioids in the preanesthetic period to provide preemptive analgesia is discussed in Chapter 7. More commonly, opioids are used in small mammals in combination with sedative agents to provide chemical restraint and analgesia for minor procedures such as suturing

| TABLE 11-4 | Anesthetic and Related Drugs for Use in Small Mammals* | | | | | |
|---|---|---|---|---|---|---|
| Anesthetic and Related Agents | Gerbil | Guinea Pig | Hamster | Mouse | Rabbit | Rat |
| Atipamezole | 1 mg/kg SC, IM, IP, IV | 1 mg/kg SC, IM, IP, IV | 1 mg/kg SC, IM, IP, IV | 1 mg/kg SC, IM, IP, IV | 1 mg/kg SC, IM, IP, IV | 1 mg/kg SC, IM, IP, IV |
| Doxapram | 5-10 mg/kg IV or IP | 5-10 mg/kg IV or IP | 5-10 mg/kg IV or IP | 5-10 mg/kg IV or IP | 5-10 mg/kg IV or IM | 5-10 mg/kg IV or IP |
| Fentanyl-fluanisone and diazepam† | 0.3 mL/kg IM + 5 mg/kg IP | 1 mL/kg IM + 2.5 mg/kg IP | 1 mL/kg IM + 5 mg/kg IP | 0.3 mL/kg IM + 5 mg/kg IP | 0.3 mL/kg IM + 2 mg/kg IP or IV | 0.3 mL/kg IM + 2.5 mg/kg IP |
| Fentanyl-fluanisone and midazolam‡ | 8 mL/kg IP | 8 mL/kg IP | 4 mL/kg IP | 10 mL/kg IP | 0.3 mL/kg IM + 2 mg/kg IP or IV | 2.7 mL/kg IP |
| Ketamine and medetomidine | — | 40 mg/kg + 0.5 mg/kg IP | 100 mg/kg + 0.25 mg/kg IP | 75 mg/kg + 1 mg/kg IP | 15 mg/kg + 0.25 mg/kg IM | 75 mg/kg + 0.5 mg/kg IP |
| Ketamine and xylazine | 50 mg/kg + 2 mg/kg IP | 40 mg/kg + 5 mg/kg IP | 200 mg/kg + 10 mg/kg IP | 80 mg/kg + 10 mg/kg IP | 35 mg/kg + 5 mg/kg IM | 75 mg/kg + 10 mg/kg IP |
| Pentobarbitone | 60-80 mg/kg IP | 37 mg/kg IP | 50-90 mg/kg IP | 40-50 mg/kg IP | 30-45 mg/kg IV | 40-50 mg/kg IP |
| Tiletamine and zolazepam (immobilizes, does not usually produce anesthesia) | 60 mg/kg IM | 40-60 mg/kg IM | 50-80 mg/kg IM | 80-100 mg/kg IM | 5-25 mg/kg IM | 20-40 mg/kg IM |

*IM*, Intramuscular; *IP*, intraperitoneal; *IV*, intravenous; *SC*, subcutaneous.

*Note that there may be considerable variation among strains, and these dose rates should be taken as a general guide only.

†These drugs cannot be mixed together and must be given separately.

‡Doses are milliliters of a combination of fentanyl/fluanisone and midazolam, prepared as 2 mL water for injection plus 1 mL of 5 mg/mL midazolam and 1 mL of "Hypnorm" (Janssen, fentanyl-fluanisone).

superficial wounds and draining abscesses. In North America a commercially prepared mixture of fentanyl and **droperidol** (Innovar Vet) was formerly available for this purpose, and a similar mixture of fentanyl and **fluanisone** (Hypnorm) is still available in Europe. A mixture of acepromazine and butorphanol is useful for getting blood samples from rabbits because it provides some sedation and analgesia and dilates the ear veins.

## GENERAL ANESTHESIA

### Induction Techniques and Agents

Although techniques similar to those used for anesthetic induction in dogs and cats can be used in small mammals, practical considerations limit the use of the intravenous route except in rabbits. A wide range of different anesthetic agents can be used in these species, and suggested dose rates are given in Table 11-4. Formulas for anesthetic mixtures used in small mammals are given in Box 11-1.

In rabbits, the subcutaneous and intramuscular routes are often used, although intravenous injection of short-acting agents is also possible in some animals. For small mammals, intraperitoneal injection is a simple and relatively painless injection route for induction agents.

The intraperitoneal route appears to be less painful than intramuscular injection, although the technique is less familiar. The technique is similar in most small rodents, in which an assistant extends the right hindlimb and injects the anesthetic into the middle of the right posterior quadrant of the abdomen. This technique avoids the bladder, which lies in the midline just in front of the pelvis. Use of the right side of the abdomen also avoids the cecum, which is large and thin-walled in rodents.

Although the technique for intraperitoneal injection is simple to carry out, administration of anesthetics by this route has important practical implications. If an anesthetic is given intravenously, the dose that is administered can be titrated to provide the required effect in that particular animal. It is therefore relatively simple to adjust the dose to account for individual, breed, and strain variation, and overdosing or underdosing is easy to avoid. When anesthetics are given intraperitoneally (or by subcutaneous or intramuscular injection), a calculated dose is given, and there is no opportunity to adjust it to suit the requirements of the particular animal. As large variations in response to anesthetics have been noted in small rodents, it is advisable to select an anesthetic regimen that has a wide safety margin (preferably one that is completely or partially reversible) if injection routes other than intravenous are used.

---

**BOX 11-1** | **Formulas for Anesthetic Mixtures for Small Mammals**

- Many of these solutions can be stored for a few days if made carefully and placed in a sterile multidose ampule. There is some risk of instability with prolonged storage, and this practice is not recommended by the manufacturers.
- If necessary, solutions can be diluted with sterile water for injection or sterile saline to provide an appropriate volume for accurate administration. The appropriate volume for mice is 0.1 mL/10 g (therefore an adult mouse would need 0.2 to 0.4 mL IP or SC). The appropriate volume for a rat is 0.2 mL/100 g (therefore an adult rat would need 0.5 to 0.8 mL IP or SC).
- See Tables 11-3 and 11-4 for doses used in each species.

**Examples**

1. To make a 2-mL mixture of ketamine (75 mg/kg) and medetomidine (0.5 mg/kg) for rats, mix together the following:

   | | |
   |---|---|
   | Ketamine (100 mg/mL) | 0.75 mL |
   | Medetomidine (1 mg/mL) | 0.5 mL |
   | Sterile saline (0.9%) | 0.75 mL |

   Administer at 0.2 mL/100 g IP.

2. To make a 5-mL mixture of ketamine (75 mg/kg) and medetomidine (1 mg/kg) for mice, mix together the following:

   | | |
   |---|---|
   | Ketamine (100 mg/mL) | 0.38 mL |
   | Medetomidine (1 mg/mL) | 0.5 mL |
   | Sterile saline (0.9%) | 4.12 mL |

   Administer at 0.1 mL/10 g IP.

*IP*, Intraperitoneal; *SC*, subcutaneous.

---

A further problem associated with use of the intraperitoneal or intramuscular route is that relatively high dose rates are required compared with those that are needed when drugs are given intravenously. One consequence is that recovery times tend to be prolonged, which is particularly undesirable in small mammals because of the high risk of hypothermia.

## Cyclohexamine Agents

When used alone, ketamine has limited effect in small mammals, even at high doses. In rodents it barely immobilizes the animal and does not provide sufficient analgesia for even superficial surgical procedures such as suturing of skin wounds. In rabbits, use of ketamine alone provides restraint, but the degree of analgesia is insufficient for surgery. Ketamine-acepromazine and ketamine-diazepam or ketamine-midazolam produces surgical anesthesia in some rabbits, but these combinations generally produce only light anesthesia in small rodents. Ketamine is most effective when combined with an alpha$_2$-agonist such as medetomidine or xylazine, because these agents have analgesic activity. Ketamine with medetomidine or xylazine produces surgical anesthesia in most rodents and rabbits, but the effects of these agents are less uniform in guinea pigs, and some animals may not be at a sufficient

depth of anesthesia for an operation to be carried out humanely. Although relatively little information is available at present concerning the use of dexmedetomidine in small mammals, experience in other species indicates it will have equivalent effects to medetomidine. As in other species, the dose required is approximately 50% of the medetomidine dose. Because ketamine has limited effects when used alone in small mammals, reversal of xylazine, medetomidine, or dexmedetomidine will considerably reduce the length of the recovery period. However, because the analgesic effects are also reversed, another analgesic should be administered to provide postoperative pain relief.

Tiletamine in combination with zolazepam (Zoletil, Telazol) produces light to medium planes of anesthesia in small rodents. It offers little advantage in comparison with ketamine combined with diazepam or midazolam, and it produces less analgesia than ketamine in combination with xylazine or medetomidine.

## Neuroleptanalgesics

As mentioned earlier, the combinations of fentanyl-droperidol and fentanyl-fluanisone provide restraint and analgesia in small mammals. Fentanyl and fluanisone also can be combined with a benzodiazepine to provide surgical anesthesia. The addition of midazolam or diazepam provides muscle relaxation and increases the depth of anesthesia. Recovery can be enhanced by reversal of fentanyl with a mixed agonist-antagonist opioid such as butorphanol or nalbuphine. This reverses the respiratory depression and some of the sedation caused by the fentanyl component of the anesthetic mixture but continues to provide postoperative analgesia. Although antagonists of benzodiazepine (e.g., flumazenil) can be administered to speed recovery, their duration of action is short, and resedation may occur.

The effects of fentanyl and droperidol together with benzodiazepines are less predictable, and this mixture is best avoided in small mammals.

## Barbiturates

Although pentobarbital has been widely used for anesthesia of small mammals, it has a very narrow safety margin and produces severe cardiovascular and respiratory depression. Recovery from pentobarbital is prolonged and can be associated with involuntary excitement. For these reasons its use is best avoided. Thiopental and methohexital can be given by intravenous injection in rabbits to produce a short period of anesthesia, and they have effects similar to those seen in dogs and cats.

## Propofol

Propofol produces short periods of surgical anesthesia in small rodents, but, because it must be given by intravenous injection, it is rarely used in these species. Propofol can be used in rabbits to provide a short period of light anesthesia, sufficient for induction of anesthesia followed

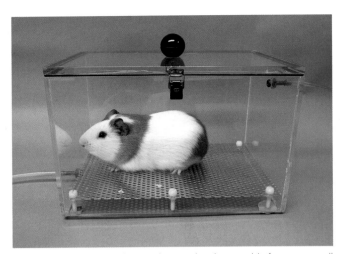

**FIGURE 11-13**    Anesthetic induction chamber suitable for use in small mammals.

by endotracheal intubation and maintenance of anesthesia with gas anesthetics. If high doses of propofol are given to rabbits in an attempt to produce a surgical plane of anesthesia, respiratory arrest often occurs. When propofol is administered to rabbits, it should be injected slowly (e.g., over 1 to 2 minutes for an induction dose in a 3-kg rabbit). When administered in this way, it rarely causes significant respiratory depression.

### Alphaxalone

The steroid anesthetic alphaxalone can be used to induce anesthesia in rabbits when given by intravenous injection. This anesthetic causes minimal cardiovascular depression, and recovery after its use is relatively rapid.

### Inhalation Anesthetics

Induction of anesthesia with inhalation agents is probably the safest and most effective means of providing anesthesia in small rodents. Although mask induction is possible, it is usually most convenient to induce anesthesia in an anesthetic chamber. Suitable chambers can be purchased commercially or can be constructed from clear plastic containers. The size of the chamber should be such that it can be filled rapidly with anesthetic vapor from the anesthetic machine. This will ensure that induction of anesthesia is rapid and smooth with a brief period of involuntary excitement. Anesthetic vapors are denser than air, so the chamber should be filled from the bottom and excess anesthetic gases removed from the top. A suitable design is shown in Figure 11-13.

Isoflurane, desflurane, and sevoflurane can all be used safely in small rodents. The concentrations required for induction and maintenance are similar to those used in dogs and cats. Provided the anesthetic chamber is filled rapidly, induction is generally complete in 2 to 3 minutes. Recovery is also rapid, with rodents recovering their righting reflex within 5 to 10 minutes after 20 to 30 minutes of anesthesia. After a further 10 to 15 minutes they will appear to be fully recovered. As in dogs and cats, induction of anesthesia and recovery are rapid with isoflurane and even more rapid with desflurane and sevoflurane.

Inhalation anesthetics should be delivered with a precision vaporizer. Induction of anesthesia in a chamber in which liquid anesthetic is placed on a gauze pad is extremely dangerous because high concentrations (>20%) of anesthetic vapor are produced.

After induction of anesthesia, the animal can be removed from the chamber and brief (<30 seconds) procedures carried out. For longer procedures it is usually more convenient to maintain anesthesia by placing a face mask on the animal. Suitable masks can be either purchased commercially or constructed from plastic syringes. As with dogs and cats it is important that waste anesthetic gases be scavenged effectively, and this is most easily achieved by using a commercial apparatus designed for this purpose.

> **TECHNICIAN NOTE**    Rabbits should be premedicated before mask or chamber induction with an inhalant anesthetic in order to avoid violent struggling and prolonged breath-holding.

The use of gas anesthetics in rabbits can be difficult because they frequently hold their breath when exposed to these agents. Breath-holding can be prolonged and is sometimes associated with marked bradycardia. If a mask is used, animals appear to resent the procedure and may struggle violently. If placed in an anesthetic chamber, they attempt to avoid inhaling the anesthetic and may make violent attempts to escape. It is therefore preferable to administer preanesthetic medication (e.g., acepromazine, diazepam, midazolam, or medetomidine) before inducing anesthesia with a face mask or chamber. After this medication has taken effect, a mask can be used to administer 100% oxygen for 1 to 2 minutes before introducing the induction agent. The animal may still hold its breath but is unlikely to struggle. If breath-holding occurs, the mask should be briefly removed and replaced when the animal commences breathing again. An alternative approach is to administer a short-acting induction agent such as propofol and maintain anesthesia with an inhalation agent.

> **TECHNICIAN NOTE**    Because of the ease of control of depth of anesthesia, the simple and convenient method of induction, and the rapid recovery, inhalation agents are often the anesthesia method of choice in small mammals.

### Summary of Recommended Techniques

Because of the ease of control of depth of anesthesia, the simple and convenient method of induction, and the rapid recovery, inhalation agents are often the anesthesia method of choice in small mammals. If injectable anesthetics are preferred, ketamine with an alpha$_2$-agonist, or fentanyl-fluanisone with a benzodiazepine are the combinations of choice. If an injectable anesthetic combination has been administered and the desired depth of anesthesia is not reached, it is possible to administer an additional drug to deepen anesthesia. However, it is often preferable to deepen anesthesia with a low concentration of an inhalation agent or alternatively to provide local analgesia by infiltrating the surgical site with local anesthetic. These techniques are also useful when dealing with high-risk patients. In these circumstances a low dose of an injectable anesthetic combination can be given to provide a light plane of anesthesia, and inhalation anesthetics or local anesthetics can be used to provide surgical anesthesia.

## Intubation and Maintenance of Anesthesia

The apparatus used to anesthetize small rodents and rabbits is similar to that used in dogs and cats, but the size of the patient limits some of the equipment that can be used. Generally, anesthetic gases are delivered with a face mask; however, in rabbits endotracheal intubation is a relatively simple technique to perform and is recommended as a routine procedure. Endotracheal intubation can be carried out by visualizing the larynx with a laryngoscope and blade created for this purpose (such as a Wisconsin or Flecknell blade) or a canine otoscope. Alternatively, a blind technique can be used. These procedures are outlined in detail in Procedure 11-1, p. 316.

Uncuffed endotracheal tubes are preferred. A typical 3-kg rabbit requires a tube with a 3- to 3.5-mm diameter. Very small rabbits (<800 g) need tubes with a diameter of less than 2.5 mm, which can be purchased from specialist suppliers. A rabbit's airway can also be maintained using a **laryngeal mask.** These are simple to use in this species and allow some control of respiration. As an alternative to intubation, a nasal catheter can be passed and positioned in the back of the pharynx. This allows oxygen supplementation during oral surgery but does not enable ventilation to be assisted effectively. Nasal catheters can also be used in small rodents to deliver oxygen or anesthetic gases (Figure 11-14). This is particularly useful when carrying out dental procedures. Waste anesthetic gases can be removed by placing an extract tube close to the animal's nose, and the potential problem reduced by using appropriately low fresh gas flows.

An anesthetic machine with an out-of-circuit precision vaporizer should be used. Open, non-rebreathing systems are preferred to closed-circuit systems because they offer less resistance and have less equipment dead space. Examples of suitable non-rebreathing systems include the Bain circuit and Ayres T-piece. With smaller rabbits, it is advisable to use low–dead space pediatric connectors to attach the endotracheal tube to the breathing circuit. Low–dead space T-piece systems designed for use in human beings are also useful for

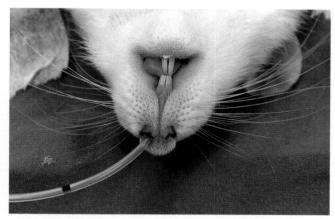

**FIGURE 11-14**   Nasal catheter being used to deliver oxygen to a rat. The catheter is an infant nasogastric feeding tube, but any suitably sized soft catheter can be used.

rabbits (Figure 11-15). Fresh gas flow rates are calculated in the same way as for dogs and cats (see Box 4-3).

### Monitoring

#### Depth of Anesthesia

Before a surgical or other painful procedure is started, it is essential to ensure that the animal is at an appropriate depth of anesthesia. The most reliable method in rodents is to assess the pedal withdrawal reflex (discussed in Chapter 5) or tail pinch reflex. To assess the tail pinch, the operator firmly pinches the tip of the tail with fingernails. It is important to pinch hard enough to produce a painful stimulus, but not so hard as to damage the tail. If the animal is too lightly anesthetized for surgery, it will flick its tail and may vocalize. The tail pinch response is usually lost at light to medium planes of anesthesia, and this is followed by a loss of the pedal withdrawal response at medium to deep planes of anesthesia. Most surgical procedures can be carried out when the pedal withdrawal reflex is absent or barely detectable. In rabbits and guinea pigs the ear pinch reflex can also be used to measure anesthetic depth.

Ocular reflexes are not as useful in small mammals as in the dog and cat. With most anesthetic regimens, the position of the eye remains fixed in rodents, and the palpebral (blink) reflex may still be present at surgical planes of anesthesia. In rabbits, there is considerable variation in loss of ocular reflexes; however, at deep planes of anesthesia the eye may rotate and protrude. Because cardiac arrest may occur shortly after the animal reaches such a deep plane of anesthesia, this appearance indicates that supportive measures should be initiated immediately and administration of anesthetic should be reduced or terminated.

---

*TECHNICIAN NOTE*   Many pieces of monitoring equipment (blood pressure monitor, electrocardiograph, pulse oximeter) are not designed to function normally within the range of heart rates (often 250 to 300) seen in small mammals.

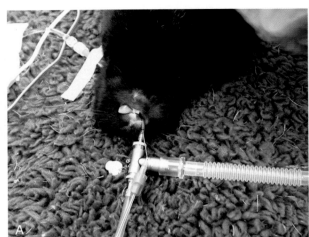
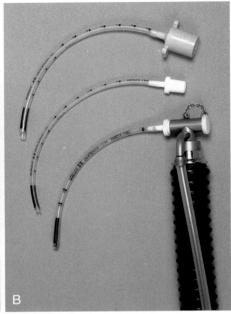

**FIGURE 11-15** **A,** Low–dead space pediatric T-piece and endotracheal connector suitable for anesthetic delivery in a rabbit. **B,** Endotracheal tube connectors. *Top,* Standard connector; *middle,* pediatric connector; *bottom,* pediatric connector and T-piece.

### Heart Rate and Rhythm

The small size of rodents and rabbits and their rapid heart rate can make it difficult to monitor heart rate and rhythm, and it is not usually possible to palpate a peripheral pulse. Auscultation of the chest wall is possible in rabbits and guinea pigs but difficult in smaller rodents. An esophageal stethoscope can be used in rabbits, and the heartbeat can be detected by palpating the chest wall in all species. However, because the heart rate often exceeds 250 beats per minute (bpm) in many of these animals, it is not possible to accurately assess the heart rate. Problems can also arise when an electrocardiograph is used, because many instruments have an upper heart rate limit of 250 or 300 bpm and may also be unable to detect the low-amplitude signals generated in small rodents.

### Capillary Refill Time

The small size of rodents usually prevents use of capillary refill time for assessment of peripheral perfusion, although it is possible to assess this in rabbits. The color of the mucous membranes can give some indication of problems associated with blood loss, cyanosis, and poor peripheral perfusion. In addition to inspection of the gingiva, the color of light reflected in the eyes can be used to detect cyanosis or pallor caused by blood loss in albino animals.

> TECHNICIAN NOTE    Loss of 1 mL of blood represents a 15% blood loss in a small mammal weighing 100 g; this puts the patient at risk for hypovolemic circulatory failure.

### Blood Loss

Because these animals are small, total blood volume is small—approximately 70 mL/kg of body weight. A 100-g hamster will have a total blood volume of only 7 mL. As in dogs and cats, loss of more than 15% (approximately 1 mL in this example) can lead to signs of circulatory failure. It is therefore critically important to monitor blood loss by carefully weighing swabs and assessing other losses at the surgical site.

### Arterial Blood Pressure

Blood pressure can be monitored in rabbits either with a catheter placed in the central ear artery or noninvasively with an oscillometric technique. The pressure cuff should be placed either on the forelimb, just proximal to the elbow, or on the hindlimb, proximal to the stifle (Figure 11-16). The success of this technique depends on both the size of the rabbit and the particular monitor. As an alternative, a Doppler probe can be placed over a suitable artery, and, if the probe is combined with use of a blood pressure cuff and sphygmomanometer, an estimate of arterial pressure can be obtained (see Chapter 5).

### Respiratory Rate and Depth

The pattern and depth of respiration can be monitored by observing the chest movements, although this becomes difficult once surgical drapes have been placed. Because of the small size of these animals, there is usually no reservoir bag in the anesthetic circuit, and respiration cannot be monitored by bag movement. It is helpful to use an electronic monitor, but as with the electrocardiograph, the small size of the animal and rapid respiratory rate can make some monitors ineffective.

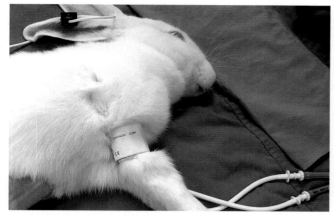

**FIGURE 11-16** Use of noninvasive blood pressure monitoring in the rabbit. A pulse oximeter probe placed on the pinna is also being used to monitor this animal.

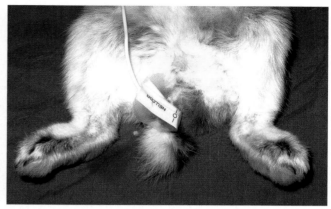

**FIGURE 11-17** Use of a pulse oximeter in a rabbit, with the probe positioned across the base of the tail.

Although the pattern and rate of respiration change during anesthesia, they can both vary greatly depending on the anesthetic regimen used. Becoming familiar with one or two regularly used regimens allows changes to be interpreted more reliably. In general, once anesthesia has been induced, respiratory rate decreases markedly, especially because most of these animals will show tachypnea before induction. Typical respiratory rates during anesthesia are 50 to 100 breaths/min for small rodents and 30 to 60 breaths/min for rabbits. A reduction to less than 50% of the estimated normal respiratory rate (see Table 11-1) should give cause for concern. As in dogs and cats, it is more common to see gradual changes in rate, rather than a sudden reduction. For this reason, it is helpful to keep a written anesthetic record when assessing the state of the animal during anesthesia.

### Pulse Oximetry

Pulse oximeters can be used to monitor both the adequacy of oxygenation and the heart rate, but not all instruments function well in small rodents. The high heart rates may exceed the upper limits of the monitor, and the low signal strength means the signal may not be detectable. A monitor with an upper limit of at least 350 bpm is needed, and it is useful to have a variety of different probe designs. A reliable signal can usually be obtained by placing the probe across the hind foot in small rodents or across a toe in larger rabbits, but the tail, tongue, and ear are also useful in some animals (Figures 11-16 and 11-17).

### Capnography

Side-stream capnographs can be used to monitor respiratory function in small animals, although the volume of gas sampled may be very large in relation to the animal's tidal volume. Mainstream capnographs introduce too much equipment dead space into the anesthetic breathing circuit and are not recommended in these species, but

low–dead space, human pediatric versions can be used successfully in rabbits.

> *TECHNICIAN NOTE* Because of their small body size, rodents and rabbits have an increased ratio of surface area to body weight, which may lead to rapid cooling during anesthesia. It is therefore critically important to monitor and maintain body temperature during anesthesia and in the postoperative period.

### Thermoregulation

It is critically important to monitor and maintain body temperature during anesthesia and in the postoperative period. Because of their small body size, rodents and rabbits have an increased ratio of surface area to body weight, which may lead to rapid cooling during anesthesia. Heat loss can be much more rapid than in dogs and cats. For example, the rectal temperature in a mouse can fall 5° to 6° C (9° to 11° F) in 5 to 10 minutes after induction of anesthesia. The following procedures help avoid hypothermia:

- Monitor rectal temperatures with an electronic thermometer rather than a glass clinical thermometer. Glass clinical thermometers can indicate a minimum temperature of only 35° C, and the animal may be colder than this when the first measurement is made.
- Adopt good standards of asepsis, but keep the area of fur that is shaved at the surgical site to a minimum, and use the minimum quantity of skin disinfectant.
- Place the animal on a warming pad as soon as it has lost consciousness, and provide additional insulation if needed.
- Always warm fluids to body temperature before administration.
- Continue measures to prevent heat loss in the recovery period (see the following section).

## POSTOPERATIVE CARE

The provision of appropriate postoperative care is critical to the successful outcome of anesthesia and surgery in small mammals. Supportive measures to maintain body temperature must be continued, and a quiet, warm, secure environment should be provided. Because heat loss can occur relatively rapidly, an appropriate recovery environment should be set up before commencement of anesthesia and an operation. The animal can then be transferred to the recovery area immediately after completion of the operation. While the animal is immobile and unconscious, an environmental temperature of approximately 35° C (95° F) should be maintained. This can be lowered to 26° to 28° C (79° to 81° F) as the animal recovers. Warm and comfortable bedding must be provided. Synthetic sheepskin is ideal, but if this is unavailable, shredded paper or tissues can be used. Sawdust is unsuitable because it tends to crust around the nose, eyes, and mouth. Good-quality hay should be provided to guinea pigs and rabbits once they have recovered their righting reflex. This type of bedding allows the animal to surround itself with insulating material, which provides both warmth and a sense of security and encourages early feeding. Small mammals of other species should also be encouraged to eat soon after recovery and should be given their preferred foods.

Animals should also be provided with water, but care must be taken that they do not spill water bowls, because the animal will lose heat rapidly if it becomes wet. The animal may also fail to drink from an unfamiliar water container, and when a case history is obtained before anesthesia it is important to find out what type of container the animal is accustomed to using. In most circumstances, it is advisable to administer warmed (37° C or 98.6° F) subcutaneous or intraperitoneal dextrose-saline (4% dextrose, 0.15% saline) at the end of the operation to provide some fluid supplementation in the immediate postoperative period.

Postoperative analgesia is discussed later in the chapter.

## ANESTHETIC EMERGENCIES

### Respiratory Depression

Changes in the depth and pattern of respiration usually precede respiratory arrest. Careful monitoring of respiratory function will usually allow corrective measures to be taken before an emergency arises. If the animal has been intubated, respiration can be assisted by delivery of 100% oxygen from the anesthetic machine. As with larger species, it is important to check that the endotracheal tube is properly positioned and has not become disconnected from the breathing circuit or obstructed. If the animal has not been intubated, respiration can be assisted by extending the head and neck and gently compressing the chest.

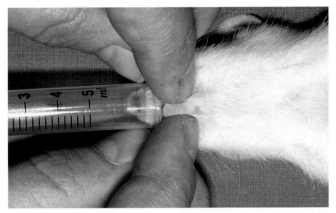

**FIGURE 11-18**  Assisting ventilation in a rat by blowing down the barrel of a syringe placed over the mouth and nose.

Attempts to assist ventilation with a face mask are usually unsuccessful. In small rodents, a soft piece of rubber tubing can be placed over the nose and mouth and the lungs inflated by gently blowing down the tube (Figure 11-18). Respiration can also be stimulated by administration of doxapram, but this drug has a relatively short duration of action (approximately 10 minutes), and repeated doses may be needed. Efforts should be made to determine the cause of the respiratory depression and to initiate corrective measures.

### Circulatory Failure

Treatment of circulatory failure and cardiac arrest is similar to that in dogs and cats, but the small size of these animals causes some practical problems. Fluid therapy is difficult because of the small size of the superficial vessels, although it is possible to place over-the-needle catheters in the tail vein of rats and the medial tarsal vein in guinea pigs. In rabbits, intravenous access is much easier, and catheters can be placed in the marginal ear veins or cephalic veins. The jugular vein is relatively mobile in the rabbit and is more difficult to locate and catheterize than in the dog and cat.

Loss of blood can be treated by transfusion from a donor animal. Fortunately, problems of incompatibility are rare on initial transfusion; however, it is likely to be more difficult to locate a suitable donor than when dealing with dogs and cats. As an alternative, a plasma volume expander such as dextran or hetastarch can be administered. All of the commonly available products can be administered safely to small mammals, providing appropriate allowance is made for their smaller circulating volumes. In smaller species in which intravenous access is not practical, intraperitoneal or subcutaneous administration of warmed electrolyte solutions can slowly replace fluid deficits or blood loss but will be of minimal benefit if rapid hemorrhage is occurring. As discussed earlier, preventing problems by minimizing hemorrhage through meticulous surgical technique is important.

| TABLE 11-5 | Dose Rates for Emergency Drugs with Typical Dilutions and Volumes Needed for an Adult Animal* | | |
|---|---|---|---|
| Drug | Concentration in Commercial Preparation | Dilution Instructions | Volume of Diluted Drug for a Typical Adult Animal |
| Doxapram | 20 mg/mL | 1 in 10 | Mouse, 0.1 mL; hamster and gerbil, 0.25 mL SC or IV |
| | | Not required | Rat, 0.1 mL; guinea pig, 0.25 mL SC or IV |
| Epinephrine | 1:1000 | 1 in 10 | Mouse, 0.03 mL; hamster and gerbil, 0.1 mL; rat, 0.3 mL; guinea pig, 0.7 mL IV or intracardiac |
| Lidocaine | 20 mg/mL | 1 in 10 | Mouse, 0.03 mL; hamster and gerbil, 0.1 mL; rat, 0.3 mL; guinea pig, 0.7 mL IV or intracardiac |
| Sodium bicarbonate | 1 mEq/mL | Not required | Mouse, 0.03 mL; hamster and gerbil, 0.1 mL; rat, 0.3 mL; guinea pig, 0.7 mL IV |

*IV*, Intravenous; *SC*, subcutaneous.
*For rabbits, dose rates are similar to those for dogs and cats.

If cardiac arrest occurs, external cardiac massage and emergency drugs such as epinephrine can be used to try to resuscitate the animal (see Chapter 12). One significant problem is the practical difficulty of rapidly calculating drug dose rates when an emergency occurs. It is much simpler to use a list of dose rates and volumes, expressed as the dose volumes for a typical adult animal of each species. This will help avoid errors and speed therapy (Table 11-5).

## POSTOPERATIVE ANALGESIA

As discussed in Chapter 7, the use of analgesics in veterinary practice has become more widespread in recent years. Although most dogs and cats now receive at least some perioperative analgesia, these drugs are often not used as frequently in small mammals. This is probably a result of a number of factors, including poor ability to recognize pain in these small animals and a lack of knowledge about the safety and efficacy of analgesic agents. However, it is critically important to provide postoperative analgesia to these patients, because most small mammals will fail to eat or drink if they are experiencing postoperative pain.

### Pain Assessment in Small Mammals

Pain assessment in dogs and cats is not always easy, but most veterinarians and veterinary technicians are relatively familiar with the normal behavior of these species. The normal behavior and general appearance of small rodents and rabbits are often less well appreciated, and as a result the signs associated with pain may be overlooked. In addition, several species of small mammals are nocturnal and may not be active when observed during normal working hours. They may also remain immobile in the presence of an observer if they perceive the

observer as a threat. It is therefore not always easy to use behavior and changes in posture to assess pain. However, it is important to overcome these difficulties so that pain can be prevented or controlled effectively in these small animals.

As in dogs and cats, an initial assessment of the animal should be made without disturbing the animal. The animal's appearance and posture may be abnormal, and it may appear hunched. Its coat may be unkempt and ruffled because of a lack of grooming and the presence of piloerection. Rats may have a blackish discharge around their eyes and nose because of a buildup of secretions from their harderian glands. It is uncertain whether this buildup of material results from reduced grooming or whether it is a response to stress, but it is a valuable indicator that the animal is not healthy and may be in pain. While it is being observed, the animal may demonstrate normal inquisitive behavior and explore its environment, but as mentioned earlier, if it remains motionless, this may be because it feels threatened rather than because it is in pain. If the animal has positioned itself in the back of its cage or pen or has hidden in bedding, this can be a sign of fear but may also indicate pain.

When encouraged to move, the animal may have an abnormal gait or posture and may show uncharacteristic signs of aggression. Rats, mice, and gerbils will usually rear when investigating what has disturbed them, and the absence of this behavior may indicate pain. When handled, rather than attempting to evade capture, animals in pain may be apathetic or may be aggressive and bite the handler. When it is examined, the animal may respond to manipulation or palpation of a painful area by vocalizing or trying to bite. Confusingly, some small mammals such as guinea pigs will also vocalize loudly when not in pain and may respond to any manipulation by tensing their muscles and remaining immobile. Similar immobility can also be seen in rabbits. Abdominal pain in rabbits, rats, and mice often produces characteristic behaviors

| TABLE 11-6 | Analgesic Agents for Use in Small Mammals* | | | | | |
|---|---|---|---|---|---|---|
| Analgesic | Gerbil | Guinea Pig | Hamster | Mouse | Rabbit | Rat |
| Buprenorphine | 0.1 mg/kg SC | 0.05 mg/kg SC | 0.1 mg/kg SC | 0.1 mg/kg SC | 0.01-0.05 mg/kg SC | 0.05 mg/kg SC |
| Butorphanol | ? | 2 mg/kg | ? | 1-5 mg/kg SC | 0.1-0.5 mg/kg SC | 2 mg/kg SC |
| Carprofen | ? | 2.5 mg/kg SC daily | ? | 5 mg/kg bid SC or PO | 1.5 mg/kg PO daily, 4 mg/kg SC daily | 5 mg/kg bid SC or PO |
| Flunixin | ? | ? | ? | 2.5 mg/kg SC bid | 1.1 mg/kg SC bid | 2.5 mg/kg SC bid |
| Ketoprofen | ? | ? | ? | ? | 3 mg/kg IM | 5 mg/kg IM |
| Meloxicam | ? | ? | ? | ? | 0.6 mg/kg SC daily | 1 mg/kg SC or PO daily |
| Meperidine (pethidine) | ? | 10-20 mg/kg SC or IM 2-3 hourly | ? | 10-20 mg/kg SC or IM 2-3 hourly | 10 mg/kg SC or IM 2-3 hourly | 10-20 mg/kg SC or IM 2-3 hourly |
| Morphine | ? | 2-5 mg/kg SC or IM 4 hourly | ? | 2.5 mg/kg SC or IM 4 hourly | 2-5 mg/kg SC or IM 4 hourly | 2.5 mg/kg SC or IM 4 hourly |
| Oxymorphone | ? | ? | ? | ? | 0.1-0.2 mg/kg IM, IV | 0.2-0.3 mg/kg SC |

Data modified from Flecknell PA, Waterman-Pearson AE, eds: *Pain management in animals*, London, 2001, Harcourt International.

*IM,* Intramuscular; *IV,* intravenous; *PO,* by mouth; *SC,* subcutaneous.

*These are only suggestions based on clinical experience and the limited published data that are available. Dose rates should be adjusted depending on the clinical response of the animal. A "?" indicates that there is insufficient information to make a firm recommendation of an appropriate dose.

involving contraction of the abdominal muscles, pressing of the abdomen to the floor, and, in rabbits and rats, arching of the back.

Rabbits and small mammals may stop eating and drinking when experiencing pain. This can be difficult to detect if food is provided ad lib, but the subsequent loss in body weight can easily be monitored. This is one of the easiest ways of following a small mammal's progress after surgery or during treatment of any disease condition. The inappetence caused by pain is a serious problem in small mammals, because failure to drink can rapidly lead to significant dehydration and lack of food intake can predispose to the development of hypoglycemia in small rodents. In rabbits, guinea pigs, and chinchillas, disturbances in food intake can lead to the development of life-threatening gastrointestinal disturbances.

As experience is gained in observing the normal behavior patterns of small mammals, abnormalities will be detected with greater confidence. Although relatively specific signs of pain such as guarding of an injured area may be seen, many of the signs are relatively nonspecific and can also occur in response to nonpainful conditions. It is therefore important to consider the appearance of the animal in relation to its case history and other clinical findings. Although it is highly desirable to try to assess pain in each individual patient so that appropriate analgesia therapy can be administered, it is not unreasonable to accept that some analgesic treatment will be needed after every surgical procedure.

## Analgesic Agents

None of the analgesics that are currently marketed for use in dogs and cats provide any product information regarding their use in small mammals. It is worth noting, however, that all of these products were originally tested for safety and efficacy in small rodents. This information provides reassurance that the drugs can be used safely to provide effective pain relief in these species. There is less information available on the use of analgesics in rabbits and guinea pigs, but extensive clinical experience indicates that most analgesics can be used safely in these animals. Suggested dose rates are listed in Table 11-6. The options for pain management are similar to those available for dogs and cats, but the small size of the animal may limit the use of techniques such as epidural administration of drugs or use of fentanyl patches.

> **TECHNICIAN NOTE** Many opioids—for example, morphine—have a shorter duration of action in small mammals compared with other species. Buprenorphine, with a duration of action of 6 to 12 hours in small mammals, is preferred.

All of the morphine-like drugs that can be used in dogs and cats can also be used in small mammals but often have a shorter duration of action in these species. Meperidine lasts for only 30 to 60 minutes in rodents, for example. Buprenorphine, which has a duration of action of approximately 6 to 12 hours in small mammals, is often preferred. Some authorities question whether partial agonists such as buprenorphine are potent enough to control severe pain; however, clinical experience suggests that this analgesic is effective after most surgical procedures in small rodents and rabbits. Buprenorphine may cause behavioral abnormalities in small rodents (such as eating sawdust bedding in rats). However, this side effect appears rare, and most animals appear to benefit from the use of buprenorphine after surgery. If other opioid analgesics are to be used, repeated administration is likely to be needed to provide effective pain relief. One useful means of avoiding the need for frequent injections of drug is to combine administration of an opioid with the use of a nonsteroidal antiinflammatory drug (NSAID) (see the following section).

### Nonsteroidal Antiinflammatory Drugs

NSAIDS (particularly the more potent NSAIDs such as carprofen, ketoprofen, and meloxicam) can provide very effective pain relief in small mammals. Considerable basic information is available from pharmaceutical companies concerning the safety and efficacy of these analgesics in small rodents. Although there have been no reports of adverse reactions to these drugs in small mammals, it seems advisable to adopt the same precautions as those in dogs and cats (see Chapter 7). Prolonged use (more than a few days) should be avoided when possible, although clinical experience suggests that meloxicam can be used for extended periods in rabbits to control dental pain. Because of the risks of renal toxicity should hypotension occur during anesthesia, only carprofen or meloxicam should be administered preoperatively. A significant advantage of the use of NSAIDs is that they appear to have a prolonged duration of action in small mammals. A single dose of carprofen, ketoprofen, or meloxicam may provide analgesia for 12 to 24 hours. Meloxicam has the additional advantage of being available in some countries as a palatable liquid preparation. This makes it easier for owners to continue analgesic administration if needed.

### Local Anesthetics

Local anesthetics can be used to provide postoperative analgesia. As in dogs and cats, they can be infiltrated around surgical wounds or administered as specific nerve blocks. Although the safety of these agents in small mammals is similar to that in dogs and cats, it is relatively easy to inadvertently overdose rodents because of their small size. Care must be taken to calculate the dose accurately (maximum recommended doses in rodents: lidocaine 10 mg/kg, bupivacaine 4 mg/kg; maximum recommended dose in rabbits: same as for cats, see Chapter 7). It is important to note that the duration of action of some local anesthetics may be shorter in rodents than in larger species, such as dogs. As mentioned earlier, the application of topical agents such as EMLA cream provides analgesia for venipuncture or placement of intravenous catheters.

### Chronic Pain

Small mammals may have a range of chronic conditions that can cause pain. Rats may have arthritis; guinea pigs, chinchillas, and rabbits may have dental disease; and neoplasia is common in many species. NSAIDs can often be used successfully to control the pain associated with these conditions, although it is necessary to carefully monitor the patient for side effects, especially during long-term use of these agents.

### Administration of Analgesics

Intravenous administration of analgesics is difficult in rodents but relatively straightforward in rabbits. Because of the small muscle mass in rodents, subcutaneous administration is preferred. Oral administration can be difficult and may require firm physical restraint that can exacerbate pain from surgical wounds. Provided the animal is eating, analgesics can be added to highly palatable food items (e.g., doughnuts for rats and mice). Analgesics for rats or mice can also be incorporated into fruit or meat-flavored gelatin. Commercial flavored gelatin should be prepared with half of the recommended quantity of water, and after the mixture is allowed to cool, a measured quantity of analgesic is added. After the gelatin has set, it can be cut into cubes of an appropriate weight. The remaining gelatin should be labeled and stored in a refrigerator, taking note of any legal requirements concerning storage of controlled drugs. Commercial gelatin mixed with beef extract may also be used, as can the commercial spread Nutella.

As in dogs and cats, preemptive administration of analgesics may provide more effective pain relief than postoperative use and may reduce the amount of anesthetic required for the surgical procedure. If volatile anesthetics are being used, opioids can be administered safely before the operation, and the concentration of anesthetic delivered can be reduced as necessary to maintain a safe level of anesthesia. For example, when buprenorphine is administered preoperatively to rodents, the concentration of isoflurane needed to provide surgical anesthesia can be reduced by approximately 25% to 50%. If injectable agents are used, preemptive analgesia is more difficult, because injectable anesthetics are often given as a single dose by the intraperitoneal or subcutaneous route and cannot be titrated according to their effect in the individual animal. Because the commonly used opioids will potentiate the actions of injectable anesthetic agents, their preoperative administration could lead to inadvertent anesthetic overdose. Because of the limited information available concerning the degree of interaction between injectable anesthetics and opioids, it is safer in this case to administer opioid analgesics at the end of the operation in small rodents, as the depth of anesthesia is becoming lighter.

Not all NSAIDs can be safely used preoperatively, because of potential adverse effects such as renal hypotension and prolonged bleeding times. Carprofen and meloxicam can both apparently be safely used for preemptive analgesia.

Although the use of analgesic drugs remains the most important technique for reducing postoperative pain, pain medication must be integrated into the overall plan for perioperative care. Animals must be provided with a postoperative recovery area appropriate to their particular needs. For example, it is stressful for a small mammal to recover in the same room as its predators (e.g., cats), and the resulting change in the animal's behavior pattern could mask signs of pain.

## PROCEDURE 11-1  Rabbit Endotracheal Intubation

1. Have ready an appropriate-size tube, local anesthetic spray, a laryngoscope or otoscope, and an introducer (Figure 1). Check that the batteries in the otoscope or laryngoscope are functioning.
2. Measure from the nares to the thoracic inlet, and trim the length of the endotracheal tube if necessary.
3. Anesthetize the animal, ensuring that it has lost the chewing reflex elicited when the mouth is opened. Place the animal on its back and administer oxygen through a face mask for 2 minutes.
4. Open the mouth and pull the tongue forward into the gap between the incisors and premolars. The incisors are sharp, so take care not to damage the tongue. Insert the blade of the laryngoscope or the otoscope speculum into the gap between teeth on the opposite side of the mouth, and advance until the end of the soft palate or the larynx is visible. In some animals the epiglottis will be positioned behind the soft palate, hiding the larynx from view. To expose the larynx, use the introducer to reposition the epiglottis and soft palate (Figure 2).
5. Spray the larynx with local anesthetic.
6. Advance the introducer through the larynx into the trachea. If an otoscope is being used, thread the introducer through the speculum, remove the otoscope, and thread the endotracheal tube onto the introducer. If a laryngoscope is being used, the tube and introducer are advanced into the mouth together and then into the larynx and trachea. The introducer is used to guide the endotracheal tube into the trachea and is then withdrawn. Although introducers are commercially available, a dog or cat urinary catheter can be used to stiffen and straighten the endotracheal tube and act as a guide.
7. When a blind intubation technique is used, place the rabbit on its chest and supply oxygen through a face mask for 2 minutes. Hold the rabbit around the base of the skull and position the rabbit so its head and

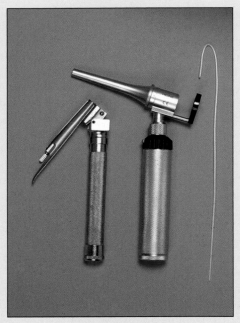

**FIGURE 1** Apparatus for endotracheal intubation in the rabbit. A laryngoscope *(left)* or otoscope *(center)* is used to visualize the larynx, and an introducer *(right)* is used to guide the endotracheal tube into the airway.

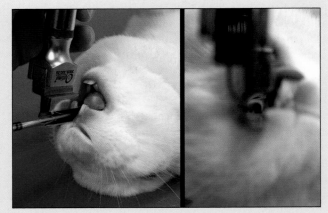

**FIGURE 2** Endotracheal intubation in a dorsally recumbent rabbit using a laryngoscope (Flecknell blade) to visualize the larynx. *Left,* Placing the endotracheal tube using an introducer. *Right,* View of the larynx through the laryngoscope blade.

## PROCEDURE 11-1 Rabbit Endotracheal Intubation—cont'd

neck are elevated (Figure 3). Introduce the endotracheal tube into the gap between the incisors and premolars and slide it into the pharynx. As it reaches the larynx, some increase in resistance is felt. The tube is then advanced into the larynx and trachea; this is usually accompanied by a slight cough. In some cases the tube passes into the esophagus and will need to be withdrawn and repositioned. The position of the tube can be monitored by listening at the end of the tube. If breath sounds can be heard, the tube is in the pharynx or the trachea.

8. Confirm successful placement of the tube by observing condensation in the tube on each expiration, by observing movement of a small piece of tissue paper or a tuft of fur placed at the end of the tube, or by using a capnograph to detect carbon dioxide. After attaching the tube to an anesthetic circuit, auscultate the chest and ensure that both sides are inflated when the reservoir bag is compressed or the expiratory limb of the circuit is occluded.

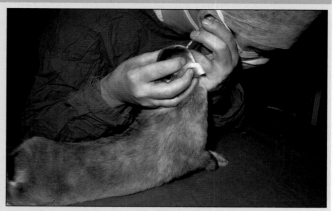

**FIGURE 3** Rabbit positioned for endotracheal intubation with a blind technique. After successful blind intubation of the trachea, the operator will hear breath sounds through the tube.

## REVIEW QUESTIONS

1. Glycopyrrolate should be used in rabbits, instead of atropine, because:
   a. Atropine is highly toxic in rabbits
   b. Many rabbits have high levels of atropinase, so atropine is relatively ineffective
   c. Rabbits are unable to metabolize atropine
   d. Atropine causes marked bradycardia in rabbits

2. Pulse oximeters can be used in small mammals, but they may not be reliable because:
   a. The heart rate of the animal may exceed the upper range of the instrument
   b. The hemoglobin absorption characteristics are different in rodents and dogs and cats
   c. Pulse oximeters do not function on animals that have dark fur
   d. Small rodents have a rapid respiratory rate

3. The position of the eye cannot be used to assess the depth of anesthesia in rodents because:
   a. The eye is too small to assess its position accurately
   b. The position of the eye does not change during anesthesia
   c. The eye rotates downward in very light planes of anesthesia
   d. The eyelids remain closed throughout anesthesia

4. An advantage of using medetomidine combined with ketamine for anesthesia of rodents and rabbits is that:
   a. It is readily absorbed from body fat
   b. It can be given by mouth to produce anesthesia
   c. It promotes gut motility and so reduces the occurrence of postoperative inappetence
   d. It can be partially reversed using atipamezole, allowing faster recovery

5. An adult mouse weighing 40 g will have a blood volume of approximately:
   a. 10 mL
   b. 3 mL
   c. 50 mL
   d. 0.2 mL

6. When fluids such as lactated Ringer's solution are given to small mammals, they should be:
   a. Used at about 4° C so that they are rapidly absorbed
   b. Administered orally, because it is not possible to use any other route
   c. Warmed to body temperature before administration, to avoid causing hypothermia
   d. Given only postoperatively, to avoid overloading the circulation

7. Anesthetic breathing circuits for use in small rabbits should:
   a. Be constructed of only plastic components because rabbits are allergic to latex
   b. Have low equipment dead space
   c. Have high equipment dead space
   d. Always include soda lime to prevent rebreathing

8. When small rodents are anesthetized with injectable anesthetics:
   a. It is not necessary to administer oxygen, because most anesthetics stimulate respiration
   b. Oxygen should be administered, because most anesthetics depress respiration
   c. Carbon dioxide should be included in the fresh gas mixture to stimulate respiration
   d. Nitrous oxide should always be used; otherwise the depth of anesthesia will be insufficient for surgery

9. Postoperative analgesic should be given to rodents and rabbits to alleviate pain, but:
   a. NSAIDs cannot be used because they cause gastric ulceration at normal therapeutic doses in these species
   b. Opioids (narcotics) cause severe respiratory depression and so must never be used
   c. Opioids must be given with care if a neuroleptanalgesic mixture has been used for anesthesia
   d. Local anesthetics cannot be used because they produce cardiac arrest even at low doses in these species

10. If postoperative pain is not alleviated in rabbits, then:
    a. They will not eat or drink normally
    b. They will recover much faster from anesthesia
    c. They will spend a great deal of time grooming themselves
    d. Porphyrin staining will appear around their eyes

## SELECTED READINGS

Flecknell PA: *Laboratory animal anesthesia*, London, 1996, Academic Press.

Flecknell PA, Waterman-Pearson AE, editors: *Pain management in laboratory animals*, London, 2001, Harcourt International.

Kohn DF, Wixson SK, White WJ et al: *Anesthesia and analgesia in laboratory animals*, San Diego, 1997, Academic.

# Anesthetic Problems and Emergencies

## K. Wayne Hollingshead

# 12

## KEY TERMS

Agonal
Ambu bag
CABDE
Functional residual
  volume
Opisthotonus
Physiologic anemia
Pleural effusion
Pneumothorax
Pulmonary contusions
Return of spontaneous
  circulation (ROSC)
Sequestration
Stertor
Thoracocentesis

## OUTLINE

Reasons That Anesthetic Problems and
  Emergencies Arise, 320
  *Human Errors That May Lead to Anesthetic
    Problems and Emergencies, 320*
  *Equipment Issues That May Lead to
    Anesthetic Problems and Emergencies, 321*
  *Adverse Effects of Anesthetic Agents, 323*
  *Patient Factors That May Lead to Anesthetic
    Problems and Emergencies, 323*

Response to Anesthetic Problems and
  Emergencies, 334
  *Role of the Veterinary Technician in
    Emergency Care, 334*
  *General Approach to Emergencies, 334*
  *Emergency Situations That May Arise
    during Anesthesia, 334*
  *Problems That May Arise in the
    Recovery Period, 341*

## LEARNING OBJECTIVES

*After completion of this chapter, the reader will be able to:*

- List the most common reasons why anesthetic emergencies occur, including problems arising from human error, equipment failure, and the adverse effects of anesthetic agents.
- Explain how anesthesia of geriatric and pediatric patients differs from anesthesia of healthy adult dogs and cats.
- Describe the problems involved in anesthetizing each of the following: brachycephalic dogs; sighthounds; obese animals; and patients affected by trauma or cardiovascular, respiratory, hepatic, or renal disease.
- Describe the role of the veterinary technician in responding to anesthetic emergencies.
- Explain the importance of oxygen supplementation in the trauma patient.
- List various ways of administering oxygen
- List the most common causes of the following anesthetic problems: inadequate anesthetic depth, excessive anesthetic depth, pale mucous membranes, prolonged capillary refill time, dyspnea, tachypnea, bradycardia, tachycardia, and cardiac arrhythmias.
- Describe the appropriate response to common emergencies, including dyspnea, respiratory arrest, and cardiac arrest.
- List the most common problems that may arise in the recovery period and the appropriate action that can be taken to prevent or treat these problems.

General anesthesia poses little risk to most patients when performed by capable personnel using an anesthetic protocol appropriate for the animal. Emergencies are uncommon, and the overwhelming majority of patients recover from anesthesia with no lasting ill effects. After successfully anesthetizing hundreds of patients, it is easy for the technician to be lulled into a false sense of security. However, it is vitally important that the anesthetist remember that every anesthetic procedure has the potential to cause the death of the animal. The anesthetist must remain watchful for problems that may arise in even the most routine anesthetic procedure.

A survey of British veterinary clinics revealed a mortality rate of one death for every 870 anesthetic procedures in healthy dogs and one death for every 552 procedures in healthy cats. The same study found a mortality rate of 1 in 30 patients where systemic disease was present. An American study of 3239 cases found the incidence of anesthetic complications to be 12% in dogs and 10.5% in cats, with a mortality rate of 0.43% (4.3 per 1000) in both dogs and cats.* A Canadian study of 16,000 anesthetized animals found the incidence of

---

*The mortality rate related to general anesthesia in human patients has been variously estimated to be as high as 1.5 per 1000 and as low as 1 per 10,000 patients.

cardiac arrest to be approximately 1 in 900 patients. Of the dogs with anesthetic complications, bulldogs, Pekingese, and other brachycephalic breeds; Weimaraners; and Jack Russell terriers were disproportionately represented. Emergency anesthesia was associated with a much greater risk than elective anesthesia.

This chapter describes problems that may arise during anesthesia, ranging from minor (such as maintaining appropriate anesthetic depth) to major (including respiratory arrest and cardiac arrest). Appropriate responses to various anesthetic emergencies are presented, and the reasons the anesthetic problems may arise (and procedures for their prevention) are emphasized. The challenges associated with anesthesia of patients with special problems such as heart disease or brachycephalic conformation are also discussed.

## REASONS THAT ANESTHETIC PROBLEMS AND EMERGENCIES ARISE

Although an awareness of the correct response to an anesthetic emergency is essential, it is even more important to understand why emergencies arise and how they may be prevented. Most anesthetic problems and emergencies are the result of one or more of the following factors: (1) human error, (2) equipment failure, (3) adverse effects of anesthetic agents, and (4) patient-related factors.

> *TECHNICIAN NOTE* Human error is one of the most common reasons for anesthetic emergencies. Examples include the following:
> - Improper calculations
> - Lack of attention to the anesthetic machine
> - Lack of proper patient evaluation
> - Incorrect use of drugs—for example, administering a drug by the incorrect route
> - Lack of knowledge of drug pharmacology

### Human Errors That May Lead to Anesthetic Problems and Emergencies

Human error is, unfortunately, a contributing cause in some anesthetic deaths. Human errors commonly encountered in veterinary practice include the following:

- Failure to obtain an adequate history or perform an adequate physical examination on the patient
- Inadequate experience with the anesthetic machine or anesthetic agents being used
- Failure to devote sufficient time or attention to the anesthetized patient
- Errors caused by fatigue
- Failure to recognize and respond to early signs of patient difficulty
- Lack of proper patient evaluation

### Failure to Obtain an Adequate History or to Perform a Physical Examination

Ideally, every patient scheduled for anesthesia should have a complete physical examination, and a thorough history should be obtained. In practice, this is not always possible. Animals are sometimes dropped off at the veterinary clinic by owners who are in a hurry and reluctant to stop and answer questions. Animals may be brought in by neighbors or friends of the owner, or by other persons unfamiliar with the animal's history. The receptionist or other person admitting the animal to the hospital may fail to ask important questions or may not transmit the information to the anesthetist or veterinarian. The physical examination is sometimes cursory or omitted entirely. The net result is that significant information may be overlooked. For example, the anesthetist may be unaware that a patient has not been fasted or that an animal scheduled for surgery is dehydrated as a result of vomiting and diarrhea. An anesthetic protocol that is safe for a healthy patient could be inappropriate for these animals, and an anesthetic problem or even death of the patient could result.

### Lack of Familiarity with the Anesthetic Machine or Anesthetic Agents

It is the responsibility of the veterinarian, and in some states or provinces a requirement of the Veterinary Association, to ensure that his or her personnel are sufficiently trained and knowledgeable to competently perform all required procedures. Although unskilled personnel working under a veterinarian's direct supervision may assist with some aspects of an anesthetic procedure, skilled tasks, such as induction of anesthesia and monitoring of anesthetized patients, must be assigned only to personnel (veterinarians or technicians) who have sufficient training, knowledge, and experience to recognize abnormalities and danger signals and to respond appropriately.

### Incorrect Administration of Drugs

Many anesthetic agents have a narrow margin of safety between therapeutic and toxic doses. The incorrect administration of drugs may have serious or even fatal consequences, and may arise from any of the following:

- Failure to weigh the patient and calculate an accurate dose.
- Mathematical errors (particularly decimal errors, which can result in an error of 10 times or 100 times in the amount of drug given).
- Use of the wrong medication (e.g., calculating a dose of atropine and drawing up acepromazine instead).
- Use of the wrong concentration of a medication. This is a common problem with drugs that are available in several different concentrations (e.g., atropine and acepromazine). Obviously, the concentration used in calculating the dose must be the same as that drawn up into the syringe.

- Administration of anesthetics by the incorrect route (e.g., administration of an intramuscular dose of ketamine by the intravenous [IV] route).
- Confusion between syringes drawn up for two different patients. This involves either a failure to label the syringes or a failure to read the labels correctly.

## Personnel Who Are Preoccupied or in a Hurry

Although efficiency is desirable in any anesthetic procedure, it is not necessary or advisable that the anesthetist feel hurried. A technician who is feeling rushed is more likely to make mistakes such as injecting barbiturates perivascularly or inserting an endotracheal tube into the esophagus. Unfortunately, it is common for the technician working in a busy practice to feel pressured and distracted. The technician responsible for anesthesia may be simultaneously called on to restrain patients for examination or procedures, answer the phone, perform laboratory tests, take radiographs, discharge animals, clean soiled kennels, and carry out other similar tasks. However, when an animal is anesthetized, the technician's top priority must be monitoring that patient, because failure to satisfactorily perform this duty may result in the death of the animal.

The technician usually does not have the luxury of being constantly by the animal's side throughout the procedure. In most work situations, periodic absences are necessary. However, the anesthetist should return to check the patient at least once every 5 minutes, or more frequently if the patient's status requires close monitoring. If necessary, other tasks must be temporarily set aside to allow the anesthetist to return to the patient.

## Fatigue

Veterinarians and technicians often become fatigued, particularly at the end of a busy day. Anesthetic emergencies may arise when personnel are tired and less alert than normal, possibly because minor problems are not detected and corrected at an early stage. If possible, surgeries that are lengthy or difficult should be scheduled early in the day.

## Inattentiveness

One of the most serious human errors in anesthesia is the failure to monitor and recognize danger signals. It is obviously better for the patient—and easier for the anesthetist—to detect and address anesthetic problems early, rather than late. For example, when anesthetic depth is excessive, an animal may show a gradually decreasing respiratory rate, from 10 to 12 breaths/min in a dog or cat to fewer than 8 breaths/min (at which point the anesthetist should consider adjusting the vaporizer to a lower setting); then to 4 breaths/min (at which point the vaporizer should be turned off and the animal bagged with oxygen); then from 4 breaths/min to 0 (at which point cardiac arrest may quickly follow if these changes are not recognized and managed).

The anesthetist's attitude toward patient care is a key factor in the safety of anesthesia. The conscientious anesthetist will monitor the animal often to ensure that the patient is not in trouble. A brief check of the patient's pulse rate, respiratory rate, and capillary refill time takes less than 1 minute and gives the anesthetist a good assessment of the patient's status. The best attitude is one of low-level anxiety that is relieved only when a quick examination of the patient reveals that all vital signs and depth indicators are within acceptable limits.

## Equipment Issues That May Lead to Anesthetic Problems and Emergencies

Equipment failure is an uncommon cause of anesthetic emergencies, but it does occur. In many cases, failure of the anesthetic machine is, in fact, caused by a failure of the operator to maintain and monitor the machine properly. The importance of a preanesthetic check of the anesthetic machine, as described in Chapter 4, cannot be overemphasized.

The following equipment problems are occasionally encountered in routine anesthesia.

### Carbon Dioxide Absorbent Exhaustion

Patients on a rebreathing system rely on the carbon dioxide absorbent to remove expired $CO_2$ from the circuit, preventing inhalation of excessive levels of this toxic gas. If $CO_2$ is not removed from the circuit, the patient will experience hypercapnia (elevated blood $CO_2$). Signs of this disorder include tachypnea (rapid respiration), tachycardia, and cardiac arrhythmias. Examination of the $CO_2$ absorbent may reveal an obvious color change, if exhausted, although this does not always occur.

### Empty Oxygen Tank

Failure to deliver oxygen to the patient is one of the most serious and yet one of the most easily preventable mistakes that an anesthetist can make. Before starting an anesthetic procedure, the anesthetist must ensure that the tank contains sufficient oxygen for the duration of the surgery. (For information on calculating the amount of oxygen present in a tank, refer to p. 108.) During the procedure, the oxygen tank pressure and flow meter should be checked every 5 minutes during anesthesia. The anesthetist must ensure that either oxygen or room air is continuously provided to the patient. At the end of a procedure, the patient should be disconnected from the machine before the oxygen flow meter is turned off.

It is important to be able to recognize when the machine is no longer delivering oxygen to the patient. If the oxygen flow meter reads zero, the patient is not receiving any oxygen, regardless of the oxygen tank pressure. Occasionally when the oxygen tank is nearly empty, the oxygen tank pressure gauge reads zero but the flow meter indicates some oxygen flow. Even though the tank is still delivering a small amount of oxygen, loss of oxygen pressure is imminent and the tank must be changed immediately.

The anesthetist must be aware of the proper response when oxygen delivery to the patient is stopped, whether because of machine malfunction or an empty tank. If the oxygen flow stops (i.e., the flow meter reads zero despite the efforts of the anesthetist to establish flow) and the patient is on a non-rebreathing system, the anesthetist should immediately disconnect the hose from the endotracheal tube, allowing the patient to breathe room air until oxygen delivery is reestablished. (If a circle system with a full reservoir bag is in use, the patient can remain connected for a short period of time.)

## Misassembly of the Anesthetic Machine

It is essential that the person handling the anesthetic machine be familiar with every connection, hose, dial, and component of the machine. Before using an unfamiliar machine, the anesthetist should take a few minutes to examine it carefully for the location of the controls and to understand the direction and path of gas flow within the machine. Every time a connection, such as a Bain circuit, is added or removed, the anesthetist must trace the flow of gas, ensuring that the correct pattern of flow is maintained and that all connections are secure. Failure to do so can result in the patient not receiving anesthetic gases or rebreathing expired $CO_2$.

## Endotracheal Tube Problems

Although the endotracheal tube is, strictly speaking, not a part of the anesthetic machine, it is a critical component of the anesthetic delivery system and is subject to many problems. Endotracheal tubes may become blocked during anesthesia, cutting off the flow of anesthetic gas and oxygen to the patient. Blockages may be the result of twisting or kinking of the tube; accumulation of material such as blood, mucus, or saliva within the tube; or inappropriate positioning of the tube (as may occur when the neck is flexed). The endotracheal tube should be premeasured from the incisor teeth to the mid-neck, and it should be advanced no further than the position of the carina. If the tube is accidentally advanced into a bronchus, the patient may become hypoxic and hypercapnic.

Endotracheal tube blockage (if complete) results in a cessation of oxygen flow to the patient and retention of carbon dioxide. The patient may become dyspneic and may develop cardiac arrhythmias. Eventually, respiratory arrest may occur. The anesthetist usually becomes aware of the problem by observing the patient's exaggerated breathing pattern or by noting that the reservoir bag no longer inflates and deflates with the patient's respirations. If a problem is suspected, the anesthetist should quickly check the endotracheal tube function in two ways:

1. Attempt to bag the patient and observe if the chest rises. If the endotracheal tube is blocked, no chest movement will be seen, and there will be considerable resistance to the passage of air into the patient.

2. Disconnect the animal from the machine. With the endotracheal tube still in place, feel for air coming out of the tube when the patient's chest is compressed. If no air movement is felt, a blockage may be present. In this case, the tube should be removed and another endotracheal tube or mask used to deliver oxygen to the patient. If blood, mucus, or similar material is causing the obstruction, suction with a 20-mL syringe and a feeding tube cut to the length of the endotracheal tube may be helpful.

## Vaporizer Problems

Each vaporizer is designed for a specific agent. A potentially disastrous problem can arise if the wrong anesthetic is put into a vaporizer. Each anesthetic liquid has its own vapor pressure (the amount of anesthetic that vaporizes at 20° C), and anesthetic vaporizers are calibrated on the basis of a particular anesthetic being used in the vaporizer with a particular vapor pressure. If an anesthetic is put into the incorrect vaporizer, it is possible that when the vaporizer is set at 1% a higher or lower concentration will be delivered because the anesthetic has a different vapor pressure than the anesthetic for which the vaporizer was designed. This leads to the patient's anesthetic depth becoming unexpectedly deep or light. Other problems involving vaporizers are as follows:

- Vaporizers should not be tipped. Tipping may lead to leakage of anesthetic into the oxygen bypass channel, resulting in higher concentrations of anesthetic reaching the patient and therefore potential overdose.
- Occasionally, a vaporizer dial may stick or become jammed. If the dial cannot be adjusted, the patient should be transferred to another machine.
- Anesthetic machines equipped with two or more vaporizers in series should be monitored carefully to ensure that both vaporizers are not turned on at the same time.
- Vaporizers should not be overfilled. If too much anesthetic is put into the vaporizer, it should be drained until the fluid level is at, or below, the indicator line.

> **TECHNICIAN NOTE** If the pop-off valve is closed and the oxygen flow rate is greater than the patient's oxygen requirement, pressure within the circuit and the patient's lungs and thoracic cavity will rapidly rise. This prevents exhalation and decreases the venous return to the heart, which decreases cardiac output and can lead to death within a short time unless recognized and corrected immediately.

## Pop-off Valve Problems

Occasionally, an anesthetist inadvertently leaves the pop-off valve in a closed position. If the pop-off valve is closed and the oxygen flow rate is greater than the patient's oxygen requirement, pressure within the circuit will rapidly rise. This can happen with use of a closed system in which the oxygen flow rate has inadvertently been set higher than the metabolic oxygen consumption (approximately 10 mL/kg/min). As pressure rises in the circuit, the reservoir bag will expand, as will the patient's lungs. This prevents exhalation and also decreases the venous return to the heart. This in turn may decrease cardiac output, cause blood pressure to fall rapidly, and can lead to death within a short time unless recognized and corrected.

To detect the problem at an early stage, the anesthetist should frequently monitor the reservoir bag size and attempt to maintain it at no more than two-thirds full of gas during anesthesia. The reservoir bag size is easily adjusted by changing the oxygen flow rate or by opening and closing the pop-off valve.

 *TECHNICIAN NOTE* Multidrug protocols are generally safer than use of only one or two drugs.

## Adverse Effects of Anesthetic Agents

Each injectable or inhalation agent has the potential to harm a patient and, in some cases, cause death. Several strategies are used to reduce this potential:

- The anesthetic protocol must be chosen to reflect the special needs of the patient. For example, acepromazine is a poor preanesthetic for patients with low blood pressure because this agent may cause vasodilation, further decreasing the blood pressure. Similarly, halothane, although rarely used now, is not the preferred inhalation agent for patients with cardiac arrhythmias because it may cause arrhythmias to worsen. Isoflurane, the common replacement for halothane, may cause a significant drop in blood pressure, and therefore blood pressure monitoring should be performed on the patient. Animals that are fearful or excited may have increased levels of epinephrine circulating throughout their bodies. Drugs such as the alpha$_2$-agonists (e.g., xylazine) should be avoided, as they will augment the arrhythmogenic effects of epinephrine. In each case the veterinarian might choose to use an alternative agent.
- The anesthetist must be familiar with the side effects and contraindications associated with each of the preanesthetic and general anesthetic agents used in the hospital. For example, the anesthetist who administers an alpha$_2$-agonist should be aware of its potential to cause bradycardia, cardiac arrhythmias, vomiting, bloating, and respiratory depression.
- Multidrug use to achieve balanced anesthesia can be safer than anesthesia with a single drug, provided that the doses of the individual drugs are appropriately reduced. For example, the concentration of isoflurane needed to anesthetize an animal is significantly reduced if the animal is premedicated with

acepromazine and butorphanol, as compared with an animal that is not premedicated. If the same isoflurane concentration were used in both situations, the multidrug regimen could be dangerous for the patient.

A detailed description of the pharmacology and physiologic effects of preanesthetic and general anesthetic agents is given in Chapter 3.

## Patient Factors That May Lead to Anesthetic Problems and Emergencies

Animals presented for anesthesia may have systemic abnormalities that considerably increase anesthetic risk. Patients with a preoperative status of class P4 or class P5 are particularly difficult to anesthetize successfully. Challenging patients routinely encountered in veterinary practice include geriatric animals, neonates, brachycephalic animals, sighthounds, and obese animals. Cesarean delivery of puppies or kittens also places unique demands on the anesthetist because the response of both the dam and the offspring to anesthetic agents must be considered. Animals that have experienced recent trauma may be presented for emergency surgery, and the anesthetist must be prepared to deal with shock, respiratory difficulties, and cardiac arrhythmias in these patients. Animals with cardiac problems such as heartworm disease or congestive heart failure may require anesthesia for diagnostic or therapeutic procedures. Similarly, animals may require anesthesia despite the presence of renal or hepatic disease. Although a detailed discussion of the anesthetic challenges posed by these and other patients is beyond the scope of this book, it is desirable that the technician be familiar with some of the special problems encountered when anesthetizing these animals. These are summarized in Table 12-1.

### Geriatric Patients

A geriatric patient is one that has reached 75% of the average life expectancy for that species and breed. In these patients the functions of critical organs such as the heart, lungs, kidneys, and liver are reduced in comparison with the healthy, young patient. Geriatric animals have less functional reserve than do younger animals, and a relatively poor response to stress. Often they are less able to adequately maintain their state of hydration than younger patients. In addition, geriatric animals are often affected by degenerative disorders such as diabetes mellitus, cancer, congestive heart failure secondary to mitral valve insufficiency, and chronic renal disease, all of which are of concern to the anesthetist. Because of the high incidence of health problems in these animals, the importance of a thorough history and physical examination cannot be overemphasized. Preoperative tests such as a blood chemistry panel, urinalysis, chest radiographs, and an electrocardiogram (ECG) may be advisable for these patients.

| TABLE 12-1 | Patient Factors That Increase Anesthetic Risk | |
|---|---|---|
| Patient Factor | Anesthetic Problems Encountered | Strategies Used to Decrease Risk |
| Geriatric patients | Reduced organ function; poor response to stress; degenerative disorders common; increased risk of hypothermia and overhydration | Reduce anesthetic doses by 30% to 50%; allow longer time for response to drugs; administer fluids at reduced rate; keep patient warm |
| Pediatric patients | Increased risk of hypothermia and overhydration; inefficient excretion of drugs; difficult intubation and intravenous catheterization | Avoid heat loss; avoid prolonged fasting; administer 5% dextrose in lactated Ringer's using accurate methods of delivery; weigh accurately; dilute injectable drugs; reduce anesthetic doses; inhalant agents preferred to injectable agents |
| Brachycephalic dogs | Conformational tendency toward airway obstruction; abnormally high vagal tone | Include anticholinergic in anesthetic protocol; preoxygenate; rapid induction using intravenous agents; delay extubation; observe closely during recovery period |
| Sighthounds | Increased sensitivity to barbiturates | Use alternative agents |
| Obese animals | Accurate dosing difficult; poor distribution of anesthetics; may have respiratory difficulties | Determine dose according to ideal weight; preoxygenate; induce rapidly; assist ventilation if necessary; delay extubation; observe closely in recovery period |
| Cesarean patients | *Dam:* increased workload to heart; respiration may be compromised; increased tendency to vomit or regurgitate; increased risk of hemorrhage<br>*Offspring:* anesthetic agents cross placenta and may reduce respiratory and cardiovascular function | *Dam:* administer intravenous fluids; clip patient before induction; preoxygenate; use lowest effective dose of general anesthetic; avoid pentobarbital and ketamine-diazepam<br>*Offspring:* use reversal agents and doxapram; administer oxygen by facemask; administer atropine for bradycardia |
| Trauma patients | Respiratory distress common; cardiac arrhythmias seen for 72 hours after incident; shock and hemorrhage common; internal injuries often present | Stabilize before anesthesia; obtain thoracic radiographs and electrocardiogram; thorough physical examination necessary to check for concurrent injuries |
| Cardiovascular disease | Circulation is compromised; pulmonary edema common; increased tendency to develop arrhythmias and tachycardia | Alleviate pulmonary edema with diuretics; preoxygenate for 5 minutes before induction; avoid agents that depress myocardium or cause arrhythmias; avoid overhydration |
| Respiratory disease | Poor oxygenation of tissues; patient may be anxious and difficult to restrain; respiratory arrest common | Avoid stress and unnecessary handling; preoxygenate; avoid nitrous oxide; induce with injectable agents; intubate rapidly and control ventilation if necessary; monitor closely during recovery |
| Hepatic disease | Delayed metabolism of anesthetic agents; decreased synthesis of blood clotting factors; may be hypoproteinemic; dehydration common; may be anemic and/or icteric | Preanesthetic blood chemistry tests; may omit preanesthetic medication; inhalation agents preferred over injectable agents; expect prolonged recovery |
| Renal disease | Delayed excretion of anesthetic agents; electrolyte imbalances common, including hyperkalemia, hyperphosphatemia, and metabolic acidosis; dehydration usually present | Rehydrate before surgery; obtain renal function test results and electrolyte values; reduce doses of anesthetic agents; use caution with barbiturates; may require intraoperative intravenous fluids |
| Urinary obstruction | Dehydration, acidosis, uremia, and hyperkalemia common; bradycardia may be present | Avoid barbiturates; treat for hyperkalemia if present |

Geriatric animals typically have reduced anesthetic requirements, and doses of anesthetic agents are often decreased by one half to one third compared with doses for healthy, young patients. In the case of barbiturates, dose requirements may be as little as one twentieth of the normal dose. Response to drugs is slower, and the technician should allow more time for IV injections to take effect. Recovery from anesthesia also may be prolonged in geriatric animals, partly because of decreased renal and hepatic function (and hence, decreased ability to excrete drugs). Geriatric patients also have a tendency to develop hypothermia because they have a reduced ability to regulate body temperature.

The use of IV fluids is generally advocated in geriatric patients because they have less tolerance for hypotension and often have reduced kidney function. Geriatric animals are, however, at increased risk for developing overhydration, so IV fluids should be given with care.

## Pediatric Patients

A veterinary patient under 3 months of age is generally considered to be at increased risk when anesthetized, compared with a mature animal. When working with these patients, the anesthetist must be aware of special considerations during the preanesthetic, anesthetic, and recovery periods.

Preoperative fasting of the pediatric patient may not be advisable because hypoglycemia and dehydration can occur after even a short period of fasting. Oral fluids are usually allowed up to 1 hour before induction. To prevent hypoglycemia during surgery, many veterinarians use 5% dextrose in lactated Ringer's for IV fluid therapy of anesthetized pediatric patients. (This can be formulated by adding 100 mL of 50% dextrose to 1 L of lactated Ringer's solution.) The fluid administration rate should not exceed 5 mL/kg/hr unless shock or dehydration is present, because these animals are prone to overhydration if fluid administration is rapid. The use of a syringe driver or pediatric microdrip administration set with a delivery rate of 60 drops/mL and a burette is helpful in preventing inadvertent overinfusion of fluid.

For calculation of drug doses, an accurate weight must be obtained. For animals weighing less than 5 kg, a pediatric or gram scale gives more reliable weights than does a conventional scale. Injectable agents may require dilution because otherwise the dose may be too small to measure or administer accurately. The dose of injectable anesthetics given to pediatric animals is often one half to two thirds of the dose given to mature animals because very young animals have less plasma protein binding of drugs and lack an efficient mechanism to metabolize drugs within the liver. Injectable anesthetic agents that require liver metabolism for inactivation (e.g., thiopental and pentobarbital) can be expected to have a prolonged effect in puppies or kittens less than 8 weeks of age and should be avoided. Renal function is also inefficient compared with the adult animal, and excretion of drugs by this route may be slow.

Many veterinarians prefer to anesthetize pediatric patients with inhalant agents (particularly isoflurane) because administration and elimination of these agents is accomplished through the respiratory tract and patient recovery tends to be rapid.

Certain anesthetic procedures such as intubation and IV catheterization can be more challenging in pediatric patients because of their small body size. The larynx may be difficult to see, and use of a laryngoscope may be required. It is often necessary to cut endotracheal tubes short to avoid bronchial intubation.

Apart from obvious differences in size, the monitoring of pediatric patients is similar to that of adults. The anesthetist should be particularly watchful for bradycardia, which is associated with poor cardiac output

in anesthetized animals under 4 weeks of age. Alpha$_2$-agonists may cause significant bradycardia and should be avoided in these patients. Premedication with atropine may not be effective because response to atropine is unpredictable in patients younger than 14 days old.

Pediatric patients are prone to hypothermia because of their lack of subcutaneous fat, their relatively large body surface area, and their reduced ability to shiver. Particular care should be taken to avoid heat loss during surgery. This is accomplished through the use of warmed IV fluids and circulating warm water heating pads or Bair Huggers. It is also essential to make sure that all air is removed from IV lines to avoid the risk of air embolism.

 *TECHNICIAN NOTE* Brachycephalic dogs pose special problems for the anesthetist.

## Brachycephalic Dogs

Technicians are often called on to anesthetize brachycephalic dogs such as the English bulldog, pug, Boston terrier, and Pekingese. Because of their conformation, these animals may have one or more anatomic characteristics that impede air exchange, including very small nasal openings, an elongated soft palate, and a small-diameter trachea. Any anesthetic agent that depresses respiration or reduces muscle tone in the pharyngeal and laryngeal area will cause increased respiratory difficulty in these animals. In some cases this may be fatal, particularly if the animal is not intubated and an open airway cannot be maintained. These problems are most evident in animals undergoing surgery to correct conformation defects in the pharyngeal region (e.g., soft palate resection), because postoperative swelling or hemorrhage may occur, increasing the risk of respiratory difficulty.

In addition to respiratory problems, many brachycephalic animals have abnormally high parasympathetic tone, which may cause bradycardia. Use of atropine or glycopyrrolate in these patients is helpful for increasing heart rates before surgery.

The induction period is particularly difficult for brachycephalic dogs. If possible, the anesthetist should preoxygenate brachycephalic patients for 5 minutes before induction. This is done by gently restraining the animal and administering oxygen through a facemask. This procedure helps maintain adequate blood oxygen levels and gives the animal an extra margin of safety during the induction period that follows. Induction should be rapid in order to gain control over the airway, and for this reason IV induction agents are generally preferred over mask induction. Agents that are rapidly metabolized (e.g., propofol, ketamine-diazepam, and methohexital) are preferred. The dog must be adequately anesthetized to allow rapid and efficient intubation. Difficulties may be encountered because of the large amount of redundant tissue in the pharynx. This reduces visibility of the laryngeal opening, and the use of a laryngoscope is helpful in these patients. The anesthetist may find that the endotracheal tube that fits the trachea is smaller than expected, considering the size and weight of the dog.

Anesthesia usually can be safely maintained through the use of an inhalation anesthetic. With the help of an endotracheal tube, breathing during anesthesia may, in fact, be superior to that of the normal awake brachycephalic animal. Agents that allow rapid recovery (particularly isoflurane or sevoflurane) are preferred because dyspnea is common in these dogs during the early recovery period.

After surgery the patient should be observed closely until it is extubated and breathing well. Vigilance is necessary well into the recovery period because patients may develop airway obstructions even after attempting to stand. The endotracheal tube should be left in place as long as possible because the animal will maintain an open airway as long as the tube is in place. It is possible to give a low dose of morphine or hydromorphone just before turning off the vaporizer. This will allow the endotracheal tube to be left in longer, as these drugs suppress the cough reflex. Oxygen should be delivered until the patient is extubated. Once the endotracheal tube has been removed, the animal's head and neck should be extended, and the animal should be watched closely for dyspnea and cyanosis. If dyspnea is seen, the mouth should be kept open with a mouth gag and the tongue pulled forward. Administration of oxygen by mask or even reinduction (with ketamine-diazepam, propofol, or other IV induction agent) and reintubation may occasionally be necessary. It is advisable to have supplemental oxygen and supplies for reintubation (i.e., a laryngoscope, new endotracheal tube, and the appropriate dose of an inducing agent) readily available in the recovery area in case dyspnea occurs after extubation.

Excitement and stress should be minimized as much as possible in the recovery period, especially if airway surgery was carried out. Some patients may require mild tranquilization or the use of opioid analgesics to reduce the rapid respirations that can worsen laryngeal swelling. Corticosteroids are also helpful in some patients.

### Sighthounds

Several canine breeds (including the greyhound, saluki, Afghan hound, whippet, and Russian wolfhound) show increased sensitivity to anesthetic agents, particularly thiobarbiturates such as thiopental. The reason for this increased sensitivity is not entirely understood, but it may involve a lack of body fat for redistribution of the drug and inefficient hepatic metabolism of many drugs. Fortunately, many induction agents (including diazepam and ketamine, methohexital, propofol, isoflurane, and sevoflurane) can be safely used as alternatives to thiobarbiturates in these animals.

### Obese Animals

Some patients presented for anesthesia have a high percentage of body fat. Because the blood supply to fat is relatively poor, anesthetics are not efficiently distributed to fat stores. Obese dogs, therefore, require lower doses of drugs on a per kilogram basis than do normal dogs. It is advisable to decrease the dose of preanesthetic and anesthetic agents so that the dose is determined according to a weight halfway between the normal breed weight and the actual weight.

Obese animals also may have some degree of respiratory difficulty, further complicating the anesthetic process. Dogs that show respiratory difficulties should receive oxygen by facemask for 5 minutes before induction. They may also require the use of induction techniques similar to those used in brachycephalic dogs and may require ventilatory support during maintenance of anesthesia (see Chapter 6).

Obese dogs and toy breeds often exhibit rapid shallow respirations during anesthesia. This breathing pattern may result in hypercapnia. The anesthetist who observes persistent rapid and shallow respirations should assume control over respiration by bagging the patient with oxygen and inhalant anesthetic, once every 5 seconds, until increased anesthetic depth and slower respirations are observed. The anesthetist can also slow down the respiratory rate by administering opioids such as hydromorphone or oxymorphone, especially if the elevated rate is a result of surgical stimulation, although occasionally opioids may cause panting.

### Cesarean Section

The parturient patient faces risks that must be dealt with by the veterinary team. These include the following:

- Aspiration of vomitus because of a partially full stomach
- Decreased lung capacity because of a diaphragm that is pushed cranially from a distended uterus
- Increased cardiac workload because of advanced pregnancy
- **Physiologic anemia** because of increased plasma volume without a corresponding increase in the number of red blood cells (this is accentuated as the number of fetuses increases)
- Poor regulation of blood pressure
- Decreased anesthetic requirements because of the effect of progesterone and its metabolites on gamma-aminobutyric acid (GABA) receptors

Essentially, all anesthetic drugs administered to the pregnant patient (with the exception of neuromuscular blocking agents and local anesthetics) will readily cross the placenta and affect the newborn. Although it is essential that the patient receive adequate anesthetic agent to provide immobilization and analgesia for the surgery, it is advisable to use minimal doses of those agents that depress respiration in the puppies or kittens.

Hemorrhage from the uterus is a common complication of cesarean surgery, and even nonhemorrhaging patients have an increased risk of shock. Therefore, an IV catheter should be placed and fluids should be administered intraoperatively to all cesarean patients.

It is helpful to do as much preparation of the cesarean patient preoperatively as possible, thereby reducing the anesthesia time. If possible, clipping and preparation should be initiated before induction. Whether the patient is awake or anesthetized, it is advisable that patient clipping and surgical preparation be done as much as possible with the patient gently restrained in left lateral recumbency rather than in dorsal recumbency. The latter position may cause the heavy uterus to compress the vena cava, decreasing venous return to the heart.

Various anesthetic techniques are used for cesarean surgeries, depending on the preference of the veterinarian:

- Epidural analgesia combined with a tranquilizer or neuroleptanalgesia is popular because this technique, once mastered, provides inexpensive but effective anesthesia with minimal depression of the patient or the neonates. IV fluids and oxygen should be administered in conjunction with epidural analgesia, and blood pressure should be monitored.
- General anesthesia using a variety of injectable and inhalant agents is also commonly used, with anesthetics given at the lowest effective dose to maintain anesthesia without unnecessarily depressing pediatric respiration. Because of the dam's increased sensitivity to medications, the dose of inhalant anesthetic required is often reduced by up to 40%. Propofol and ketamine are commonly used.
- Preoxygenation is helpful, regardless of the anesthetic protocol.
- Opioid agents are favored by some veterinarians for cesarean anesthesia because they are reversible in both the dam and the neonates through the use of naloxone or another reversal agent.
- Use of diazepam should be avoided because this agent is poorly metabolized by pediatric animals.

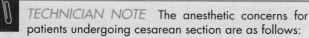

**TECHNICIAN NOTE** The anesthetic concerns for patients undergoing cesarean section are as follows:
- Hypoxemia
- Hypercarbia
- Hypotension
- Bleeding
- Acid-base imbalance
- Tissue trauma
- Arrhythmias

In the cesarean patient the stomach empties more slowly, and the queen or bitch is more likely to eat small meals frequently, increasing the risk of food within the stomach. As time permits, the patient should be given appropriate premedication with an agent that can decrease vomiting, such as an anticholinergic. Induction should allow for quick intubation, and therefore the IV route is preferred over mask induction. During the postanesthetic period, the veterinary technician should ensure that the patient has a good swallowing reflex before extubation is performed. The technician should ensure that the patient is in a sternal position, to reduce the risk of any aspiration of vomitus. If the patient does vomit after extubation, the patient must immediately have its head lowered below the rest of the body, and suction of the oropharynx should commence immediately. Once the oropharyngeal area is clear, the patient should be placed back in sternal recumbency and may require a short period of oxygenation. The patient should be monitored for the next 24 to 48 hours for pneumonia (signs of which include pyrexia, dyspnea, hyperpnea, and depression), and the veterinarian may prescribe a course of antibiotics.

The distended uterus of the parturient patient causes lung capacity, **functional residual volume,** and tidal volume ($V_T$) to decrease. In the parturient patient there is also an increased demand for oxygen. With such patients the need for supplemental oxygen before and during induction becomes important to reduce the risk of oxygen desaturation should intubation become difficult. Induction should be done as quickly as possible; mask induction is not advisable.

Hypotension is also a potential problem for the cesarean patient. It is important that large bore catheters be used, and in some situations, such as dogs over 20 kg, it may be advantageous to have two catheters in place to ensure that rapid volume infusion is possible. Drugs chosen should help maintain blood pressure or at least not cause significant variation from normotension.

Because of physiologic anemia, the veterinary team must work with a patient that has a decreased ability to get oxygen to the necessary parts of the body. Oxygen delivery may be further compromised by an inability to control blood pressure as noted earlier. Such patients must be preoxygenated before and during the induction procedure to reduce the chance of hypoxemia and anaerobic glycolysis. Either or both of these situations can result in arrhythmias or acid-base imbalance.

Puppies or kittens delivered by cesarean section often show signs of reduced respiratory and cardiovascular function when first delivered. If respiration appears inadequate or if cyanosis is present, oxygen should be administered by facemask. If necessary, the newborn animal can be intubated with a 16- or 18-gauge IV catheter and gently bagged with oxygen every 5 seconds. Aspiration of fluid from the mouth and nose with an eyedropper or bulb syringe may also be useful. The use of reversal agents and doxapram (1 to 2 drops delivered under the tongue or 0.1 to 0.2 mL injected into the root of the tongue) is common. If bradycardia is present, a drop of dilute atropine (0.25 mg/mL) can be administered under the tongue or injected into the tongue. Gentle cardiac massage and oxygen may also be helpful.

The newborn should be allowed to nurse as soon as the mother appears to be recovered from anesthesia (or, with supervision, during the recovery period). The dam may be disoriented and should be closely watched to ensure the safety of the newborn puppies or kittens. Anesthetic agents excreted in the milk appear to have little effect on nursing or viability of the neonates. Postoperative analgesics such as butorphanol or buprenorphine assist the mother's recovery.

## Trauma Patients

Animals that have recently undergone trauma, such as being hit by a car, may have numerous ailments that greatly increase anesthetic risk. Respiratory difficulties are common and may be the result of **pneumothorax, pulmonary contusions,** hemorrhage, or diaphragmatic hernia. Any one of these decreases the $V_T$ of the patient and therefore can cause a decrease in oxygenation. Lack of adequate oxygen exchange will lead to hypoxemia, which will lead to myocardial hypoxia and therefore arrhythmias, cell death, and acid-base imbalances. Increased $CO_2$ levels caused by lack of proper ventilation will also lead to acid-base imbalances and arrhythmias. Loss of blood or **sequestration** of fluid will result in changes in blood pressure, which must be corrected before anesthesia. Fluid sequestration can result from such situations as burns, where serum (fluid) oozes from the blood vascular system into the burn site. This causes a decrease in circulating volume and therefore a change in blood pressure.

Anemia may be present in the traumatized patient as a result of loss of blood directly or sequestration of blood into the trauma site. It has been shown in human medicine that a pelvic fracture can sequester as much as 40% of the circulating blood volume.

Details of these various issues are further described in this chapter.

### Changes in Blood Pressure

Any change in cardiac output or vascular tone will have an effect on blood pressure. The veterinary technician is reminded that depth of anesthesia will affect both of these parameters. Therefore depth of anesthesia should always be considered in the anesthetized patient when blood pressure decreases. Inadequate blood pressure decreases tissue perfusion. This will result in tissue hypoxia or anoxia leading to tissue glycolysis via the anaerobic method, with the production of lactic acid and therefore an acid-base imbalance. It is therefore important that blood pressure be properly monitored. Either the Doppler or oscillometric method can be used, along with adequate digital palpation of the pulse in an extremity as well as core arteries (lingual or femoral). A poor or weak pulse along with slow capillary refill (>2 seconds) is suggestive of hypotension, and mean arterial blood pressure of less than 60 mm Hg indicates inadequate tissue perfusion. Once it has been determined that the blood pressure is abnormal, the veterinary technician should alert the veterinarian in charge (VIC).

Hypotension may be addressed by crystalloid fluid administration at rates of 10 to 20 mL/kg/hr. In the short term, it may be necessary to give small fluid boluses of 10 to 20 mL/kg over 15 minutes for cats (approximately 1 mL/kg/min) and 20 to 40 mL/kg over 15 minutes for

dogs (approximately 2 mL/kg/min) to help improve blood pressure quickly. One must remember that most crystalloids will be gone from the intravascular fluid space in less than 2 hours. Fluid overload, especially in the cat, should always be closely monitored. During fluid administration the technician should monitor the heart rate, blood pressure, mucous membrane color, and capillary refill time. Signs of fluid overload in the awake patient may include the following:

- Crackles or wheezes on lung auscultation
- Serous nasal discharge
- Bulging eyes (chemosis)
- Increased ventilatory rate or effort or both
- Coughing
- Vomiting or diarrhea
- Restlessness
- Increased urine output

Most of these clinical signs are not evident in the anaesthetized patient, and so it becomes prudent to auscultate the lungs in all four quadrants if fluids are being administered rapidly (Figure 12-1).

Colloids are often beneficial if blood pressure cannot be maintained, especially if the plasma protein is less than 3.5 g/dL. As colloids are large macromolecules, they remain within the vascular system for a longer period of time than crystalloids. Colloids will increase the colloidal osmotic pressure and hence help stabilize blood pressure before and/or during anesthesia. Colloids include the following:

- Hetastarch
- Dextran 40 or 70
- 10% Pentastarch
- Plasma
- Whole blood

Colloids are given in much smaller volumes than crystalloids and should always be given in concert with crystalloids. Results of colloid administration include increased cardiac output and blood pressure. Doses for colloids vary depending on the type that is used, but in

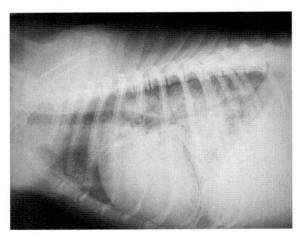

**FIGURE 12-1**    Pulmonary edema secondary to fluid overload in a cat. (From Battaglia AM: *Small animal emergency and critical care for veterinary technicians,* ed 2, St Louis, 2007, Elsevier.)

general, for dogs one uses 10 to 20 mL/kg, and for cats 5 to 10 mL/kg.

If drugs are required to stabilize blood pressure, the veterinarian may choose one or more of various medications such as dopamine (1 to 5 mcg/kg/min) if the heart rate is low or dobutamine (1 to 5 mcg/kg/min) for the patient with normal heart rate but decreased blood pressure.

### Respiratory Problems in the Trauma Patient

The trauma patient may have a compromised respiratory system owing to chest trauma. Direct trauma to the chest wall may cause an inability for the bellows system of lung inflation to work resulting from air or fluid entering the chest cavity, or fluid or blood entering the lung parenchyma. In the former situation the lung tissue collapses owing to the lack of negative pressure in the chest cavity, and in the latter the alveoli are unable to exchange $CO_2$ and $O_2$ because of the presence of fluid in the alveoli. It is imperative that any air or fluid within the chest cavity be removed before the anesthetic procedure via a chest tap. Fluid within the lung parenchyma will need to be removed with a diuretic provided that there is an absence of lung contusions. During these procedures the animal should be receiving oxygen by one of the following methods.

**Oxygen delivery methods**

*Flow-by oxygen.* Flow-by oxygen involves using an oxygen source with a pressure-reducing valve and an oxygen line, which is held in front of the patient's nose. Alternatively the technician may choose to use a breathing circuit (preferably one that has not had anesthetic gases pass through it recently) directed at the patient's nose. In either case it is important that the oxygen hose or circuit not be held too close to the patient, as this may cause some distress. Flow rates of 50 to 100 mL/kg/min will provide inspired oxygen levels of 40% to 50%.

*Nasal catheters.* The nasal catheter technique involves insertion of either a nasal cannula, as is used in human medicine, or a nasal catheter (Figure 12-2). Before insertion of either a cannula or a nasal catheter, a topical lubricant should be applied to the tube. A nasal catheter is measured from the nasal meatus to the angle of the mandible, or medial canthus of the eye. The diameter of a cannula that can be inserted is limited by the size of the nasal meatus. The diameter of a catheter is limited by the size of the nasal meatus as well as the nasal passage, which in a cat is a maximum of approximately 4 to 5 French units and in a dog is a maximum of 10 to 12 French units. Oxygen flow rates for this technique are approximately 10 mL/kg/min.

*Oxygen collars.* It is possible to supply oxygen with the use of an Elizabethan collar and clear plastic wrap placed across the lower two thirds to three quarters of the opening, and an oxygen tube entering at the base of the neck (Figure 12-3). As oxygen is heavier than room air, it will remain in the lower portion of the E-collar. The upper uncovered portion allows for the escape of heat and $CO_2$.

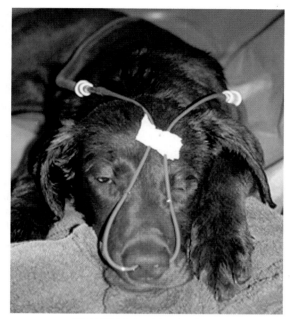

**FIGURE 12-2** Nasal catheter.

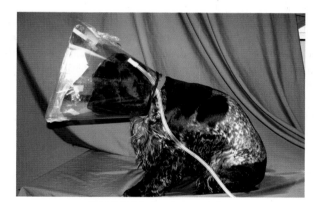

**FIGURE 12-3** Oxygen collar.

*Thoracocentesis.* **Thoracocentesis** (or chest tap) may be required to remove air (pneumothorax), blood, or other fluid (**pleural effusion**) from the chest cavity. This will normally be done by a veterinarian, but the veterinary technician should be familiar with the equipment and procedure. If there is an external wound in the chest wall, then a temporary bandage should be securely placed over the defect to stop additional air from entering the chest cavity until it can be surgically repaired. If time permits, the lateral chest wall from the seventh to ninth intercostal spaces (caudal to the point of the elbow) should be shaved and aseptically prepared (approximately a 4 cm × 4 cm area). The animal will probably be most comfortable in a sternal or standing position during this procedure. For trauma to the lung parenchyma to be reduced, a 20- to 22-gauge, 1- to 1½-inch IV catheter should be used, although some practitioners prefer a winged infusion set. A three-way stopcock and large syringe are also required.

If air is present in the chest, the catheter will be inserted dorsal to the costochondral junction. If fluid is present within the chest cavity the catheter will need to be inserted below the costochondral junction. The catheter is inserted at the seventh to ninth intercostal space, keeping the needle or catheter toward the cranial aspect of the rib. The artery, vein, and nerve pass along the caudal aspect of each rib and should be avoided. The catheter or needle will pass through the various tissue layers fairly readily, until it encounters the pleura of the chest cavity. Extra force is usually required to enter into the chest cavity at this point, and a "pop" may be felt as the catheter or needle passes into the chest cavity. At this time the stylette of the catheter is removed and a three-way stopcock and syringe (at least 6 to 60 mL) are attached to the catheter (syringe size will be determined by the VIC, as will the type of procedure being done—collection of a sample versus emergency thoracocentesis to remove fluid or air). The needle or catheter should now be directed so it is parallel to the chest wall, to reduce the risk of trauma to the lung parenchyma as the patient breathes. The fluid or air should now be quickly withdrawn from the chest cavity, using the three-way stopcock to expel any fluid or air that accumulates in the syringe. The total volume and character of the fluid or air that is removed from the chest cavity should be noted. Some of the fluid should be kept for analysis. Once the animal shows clinical signs that it can breathe more comfortably, then the anesthetic procedure may be started if required. Oxygen support should be available during the induction phase (i.e., facemask) and intubation, which should proceed quickly. The ability to support ventilation should also be an option if required.

Cardiac arrhythmias are common in the first 12 to 72 hours after chest trauma. The veterinarian may request an ECG as part of the preanesthetic workup because cardiac arrhythmias may be seen as long as 3 days after chest trauma. Shock is also common in animals that have undergone significant trauma, particularly if hemorrhage has been severe. Serious internal injuries such as fractures and herniated or ruptured organs may pose further difficulties for the veterinarian and anesthetist.

Very few trauma patients require anesthesia immediately after the accident, and as a general rule it is wise to stabilize these animals before anesthesia. Delaying anesthesia offers two advantages: (1) it allows time for a thorough workup to assess the extent of the injuries, and (2) it provides some time to stabilize the animal's condition (which reduces anesthetic risk). The patient should be closely monitored for signs of dyspnea, cardiac arrhythmias, or altered mentation. It is advisable to obtain thoracic radiographs before anesthesia for repair of internal injuries (such as fractures) resulting from trauma. Studies have shown that one third of patients with traumatic forelimb, hindlimb, or pelvic injuries have concurrent thoracic injuries that could jeopardize the safety of anesthesia. It is obviously advisable to identify and treat a disorder such as pneumothorax before anesthetizing an animal for the repair of a fractured femur. Fortunately, many thoracic injuries improve with cage rest, and if anesthesia can be delayed for 24 to 72 hours after the traumatic incident, the anesthetist usually encounters fewer problems.

## Cardiovascular Disease

Common cardiovascular disorders in patients scheduled for anesthesia include anemia, shock, cardiomyopathy (primary, or secondary to hyperthyroidism), and congestive heart disease (secondary to mitral valve insufficiency). In endemic areas, heartworm disease is also common.

Hypoxia, hypercapnia, electrolyte imbalance, hypothermia, vagal stimulation, and anesthetic overdose can all lead to cardiac dysfunction. Preanesthetic evaluation and laboratory evaluation can help rule out many of these abnormalities, or at least alert the veterinary anesthetist of potential problems. Evaluation of heart rate and synchrony with the pulse is also an important aspect of cardiovascular evaluation.

> **TECHNICIAN NOTE** The most common cardiovascular problem seen by the veterinary anesthetist is bradycardia.

The most common cardiac problem seen by the veterinary anesthetist is bradycardia. This is commonly caused by various drugs, either preanesthetics or general anesthetics, which are used as part of the anesthetic protocol. It is important for the veterinary technician to know the normal ranges for the heart rate for various species (please refer to Table 5-2). Heart rates below these values will result in decreased cardiac output and therefore decreased perfusion and blood pressure. The following equation is one of which every veterinary technician should be aware:

$$ABP = CO \times SVR, \text{ with } CO = HR \times SV$$

- ABP: Arterial blood pressure
- CO: Cardiac output
- SVR: Systemic vascular resistance (the degree of systemic arterial dilation or constriction)
- HR: Heart rate
- SV: Stroke volume (the volume of blood the heart pumps out with each contraction; influenced by the volume of venous blood returning to the heart and the contractile force of the heart muscle)

Anesthetic drugs may decrease not only heart rate but also force of contraction, and may decrease blood return to the heart (also known as *preload*). The decision to treat bradycardia will ultimately be the choice of the veterinarian, but the veterinary technician should be ready to give the appropriate dose of anticholinergic such as atropine or glycopyrrolate, although the former has a quicker onset of action (1 to 2 minutes intravenously) than the latter (up to 15 minutes). It should be remembered that anticholinergics might be selected by the attending veterinarian for treating bradycardia caused by increased vagal tone. However, many veterinary anesthesiologists no longer recommend the routine use of anticholinergics, and certainly these drugs do not work well for other types of bradyarrhythmias. Drugs that may cause an increase in parasympathetic tone include the alpha$_2$-agonists (medetomidine or dexmedetomidine, xylazine), the opioids, and occasionally the phenothiazines. When bradycardia is caused by anesthetic drugs that do not increase vagal tone, it is best treated with catecholamine drugs such as dopamine (1 to 5 mcg/kg/min). If the heart rate has dropped to 50% of normal value and/or blood pressure has dropped to dangerously low levels, then epinephrine becomes a drug of choice (0.01 mcg/kg).

Alternatively, reassessing the depth of anesthesia and turning the patient anesthetic level down, if appropriate, might be all that is needed. The temperature of the patient should also be assessed, as this can be another reason for bradycardia.

Arrhythmias may result from a variety of physiologic causes including the following:
- Anoxia, hypercarbia
- Poor perfusion
- Acid-base imbalance
- Damaged myocardial tissue

Clinically it may be difficult to discern on physical examination if a patient is having arrhythmias. However, the veterinary technician can detect some arrhythmias by auscultating the heart while palpating the pulse and checking for a lack of coordination between the two, which is often called "dropped beats." If dropped beats are discernible, an ECG should be obtained to determine what type of arrhythmia is present and what precautions may need to be taken. The only real way to determine the presence of arrhythmias is with an ECG recording.

As a veterinary paraprofessional there are certain arrhythmias that may require immediate attention by the veterinarian. It is therefore important for the veterinary technician to recognize the normal ECG so that he or she can advise the veterinarian that there may be some abnormality present. Following are some of the arrhythmias that may be encountered in trauma patients or anesthetized patients:
- Premature ventricular contractions
- Atrial fibrillation
- Ventricular fibrillation
- First- and second-degree heart block (which is normal in the equine species)
- Ventricular tachyarrhythmias
- Sinus arrest with escape beats

See Figures 5-6 to 5-15 for examples of commonly encountered arrhythmias.

The veterinarian must be informed immediately about any of the listed arrhythmias because each could be life-threatening. Various drugs such as beta blockers or lidocaine may be indicated in tachyarrhythmias, and atropine may be indicated to treat atrioventricular (AV) heart block. The veterinarian will decide what is the most appropriate drug to use.

Tachyarrhythmias may be treated either with lidocaine in dogs or with beta blockers or calcium channel blockers in cats, as lidocaine tends to be more toxic in the cat. It may be necessary to treat with a constant rate infusion (CRI) if the arrhythmia continues, as lidocaine has a very short half-life. However, a variety of different causes of and specific treatments for tachyarrhythmias exist, and discussion of them is beyond the scope of this book. On a short-term basis while drugs are being prepared, it may be necessary to slow the heart down by applying pressure to the eyeballs or massaging the carotid sinus. Either will increase parasympathetic stimulation.

Many animals with heart disease have concurrent pulmonary disease, particularly pulmonary edema, which further complicates anesthesia. Diuretics such as furosemide may be helpful in alleviating pulmonary edema before anesthesia.

As with patients that have undergone recent trauma, before initiating anesthesia it is generally advisable to stabilize the patient's condition by treating cardiovascular and respiratory disease to alleviate the signs as much as possible. Preoxygenation using a facemask or oxygen chamber for 5 minutes immediately before induction is also extremely helpful in reducing anesthetic risk in animals with cardiovascular or respiratory difficulties.

The veterinarian and anesthetist should ensure that anesthetic agents that depress the myocardium or that exacerbate arrhythmias (e.g., alpha$_2$-agonists and halothane) are avoided as much as possible in these animals. Opioid agents, diazepam, and isoflurane or sevoflurane offer the advantage of relative lack of toxicity to the heart.

When anesthetizing animals with cardiovascular problems, the anesthetist should be aware of the increased risk of overhydration through excessive or rapid administration of IV fluids. Even the standard infusion rate of 10 mL/kg/hr may be dangerous for these animals. Therefore it is advisable to frequently monitor these patients for signs of pulmonary edema such as ocular or nasal discharge, increased lung sounds, and increased respiratory rate. Central venous pressure monitoring, if available, is useful for detection of overhydration.

## Respiratory Disease

Of all the animals to undergo anesthesia, those with respiratory problems are perhaps the most challenging for the anesthetist. Examples of these patients include animals with pleural effusion (i.e., free fluid present in the chest cavity), diaphragmatic hernia, pneumothorax, pulmonary contusions resulting from trauma, pneumonia, tracheal collapse, and pulmonary edema. Poor oxygenation is often present in these animals, and many show signs of tachypnea, dyspnea, and cyanosis. If possible, anesthesia should be delayed until respiratory function has improved. If surgery is absolutely required (e.g., to place a chest tube), local analgesia and gentle manual restraint may be preferable to general anesthesia. Administration of oxygen via previously described techniques is helpful for patients with respiratory compromise. Nitrous oxide should be avoided in patients with respiratory distress because the administration of 100% oxygen is usually necessary to maintain adequate oxygenation.

Before anesthesia, it is important to thoroughly evaluate the animal and, if possible, to find the cause of the respiratory distress. Patients that are presented for anesthesia should be assessed as to their ability to move air into and out of the lungs. Such patients as brachycephalics or those with collapsing trachea can be compromised with regard to their ability to adequately move air even when they are awake. These patients should be preoxygenated during the preanesthetic period and may also need assisted ventilation during the anesthetic procedure.

An animal under anesthesia will frequently have a reduced $V_T$ and decreased respiratory rate. Even when standard anesthetic protocols are used, it is common for the $V_T$ to be decreased by 25% to 40% and for the respiratory rate to drop to 8 to 12 breaths/min. During this time there can be an increase in the $CO_2$ levels, which can result in acid-base imbalances. Such changes may also lead to hypoxemia unless the patient is breathing 100% oxygen. The technician must remember that the inspired air is divided into two portions. Dead space ventilation ($V_D$) is a relatively constant portion of inspired air that fills the upper airways and bronchi. This portion of ventilation is not involved in gas exchange. Some drugs such as anticholinergics may increase dead space. Alveolar ventilation ($V_A$) is the inspired air that fills the alveoli, where oxygen and $CO_2$ are exchanged at the capillary level. Thus the total or tidal volume of air taken in ($V_T$) is the sum of the dead space air plus alveolar air. $V_D$ will always be the first air that is inspired, but because $V_D$ is a relatively constant volume and cannot be changed, any decrease in $V_T$ will result in a decrease in alveolar gas exchange.

One can then see how levels of $CO_2$ may increase and levels of $O_2$ may decrease. These changes can come about from either decreased ventilation or apnea. Generally drugs are not used to improve the ventilatory rate or volume, because drugs such as doxapram will result in only a period of increased ventilatory rate followed by apnea. There will also be a corresponding increase in oxygen demand by the central nervous system with this drug. The technician should properly assess the depth of anesthesia and lighten it if possible. If this is not possible, the technician should provide intermittent ventilation at a volume of 12 to 15 mL/kg per breath. During the anesthetic protocol it is also important that the anesthetist remember to sigh the patient every 5 to 10 minutes to reduce these issues of hypoventilation, atelectasis, and/or apnea.

Patients that are presented for anesthesia should also be assessed as to their oxygen-carrying capabilities by evaluating the packed cell volume (PCV) and the oxygen saturation with a pulse oximeter or a blood gas analysis machine such as the i-STAT if either of these monitors is available. Patients that have a perceived or real decrease in PCV (hematocrit) or an oxygen saturation below 92% should receive oxygen supplementation before the anesthetic protocol for a minimum of 5 minutes. This will ensure saturated oxygen levels within the blood vascular system and the tissues, thus reducing the chance of arrhythmias or hypoxic events.

### Respiratory Problems during Anesthesia

In spite of all of the precautions taken it is possible for the veterinary anesthetist to have respiratory problems with patients. Clinical signs may include dyspnea or cyanosis. When assessing these patients, the anesthetist should determine the following:

- The patient's respiratory character (short and shallow, or deep and exaggerated) and volume
- The depth of anesthesia (not too light or too deep)
- Whether the abnormal breathing is associated with pain (inadequate depth of anesthesia or pain control)
- Whether the endotracheal tube is placed correctly—not too far in (bronchial intubation) or out of the trachea
- Whether the endotracheal tube is partly occluded with mucus or blood
- The oxygen saturation with pulse oximetry or blood gas analysis
- If available, arterial or end-tidal $CO_2$

The cause of the respiratory dysfunction will determine what should be done. However, intermittent positive pressure ventilation (IPPV; see Chapter 6) is usually performed (with the vaporizer turned down) while the cause of the respiratory dysfunction is determined. The technician must ensure that adequate pressures are being achieved during IPPV (15 to 20 cm $H_2O$ in small animal patients and 35 to 40 cm $H_2O$ in large animal patients) to allow for adequate inflation of the alveoli. Occasionally it may be necessary to reintubate the patient to rule out a partial blockage or misplacement of the endotracheal tube.

Radiographs and thoracocentesis are particularly helpful. Thoracocentesis not only is useful in diagnosis, but also may be therapeutic if large volumes of air or fluid can be removed from the chest.

### Diaphragmatic Hernia

One of the most common procedures requiring anesthesia of an animal in respiratory distress is surgical repair of a diaphragmatic hernia. When preparing to anesthetize these patients, as with all patients showing signs of dyspnea, it is advisable to preoxygenate for 5 to 10 minutes before surgery. Head-down positions should be avoided before and during anesthesia because they may result in further movement of abdominal contents into the thorax. If possible, an induction method that allows rapid intubation (i.e., use of an injectable agent) is preferred over mask induction. After induction, some patients may show signs of respiratory depression and even respiratory arrest, and the anesthetist must be prepared to intubate rapidly and assist or control ventilation. Nitrous oxide should not be used because it can cause diffusion of the gas into the displaced stomach and intestines and further distend these organs. Ventilatory assistance must be provided by manual "bagging" of the patient, or a ventilator may be used. The animal should be closely observed for cyanosis. Pulse oximetry, capnography, and arterial blood gas determination are helpful aids for assessing ventilation. Blood gas levels can be evaluated with many blood machines such as the Heska i-STAT hand-held analyzer or the IRMA TRUpoint portable analyzer (Figure 12-4).

These patients require close observation during the recovery period. Administration of oxygen may be necessary if signs of respiratory distress are seen. Pneumothorax is common after chest surgery, and affected patients

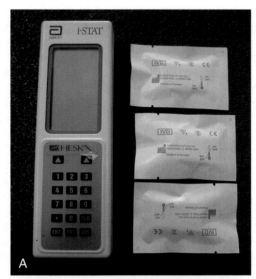

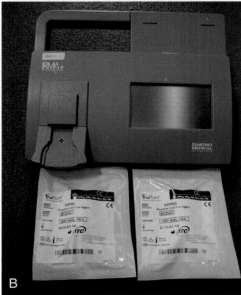

**FIGURE 12-4** Blood gas machines. **A,** Heska i-STAT hand-held analyzer. **B,** IRMA TRUpoint portable analyzer.

may require chest tube placement or removal of air from the pleural space using a syringe and needle.

## Hepatic Disease

Animals with liver disease are subject to increased anesthetic risk because of the central role that organ plays in drug metabolism, synthesis of blood clotting factors and other serum proteins, and carbohydrate metabolism. Some animals with liver disease are hypoproteinemic, which may lead to increased potency of barbiturate agents. Patients with chronic liver failure are also commonly dehydrated, thin, and icteric and may be anemic.

Preanesthetic medication should be given with care or omitted from the protocol because most of these agents require hepatic metabolism before they can be excreted. Acepromazine in particular may have long-lasting effects in patients with compromised hepatic function. Agents that can be reversed are preferred. Use of ketamine and diazepam should also be avoided. Induction and maintenance of anesthesia is best achieved using isoflurane or propofol, which require little or no hepatic function for elimination.

## Renal Disease

The kidneys are the organs most involved in maintaining the volume and electrolyte composition of body fluids. This helps explain why animals with renal disease are often dehydrated and may have severe electrolyte and acid-base imbalances, including metabolic acidosis and hyperkalemia. General anesthesia may be particularly stressful for these patients because renal blood flow is decreased during anesthesia and renal function may be further compromised, particularly if the animal is hypotensive. Use of injectable nonsteroidal antiinflammatory agents such as ketoprofen during anesthesia may reduce renal perfusion even further.

Renal function tests such as urine specific gravity, blood urea nitrogen (BUN), and creatinine may be useful in obtaining an accurate picture of renal function. Preoperative water deprivation may not be advisable in some patients with renal disease because dehydration can occur rapidly after withdrawal of oral fluids. Water should be offered up to 1 hour before premedication. The patient with renal disease should be rehydrated as much as possible before surgery, and electrolyte problems should be identified and addressed. Administration of IV fluids is often continued throughout the anesthetic and postanesthetic periods until the animal is fully hydrated and able to drink unassisted.

Many preanesthetic and anesthetic agents and their metabolites are eliminated from the body by renal excretion. For this reason, animals with compromised renal function may show prolonged recovery after anesthesia if conventional doses are used. It is prudent to reduce doses of anesthetic drugs (including acepromazine, xylazine, diazepam, ketamine, and barbiturates) in these patients. Barbiturates, in particular, have increased potency in acidotic and uremic animals and should be used with great caution in patients with renal disease. Inhalation agents (particularly isoflurane) have some advantages over injectable agents, although halothane can produce fluoride ions, which are damaging to the kidneys.

Animals with urinary blockages (including male cats with urethral obstructions caused by struvite or calcium oxalate crystals) pose similar problems to the anesthetist. Many of these cats are depressed, dehydrated, uremic, acidotic, and hyperkalemic. Hyperkalemic animals are at particular risk for cardiac arrest. Hyperkalemia may sometimes be suspected during auscultation because bradycardia is often seen if plasma potassium levels exceed 6 mEq/L. Some blood chemistry analyzers are capable of measuring electrolytes quickly and easily. Treatment of hyperkalemia may require the use of sodium bicarbonate, 10% calcium gluconate, and/or dextrose and should be done only with close supervision and guidance from the veterinarian. Conditions stressful to the animal should be avoided as much as possible because the release of epinephrine from the adrenal glands may potentiate cardiac arrhythmias.

The administration of inhalation agents (particularly isoflurane) to cats with urinary blockages may be less hazardous than the use of injectable drugs because minimal renal excretion is required for patient recovery. Propofol or ketamine-diazepam may be used intravenously with caution and at reduced doses, provided normal kidney function is present. Cats with obstructions showing extreme depression may not require general anesthesia, particularly if a local anesthetic such as lidocaine gel is administered as part of the urethral catheterization procedure.

 *TECHNICIAN NOTE* Emergencies during anesthesia include the following:
- Too lightly or too deeply anesthetized
- Hypotension
- Cyanosis
- Dyspnea, tachypnea
- Lack of normal heart rate or rhythm
- Respiratory arrest
- Cardiac arrest

## RESPONSE TO ANESTHETIC PROBLEMS AND EMERGENCIES

Despite every precaution, the veterinary technician is likely to encounter anesthetic problems and emergencies throughout the course of a career. The nature of the technician's response may mean the difference between life and death for the anesthetized patient.

### Role of the Veterinary Technician in Emergency Care

Ideally, emergency response is a team effort involving the veterinarian, technician, and other hospital staff. Normally the veterinarian acts as the team leader, directing the staff in emergency procedures. However, the veterinarian may be performing surgery on the patient when an anesthetic emergency arises and therefore may have other pressing concerns. The technician must be prepared to take an active role in resuscitating his or her patient and not rely solely on the already-busy veterinarian. Constant communication between the veterinarian and the technician is obviously important under these circumstances.

It is a good idea to conduct periodic "dress rehearsals" or mock resuscitations in which all staff members participate. Everyone in the hospital should be familiar with the location of the crash kit and IV fluids. Procedures such as warming towels in a clothes dryer, making up hot water bottles, and drawing up drugs into a syringe can be readily taught to hospital staff, which, once the staff has mastered these tasks, will free the veterinarian and technician to perform more demanding tasks.

Occasionally an emergency arises when the veterinarian is absent from the hospital or unavailable to assist. For example, seizures may occur in the postoperative recovery period. Most provincial and state regulations allow the technician to undertake emergency care if the veterinarian is absent. To protect the veterinarian and technician from liability, however, it is advisable to discuss in advance the procedures that the veterinarian will authorize the technician to do in an emergency. It is helpful to have written instructions available in the form of an emergency protocol authorized by the veterinarian.

### General Approach to Emergencies

It cannot be assumed that every anesthetic emergency should be treated in the same way. For example, the veterinarian and animal owner may elect not to resuscitate a severely ill or debilitated animal that undergoes cardiac arrest during anesthesia. Cost considerations may influence treatment in some cases, because emergency care is labor-intensive, and treatment costs may be considerable. Most veterinarians, however, will not stop to consider cost if the emergency arises during a routine surgery, such as a spay, and will do everything possible to revive the animal.

When responding to an emergency, the technician should bear in mind the principles of emergency care listed in Procedure 12-1, p. 345.

### Emergency Situations That May Arise during Anesthesia

Although anesthetic emergencies are by their nature unpredictable, certain problems occur with some frequency. The following situations will be addressed in detail:
- Animals that will not stay anesthetized
- Animals that are too deeply anesthetized
- Pale mucous membranes
- Prolonged capillary refill time
- Cyanosis and dyspnea

- Tachypnea
- Abnormalities in cardiac rate and rhythm
- Respiratory arrest
- Cardiac arrest

## Animals That Will Not Stay Anesthetized

Occasionally, the anesthetist will have difficulty in maintaining a patient at sufficient anesthetic depth. Often the veterinarian becomes aware of the problem when the patient shows signs of movement in response to surgical stimulation. If depth appears inadequate, the anesthetist should check the following:

- Has the vaporizer been turned off, or is the setting too low to maintain an adequate depth of anesthesia?
- Does the vaporizer contain anesthetic?
- Is the endotracheal tube in the trachea? This can be easily determined by checking to see if the reservoir bag expands and contracts as the animal breathes. If so, the endotracheal tube is in the trachea. Movement of the reservoir bag also tells the anesthetist that the endotracheal tube is connected to the Y-piece and that the tube is not blocked. Other procedures used to determine the location and patency of the endotracheal tube include palpation of the neck, and compression of the reservoir bag to see if the chest expands.
- Is air leaking around the endotracheal tube? If so, the patient is probably inspiring some room air, which dilutes the anesthetic gas entering the lungs. Air leakage can be detected by closing the pop-off valve, inflating the reservoir bag, and gently pressing on the bag while listening for the sound of air escaping from the animal's mouth. A soft hiss of escaping air is acceptable at a pressure manometer reading of 20 cm $H_2O$, but a large gush of exiting air should alert the anesthetist that either the endotracheal tube is too small or the cuff is not sufficiently inflated. If this is the case, the cuff can be further inflated or the pharyngeal area can be packed with damp gauze.
- Is the patient apneic? This is most commonly seen immediately after the intubated animal is connected to the machine, particularly if propofol or thiopental was used for induction. Prolonged apnea may lead to arousal from anesthesia because adequate quantities of vaporized anesthetic will not enter the lungs or the bloodstream. If arousal appears imminent, it may be necessary to periodically bag the animal with a mixture of oxygen and anesthetic until anesthetic depth is adequate.
- Are the patient's respirations too shallow to draw sufficient anesthetic into the lungs? Rapid, shallow respiration, commonly seen in toy dogs and obese animals, may be associated with insufficient anesthetic depth. The anesthetist should assist ventilation by bagging these patients (with the vaporizer on) every 5 to 10 seconds.

- Is the anesthetic machine assembled correctly, and are all connections tight? Occasionally, hoses become detached from the machine or the endotracheal tube, in which case the patient will not receive any anesthetic from the machine.
- Is the oxygen flow rate adequate to vaporize the anesthetic? For most precision vaporizers, a minimum flow rate of at least 500 mL/min is necessary for accurate delivery of anesthetic. Very high oxygen flow rates or excessive use of the oxygen flush valve may also result in unpredictable vaporization of anesthetic.
- Is the anesthetic machine functioning correctly? Repeated episodes of awakening during anesthesia may indicate poor vaporizer function. If a halothane or isoflurane vaporizer setting of 3% to 4% seems necessary to maintain anesthesia in many patients, cleaning and recalibration of the vaporizer are probably necessary.
- Is the exaggerated respiratory movement actually an **agonal** (near death) phenomenon, indicating dangerous anesthetic depth rather than a light plane?

If none of these reasons can explain the patient's arousal, the anesthetist should consult with the veterinarian. It may be necessary to increase the vaporizer setting, administer an analgesic, or switch to a different anesthetic in order to achieve the desired anesthetic depth.

## Animals That Are Too Deeply Anesthetized

An animal that is too deeply anesthetized will usually show the following signs:

- A respiratory rate of 6 breaths/min or fewer; shallow respirations, or dyspnea.
- Pale or cyanotic mucous membranes.
- Capillary refill time greater than 2 seconds.
- Bradycardia.
- Weak pulse; systolic blood pressure less than 80 mm Hg (indirect measurement).
- Cardiac arrhythmias may be present; irregular QRS complexes (ventricular complexes) on the ECG, or abnormal complexes such as ventricular premature complexes (VPCs) may be present.
- Cold extremities; body temperature is often less than 35° C.
- Absent reflexes, including palpebral and corneal reflexes.
- Flaccid muscle tone.
- Dilated pupils; absent pupillary light reflex.

The anesthetist should use judgment in interpreting the signs listed. The presence of one or two signs may not indicate excessive depth, provided the other signs are absent. Vital signs also vary depending on the preanesthetic and general anesthetics used (e.g., atropine may affect heart rate and pupil dilation). The more parameters that the anesthetist considers, the more accurate the depth assessment is likely to be.

There are several reasons why anesthetic depth may be excessive. In most cases the vaporizer setting is too high for the patient being anesthetized or, in the case of injectable agents, too high a dose has been given. Occasionally the animal may have a preexisting problem such as shock or anemia that increases susceptibility to anesthetic overdose (Procedure 12-2, pp. 345).

## Pale Mucous Membranes

Pale mucous membranes may arise from several causes. Some patients have preexisting anemia secondary to diseases such as feline leukemia, hemolytic anemia, bleeding disorders, neoplasia, or chronic renal disease. In other cases blood loss may have occurred during surgery. Some anesthetic agents (particularly inhalation agents, propofol, and acepromazine) cause vasodilation and decrease blood pressure, resulting in poor perfusion of capillary beds and pale mucous membranes in some animals. Hypothermia or pain can also reduce blood supply to the tissues and can cause pale mucous membranes.

If pale mucous membranes are observed during surgery, follow Procedure 12-3, p. 345.

## Prolonged Capillary Refill Time

The observation of a capillary refill time greater than 2 seconds suggests that blood pressure is inadequate to perfuse superficial tissues. The presence of hypotension should be suspected in any animal with a slow capillary refill time. Hypotension was the most common anesthetic complication found in one study of dogs and cats (Gaynor and colleagues, 1999). Hypotension may be present before the induction of anesthesia, as in the case of animals undergoing emergency surgery after trauma. Hypotension or shock also may develop secondary to blood loss during surgery or may occur in patients that are at a very deep plane of anesthesia. Acepromazine and the inhalation agents may also cause hypotension in susceptible patients. Follow Procedure 12-4, p. 345, if a prolonged capillary refill time is observed. The treatment for shock in the anesthetized patient is similar to that in the conscious patient and should be performed under the supervision of a veterinarian (Procedure 12-5, p. 346).

## Dyspnea and/or Cyanosis

Any patient showing dyspnea or cyanosis during the administration of an anesthetic should be immediately brought to the veterinarian's attention. The presence of dyspnea indicates that the animal is unable to obtain sufficient oxygen or remove adequate $CO_2$ with normal respiratory movements. Cyanosis indicates that tissue oxygenation is inadequate. Dyspnea and cyanosis often are seen together and if not managed quickly may be followed by respiratory arrest, in which respiratory efforts cease and the amount of oxygen available to the tissues rapidly declines.

The most common sources of respiratory distress during anesthesia are as follows:

- The animal is unable to obtain oxygen from the anesthetic machine because the oxygen supply has run out, the flow meter has been turned off, or the anesthetic circuit or endotracheal tube is blocked.
- The animal is unable to breathe normally because of airway obstruction or respiratory pathology. Causes of airway obstruction include endotracheal tube blockage, excessive flexion of the head and neck, laryngospasm, bronchoconstriction, aspiration of stomach contents after vomiting or regurgitation, and brachycephalic conformation. Common causes of respiratory pathology include pneumothorax, pulmonary edema, diaphragmatic hernia, and pleural effusion. Use of heavy surgical drapes or constricting bandages also may impair normal respiration.
- The animal is too deeply anesthetized, to the point that respiration and other vital functions are adversely affected.

Respiratory problems are life-threatening and should be addressed as discussed in Procedure 12-6, p. 346.

## Tachypnea

Tachypnea, or rapid respirations, must be differentiated from dyspnea, in which respiratory distress is present. Tachypnea may arise at any time during anesthesia and may be disconcerting to the anesthetist. It is particularly common during procedures using opioids. Tachypnea also may be seen if anesthetic depth is inadequate, in which case it is often accompanied by tachycardia and spontaneous movement. Paradoxically, tachypnea also may occur in deep anesthesia as a response to low blood oxygen and high blood carbon dioxide levels. Tachypnea is also seen in hyperthermic patients, including animals with malignant hyperthermia.

If tachypnea is seen, follow Procedure 12-7, p. 346.

## Abnormalities in Cardiac Rate and Rhythm

Tachycardia, bradycardia, and cardiac arrhythmias are commonly seen in anesthetized patients.

Tachycardia is present if the heart rate during stage III anesthesia is greater than 140 bpm for a large dog, 160 bpm for a small dog, 200 for a cat, 60 for a horse, or 100 for a cow. It may result from the administration of drugs such as atropine, ketamine, or epinephrine. Tachycardia may also be a preexisting condition in animals with hyperthyroidism, shock, congestive heart failure, and other conditions. An elevation in heart rate is also a common response to surgical stimulation, although it does not necessarily indicate insufficient anesthetic depth unless accompanied by rapid respiration, spontaneous movement, or active reflexes.

Not all cases of tachycardia require treatment (e.g., those in patients with otherwise normal cardiac function), but the anesthetist should notify the veterinarian before assuming that tachycardia is not significant. It is also important to check the vaporizer setting and anesthetic depth and adjust them if necessary.

Bradycardia can be defined as a heart rate less than 60 to 70 bpm in a dog, <100 bpm in a cat, <25 bpm in a horse or <40 bpm in a cow. Bradycardia may be secondary to the administration of alpha$_2$-agonists, or opioids, particularly if anticholinergics were not administered preoperatively. Bradycardia also may result from increased activity of the vagus nerve in response to endotracheal intubation, ocular surgery, or handling of the viscera by the surgeon. Bradycardia may also occur if the animal is very deeply anesthetized, and when seen in this context it is a warning that respiratory and cardiac arrest may be imminent. Other causes of bradycardia include hypertension, hyperkalemia, hypothermia, and hypoxia.

Not all cases of bradycardia require treatment. If capillary refill, pulse oximeter readings, blood pressure, and pulse strength appear normal, tissue perfusion may be adequate and treatment may be unnecessary. The veterinarian should be consulted and should direct treatment. If anesthetic depth is excessive, the vaporizer setting should be adjusted, and bagging with 100% oxygen (empty the breathing bag into the scavenging system and refill it with pure oxygen) may be helpful. Bradycardia as a result of the administration of drugs or because of excessive vagal stimulation may be treated with anticholinergics, reversal agents, or a change in the anesthetic protocol.

The term *cardiac arrhythmia* (or *cardiac dysrhythmia*) refers to any one of a number of electrocardiographic abnormalities, including "dropped beats," VPCs arising spontaneously from individual heart muscle cells, and sustained episodes of tachycardia. These abnormalities are most easily detected through the use of an ECG. The alert technician also may note that a pulse deficit is present in animals with some types of arrhythmias.

Cardiac arrhythmias commonly arise in animals given arrhythmogenic drugs such as barbiturates, alpha$_2$-agonists, and halothane. Such arrhythmias are often of short duration and well tolerated in young, healthy patients but may be a significant problem in animals with preexisting heart disease and in geriatric patients. Arrhythmias are particularly common during induction and light anesthesia. They may also be the result of respiratory depression and subsequent hypoxia. Other causes of cardiac arrhythmias include preexisting heart disease, electrolyte and acid-base disturbances, gastric volvulus, thoracic surgery, endotracheal intubation, and hypercapnia. Hypercapnia may arise from poor anesthetic technique, including exhaustion of the $CO_2$ absorber crystals or inadequate oxygen flow rates. Cardiac arrhythmias should be treated in consultation with the veterinarian (Procedure 12-8, p. 346).

### Respiratory Arrest

Respiratory arrest is the cessation of respiratory efforts by the patient. It may lead to cardiac arrest and is therefore potentially fatal. Not all cases of respiratory arrest require immediate action by the anesthetist. Respiratory efforts may temporarily cease after the IV injection of ketamine, barbiturates, propofol, and other respiratory depressants. Minimal respiratory efforts may also be seen after a period of prolonged bagging with oxygen and in this case reflect low blood carbon dioxide and high blood oxygen levels. Whether respiratory arrest is the result of drug administration or excessive bagging with oxygen, the anesthetist must be sure that other vital signs, particularly heart rate and mucous membrane color, are normal. If the heartbeat is regular, the heart rate is greater than the minimum acceptable rate (see Table 5-2), the pulse is strong, and mucous membranes are pink, the patient does not usually require immediate treatment for respiratory arrest. Pulse oximeter readings are helpful in indicating if the patient's oxygenation status is adequate (i.e., a reading greater than 95% usually indicates that bagging is not necessary). To be safe, occasional "breaths" of oxygen (one every 30 seconds) can be delivered to the patient during this period to prevent hypoxia. However, premature bagging with oxygen may extend the period of apnea by removing carbon dioxide from the blood, which is a stimulus for the patient to resume breathing. The anesthetist who suspects that respiratory efforts have temporarily ceased because of administration of drugs or ventilation with oxygen should closely monitor the patient's heart rate and mucous membrane color for 1 to 2 minutes before assuming that a serious condition exists. If spontaneous respiration does not resume within this time, the veterinarian should be consulted, and it may be advisable to begin bagging the patient with oxygen.

True respiratory arrest is much more serious and requires immediate attention. This condition may arise because of anesthetic overdose, cessation of oxygen flow, or preexisting respiratory disease such as pneumothorax or diaphragmatic hernia. Affected animals may show warning signs such as dyspnea and/or cyanosis before respiratory arrest occurs. Other vital signs, such as heart rate, capillary refill time, pulse strength, and pupil size, are often abnormal. Pulse oximetry values rapidly fall below 90%. The treatment of respiratory arrest involves the steps shown in Procedure 12-9, p. 347.

Bagging should continue until the heart rate, mucous membrane color, and pulse oximeter values have been restored to normal. Once this is achieved, the anesthetist should discontinue bagging for 15 to 30 seconds and closely observe the patient for respiratory efforts. If none are seen, bagging should resume. On occasion, the anesthetist may be faced with a patient in respiratory arrest in the absence of an anesthetic machine. It is possible to substitute an **Ambu bag** (Figure 12-5) or even institute mouth-to–endotracheal tube or mouth-to-muzzle resuscitation in these cases.

### Cardiac Arrest

Cardiac arrest may occur at any time during anesthesia. In most cases the anesthetist receives some warning that arrest is imminent, in the form of a short period in

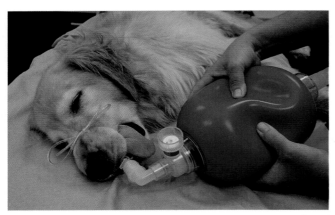

**FIGURE 12-5**   Use of an Ambu bag to deliver room air to an intubated patient.

which cyanosis, dyspnea or respiratory arrest, and prolonged capillary refill are evident, often accompanied by an arrhythmia. If cardiac arrest appears imminent, the anesthetist should immediately alert the veterinarian and the hospital staff while continuing to monitor the heart by auscultation, by palpation of the chest, or through the use of an ECG. A patient experiencing cardiac arrest rapidly develops the following signs:

- No heartbeat can be auscultated or palpated, and normal QRS complexes are absent from the ECG tracing.
- There is no palpable arterial pulse, and blood pressure readings (if available) are 25 mm Hg or less.
- Mucous membranes are gray or cyanotic, and capillary refill may be prolonged.
- Pupils are widely dilated with no response to light, and corneal reflex is absent.
- Respiration is absent except for intermittent, abrupt gasps (agonal breaths).

Coordinated action by all hospital staff members is essential to reverse cardiac arrest by performing cardiopulmonary cerebrovascular resuscitation (CPCR). Once arrest occurs, permanent brain damage may result if oxygen delivery to the brain is not reestablished within 4 minutes, by either cardiopulmonary resuscitation (CPR) or restoration of cardiac function. Ideally, at least five staff members should participate in the resuscitative efforts as follows: one person performs chest compressions, the second person bags the animal, the third assesses the pulse during compressions and checks the pulse or ECG when compressions are temporarily suspended, the fourth draws up and administers drugs on the veterinarian's orders, and the fifth maintains a record of patient status and resuscitative treatments. The minimum number of people required is three, with compressions performed by one person, tasks two and five by a second person, and tasks three and four by a third.

The essential steps in performing CPCR have traditionally been summarized by the mnemonic ABCDE, which stands for *a*irway, *b*reathing, *c*irculation, *d*rugs, *E*CG. Of these, the single most important one is circulation.

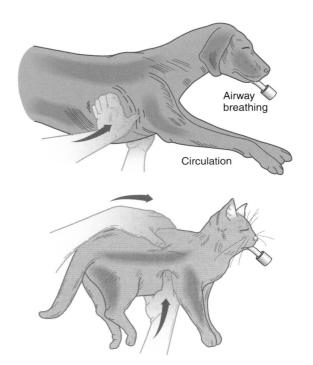

**FIGURE 12-6**   Correct location for cardiac compressions for a medium-sized dog or a cat. In the case of dogs undergoing a laparotomy at the time of arrest, the surgeon may immediately initiate internal compressions by opening the diaphragm, entering the thorax, and compressing the heart.

Current evidence suggests that initiating steps to generate circulation of blood should be done first, particularly if the patient arrests under anesthesia and is correctly intubated, thus **CABDE.**

### Circulation

Cardiac compressions should be initiated immediately, as they have been shown to be the single most important factor in successful **return of spontaneous circulation (ROSC).** The animal should be turned on its right side with its feet toward the person doing compressions and the head tilted down, if possible.

- *Cardiac compressions for a large dog, a foal, or a small ruminant:* A firm object such as a book, sandbag, or rolled-up towel should be placed under the animal's chest just behind the elbow. The heel of the compressor's hand should compress the chest against this object, with the pressure applied at the point where the chest is widest. Both hands should be used to compress the chest. The chest wall should be allowed to bounce back rapidly after each compression.
- *Cardiac compressions for a medium-sized dog:* One hand should be placed under the chest and the other hand at the fifth intercostal space, just over the heart itself (Figure 12-6). The chest is then compressed between the two hands.
- *Cardiac compressions for a cat or small dog:* Compression may be done by using the thumb to compress the chest against the fingers of the same hand.

- *Note*: Attempting to perform compressions in adult cattle and horses does not produce effective circulation. CPCR is limited to drug administration and ventilation in these patients.

The rate of compressions should be one to two times per second to generate a heart rate of approximately 100 bpm. The chest should be compressed by approximately one third of the diameter of the chest wall. The aim of the compressions is to manually force blood through the heart and, ultimately, to the tissues. It is believed that compressions also may assist circulation by increasing pressure in the chest, indirectly inducing blood flow. Each compression should result in a palpable femoral pulse, which should be periodically monitored by another staff member, if possible. If a pulse is not detected and the mucous membrane color does not improve, the method of compression should be adjusted by changing the rate or intensity, by repositioning the patient, or by assigning the compression task to another staff member. A Doppler probe placed on the cornea may also be useful in detecting pulses from effective compressions.

If two people are administering CPR, one person should bag every 10 to 12 seconds while the other compresses the chest. Bagging and compressions should be delivered simultaneously. In the case of a technician working alone, compressions should be given priority—as long as the patient has a patent airway or endotracheal tube, the compressions will result in some gas exchange. Once CPR is initiated, it should not be discontinued for longer than 3 to 5 seconds at a time.

If external cardiac compressions are not effective, as shown by failure to achieve a palpable pulse or pink mucous membranes within 2 minutes, internal compressions may be attempted. In the case of dogs weighing over 20 kg, some authorities suggest that internal compressions should be initiated immediately after cardiac arrest is identified. Investigators have shown that external chest compression in dogs weighing more than 20 kg results in less than 30% of normal cardiac output, whereas internal massage results in outputs of up to 70% of normal. There is understandable reluctance on the part of many veterinarians and technicians to enter the chest to perform internal massage; however, controlled studies have demonstrated that the success rate for resuscitation of large dogs is much greater if internal cardiac massage is performed.

For performance of internal compressions, the lateral thorax is quickly clipped and rinsed with alcohol, a self-adhering sterile drape is applied to the prepared area, and a skin incision is made between the seventh and eighth ribs, using a scalpel. The incision is extended through the muscle until the chest cavity is encountered. Care should be taken to avoid incising lung tissue, which lies immediately below the pleura. The operator's hand is inserted between the ribs (the use of a retractor may be necessary to separate the ribs adequately). The heart is grasped, and gentle but firm pressure is applied to the ventricles at a rate of 100 times per minute. If resuscitation efforts are successful, a palpable heartbeat may return within seconds or minutes. Surgical closure and antibiotic therapy are essential after reestablishment of cardiac function by internal compression.

When doing compressions, it is necessary to stop periodically to determine whether the heart has resumed spontaneous contractions. This is easy to ascertain by palpation when doing internal compressions, but more difficult with external compression methods. Spontaneous contractions can be detected by discontinuing external compression and either palpating for a spontaneous pulse or observing an ECG for QRS complexes. Auscultation may also be useful. The presence of increasing $ET_{CO_2}$ concentrations on a capnograph also indicates ROSC.

If spontaneous contractions are not observed, external or internal compressions can be resumed, although after 15 minutes they are unlikely to be successful in establishing a heartbeat. Use of a defibrillator is helpful in some situations but should be authorized and directly supervised by a veterinarian.

If spontaneous contractions are observed, cardiac compressions should be discontinued, although bagging must be maintained until spontaneous breathing is established, which may require up to several hours. The anesthetist should periodically check the capillary refill time, mucous membrane color, and heart rate and should discontinue bagging only if these vital signs appear normal. If mucous membrane color deteriorates or if spontaneous respiration does not occur within 1 minute after bagging has been discontinued, bagging should be resumed.

### Airway and Breathing

If the animal is intubated and connected to an anesthetic machine, one staff member should note the time of arrest and immediately initiate respiratory support by turning off the vaporizer and nitrous oxide flow and bagging the animal with 100% oxygen at the rate of one breath every 10 to 12 seconds. Mask administration of oxygen is inadequate; if an endotracheal tube is not present, it is essential that the animal be intubated immediately. In addition, the anesthetist must ensure that the patient's chest rises slightly during bagging, indicating that the airway is not blocked or the tube is not placed in the esophagus.

### Drugs

Drugs are commonly administered to aid recovery. In all cases, the veterinarian, if present, should authorize the dosage, route, and nature of drugs to be administered.

If an IV catheter is present, the drugs are normally given through it, followed by IV fluids at a dosage of 20 mL/kg (cats) or 40 mL/kg (dogs) as rapidly as possible. Caution should be used when administering fluids to patients in cardiac arrest because overhydration and pulmonary edema are common sequelae. If IV access is difficult, drugs may be given by injection into the base of the tongue or by intratracheal administration. Intratracheal

| TABLE 12-2 | **Drugs Used in Treating Anesthetic Emergencies in Cats and Dogs** | |
|---|---|---|
| Drug | Dose for Intravenous Use | Indications for Use |
| Atipamezole | 0.1-0.2 mg/kg | Reversal agent for dexmedetomidine |
| Atropine | 0.025 mg/kg, can give 2-3 × dose intratracheally | Treatment for bradycardia |
| Dexamethasone | 4-8 mg/kg | Corticosteroid used in treatment of shock |
| Diazepam | 0.2-1 mg/kg | Treatment of seizures |
| Dobutamine | 1-10 mcg/kg/min infusion in 5% dextrose | Increases force of myocardial contractions |
| Dopamine | 5-10 mcg/kg/min infusion in lactated Ringer's | Increases force of myocardial contractions, increases heart rate |
| Doxapram | 1-4 mg/kg | Respiratory and central nervous system stimulant |
| Epinephrine | 0.1-0.2 mg/kg, can give 2-3 × dose intratracheally | Increases rate and force of cardiac contractions, increases systemic vascular resistance |
| Lidocaine without epinephrine | 2 mg/kg (dog, horse) 0.5 mg/kg (cat) can give 2-3 × dose intratracheally | Antiarrhythmic agent for treating ventricular tachycardia and ventricular premature complexes |
| Naloxone | 0.01-0.02 mg/kg | Opioid antagonist |
| Prednisolone sodium succinate | 10-30 mg/kg | Corticosteroid used in treatment of shock |
| Sodium bicarbonate | 1-2 mEq/kg | Treatment of metabolic acidosis |
| Vasopressin | 0.8 U/kg | Increases rate and force of cardiac contractions, increases systemic vascular resistance |
| Yohimbine | 0.1 mg/kg | Reversal agent for xylazine |

| TABLE 12-3 | **Doses of Emergency Drugs Used in Cardiopulmonary Resuscitation of Cats and Dogs** | | | | | | | | | |
|---|---|---|---|---|---|---|---|---|---|---|
| | | Patient Weight | | | | | | | | |
| Emergency Drug | Dose | 3 kg 6.6 lb | 5 kg 11 lb | 10 kg 22 lb | 15 kg 33 lb | 20 kg 44 lb | 25 kg 55 lb | 30 kg 66 lb | 40 kg 88 lb | 50 kg 110 lb |
| Epinephrine (1 mg/mL) | 0.1 mg/kg | 0.3 mL | 0.5 mL | 1 mL | 1.5 mL | 2 mL | 2.5 mL | 3 mL | 4 mL | 5 mL |
| Vasopressin (20 U/mL) | 0.8 U/kg | 0.12 mL | 0.2 mL | 0.4 mL | 0.6 mL | 0.8 mL | 1 mL | 1.2 mL | 1.6 mL | 2 mL |
| Atropine (0.4 mg/mL) | 0.05 mg/kg | 0.3 mL | 0.5 mL | 1 mL | 1.5 mL | 2 mL | 2.5 mL | 3 mL | 4 mL | 5 mL |
| Lidocaine (dog) (20 mg/mL) | 2 mg/kg | 0.3 mL | 0.5 mL | 1 mL | 1.5 mL | 2 mL | 2.5 mL | 3 mL | 4 mL | 5 mL |
| Sodium bicarbonate (1 mEq/mL) | 1 mEq/kg | 3 mL | 5 mL | 10 mL | 15 mL | 20 mL | 25 mL | 30 mL | 40 mL | 50 mL |
| Prednisolone sodium succinate | 30 mg/kg | 90 mg | 150 mg | 300 mg | 450 mg | 600 mg | 750 mg | 900 mg | 1200 mg | 1500 mg |

administration may involve injection of the drug directly into the tracheal lumen, or the drug may be administered by means of a urinary catheter passed through the endotracheal tube. For intratracheal administration, the dose of emergency drug given should be twice the recommended IV dose.

Intracardiac injections should be avoided if possible because injections by this route require the interruption of cardiac compressions and have some potential to damage the myocardium or lacerate coronary blood vessels. As a last resort drugs may be injected into the left ventricle.

Agents that are commonly administered to assist with ROSC are epinephrine, vasopressin, atropine, dopamine, and dobutamine. The current recommended doses of emergency drugs are given in Tables 12-2 and 12-3.

Epinephrine is the drug most commonly used for initial treatment of cardiac arrest. The currently recommended dose is 1 mL/10 kg—thus 0.5 mL for cats, 1 mL for small dogs, 2 mL for medium-sized dogs, and 3 mL for large dogs, all drawn up from a 1:1000 solution. Epinephrine is administered every 3 to 5 minutes.

Vasopressin may be used in place of epinephrine or alternated with doses of epinephrine. The recommended dose is 0.4 mL/10 kg. Like epinephrine, vasopressin is administered every 3 to 5 minutes.

Atropine is frequently indicated with anesthesia-related cardiac arrest in order to decrease parasympathetic tone and can be administered every 15 to 20 minutes.

Dopamine or dobutamine infusions are also advised by many authorities because these drugs increase the force and rate of cardiac contractions.

Bicarbonate administration is no longer recommended unless the animal is hyperkalemic.

Calcium injections are also no longer advocated, except in hyperkalemic or severely hypocalcemic animals.

### Electrocardiogram

Placement of ECG leads can give the CPCR team information regarding the underlying "rhythm" of the patient. Compressions should not be halted in order to place leads. It is imperative that alcohol *not* be used to wet lead-patient contacts if a defibrillator is available, as it could result in an explosion. Compressions should be stopped for only a few seconds to allow the ECG to be evaluated. One of three rhythms may be observed:

- Asystole: no electrical activity ("flatline")
- Ventricular fibrillation: coarse vertical zigzag lines that do not resemble normal complexes
- Pulseless electrical activity: organized electrical activity that frequently resembles normal or near-normal complexes

Asystole, in which the heart has no electrical or mechanical activity, is most likely to respond to the CPCR technique described earlier (compressions, ventilation, drugs).

Ventricular fibrillation represents disorganized muscular activity of the heart (see Figure 5-15). During open-chest CPCR the heart muscle "writhes" and has the appearance of a bag of worms. This type of cardiac arrest is best treated by electrical defibrillation (Procedure 12-10, p. 347).

Pulseless electrical activity (also known as *electromechanical dissociation* [EMD]) is the hardest situation to treat. Patients with this type of cardiac arrest may respond to standard CPCR (Figure 12-7).

### Aftercare

After ROSC the patient requires intensive monitoring of cardiovascular and respiratory function, as well as an assessment of brain function. It is very common for patients to experience another cardiac arrest within 24 hours of successful CPCR. Monitoring may include blood pressure (indirect or direct), blood gases, pulse oximetry, continuous ECG, and capnography. Decisions regarding treatment with fluids and infusions are often made on a minute-to-minute basis as patient status changes rapidly in one direction or the other. In an ideal situation, cardiovascular, ventilatory, and neurologic status will improve, infusions will be decreased and finally discontinued, and the patient will be discharged. Drugs commonly used in the postresuscitation period include lidocaine to treat ventricular arrhythmias, inotropes (dobutamine, dopamine), fluids, sodium bicarbonate, corticosteroids, furosemide, and mannitol.

Unfortunately, many patients that sustain cardiac arrest cannot be revived. In the case of those patients in which cardiac function is reestablished, conditions such as pulmonary edema and cerebral edema may occur. Cerebral edema is manifested by seizures, failure to return to consciousness, and temporary or permanent neurologic damage.

## Problems That May Arise in the Recovery Period

### Regurgitation during Anesthesia and Postanesthesia Vomiting

Regurgitation is a passive phenomenon that may occur even during deep anesthesia. In a regurgitating animal, stomach contents exit through the cardiac sphincter, move up the esophagus, and enter the pharynx, nasopharynx, and oral cavity. Once in the pharynx, stomach contents may be aspirated into the respiratory tract. Regurgitation is most common in animals placed in a head-down position during surgery, because this causes increased pressure on the stomach, and in ruminants. Unlike vomiting, regurgitation is not accompanied by retching or other outward signs, and in fact the only sign apparent to the anesthetist may be a small amount of fluid draining from the animal's mouth or nose. Treatment of regurgitation involves immediate intubation (if a cuffed endotracheal tube is not already present) and removal of as much regurgitated material as possible through suction.

Vomiting during or after anesthesia is a relatively common phenomenon, particularly in brachycephalic

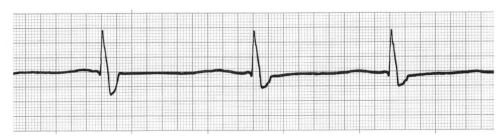

**FIGURE 12-7**   This electrocardiogram (ECG) pattern, accompanied by lack of palpable pulses, is called *pulseless electrical activity,* or *electromechanical dissociation.*

dogs. Unlike regurgitation, vomiting is an active phenomenon, often accompanied by retching. Vomiting usually occurs as the animal is losing consciousness during induction or as it is returning to consciousness during anesthetic recovery. Vomiting is potentially most dangerous if the animal is unconscious and the airway is not protected with an endotracheal tube. In this situation, the vomitus may be easily aspirated into the trachea. Aspiration of vomitus may cause immediate signs of dyspnea and cyanosis as a result of airway obstruction and bronchospasm. If the patient survives this episode, signs of aspiration pneumonia (including fever, increased respiratory rate, and increased lung sounds) may appear over the next 24 to 48 hours. It is imperative, therefore, that the anesthetist prevents the accumulation of vomitus within the oral cavity of the unconscious patient and the subsequent aspiration of the material into the air passages.

To do this, an endotracheal tube should be immediately inserted if time and level of consciousness of the patient allow. If this cannot be achieved, the animal's head should immediately be placed at a lower level than the rest of its body (e.g., over the edge of the surgery table). This helps prevent passive flow of liquid material into the trachea. When the vomiting stops, it may be necessary to manually clean the oral cavity, using suction if available. If respiratory arrest occurs because of airway blockage, the animal should be intubated and bagged with oxygen.

Unconscious animals have a low risk of aspiration if a cuffed endotracheal tube is already in place during the vomiting episode. It is for this reason that the endotracheal tube is customarily left in place until the patient regains the swallowing reflex and is close to consciousness. If vomiting is seen in an unconscious animal that has a cuffed endotracheal tube in place, the anesthetist should ensure that the cuff of the tube is inflated and position the animal's head lower than the rest of its body to prevent accumulation of vomitus within the oral cavity.

Occasionally, an animal may regurgitate after esophageal intubation. If this occurs the tube should be left in place to direct the contents away from the pharynx. Another endotracheal tube should be placed in the trachea, if possible, while the first tube is still in place. Fortunately, most vomiting episodes occur after the animal has regained consciousness and the ability to swallow. It is not usually necessary to intubate conscious animals during a vomiting episode; however, the anesthetist should ensure that the head is kept extended and as low as possible.

Occasionally the technician may be called on to anesthetize an animal that has not been fasted before induction. These patients may be at risk of vomiting and/or regurgitation during induction, maintenance, and recovery. The anesthetist can help avoid problems by ensuring that rapid induction and intubation techniques are used. For this reason, an injectable agent is preferred over masking in these patients. A cuffed endotracheal tube with adequate diameter is essential. If possible, head-down positions should be avoided during surgery to prevent excessive pressure on the stomach. The anesthetist should also ensure that suction is readily available in case of regurgitation or vomiting. Use of antiemetic drugs such as metoclopramide may be helpful in some cases.

## Postanesthesia Seizures and Excitement

Seizures are occasionally seen in animals recovering from anesthesia. Seizures may be caused by the administration of ketamine, by diagnostic procedures such as myelography, or by patient disorders such as epilepsy or hypoglycemia.

It is important that the anesthetist differentiate between seizures and excitement during recovery. Excitement usually occurs after barbiturate anesthesia (particularly after the use of pentobarbital to treat status epilepticus) and most often appears as spontaneous paddling of the limbs and occasionally as vocalization. Geriatric animals may also vocalize and appear confused after anesthesia. Usually, treatment is unnecessary other than the calm reassurance of the patient. Sedatives can be helpful, especially if the patient did not receive a sedative in the preanesthetic period. Occasionally, excitement or dysphoria may be seen after the administration of high doses of opioids to animals that have not been tranquilized (particularly cats). Treatment with naloxone to partially reverse the opioid or a tranquilizer to reduce the dysphoric effects may be helpful in these animals. Excitement is rarely observed in animals that receive opioids for moderate or severe pain.

In contrast, seizures appear as spontaneous twitching or uncontrolled movements of the head, neck, and limbs and are often triggered by a stimulus such as sound or touch. Animals given ketamine may show stiff forelimbs, **opisthotonus,** and exaggerated responses to touch or noise.

Animals undergoing postoperative excitement or seizures should be brought to the veterinarian's attention. Elimination of stimuli such as light, sound, and touch may be adequate to resolve the episode. Adequate postoperative analgesia should be provided. If seizures are present, many animals respond well to administration of IV or rectal diazepam at a rate of 0.2 to 0.4 mg/kg. If diazepam is not effective or is unavailable, the animal may be anesthetized with propofol in sufficient quantity to induce sedation and eliminate seizures.

Animals manifesting seizures or excitement during recovery require surveillance and nursing care to prevent self-injury. In the case of cats recovering from ketamine anesthesia, it may be necessary to trim the front claws or to bandage the paws to prevent the animal from scratching its face.

All animals experiencing seizures should be monitored for hyperthermia and cyanosis. Hyperthermia can be treated by the application of cool wet towels. Cyanosis should be treated by the administration of oxygen by facemask or by endotracheal tube (if unconscious).

### Dyspnea during the Recovery Period

Dyspnea resulting from upper airway obstruction is the most common cause of death in the postanesthetic period. Dyspnea in cats is usually caused by laryngospasm, whereas dyspnea in dogs is most commonly associated with breed-related (e.g., brachycephalic) obstruction of the entrance to the trachea.

Laryngospasm is a condition in which the cartilages in the laryngeal area become so tightly closed that air is unable to enter the trachea. This condition commonly arises in cats because of this species' extremely active laryngeal reflex. In some recovering cats, the removal of the endotracheal tube initiates reflex closure of the airway. This reflex is normally useful to the cat in that it prevents the aspiration of food or water into the larynx in the conscious animal; however, in the unconscious animal it may well result in complete airway blockage. Laryngeal edema may result from repeated attempts to intubate during light anesthesia. Clinically, this resembles laryngospasm.

Cats undergoing laryngospasm or laryngeal edema may breathe with an audible **stertor** or wheeze. They typically show exaggerated thoracic movements, gasping, and upward movement of the head during inspiration. If conscious, the animal usually appears anxious or excited. Laryngospasm must be differentiated from growling, which is common in cats recovering from anesthesia. In the case of growling, the noises are particularly evident on expiration, whereas in laryngospasm the respiration is labored and the noise is most evident during inspiration.

If a cat shows signs of laryngospasm during recovery from anesthesia, the anesthetist should check the mucous membrane color and pulse oximeter readings (if available). If the cat's mucous membranes appear pink and the $SaO_2$ is greater than 90%, the obstruction is likely partial rather than complete. In this case, the situation may resolve without treatment, although administration of oxygen by facemask may be helpful, provided it does not stress the cat. It may be helpful to extend the neck and hold the tongue rostrally. If cyanosis is present or $SaO_2$ readings are less than 90%, and the cat is losing consciousness—and if these signs are not alleviated by the administration of oxygen by facemask—the animal must be intubated. If intubation is impossible, the veterinarian may elect to perform a tracheotomy to reestablish airflow. The animal should be kept anesthetized for 2 hours and given furosemide and corticosteroids to reduce swelling. The cat can be extubated once the cords appear less rounded and swollen. Nasal oxygen is useful during extubation.

Laryngospasm is easier to prevent than to treat. When cats are being anesthetized, gentle intubation technique is essential to avoid unnecessary laryngeal trauma. Use of lidocaine spray and/or gel is also helpful during intubation. Early extubation is recommended in cats so that the tube is removed before the laryngeal reflex returns.

Dyspnea in brachycephalic breeds of dogs usually occurs because the airway is obstructed by the soft palate or by other redundant tissue in the pharynx. However, there are many other potential causes of obstruction, including foreign objects such as blood clots, gauze sponges, or even extracted teeth. Animals that have undergone surgery of the pharynx or larynx often undergo postoperative tissue swelling that may lead to airway obstruction.

However it arises, airway obstruction will usually not become evident until after the endotracheal tube has been removed. Strategies to prevent and treat postoperative dyspnea in brachycephalic dogs are outlined on p. 325.

A patient that requires supplemental oxygen during the recovery period can have it administered by one of four routes: facemask, nasal cannula, E-collar, or oxygen cage or tent, all as previously described in this chapter. As a general rule, the flow rate should be at least 100 mL/kg/min. If possible, oxygen being delivered to an awake animal should be humidified (e.g., by directing the flow of oxygen through a bottle of distilled water before delivery to the patient).

### Prolonged Recovery from Anesthesia

Animals experiencing prolonged recovery from anesthesia should be examined by the veterinarian. There are many possible reasons why a patient may be slow to recover, including impaired renal or hepatic function, hypothermia, individual susceptibility to a particular anesthetic, breed variation (particularly sighthounds), or the presence of a disorder such as shock or hemorrhage. Excessive anesthetic depth or prolonged anesthesia may also result in delayed recovery. Use of certain agents (including intramuscular ketamine, or repeated injections of barbiturates) may be associated with prolonged recovery even in healthy animals. In the cat it is known that hypothermia in itself can cause significant delay in recovery even if all other organs are functioning properly.

Recovery may be hastened in several ways (Procedure 12-11, p. 347).

## KEY POINTS

1. Although anesthetic complications are uncommon, the technician must be able to anticipate and respond to emergencies in an efficient and knowledgeable fashion.

2. Human error may result in anesthetic problems. Such errors may include the failure to obtain an adequate history or perform a physical examination, errors related to a lack of familiarity with the anesthetic machine or drugs used, the incorrect administration of drugs, and errors related to fatigue, inattentiveness, or distraction.

3. Examples of equipment failure or operator carelessness include carbon dioxide absorber exhaustion, failure to deliver sufficient oxygen to the patient, misassembly of the anesthetic machine, failure of the vaporizer or pop-off valve, or endotracheal tube problems.

4. Anesthetic agents may cause problems during anesthesia, and the anesthetic protocol must be chosen to reflect the special needs of each patient. The anesthetist must be familiar with the adverse side effects associated with the use of each agent in the anesthetic protocol.

5. Some patients are at increased risk for anesthetic complications because of preexisting factors such as old age, organ failure, recent trauma, or breed-related conformation.

6. Geriatric patients have less reserve than younger patients and have reduced anesthetic requirements. Pediatric patients also require reduced doses of injectable agents and are prone to hypothermia and hypoglycemia.

7. Brachycephalic dogs have anatomic characteristics that make respiration difficult, particularly during the recovery period. Preoxygenation before induction, rapid induction and intubation, and close monitoring during recovery are essential.

8. Thiobarbiturates should be used with extreme care in sighthounds. Alternative agents are preferable in most situations.

9. Obese animals should receive anesthetic doses according to their ideal body weight.

10. Pregnant animals presented for cesarean section are at increased anesthetic risk. Various anesthetic techniques (including epidural anesthesia, balanced anesthesia, and neuroleptanalgesia) are sometimes used as alternatives to inhalation anesthesia in these patients. Almost all anesthetic agents may cause depression of fetal respiration and/or circulation, and the use of reversing agents may be advisable.

11. If possible, patients that have undergone recent trauma should be stabilized and thoroughly evaluated before anesthesia.

12. Animals with cardiovascular or respiratory disease may require special anesthetic techniques such as preoxygenation and manual control of ventilation.

13. Hepatic or renal disease may delay excretion of injectable agents, and prolonged recovery times may be seen.

14. Emergency care is ideally a team effort involving all hospital personnel. It is helpful to have preauthorized emergency protocols and periodic "dress rehearsals."

15. It may be difficult to maintain adequate anesthetic depth in some patients. Incorrect placement of the endotracheal tube, incorrect vaporizer setting, inadequate endotracheal tube size, and many other factors may contribute to this problem.

16. Excessive anesthetic depth may result from excessive administration of anesthetic agents or from preexisting patient problems. It may be necessary to bag the patient with 100% oxygen to achieve a lighter plane of anesthesia.

17. Pale mucous membranes may be the result of anemia, hemorrhage, or poor perfusion. Prolonged capillary refill time suggests that hypotension (or, if severe, shock) is present.

18. Cyanosis is a critical emergency and arises because of insufficient delivery of oxygen to the tissues. It may result from a machine problem, airway or endotracheal tube blockage, or respiratory difficulties resulting from excessive depth, pneumothorax, or respiratory disease. Oxygen delivery to the patient must be reestablished through masking, intubation, or tracheostomy.

19. Abnormalities in cardiac rate and rhythm may result from the administration of anesthetic agents, electrolyte abnormalities, hypercapnia, hypoxia, and many other factors.

20. Respiratory arrest that is accompanied by cyanosis and/or bradycardia is an emergency and must be treated by ventilation with 100% oxygen.

21. Cardiac arrest should be treated according to the principles of ABCD: establish a patent airway, bag the patient with 100% oxygen, initiate internal or external cardiac massage, and administer epinephrine and other drugs. The current trend for an intubated patient is to start with cardiac massage, thus following a CABD approach.

22. Regurgitation and/or vomiting may be dangerous in the anesthetized animal because of the danger of airway obstruction and aspiration pneumonia.

23. Postanesthesia seizures may be treated by eliminating external stimuli and administering diazepam.

24. Dyspnea caused by laryngospasm or brachycephalic airway obstruction may be treated by administration of oxygen by mask, reintubation of the patient, or tracheostomy.

25. Animals experiencing prolonged recovery from anesthesia require close observation and nursing care. An effort should be made to determine the reason for delayed arousal of each patient.

## PROCEDURE 12-1   Responding to an Emergency

1. The technician should take a few seconds to think before doing anything. After consulting with the veterinarian, the technician should mentally list the most important things to be done and undertake them in order of priority.
2. Every veterinary practice should have a well-stocked crash kit for use in emergency situations within the hospital. A list of supplies that may be useful in a crash kit is given in Appendix F.
3. Useful emergency drugs are listed in Tables 12-2 and 12-3. Doses for emergency drugs should be posted or listed on a paper kept in the crash kit. Emergency drugs kept in the crash kit should be periodically checked to ensure that they have not expired. In particular, epinephrine has a short shelf life and should not be used if a brown discoloration is present.
4. Above all, the technician should do no harm. In an emergency it is easy to panic and do things that are not only unnecessary but also potentially harmful to the animal, including performing cardiac compressions on an animal whose heart is still beating. Sometimes the best course of action is to watch, monitor, and wait.
5. After an anesthetic emergency, the technician, veterinarian, and hospital staff should discuss the reasons why the emergency arose and determine what could be done to prevent the same thing from happening again. The adequacy of the resuscitation efforts should be analyzed, and if a problem exists, it should be addressed.

## PROCEDURE 12-2   Treating Excessive Anesthetic Depth

1. After concluding that the anesthetic depth is excessive, the anesthetist should immediately decrease the vaporizer setting (to zero, if necessary) and inform the veterinarian.
2. If the veterinarian decides that the animal's condition has deteriorated so that resuscitation efforts are warranted, the anesthetist should begin to bag the animal with pure oxygen. (This assumes that the patient is intubated and is undergoing gas anesthesia. If an injectable agent has been used, intubation and oxygen delivery by means of an anesthetic machine should be initiated immediately.)
3. To bag the animal, the pop-off valve is closed, the reservoir bag is filled with oxygen, and the bag is gently squeezed until the animal's chest rises slightly.
4. This procedure should be repeated every 5 seconds until the animal shows signs of recovery (such as increased heart rate, stronger pulse, and improved mucous membrane color and refill).
5. The use of intravenous fluids, external heat, and drugs such as doxapram and specific reversing agents (such as yohimbine or naloxone) may also expedite recovery.
6. Occasionally the anesthetist may be unsure of whether a patient's anesthetic depth is excessive. If the veterinarian is not immediately available to advise on the patient's condition, it is safest to assume that the animal's anesthetic depth is too deep and to decrease the vaporizer setting while observing the animal carefully for signs of arousal.

## PROCEDURE 12-3   Treating Pale Mucous Membranes

1. The anesthetist should ascertain the animal's anesthetic depth and monitor vital signs including heart rate, respiration, pulse strength, and capillary refill time.
2. The anesthetist should rule out other possible causes including hypothermia, hypotension, and blood loss.
3. The veterinarian should be consulted because it may be necessary to initiate intravenous fluid therapy or a blood transfusion to stabilize the patient's condition.

## PROCEDURE 12-4   Treating Prolonged Capillary Refill Time

1. The anesthetist who observes a prolonged capillary refill time should immediately check the animal's pulse and blood pressure reading (if available). A mean arterial pressure under 60 mm Hg indicates hypotension and poor perfusion.
2. If blood pressure readings are not available, the anesthetist can roughly estimate the systolic pressure by palpating a peripheral pulse. As a general rule, the absence of a palpable pulse at the metatarsal artery indicates a systolic pressure under 60 mm Hg, and the absence of a palpable pulse at the femoral artery indicates a systolic pressure under 40 mm Hg.
3. If pulse pressure is reduced, the anesthetist should closely observe the animal for other signs of shock, including hypothermia and tachycardia (or bradycardia in later stages of shock). As circulation to the extremities deteriorates, the surface temperature of the ears and paws is reduced. The heart may respond to the fall in blood pressure by increased rate and force of contraction, although this effect may not be present in deep anesthesia.

## PROCEDURE 12-5    Treatment of Shock

1. Intravenous fluids should be administered at a rapid rate. Over the first 15 minutes, 20 mL/kg should be given, and the animal should be observed closely for a response. The maximum fluid administration rate is 90 mL/kg for the first hour in the dog (or 55 mL/kg in the cat). The use of colloid therapy or blood transfusions may be appropriate in some situations.
2. Anesthetic depth should be reduced, if possible, and 100% oxygen should be administered.
3. The patient must be kept warm through the use of supplemental heat in the form of warm towels, circulating warm water heating pads, hot water bottles, or similar devices.
4. Various drugs are recommended for the treatment of shock, including corticosteroids (prednisone sodium succinate, dexamethasone), sodium bicarbonate, and cardiac inotropes such as dopamine, ephedrine, or dobutamine.

## PROCEDURE 12-6    Treating Respiratory Problems

1. The anesthetist must first ensure that oxygen is being delivered to the patient. If the oxygen tank has run out, the patient must be disconnected from the machine until another oxygen source can be secured. If the endotracheal tube is blocked, it must be removed and replaced. Suspected endotracheal tube blockage can be confirmed by disconnecting the endotracheal tube from the Y-piece and feeling for air passage through the tube when the patient breathes or the chest is gently compressed. Capnography, if available, will confirm if blockage has occurred.
2. Once oxygen flow has been established, the vaporizer should be turned off and the animal should be bagged with 100% oxygen. If the anesthetic machine is unavailable, an Ambu bag (see Figure 12-5) can be used to deliver room air to the patient. While initiating bagging, the anesthetist should observe the chest for movement. If the chest does not rise when the animal is bagged, the endotracheal tube or airway may be blocked, and the blockage must be relieved. If the chest does rise when the reservoir bag is squeezed, oxygen is being delivered to the lungs and bagging should be continued until the mucous membrane color improves or pulse oximeter readings rise to 95%. It is best to watch the anterior thorax for chest rise movement in the area of the heart, so as not to be misled by passive movement of the chest because of distention of the stomach by a misplaced endotracheal tube.
3. On rare occasions, dyspnea and cyanosis may be secondary to complete airway obstruction. If intubation is not possible under these circumstances, the veterinarian may elect to perform an emergency tracheostomy, a surgical opening of the trachea to allow the insertion of a breathing tube. Alternatively, a 14-gauge intravenous catheter can be placed through the cricothyroid membrane and into the trachea. The catheter is connected to the barrel of a 3-mL syringe, which is in turn attached to the Y-piece of an anesthetic machine for oxygen delivery.
4. Administration of intravenous fluids or emergency drugs such as doxapram may be helpful in reviving patients experiencing respiratory depression or arrest.
5. It is important that the anesthetist closely observe the patient during resuscitative efforts to ensure that cardiac arrest does not occur. If a pulse or heartbeat cannot be detected, cardiac compressions should be initiated in conjunction with continued bagging.
6. If necessary, supplemental oxygen should be continued into the recovery period, using a mask, oxygen cage, or intranasal insufflation.

## PROCEDURE 12-7    Treating Tachypnea

1. The anesthetist should assess the anesthetic depth and check the $CO_2$ absorber crystals of the capnogram if available to ensure that hypercapnia is not present.
2. If anesthetic depth, body temperature, and vital signs appear to be within acceptable limits, the anesthetist should refrain from changing the vaporizer setting because the condition will usually correct itself within 1 to 2 minutes.
3. If tachypnea arises as a result of surgical stimulation and the perception of pain, intravenous injection of an analgesic such as oxymorphone, hydromorphone, or butorphanol may be helpful.
4. Obese patients are prone to tachypnea, which may result in inefficient ventilation. It may be necessary to assist or control ventilation in these patients.

## PROCEDURE 12-8    Treatment of Cardiac Arrhythmias

1. The anesthetist should rule out inadequate oxygen flow or carbon dioxide accumulation within the circuit.
2. Ventilation should be increased by periodic bagging or use of a ventilator.
3. In some cases, antiarrhythmic drugs such as atropine or lidocaine (without epinephrine) may be administered on the veterinarian's orders.

## PROCEDURE 12-9  Treatment of Respiratory Arrest

1. Inform the veterinarian.
2. If the patient is not intubated, an endotracheal tube should be immediately inserted and the patient connected to an anesthetic machine delivering 100% oxygen.
3. Check the heart rate to ensure that cardiac arrest has not occurred.
4. Turn off the anesthetic vaporizer and nitrous oxide flow.
5. Ensure oxygen flow is adequate by checking the tank pressure gauge and flow meter.
6. Ensure the airway is not obstructed by bagging the patient and observing that the chest rises on "inspiration."
7. Bag with oxygen at a rate of once every 3 to 5 seconds. Continue bagging until vital signs improve (particularly mucous membrane color, heart rate, and pulse oximeter readings).
8. If an intravenous catheter is present, administer IV fluids at a rate suitable for treatment of shock.
9. The veterinarian may advise that doxapram, reversal agents, or other drugs be given.
10. Ensure that the patient is kept warm.

## PROCEDURE 12-10  Defibrillation

1. Cardiac compressions should be carried out for at least 2 minutes before defibrillation and should be continued at all times unless the patient is being actively defibrillated.
2. The defibrillator should be turned on. Many modern defibrillators require use of the defibrillator's ECG component in order to function correctly.
3. An assistant sets the appropriate amount of joules as directed by the veterinarian. Typically the first shock uses the lowest setting for the size of patient.
   External defibrillation: 2 to 5 J/kg.
   Internal defibrillation: 0.2 to 0.5 J/kg
4. If external defibrillation is being used, the paddles are coated with conducting gel. If the thorax is open, sterilized internal paddles should be opened using sterile technique, taken by the person performing internal cardiac massage, then soaked with sterile saline. The assistant will have to connect the internal paddles to the defibrillator.
5. The operator then places the external paddles according to the directions on the paddles (usually on the sternum and the left thorax); internal paddles are placed on either side of the heart.
6. The defibrillator either makes a "ready" sound or shows that it is ready on a light-emitting diode (LED) display.
7. The operator clearly announces the word "Clear!" which warns other personnel that an electrical shock is about to be delivered and that they should stand away from the patient and the table or surface on which the patient is lying.
8. The operator then discharges the paddles by simultaneously depressing the buttons on both handles.
9. Unless there is immediate ROSC, cardiac compressions should continue for 2 minutes while the defibrillator recharges.

## PROCEDURE 12-11  Expediting Recovery from Anesthesia

1. The patient should be placed in a location where frequent observation is possible. If possible, emergency and monitoring equipment and oxygen should be available in the immediate area.
2. It is often helpful to administer intravenous fluids, which hasten renal and hepatic elimination of anesthetics and support circulation. The recommended rate of fluid administration for most intensive care patients is 3 to 5 mL/kg/hr.
3. Good nursing care is important. The patient should be turned frequently and kept warm. If the patient's temperature is less than 37° C, active warming procedures should be instituted, including the use of fan heaters, reflective blankets, circulating warm water pads, heat-producing "oat bags," chemical warmers, Bair huggers, or towels warmed in a dryer.
4. The animal must be periodically monitored for vital signs, reflexes, and urine production (which should be at least 2 mL/kg/hr).
5. Reversal agents and analeptics are used occasionally to hasten anesthetic recovery. However, the anesthetist whose patients consistently demonstrate slow recoveries should not rely on pharmacologic solutions to solve what may be a problem of technique. The anesthetist should reexamine the anesthetic protocol and consult with the veterinarian to determine whether more appropriate agents or means of administration should be used. It is important to ensure that animals are not maintained at excessively deep levels of anesthesia for routine procedures.

## REVIEW QUESTIONS

1. When an animal scheduled for a surgical procedure is brought in by a neighbor who is in a hurry, the best thing to do is:
   a. Instruct the receptionist to have the neighbor sign the consent form
   b. Ask the neighbor to take the animal back home
   c. Ask the neighbor some quick questions about the animal
   d. Have the neighbor sign the consent form and ensure that the owner is called before the procedure is initiated

2. In preparation for an anesthetic procedure, you have drawn up a syringe of barbiturate and an identical syringe of saline. You are then called to the examination room to assist the veterinarian. About 10 minutes later you return to prepare the animal for induction. With the IV catheter in place, you are just about to inject some saline into the animal when you realize that you are not sure if the syringe contains saline. The best thing to do would be to:
   a. Inject a small amount of the solution and see what effect it has
   b. Discard both syringes and start over
   c. Ask the person who was holding the animal which syringe had saline in it
   d. Discard both syringes, label some new syringes, and start over

3. You are about to use the anesthetic machine and notice that although the flow meter is working, the pressure gauge on the oxygen tank reads close to zero. The best thing to do would be to:
   a. Assume that the pressure gauge may be faulty and wait and see if the flow meter stops working
   b. Change the oxygen tank
   c. Call the repair person to have the pressure gauge checked
   d. Use low-flow anesthesia techniques and ignore the pressure gauge reading

4. While monitoring a patient on an anesthetic machine, you realize that the oxygen tank has become empty. The best thing to do would be to:
   a. Disconnect the patient from the circuit, put on a new oxygen tank, and then reconnect the patient to the circuit
   b. Remove the circuit from the patient to allow it to breathe room air for the remainder of the procedure
   c. Resuscitate the patient with an Ambu bag
   d. Switch to an injectable anesthetic

5. If the pop-off valve is inadvertently left shut, it will:
   a. Stop the oxygen flow from entering the circuit
   b. Convert the circuit to low-flow anesthesia
   c. Cause a significant rise of pressure within the circuit
   d. Cause the flutter valves to malfunction

6. You look at the oxygen tank and note that 1000 psi of pressure is left in the tank, but the flow meter now reads zero and you cannot obtain a flow by twisting the knobs. The best thing to do would be to assume:
   a. The oxygen tank pressure gauge is malfunctioning and you need to recheck the flow meter
   b. The oxygen pressure is adequate and the flow meter is simply not registering the flow
   c. The animal is not getting oxygen, and you need to remove the animal from the circuit until a new machine is found or the problem is corrected

7. A geriatric patient is considered to be one that:
   a. Is greater than 10 years old
   b. Is greater than 15 years old
   c. Has reached 50% of its life expectancy
   d. Has reached 75% of its life expectancy

8. Brain damage may occur when there is inadequate oxygenation of the tissues for longer than ___ minutes.
   a. 2
   b. 4
   c. 6
   d. 8
   e. 10

9. When a technician is performing CPR alone, the ratio of cardiac compressions to ventilation should be:
   a. 5:1
   b. 10:1
   c. 5:2
   d. 10:2

10. To ensure that the benefit an animal obtains from CPR is not lost, one should not discontinue cardiac compressions for longer than:
    a. 3 to 5 seconds
    b. 5 to 20 seconds
    c. 20 to 60 seconds
    d. 60 to 90 seconds

11. Respiratory arrest is always fatal.
    True            False

For the following questions, more than one answer may be correct.

12. One may suspect that the endotracheal tube is malfunctioning even if it is in the trachea because:
    a. Compression of the reservoir bag does not result in the raising of the chest
    b. The animal is dyspneic
    c. The animal cannot be kept at an adequate plane of anesthesia
    d. The reservoir bag is not moving or is moving very little

13. One may suspect that the pop-off valve has been closed or that it is malfunctioning if the:
    a. Reservoir bag is distended with air
    b. Patient has difficulty exhaling
    c. Patient wakes up
    d. Flow rate starts to drop

14. Administration of the normal rate of fluids (10 mL/kg/hr) during an anesthetic procedure may result in overhydration in the:
    a. Patient with cardiac disease
    b. Obese patient
    c. Pediatric patient
    d. Brachycephalic patient

15. Brachycephalic dogs may be at increased anesthetic risk because of their:
    a. Physical size
    b. Excess tissue around the oropharynx
    c. Increased vagal tone
    d. Small trachea in comparison with their physical body size
    e. Increased susceptibility to barbiturates

16. To decrease the anesthetic risk associated with a brachycephalic dog, the anesthetist may elect to:
    a. Use atropine as part of the anesthetic protocol
    b. Preoxygenate the animal before giving any anesthetic
    c. Use an injectable anesthetic to hasten induction rather than masking
    d. Ensure intubation is done quickly after induction

17. Animals that undergo cesarean section are at increased risk during anesthesia because of:
    a. Decreased respiratory function
    b. Increased chance of aspiration vomitus
    c. Increased chance of hemorrhage
    d. Increased workload of the heart

18. Anesthetic agents or drugs that one may want to avoid in the animal with cardiovascular disease include:
    a. Halothane
    b. Isoflurane
    c. Xylazine
    d. Opioids

19. An animal that has liver dysfunction may be hypoproteinemic and therefore requires _____ for induction compared with that needed for a normal dog.
    a. More barbiturate
    b. Less barbiturate
    c. The same amount of barbiturate

20. Too light a plane of anesthesia may be the result of:
    a. A flow rate that is too low
    b. An incorrect vaporizer setting
    c. Incorrect placement of the endotracheal tube
    d. Use of an anesthetic with a low MAC

21. Tachypnea may result from:
    a. Increased levels of arterial oxygen
    b. Increased levels of arterial $CO_2$
    c. The use of ketamine
    d. Too light a plane of anesthesia

22. When the blood pressure drops the veterinarian may ask the technician to infuse a colloid. Which of the following is not a colloid?
    a. Hetastarch
    b. Hypertonic saline
    c. Dextran
    d. Plasma

23. Laryngospasm is more common in the dog than in the cat.
    True          False

24. Treatment of bradycardia can always be reversed with an anticholinergic.
    True          False

25. Tachyarrhythmias in the cat are best treated with:
    a. Lidocaine
    b. Saline
    c. Propranolol
    d. Glycopyrrolate

## SELECTED READINGS

Battaglia AM: *Small animal emergency and critical care for veterinary technicians,* ed 2, St Louis, 2007, Elsevier.

Carroll G: *Small animal anesthesia and analgesia,* Ames, Iowa, 2008, Wiley-Blackwell.

Clarke KW, Hall LW: A survey of anaesthesia in small animal practice: AVA/BSAVA report, *J Assoc Vet Anaesth* 17:4-10, 1990.

Dodman NH, Lamb LA: Survey of small animal anesthetic practice in Vermont, *J Am Anim Hosp Assoc* 28:439-445, 1992.

Dyson DH, Mathews K: Recommendations for intensive care management in small animals following anaesthesia, *VCOT* 5:66-70, 1992.

Dyson DH, Maxie MG: Morbidity and mortality associated with anesthetic management in small animal veterinary practice in Ontario, *J Am Anim Hosp Assoc* 34(4):325-335, 1998.

Gaynor JS, Dunlop CI, Wagner AE, et al: Complications and mortality associated with anesthesia in dogs and cats, *J Am Anim Hosp Assoc* 35(1):13-17, 1999.

Harvey RC, Paddleford RR: Management of anesthetic emergencies and complications, *Vet Tech* 12(3):237-242, 1991.

Haskins SC: *Opinions in small animal anesthesia, Vet Clin North Am (Small Anim Pract) 22(2),* Philadelphia, 1992, Saunders.

Holland M: Anesthesia for feline cesarean section, *Vet Tech* 12(5): 397-402, 1991.

Mathews K: *Veterinary emergency and critical care manual,* New York, 1996, Lifelearn.

Muir WW III: Anesthetic emergencies and disaster prevention. In Eighth International Veterinary Emergency and Critical Care Symposium, San Antonio, 2002, pp. 40-45.

Paddleford RR: *Manual of small animal anesthesia,* ed 2, St Louis, 1999, Elsevier.

Sawyer DC: Anesthesia for problem and high-risk patients, *Vet Tech* 15(2):61-69, 1994.

Seymour C, Duke-Novakovski T: BSAVA Manual of Canine and Feline Anaesthesia and Analgesia, *Br Small Anim Vet Assoc* , 2007.

Wittnich C, Belanger MP, Salerno TA, et al: Canine cardiopulmonary resuscitation: external versus internal cardiac massage, *Compendium* 13(1):50-56, 1991.

Welsh E: *Anaesthesia for veterinary nurses,* Oxford, UK, 2003, Blackwell.

# Workplace Safety
*Diane McKelvey*

**13**

## KEY TERMS

Activated charcoal
  cartridge
National Institute for
  Occupational Safety
  and Health (NIOSH)
Occupational Safety
  and Health Adminis-
  tration (OSHA)
Scavenging system
Waste anesthetic gas

## OUTLINE

Hazards of Waste Anesthetic Gas, 351
  *Short-Term Effects, 352*
  *Long-Term Effects, 352*
  *Assessment of Risk, 353*
  *Reducing Exposure to Waste Anesthetic*
    *Gas, 356*
  *Monitoring Waste Gas Levels, 359*

Safe Handling of Compressed Gases, 359
  *Fire Safety Precautions, 359*
  *Use and Storage of Compressed Gas*
    *Cylinders, 359*
Accidental Exposure to Injectable
  Agents, 360

## LEARNING OBJECTIVES

*After completion of this chapter, the reader will be able to:*
- Describe both the short-term and long-term effects of waste anesthetic gas on persons working in health care environments.
- Recognize ways in which the release of waste anesthetic gases may be minimized.
- Describe proper procedures for handling and transporting compressed gas cylinders.
- Outline the precautions necessary for handling potentially hazardous injectable agents.

Veterinary technicians may participate in the anesthetic management of several thousand animals during the course of their careers. It is therefore essential that the technician be familiar with the human safety considerations involved in veterinary anesthesia. These can be divided into three categories: (1) hazards of waste anesthetic gas, (2) safety considerations for handling compressed gas cylinders, and (3) hazards associated with potent injectable agents.

This chapter outlines the precautions that the anesthetist can take to reduce, as much as possible, the health risks of working with anesthetic equipment, injectable drugs, and compressed gases.

## HAZARDS OF WASTE ANESTHETIC GAS

Concerns have been raised regarding the possible adverse effects resulting from exposure of hospital personnel to waste anesthetic gas and vapors. The term **waste anesthetic gas** refers to nitrous oxide, halothane, isoflurane, and other anesthetic vapors that are breathed out by the patient or that escape from the anesthetic machine. These vapors are breathed inadvertently by all personnel working in areas where animals are anesthetized or are recovering from inhalation anesthesia. Significant exposure to anesthetic vapors can also occur when emptying or filling anesthetic vaporizers. In addition, short-term exposure to high levels of anesthetic vapors can occur because of an accidental spill of liquid anesthetic.

Waste gas concentrations are usually expressed in parts per million (abbreviated ppm). If the concentration of halothane in room air is 33 ppm, this means that out of every 1 million molecules of air, 33 are halothane. (The rest are chiefly nitrogen, oxygen, and carbon dioxide.) Although at first glance 33 ppm appears to be a small amount, this is the level at which the average person can smell the odor of halothane in room air. It is also more than 15 times the recommended maximum concentration that should be present in a veterinary hospital.

TECHNICIAN NOTE The concentration of waste anesthetic gas that is hazardous to humans is surprisingly difficult to determine with exactness.

The concentration of waste anesthetic gas that is hazardous to humans is surprisingly difficult to determine with exactness.

Since the first study of waste anesthetic gas was published in 1967, many investigators have investigated the toxic effects of isoflurane, halothane, methoxyflurane, nitrous oxide, and other anesthetic agents on operating room personnel. Although some of the evidence is contradictory, it is suspected that exposure to high levels of waste anesthetic gas is associated with a higher than normal incidence of some health problems. The suspected health hazards can be divided into two categories: (1) short-term problems that occur during or immediately after exposure to these agents and (2) long-term problems that may become evident days, weeks, or years after exposure.

## Short-Term Effects

The short-term problems associated with breathing waste gas appear to arise from a direct effect of anesthetic molecules on brain neurons. Persons working in environments with a high level of waste gas have reported symptoms such as fatigue, headache, drowsiness, nausea, depression, and irritability. Although these symptoms usually resolve spontaneously when the affected person leaves the area, the frequent occurrence of these symptoms may indicate that excessive levels of waste gas are present and that a potential for long-term toxicity exists.

## Long-Term Effects

Long-term inhalation of air polluted with waste gas may be associated with serious health problems, including reproductive disorders, liver and kidney damage, bone marrow abnormalities, and chronic nervous system dysfunction. Although current evidence suggests that the risk of these disorders is not high in normal veterinary practice settings, every person working in an environment in which waste gas is present should be informed of the potential for adverse health effects.

The mechanism of long-term anesthetic gas toxicity is not fully understood but is thought to be the result of toxic metabolites produced by the breakdown of anesthetic gases within the liver and their subsequent excretion by the kidneys. These metabolites include inorganic fluoride or bromide ions, oxalic acid, and free radicals, all of which are known to have harmful effects on animal tissues. It is widely accepted that anesthetic agents that are retained by the body and metabolized are likely to have greater long-term toxicity than those that are quickly eliminated through the lungs. For this reason, isoflurane is thought to be the least toxic inhalation agent in common

use (0.2% of the amount inhaled is retained and metabolized), followed by sevoflurane (approximately 3% is retained and metabolized). In contrast, approximately 15% to 20% of the halothane and 40% to 50% of the methoxyflurane administered to a patient or inhaled by the anesthetist are retained within the body fat, to be metabolized in the liver and excreted through the kidneys over the next few hours to days. Metabolites of halothane have been recovered from the urine of human patients as long as 20 days after anesthesia. Human patients who inhale 50% nitrous oxide for 1 hour have been shown to have more than 100 ppm nitrous oxide in their expired breath for the next 3 hours. In the same way, the anesthetist who inhales waste anesthetic gas may retain the gas or its metabolites for a considerable period. For example, anesthetists may show traces of halothane in their breath 64 hours after administering this gas to a patient.

TECHNICIAN NOTE It is widely accepted that anesthetic agents that are retained by the body and metabolized are likely to have greater long-term toxicity than those that are quickly eliminated through the lungs. For this reason, isoflurane is thought to be the least toxic inhalation agent in common use, followed by sevoflurane.

Although it is generally accepted that exposure to isoflurane or sevoflurane is associated with fewer health risks than exposure to other halogenated anesthetics, safety concerns (including **National Institute for Occupational Safety and Health [NIOSH]** recommendations and **Occupational Safety and Health Administration [OSHA]** regulations) apply to all anesthetics.

### Effects on Reproduction

There is some evidence that high concentrations of waste anesthetic gas can adversely affect the reproductive system. In a comprehensive survey of nurse and physician anesthetists, the American Society of Anesthesiologists found that the risk of spontaneous abortion in this group was 1.3 to 2 times that of the normal population. Another study showed that the frequency of spontaneous abortion among working hospital anesthetists (18.2%) was higher than that observed among nonworking anesthetists (13.7%) and a control group (14.7%). The same study showed that 12% of the working anesthetists interviewed were infertile, compared with 6% of the control group. A more recent study (Shirangi and colleagues, 2008) showed a twofold increase in the risk of spontaneous abortion in women exposed to *unscavenged* waste gas for 1 or more hours per week. In contrast, a very large study of 11,000 operating room personnel showed no correlation between hours worked in the operating room and miscarriage (Spence and colleagues, 1977). Studies of veterinary personnel (Shuhaiber and co-workers, 1999; Johnson and co-workers, 1987; and Schenker and co-workers, 1990) made similar findings.

Some studies have suggested a link between exposure to anesthetic gases and an increased risk of congenital abnormalities in the children of pregnant operating room personnel. One study reported a 16% incidence of congenital abnormalities in children of practicing nurse-anesthetists, compared with a 6% incidence in a control group. Reported problems included microcephaly, mental retardation, low birth weight, and heart defects. Other studies have failed to show a statistically significant correlation between waste gas exposure and an increased incidence of congenital abnormalities, and the evidence linking waste gas exposure and congenital anomalies is generally weaker than that linking waste gas exposure to spontaneous abortion. One report (Hoerauf and colleagues, 1999) suggests that exposure to even trace levels of waste anesthetic gas could cause genetic damage, as indicated by an increased incidence of sister chromatid exchanges. However, the study group was small, and other recent studies have so far failed to confirm these findings.

Interpreting or comparing the results obtained by these and other studies is difficult because there are wide variations in the types of anesthetics used, the amount of waste gas exposure, and the availability of control measures (such as scavengers). In most cases, operating room personnel were exposed to several agents simultaneously, and it is difficult to determine which agent or combination of agents was responsible for the adverse effects. It appears, however, that nitrous oxide is a potential reproductive hazard, because rats with prolonged exposure to high levels of nitrous oxide had abnormalities in sperm morphology, reduced ovulation, fetal resorption, and abnormal fetal development.

## Oncogenic Effects

Given that waste anesthetic gases may exert their adverse reproductive effects by altering DNA, investigators have attempted to determine whether these agents have the potential to cause other DNA-related changes, such as neoplasia. Several studies undertaken in the 1970s appeared to suggest that operating room personnel have an increased incidence of some types of cancer. These studies, however, have been criticized for inappropriate data collection and statistical analysis, and it is now generally thought that none of the commonly used inhalant anesthetic agents (isoflurane, halothane, sevoflurane) is carcinogenic at the levels found in veterinary hospitals.

> TECHNICIAN NOTE  It is now generally thought that none of the commonly used inhalant anesthetic agents (isoflurane, halothane, sevoflurane) is carcinogenic at the levels found in veterinary hospitals.

## Effects on the Liver

Several studies have investigated the incidence of liver disorders in personnel exposed to waste anesthetic gas. Halothane, in particular, is recognized as being potentially hepatotoxic. Metabolism of halothane in certain rare anesthetized individuals produces toxic by-products that may result in massive hepatic necrosis, termed *halothane hepatitis*.

The possible adverse effects of waste anesthetic gas on the liver were suggested by a study showing that the risk of liver disease in hospital operating room personnel is 1.5 times that of the general population. However, it is difficult to say with certainty whether the increased incidence of liver disease is associated with exposure to halothane or other waste anesthetic gas or the result of other occupational hazards, such as viral hepatitis.

## Effects on the Kidney

It is well established that methoxyflurane has the potential to cause renal toxicity in human beings anesthetized with this agent, but the risk to operating room personnel has been more difficult to assess. Studies have indicated that there is a 1.2- to 1.4-fold increase in renal disease in female operating room personnel and a 1.2- to 1.7-fold increase in renal disease in female dental assistants compared with the general population. It has not been determined whether this increase is the result of the effect of methoxyflurane, nitrous oxide, other anesthetic agents, or other occupational factors working alone or in combination.

## Neurologic Effects

Because the mechanism of action of anesthetic agents involves their effect on neurons, various studies have investigated the effect of waste anesthetic gas on the central nervous system. It has been suggested that exposure to high levels of anesthetics produces a decline in performance of motor skills and short-term memory. However, the threshold at which they begin to affect performance has not been established.

Some studies have indicated that exposure to even low concentrations of anesthetic gas mixtures (e.g., nitrous oxide 500 ppm and halothane 15 ppm for a period of 4 hours) results in decreased cognitive and motor skills. Chronic exposure to nitrous oxide has been associated with increased risk of neurologic disease: a study of female dental assistants exposed to high levels of nitrous oxide showed them to have a 1.7- to 2.8-fold increase in the incidence of neurologic disease compared with the normal population. Dentists and dental assistants exposed to high levels of waste nitrous oxide reported muscle weakness, tingling sensations, and numbness.

## Hematologic Effects

In one study, exposure to high levels of waste nitrous oxide has been associated with bone marrow abnormalities in dentists who administer this gas.

## Assessment of Risk

Despite the alarming list of potential health hazards, the average veterinary technician working in a veterinary clinic is not necessarily at high risk. It is difficult to determine a clear-cut assessment of risk for several reasons, including the following:

- Caution must be used in interpreting the epidemiologic evidence provided by these studies. The evidence produced by various studies (or within one study) is sometimes contradictory. For example, some studies have failed to show any association between the incidence of spontaneous abortion or congenital abnormalities and a history of exposure to waste gas, whereas other studies suggest the opposite. This discrepancy may arise from inconsistencies in the way in which the studies were conducted. Studies vary widely in the type of anesthetics to which the personnel are exposed, the duration and level of waste gas exposure, and the control measures available (such as a **scavenging system**). Most anesthetists surveyed had been exposed to several different agents, and the investigators were unable to determine which agent(s) were responsible for the observed adverse health effects.
- Although many epidemiologic studies indicate an increased incidence of health problems in persons working in an environment where exposure to waste gas occurs, it does not necessarily follow that the anesthetic gases themselves are the causative agents. Other chemicals such as ethylene oxide, or exposure to x-radiation, or other factors present in the operating room or dentist's office may contribute to increased incidence of health disorders.
- Many of the early studies have been faulted for low response rates, lack of verification of reported outcomes, and the possibility of bias. Some commentators have observed that the increased risks observed are small and could be a result of uncontrolled variables.
- Most studies of the adverse effects of waste anesthetic gases do not measure the level of waste gas present in the working environment. Epidemiologic studies do not give information about the use of scavengers and procedures that reduce waste gas pollution. Without this information, interpretation of the findings of any study is difficult.

> **TECHNICIAN NOTE**  The American Society of Anesthesiologists Task Force on Trace Anesthetic Gases (1999) suggests that although adverse health effects are associated with chronic exposure to high levels of waste anesthetic gas, studies have failed to demonstrate an association between the low levels of waste anesthetic gas normally found in scavenged hospitals and adverse effects on hospital employees.

The American Society of Anesthesiologists Task Force on Trace Anesthetic Gases (1999) suggests that although adverse health effects are associated with chronic exposure

to high levels of waste anesthetic gas, studies have failed to demonstrate an association between the low levels of waste anesthetic gas normally found in scavenged hospitals and adverse effects on hospital employees. The Task Force concluded that even at the maximum allowable dose of isoflurane, halothane, or nitrous oxide, there was no evidence of significant damage to the gonads, liver, kidney, or other organs, even in long-term studies. No data suggest that waste anesthetic gases are a danger to hospital employees (including pregnant women) working in an effectively scavenged environment.

> **TECHNICIAN NOTE**  After reviewing the available literature, NIOSH recommended that the concentration of any volatile gas anesthetic (including halothane, methoxyflurane, and isoflurane) not exceed 2 ppm when used alone and not exceed 0.5 ppm when used with nitrous oxide. It is also suggested the nitrous oxide concentration not exceed 25 ppm.

Most authorities and regulatory agencies agree that exposure to high levels of waste anesthetic gas should be avoided and that controls should be introduced to reduce exposure. After reviewing the available literature, NIOSH recommended that the concentration of any volatile gas anesthetic (including halothane, methoxyflurane, and isoflurane) not exceed 2 ppm when used alone and not exceed 0.5 ppm when used with nitrous oxide. It is also suggested the nitrous oxide concentration not exceed 25 ppm. These levels were chosen because they were thought to be the lowest levels realistically achievable given current technology. The British Government Health Service Advisory Committee (1991) recommends a maximum of 100 ppm nitrous oxide, 50 ppm isoflurane, and 10 ppm halothane (average reading over an 8-hour period).

## Measurement of Waste Gas Levels

Surveys of human and veterinary hospitals reveal a wide variation in the levels of waste anesthetic gas present in different locations within the clinic (Tables 13-1 and 13-2). The halothane concentration in the air of unscavenged surgery suites in human hospitals has been reported to be as high as 85 ppm, and concentrations of nitrous oxide have been measured as high as 7000 ppm. Veterinary hospitals using scavengers usually have isoflurane or halothane levels of 1 to 20 ppm and nitrous oxide levels of 50 to 200 ppm. Higher levels may be present if scavengers are not in use. As expected, air samples taken from surgery suites, surgical preparation rooms, and anesthetic recovery rooms are more likely to contain waste gas than samples taken elsewhere in the clinic. During the anesthetic period itself, the level of waste gas is highest immediately adjacent to the anesthetic machine, but the actual level varies according to the following factors.

| TABLE 13-1 | Waste Anesthetic Gas (Halothane) Concentrations in Various Locations within the Veterinary Hospital (Semiclosed Circuit, 1 L/Min Oxygen Flow) |
|---|---|
| **Sampling Site** | **Level of Contamination (ppm)** |
| Personnel breathing zone | |
|   With scavenging | 1.45 |
|   No scavenging | 2 |
| Nose and mouth of patient just removed from anesthetic chamber | 10 |
| Air around unscavenged anesthetic chamber | 10 |
| Nose and mouth of anesthetized patient | |
|   Intubated, cuff inflated | 3.25 |
|   Intubated, cuff not inflated | 6.10 |
| Air outside recovery cage door | 1.07 |
| Nose of patient in recovery cage | 5.43 |

Modified from Short CE, Harvey RC: Anesthetic waste gases in veterinary medicine, *Cornell Vet* 73:363, 1983.

## Duration of Anesthesia

The longer the anesthetic machine is in use, the higher the waste gas concentration in the room air. For example, if a surgery room is used for several procedures in one morning, the waste gas levels may slowly increase, reaching a peak at the end of the final surgery.

## Flow Rate of Carrier Gas

Higher flow rates may lead to more waste gas pollution. For example, if the oxygen flow rate is 2 L/min, the room will contain more waste gas than if the flow rate were 500 mL/minute, unless a very effective gas scavenger is in use.

## Anesthetic Machine Maintenance

Leak testing and periodic maintenance of the anesthetic machine are important in reducing the escape of anesthetic gas from the machine, which contributes to room air pollution.

## Use of an Effective Scavenging System

When a circle system (rebreathing system) with no scavenging system is used, anesthetic gas mixed with oxygen is vented through an open pop-off valve at a rate approximately equal to the oxygen flow rate (usually 500 mL to 3 L per minute). If a non-rebreathing system such as a Bain circuit is in use, the gas exits through the relief valve or reservoir bag outlet. Either way, in the absence of a scavenging system, all of the waste gas enters the room air.

## Anesthetic Techniques Used

Mask inductions and anesthetic chambers may release high levels of waste gas, as a considerable quantity of air can leak around the mask or be released when an anesthetic chamber is opened.

## Room Ventilation

Room ventilation is the only means of eliminating waste gases that leak from anesthetic machines or are exhaled around an endotracheal tube or mask (scavengers are

| TABLE 13-2 | Sources of Anesthetic Gas Contamination |
|---|---|
| **Technique or Situation** | **Level of Contamination (ppm)** |
| Room air when filling vaporizer | 10 |
| Reservoir bag emptied into room air | 2.5->10 |
| Room air after spill of agent | 10 |
| Hands of personnel filling vaporizer | 2.5->10 |
| Hands after washing | 0 |
| Clothing of personnel filling vaporizer | 5.0-8.75 |
| Residues in unwashed rubber components | 1.8->10 |

Modified from Short CE, Harvey RC: Anesthetic waste gases in veterinary medicine, *Cornell Vet* 73:363, 1983.

unable to retrieve these gases once they enter the air). Rooms with a ceiling fan, wall fan, or other ventilating device generally have lower levels of waste gas. It is advised that all rooms in which anesthetic gases are released have at least 15 air changes per hour (20 air changes is the preferred number). Open windows and doors also reduce waste gas levels in surgery rooms, although this may not be consistent with principles of hospital design and sterile technique.

> *TECHNICIAN NOTE* It is advised that all rooms in which anesthetic gases are released have at least 15 air changes per hour. A rate of 20 air changes per hour is preferred.

## Anesthetic Spills

The highest levels of waste gas contamination are associated with spills of anesthetic liquids. Liquid anesthetic rapidly evaporates when it is poured or spilled, and this produces a very large amount of concentrated anesthetic vapor that rapidly mixes with room air. Accidental spillage of only 1 mL of liquid halothane, for example, will evaporate to form 200 mL of vapor, with a concentration of 1,000,000 ppm. Liquid anesthetic spilled on the skin can also be absorbed into the circulation.

## Reducing Exposure to Waste Anesthetic Gas

Given the potential health hazards associated with exposure to high levels of waste anesthetic gas, it is in the technician's best interest to minimize exposure as much as possible. The American College of Veterinary Anesthesiologists recommends that any veterinary facility using inhalant anesthetics should institute and maintain a control program for waste anesthetic gases.

> *TECHNICIAN NOTE* If proper equipment, techniques, and procedures are used, it is possible to reduce waste gas exposure to a level well below the NIOSH standards. This can be achieved through several means, including using a gas scavenging system, testing equipment for leaks, and using techniques and procedures that minimize exposure to waste gas.

If proper equipment, techniques, and procedures are used, it is possible to reduce waste gas exposure to a level well below the NIOSH standards. This can be achieved through several means, including using a gas scavenging system, testing equipment for leaks, and using techniques and procedures that minimize exposure to waste gas.

## Use of a Scavenging System

A scavenger consists of tubing attached to the anesthetic machine pop-off valve (or in the case of a non-rebreathing system, to the outlet port or tail of the reservoir bag). The function of a scavenger is to collect waste gas from the machine and conduct it to a disposal point outside the building. The installation and consistent use of an effective gas scavenging system are the most important steps in reducing waste gas exposure. A 1982 survey of veterinary hospitals showed that scavenging reduced waste halothane concentrations in the hospitals surveyed by 64% to 94%.

From the regulatory perspective, OSHA's Hazard Chemical Standard (1910.1200) requires the employer to install adequate engineering controls to ensure that occupational exposure to any chemical never exceeds the permissible exposure limit. In the case of waste anesthetic gas, this is difficult or impossible to achieve in a veterinary clinic unless a waste anesthetic gas scavenger or activated charcoal canister is used on every anesthetic machine. Scavenging should include the exhaust not only from the anesthetic machine but also from ancillary equipment including non-rebreathing systems such as the Bain

circuit or Ayre's T-piece, ventilators, anesthetic chambers, and capnometers.

Ideally, scavenging systems should be professionally installed when the veterinary clinic is built. However, it is not difficult to assemble and install an effective scavenging system in an established veterinary hospital. Scavenger parts may be purchased or can be readily assembled with simple materials. The hose or tubing of the scavenger may be constructed from plastic tubing, polyvinyl chloride (PVC) pipe, or other gas-impermeable material. Most modern anesthetic machines have fittings that allow easy connection to a scavenging system. Older machines can be retrofitted with adapters that can be connected to a scavenger hose. It is important to choose the type of pop-off connection that matches the type of scavenging system used (high vacuum, low vacuum, or passive). The international standard for scavenger system attachments for anesthetic machines is 30 mm.

Scavenging systems may be passive or active (Figures 13-1 and 13-2). An active system uses suction created by a vacuum pump or fan to draw gas into the scavenger, whereas a passive system uses the positive pressure of the gas in the anesthetic machine to push gas into the scavenger. The most commonly used type of passive system discharges waste gas to the outdoors through a hole in the wall. This system is best suited for rooms adjacent to the exterior of the building and is ineffective for interior rooms where the distance to the outlet is more than 20 feet (7 m).

> *TECHNICIAN NOTE* A passive scavenging system is best suited for rooms adjacent to the exterior of the building and is ineffective for interior rooms where the distance to the outlet is more than 20 feet (7 m).

Although both active and passive scavenging systems appear to be effective when correctly assembled and operated, the most efficient system appears to be an active one with a dedicated vacuum pump. However, active scavenging systems are more costly to install than passive systems, they require more maintenance, and the operator must remember to turn on the system each day.

Once the waste gas has been collected by an active or passive system, it must be expelled outside of the building, away from doors, windows, and air intakes. Waste gas collected in the tubing should be totally confined within the scavenger hose from the pop-off valve to the point of discharge and must not be recirculated into the building air. Scavenger hoses that discharge gas on the floor of the surgery room or into an attic or a basement, or that conduct the waste gas into a recirculating central vacuum system or recirculating ventilation exhaust, merely contaminate all building rooms with the waste gas.

Normally, use of a scavenging system with an anesthetic machine does not alter the operation of the machine. The anesthetist should, however, be aware of two potential

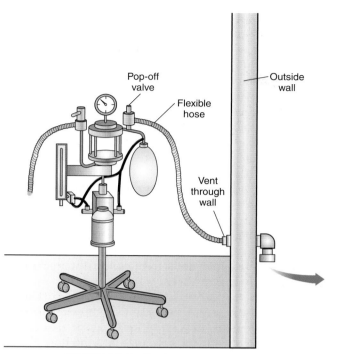

**FIGURE 13-1** Passive scavenging system.

difficulties that can occur when a scavenging system is present:

1. When an active scavenging system is used, the anesthetist should prevent the negative pressure (vacuum) from the scavenger from being excessively applied to the breathing circuit. If this is allowed to occur, the reservoir bag will collapse. Many anesthetic machines are equipped with a negative pressure relief valve, adjacent to the pop-off valve, which opens automatically if negative pressure is detected in the circuit. The open valve admits room air to the circuit, thereby ensuring that a vacuum does not develop. When a machine that is not equipped with a negative pressure relief valve is used, the anesthetist should ensure that the reservoir bag is at least partially inflated with air or oxygen at all times.

2. If either a passive or active scavenging system is in use, the anesthetist must be aware that an obstruction may occur and block waste gas entry into the system. If this happens, gas will accumulate within the anesthetic circuit. This situation is analogous to operating a machine with a closed pop-off valve and may result in excessive pressure developing within the circuit and the patient's lungs. To avoid this, many machines have scavenger interfaces that are equipped with a

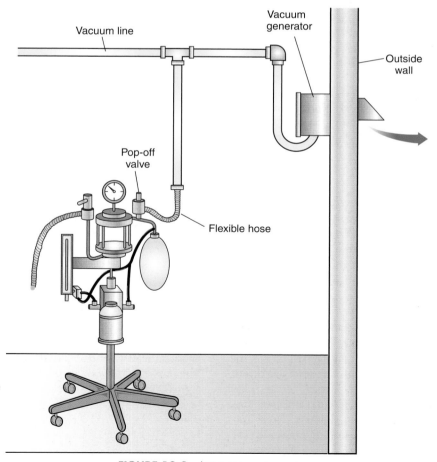

**FIGURE 13-2** Active scavenging system.

positive pressure relief valve that opens automatically if excessive pressure builds up within the circuit.

It is sometimes impractical to use a scavenger when it is in a specialized room such as the x-ray room or when a mobile anesthetic machine is used. In these situations, either anesthesia can be maintained with an injectable agent, or an anesthetic machine with an **activated charcoal cartridge** can be used (e.g., F/Air canister, AM Bickford, Inc). To effectively absorb anesthetic vapors, however, these cartridges must be replaced after 12 hours of use or after a weight gain of 50 g. Additional drawbacks of these units are their inability to absorb nitrous oxide and their relative inefficiency at flow rates greater than 2 L/min.

> *TECHNICIAN NOTE*   To effectively absorb anesthetic vapors, activated charcoal cartridges must be replaced after 12 hours of use or after a weight gain of 50 g. Additional drawbacks of these units are their inability to absorb nitrous oxide and their relative inefficiency at flow rates greater than 2 L/min.

For additional protection, masks with activated charcoal filters can be worn by personnel who are at special risk (such as pregnant workers). Like the activated charcoal canister for anesthetic machines, these are not effective in filtering out nitrous oxide vapors; however, organic vapor cartridges effectively absorb isoflurane, sevoflurane, halothane, and other anesthetic gases and vapors. Masks with cartridges designed for particulate matter do not absorb anesthetic vapors and should not be used.

> *TECHNICIAN NOTE*   Gas leaks from anesthetic machines are a significant source of operating room pollution and are not reduced by a scavenging system.

## Equipment Leak Testing

Although the installation of a scavenging device is the most important step in reducing anesthetic gas pollution, there are many other procedures and techniques that significantly reduce the anesthetist's risk of exposure. One of these is leak testing of anesthetic machines. Gas leaks from anesthetic machines are a significant source of operating room pollution and are not reduced by a scavenging system. A 1988 study of veterinary hospitals showed that 55% of the anesthetic machines tested had significant leaks. Leakage may occur from any part of the machine in which nitrous oxide or gas anesthetic is present.

The most common problems that can result in waste gas leakage are the following:

- The connections for nitrous oxide gas lines are not tightly secured.
- Rings, washers, and other seals joining nitrous oxide gas tanks to the machine hanger yokes are missing, worn, or out of position.
- The covering over a unidirectional valve is not tightly closed.
- The carbon dioxide absorber canister is not securely sealed. Leaks are often caused by improper positioning of the canister or by the presence of absorbent granules on the seals around the canister.
- The connection between the pop-off valve and scavenger is not airtight.
- Breathing hoses, the reservoir bag, or the endotracheal tube have holes or are not securely connected to the machine.
- The vaporizer cap was not replaced after the vaporizer was last filled.

In some cases the presence of a leak is obvious—there may be an audible hiss, the odor of anesthetic, or a jet of air coming out of the reservoir bag or hose. However, small leaks are often undetected unless the anesthetist regularly performs a leak test.

Two types of leak tests are commonly done in veterinary clinics: high-pressure tests and low-pressure tests.

1. High-pressure tests check for high-pressure leaks arising between the gas tanks and the flow meter, where the pressure is 50 pounds per square inch (psi) or greater. These leaks release only pure oxygen or nitrous oxide, without volatile anesthetic.
2. Low-pressure tests check for anesthetic gases that escape from the anesthetic machine itself, where the pressure of gas within the machine is approximately 15 psi. Low-pressure leaks may arise in any part of the anesthetic machine or breathing circuit that does not fit together tightly or that develops a hole. Low-pressure leaks release waste anesthetic gas as well as oxygen (and nitrous oxide, if in use).

The type of leak test used on an anesthetic machine depends on the type of carrier gas used: if both nitrous oxide and oxygen are used, both a high-pressure and a low-pressure test should be done. If oxygen alone (without nitrous oxide) is used, it is necessary to do only a low-pressure test. Release of oxygen into the room through a high-pressure leak does not affect the air quality, although it wastes oxygen and may empty the tank prematurely.

Low-pressure tests should be performed before use of the machine each day. High-pressure tests on nitrous oxide tanks should be performed once weekly and whenever the nitrous oxide tank is changed. Details of high- and low-pressure tests are given in Procedure 13-1, p. 361.

> *TECHNICIAN NOTE*   The type of leak test used on an anesthetic machine depends on the type of carrier gas used: if both nitrous oxide and oxygen are used, both a high-pressure and a low-pressure test should be done. If oxygen alone (without nitrous oxide) is used, it is necessary to do only a low-pressure test. Low-pressure tests should be performed before use of the machine each day. High-pressure tests on nitrous oxide tanks should be performed once weekly and whenever the nitrous oxide tank is changed.

For both non-rebreathing and rebreathing systems, the location of leaks may be determined by listening for the hiss of escaping air or by using a detergent solution as described in Procedure 13-1. It is important to never try to stop the flow of gas from a high-pressure leak by putting a hand over the leaking part. Once the source of a leak has been identified, it can often be fixed by tightening a connection or replacing a part. If the leak cannot be fixed, the machine should not be used until it is serviced by qualified personnel. Frequent, routine servicing of the anesthetic machine and breathing circuit by qualified personnel is helpful in detecting equipment problems that can lead to leaks but is not an adequate substitute for daily leak testing of the machine by the anesthetist.

## Anesthetic Techniques and Procedures

The anesthetist, by his or her choice of anesthetic techniques, has considerable control over the amount of waste gas released into the room air. One survey of human hospitals found that faulty work practices accounted for 94% to 99% of waste anesthetic gas released in scavenged operating rooms.

The steps in Procedure 13-2, p. 362, are recommended to minimize waste gas release.

## Monitoring Waste Gas Levels

It is advisable to periodically monitor waste anesthetic gas levels to ensure that the NIOSH-recommended levels are not exceeded. Monitoring waste gas levels is particularly important if a hospital employee becomes pregnant and is still working around anesthetized animals. Waste gas monitoring is also advisable if hospital employees frequently detect the odor of anesthetic gas, or if there are special concerns about waste gas levels (e.g., if the clinic is using induction chambers). If professional monitoring is required, an accredited industrial hygiene laboratory can be contacted for assistance. (Industrial hygienists are found in the yellow pages of the telephone directory under "occupational safety.") An occupational hygienist will usually visit the hospital to evaluate ventilation and scavenging techniques and to interview the anesthetist regarding procedures used to minimize waste gas release. Air samples should be collected from all areas in which anesthetics are used, and the level of waste gas in the collected air should be determined with an infrared spectrometer. The cost of such a visit ranges from $250 to $700.

Professional monitoring services are not always necessary. Clinic employees can inexpensively monitor waste gas levels using detector tubes or badges. Badges may detect only one chemical, such as halothane, isoflurane, or nitrous oxide, or may be sensitive to all halogenated anesthetics. The badges (called *passive dosimeters*) are uncapped at the beginning of the exposure period, then worn by personnel in the surgical preparation room, operating room, or recovery area for a timed period when anesthetic gases are being used (usually an exposure time of 2 to 8 hours is chosen). Alternatively, the badge may be placed in a room for area monitoring. After exposure, the badge is recapped and returned to the supplier (usually an industrial health and safety supply house or a company specializing in OSHA compliance) for analysis. Results are given as a time-weighted average in parts per million. Cost, including analysis, is approximately $50 to $70 per badge.*

> **TECHNICIAN NOTE**  It is advisable to periodically monitor waste anesthetic gas levels to ensure that the NIOSH-recommended levels are not exceeded, especially if a hospital employee becomes pregnant and is still working around anesthetized animals. Waste gas monitoring is also advisable if hospital employees frequently detect the odor of anesthetic gas or if there are special concerns about waste gas levels (e.g., if the clinic is using induction chambers).

## SAFE HANDLING OF COMPRESSED GASES

### Fire Safety Precautions

There is a potential for fire in any room where oxygen or nitrous oxide is used. Oxygen and nitrous oxide are not flammable; however, both support combustion and cause fuels to burn more readily. Even static electricity can cause fires in areas in which oxygen and flammable materials are used together. (This is one of the reasons why ether, which is extremely flammable, is no longer used in anesthesia.) It is recommended that no flames or sources of ignition (e.g., matches, lighters, or Bunsen burners) be present in any room in which oxygen or nitrous oxide cylinders are stored or used. For obvious reasons, smoking also must be prohibited in all rooms in which oxygen is stored or used.

### Use and Storage of Compressed Gas Cylinders

Tanks of compressed gas can be viewed as a storehouse of tremendous amounts of energy, waiting for release. If gas is released too quickly, nearby personnel may be injured. Persons connecting compressed gas cylinders to an anesthetic machine or gas piping system should wear impact-resistant goggles to protect their eyes from jets of gas. If a cylinder leak occurs, never use your hand to try to stop the leak.

Gas may also be suddenly released when the tank is turned on. When turning on a compressed air tank that is connected to the anesthetic machine, use the appropriate wrench and turn the valve slowly to the full open position.

---

*Current suppliers include Lab Safety Supply (1-800-356-2501), Assay Technology (1-800-833-1258), and Vetamac (1-800-334-1583).

Keep your head and face away from the valve outlet, pressure gauge, and pressure relief device.

If a cylinder is damaged, the sudden release of gas can have catastrophic consequences. If, for example, a cylinder is punctured or is knocked over and the regulator (the metal attachments at the top of the tank) or cylinder neck is broken off the tank, the force of the gas suddenly escaping from the tank may cause it to move like a rocket through a wall or roof. To prevent this occurrence, chain or belt large cylinders to a wall and always store them in an upright position. Valve caps should be used on all large cylinders that are not connected to gas lines to protect the valves from damage.

Gas cylinders should be stored away from emergency exits or areas with heavy traffic. If a large cylinder must be moved to another location, a handcart should be used; do not drag or roll the cylinder.

Full tanks should be kept separate from empty tanks and also should be clearly labeled for quick identification. The use of tear-off labels helps eliminate confusion regarding the empty, in-use, or full status of a given compressed air cylinder. The current status of the tank is given on the outermost section of the label (see Figure 4-23). Cylinders should be used in the order in which they are received (i.e., first in, first out).

## ACCIDENTAL EXPOSURE TO INJECTABLE AGENTS

All anesthetic agents are potentially toxic to personnel handling them. Skin exposure, eye splash, or oral ingestion of injectable drugs or inhalation agents may be hazardous (or even fatal).

The injectable drugs of most concern are the opioids used for the restraint and capture of wildlife, including etorphine (Immobilon, M99) and carfentanil (Wildnil). Etorphine has 10,000 times the potency of morphine and is absorbed readily through mucous membranes or broken skin. Exposure may also occur through accidental injection, eye splash, or oral ingestion.

Human exposure to even a minute amount of these agents by any route can cause rapid onset of unconsciousness, respiratory failure, and death. The following precautions should be taken:

- Never handle potent opioids such as etorphine unless you have been adequately trained in their safe use, potential adverse effects, and treatment in case of exposure.
- Never work alone when using potent opioids.
- Wear gloves. If exposure occurs, immediately wash skin and clothing with cold water.
- A reversal agent (diprenorphine, naloxone, naltrexone) must be drawn up and ready for use. Note that up to three bottles (12 mg) of naloxone may be necessary to antagonize a single drop of these opioids. It is advisable to have a prearranged plan for on-site treatment of exposed personnel, including provision for cardiovascular and respiratory support.
- Dispose of needles and syringes in a closed container immediately after use.

Other injectable agents that may be hazardous include the cyclohexamines (ketamine, tiletamine), which have been reported to cause disorientation, excitement and other behavioral changes, dizziness, and unconsciousness after an accidental eye splash. Human exposure to $alpha_2$-agonists (e.g., xylazine, detomidine, medetomidine, or dexmedetomidine) by injection or skin contact may cause profound sedation, hypotension, bradycardia, respiratory depression, and coma.

Safety precautions for prevention of exposure to any injectable agent include the use of personal protective equipment if there is a risk of spillage or eye splash, careful loading of syringes, and proper disposal of used needles and syringes. If accidental exposure occurs, the exposed person should receive prompt first aid (eye wash, flushing of exposed skin with large amounts of water, respiratory support) and subsequent transport to a medical center.

## KEY POINTS

1. Anesthesia presents several potential health risks to hospital personnel, including exposure to waste anesthetic gas and hazardous injectable agents and accidents associated with handling of compressed gas cylinders.
2. Waste anesthetic gases and vapors are breathed by all personnel working in areas in which animals are anesthetized or are recovering from inhalation anesthesia. Filling or emptying vaporizers and the cleanup of accidental spills also may result in significant exposure.
3. Exposure to waste anesthetic gas is associated with short-term problems such as fatigue, headache, drowsiness, nausea, depression, and irritability.
4. Long-term exposure to waste anesthetic gases may be associated with reproductive disorders, liver and kidney damage, and nervous system dysfunction, although the evidence of epidemiologic studies is sometimes contradictory and difficult to interpret. Most authorities recommend that exposure to high levels of waste anesthetic gas be avoided, particularly by pregnant women.
5. Anesthetics such as methoxyflurane and halothane, which undergo significant hepatic metabolism and renal excretion, are considered to be a greater hazard than anesthetics that are minimally eliminated by these routes (isoflurane, sevoflurane).

6. Volatile waste anesthetic gases apparently do not have oncogenic (cancer-causing) effects.

7. The National Institute for Occupational Safety and Health (NIOSH) recommendations for waste anesthetic gas concentrations limit exposure to 2 parts per million (ppm) or less for halogenated anesthetics (0.5 ppm or less if nitrous oxide is concurrently used). Surveys of veterinary clinics show wide variations in waste gas levels, depending on the sampling site, scavenging system, and anesthetic techniques used.

8. Installation and use of an effective gas scavenging system greatly reduces waste gas exposure. Caution should be used to prevent the scavenger from applying negative pressure to the breathing circuit.

9. Equipment leak testing should be done on a daily basis to detect and allow correction of leakage from the anesthetic machine and compressed air cylinders. Tests should be done on both the high-pressure and low-pressure components of the machine.

10. Certain anesthetic techniques are associated with excessive release of waste gas. These include the use of anesthetic chambers, masks, and uncuffed endotracheal tubes. Procedures such as turning off the vaporizer before disconnecting the animal from the machine are helpful in reducing waste gas contamination of hospital air.

11. Vaporizers should be filled and emptied with care, using appropriate equipment and protective clothing.

12. Waste gas levels may be monitored by professional occupational hygienists or by the use of detector badges.

13. Compressed air cylinders should be transported, used, and stored with care. Special hazards include risk of fire in areas in which cylinders are stored and the risk of sudden release of pressurized gas from damaged cylinders.

14. Potent injectable opioids such as etorphine have considerable potential to cause serious, even fatal reactions. Special training is necessary to safely handle these agents, and a narcotic reversing agent must be readily available in case of human exposure.

---

## PROCEDURE 13-1  Equipment Leak Testing

### High-Pressure System Test

1. One test of the high-pressure system is to turn the nitrous oxide tank on and place a 1:1 solution of water and dishwashing liquid on all tank connections and joints. Each location is then observed for bubble formation, which indicates a leak.

2. Another useful high-pressure test is conducted by first turning on the nitrous oxide cylinder, noting the reading on the tank pressure gauge, and then turning the cylinder off. Throughout this procedure the flow meter is set to zero, maintaining the pressure in the system (i.e., line pressure is not evacuated). The tank pressure gauge should be checked again in 1 hour. If the pressure gauge reading is unchanged or has decreased by no more than 50 lb/in$^2$, the high-pressure system is leak free. If the pressure is at or near zero, there is a leak somewhere between the cylinder and the flow meter, and nitrous oxide is escaping into the room air. The most likely location of the leak is at the connection of the cylinder to the machine yoke.

3. It is also possible to check for high-pressure leaks of oxygen by following the same procedure as that outlined previously for the nitrous oxide. Although the escape of small amounts of oxygen poses little or no risk of health problems to the anesthetic machine operator, it may lead to premature emptying of the oxygen tank.

### Low-Pressure System Test: Rebreathing Systems

One easy way to do a low-pressure test is to close the pop-off valve and place one hand (or preferably a stopper) over the Y-piece. This closes off all avenues of gas escape from the machine. The oxygen tank is turned on and the flow meter adjusted to supply a flow rate of 2 L/min. The reservoir bag will gradually fill with oxygen. When the bag is full and tight, the flow rate is reduced to 200 mL/min or less. The anesthetist should be able to squeeze the bag with significant pressure without causing escape of air from the bag (it remains tight and full). If the anesthetist is able to push air out of the bag, a leak is present or the pop-off valve or Y-piece is not completely occluded. The circuit should maintain a pressure of 30 cm (as indicated by the pressure manometer) for 30 seconds during the test, at a flow meter setting of 200 mL/min.

### Low-Pressure System Test: Non-rebreathing Systems

Non-rebreathing systems such as the Bain apparatus can also be checked for leaks. The external hose of the Bain circuit can be checked by attaching the apparatus to the inspiratory hose, occluding the patient port, and closing the pop-off valve. Oxygen is introduced into the system until the reservoir bag fills. When the pressure gauge reads 20 cm H$_2$O, the flow meter is turned off, and the pressure is observed for the next 20 seconds. A significant decrease in pressure indicates that a leak is present. For a test of the internal hose, the fresh gas hose from the anesthesia machine is attached to the Bain circuit, the oxygen flow is set at 2 L/min, and the outlet port of the internal hose is occluded by a 3-mL syringe or with a finger while the flow meter is observed. If there is no leak, the bobbin in the oxygen flow meter should drop to zero, indicating adequate back pressure.

## PROCEDURE 13-2    Procedures for Minimizing Waste Gas Release

1. Anesthetic chambers are a significant source of anesthetic waste gas pollution in veterinary facilities. Unless a scavenging system is connected to the chamber, significant amounts of waste gas are released when the chamber is opened. In addition, the fur of the patient is saturated with anesthetic during the induction and gives off waste gas vapor when the animal is removed from the chamber. Chambers should be used only in a well-ventilated room with a non-recirculating ventilation system, or under a fume hood. They must be tightly sealed to avoid leaks. The chamber should have two inlet holes to which the breathing hoses from the anesthetic machine can be attached, once the Y-piece has been removed. With this setup the anesthetic machine scavenger will be able to remove the exhaust vapors. Alternatively, the hose from a Bain system can be attached to one inlet, and the scavenger system can be directly attached to the other inlet. Either way, the chamber should be closed immediately after the patient has been removed, and the oxygen flow should be continued for several minutes to purge waste gas into the scavenger, rather than releasing waste gas into the room air. Anesthetic chambers should be washed with soap and water after each use to remove residual anesthetic and contaminants from the animal.

2. Avoid using masks to maintain anesthesia. Significant amounts of anesthetic gas may escape from around the diaphragm of the mask and enter the room air. It has been suggested that waste gas concentrations around the patient's head can be reduced by 50% if an endotracheal tube is used instead of a mask. If the situation dictates the use of a mask, it should be fitted tightly over the animal's face. Face masks are available in a variety of sizes and should be chosen to fit the patient snugly but comfortably. When a mask is used, the sequence of events is the same as for an endotracheal tube: turn the oxygen on, place the mask on the patient, then turn the vaporizer on. This order should be reversed when ending the procedure. If mask inductions are required, ideally the animal should be intubated when it reaches an appropriate depth.

3. Use cuffed endotracheal tubes when possible. To be effective the tube must be of adequate size, and the cuff must be inflated and in good repair. Before use, inflate cuffs with air to check for leaks. After intubation of the patient, check the fit of the endotracheal tube within the trachea by closing the pop-off valve and gently squeezing the reservoir bag. The cuff should not leak up to an airway pressure of 20 cm $H_2O$ but should leak at 20 cm $H_2O$. Leakage at pressures over 20 cm is necessary to reduce the risk of barotrauma in case the pop-off valve is closed and accidentally forgotten. (Note: To prevent overinflation of the patient's lungs, ensure that the circuit pressure displayed on the manometer does not exceed 20 cm of water when applying pressure to the bag to check the cuff.)

4. When using a rebreathing system, ensure that the reservoir bag inflates and deflates synchronously with the patient's respirations (in other words, inflates on expiration and deflates on inspiration, with the volume of movement approximately equal to the animal's tidal volume). If this does not occur, one should suspect either air leakage around the endotracheal tube or esophageal intubation. Significant release of waste gas can occur in either case. (It is also likely that the patient will wake up because a significant amount of room air enters the lungs in either case.)

5. The use of closed rebreathing systems may help minimize waste gas pollution. Anesthesia with open systems and high gas flows (i.e., greater than 3 L/min) is associated with greater release of waste gas, particularly if effective scavenging is unavailable.

6. When working with an anesthetic machine designed for use in dogs and cats, do not turn the vaporizer or flow meters on until the anesthetic machine is connected to the endotracheal tube and the cuff is inflated. The practice of filling the machine and reservoir bag with anesthetic gas before connecting the machine to a dog or cat should be discouraged. This practice is acceptable when working with large animals, and in this case the Y-piece should be occluded with a rubber plug. When it is time to attach the circuit to the intubated patient, the connection should be made quickly. Once the anesthetic procedure is under way, avoid disconnecting the patient from the breathing circuit unnecessarily. If the patient is to be disconnected from the machine, the vaporizer setting and flow meters should be turned to zero.

7. Do not release the contents of the reservoir bag into the room air. If it is necessary to empty the reservoir bag, leave it attached to the machine and evacuate the contents into the scavenger.

8. After the vaporizer has been shut off, maintain the connection between the animal and the machine, having the animal breathe pure oxygen at 2 to 3 times the maintenance flow rate for several minutes. Periodically flush the system with oxygen by emptying the reservoir bag through the pop-off valve. If possible, leave the patient attached to the machine until extubation occurs. This allows expired anesthetic to enter the scavenging system rather than the room air.

9. Ensure that all rooms in which anesthetic gases are released (e.g., surgical preparation room, operating room, recovery room, and radiography room) have adequate ventilation that provides at least 15 air changes per hour. A properly designed ventilation system helps eliminate residual waste gases not collected by the scavenging system (e.g., those that arise from leaks or improper work practices).

10. One study found that concentrations of halothane and nitrous oxide were higher in recovery areas than in scavenged operating rooms. For the reduction of waste gas levels, it is usually necessary to have an exhaust fan or non-recirculating ventilation system operating in the room where patients are recovering from anesthesia. Whenever possible, avoid being closer than 3 feet from the nose of an animal recovering from anesthesia.

## PROCEDURE 13-2  Procedures for Minimizing Waste Gas Release—cont'd

11. Have anesthetic machines serviced at least biannually by a qualified service technician to ensure minimal leakage through machine components. A log of evaluation and maintenance procedures and leakage testing should be maintained for each anesthetic machine, ventilator, and vaporizer.

12. Inspect equipment often, and perform necessary maintenance. The routine maintenance procedures for anesthetic machines are usually outlined in the operations manual. Hoses, reservoir bags, and endotracheal tubes that are cracked or worn should be discarded. Endotracheal tubes with nonfunctional or leaking cuffs should not be used.

13. After each procedure, wash hoses, reservoir bags, masks, endotracheal tubes, and all other rubber components of the anesthetic circuit with soap and water, flush well with water, and allow them to air dry. These components may absorb considerable amounts of anesthetic during use. Washing not only removes absorbed waste gas, but also reduces transfer of microorganisms between patients.

14. Emptying and filling vaporizers may release significant amounts of anesthetic vapor into the surrounding air. If possible, pregnant personnel should not be involved in this task. Anesthetics may also be spilled onto the technician's hands and clothing (see Table 13-2). Ideally, vaporizers should be filled at the end of the workday, as personnel are leaving the hospital. Use a filling device (a specialized attachment that transfers anesthetic directly into the vaporizer) rather than pouring from a bottle to replenish liquid anesthetic in the machine. Agent-specific keyed filler systems are preferred. If no filling device is available, use a bottle adapter with a spout to prevent spillage (see Figure 4-31). Fill vaporizers in a well-ventilated area (ideally, outside of the building), and after filling a vaporizer, be sure that the filling port is properly closed. Use of an approved organic cartridge respirator (a device that fits over the mouth and nose and filters anesthetic gas out of incoming air), vinyl or plastic gloves, a lab coat or plastic apron, and other protective equipment will also minimize exposure to anesthetic liquid or vapors. The gloves should be removed and the hands washed immediately after the vaporizer is filled, as liquid anesthetics are readily absorbed through intact skin.

15. Vaporizers should be turned off when not in use.

16. If liquid anesthetic is spilled, high concentrations of anesthetic vapor will be present in the immediate area of the spill. If a spill occurs, increase ventilation as much as possible during the cleanup by opening windows or using fans. Close doors to the rest of the building and turn off the central vacuum system to avoid spreading the fumes throughout the building. For anything other than a small spill, all personnel not involved in the cleanup should leave the area, and the remaining staff should wear approved protective clothing, vinyl or plastic (not latex or rubber) gloves, and organic cartridge respirators. Remove all contaminated articles, including lab coats. Pour absorbent material such as kitty litter on the spill so that the liquid is completely absorbed. Dispose of the litter in an airtight container outside the clinic. If the spill is large or if protective equipment is unavailable, all personnel should leave the building and the local fire department should be notified.

17. Cap empty anesthetic bottles before discarding them because residual anesthetic in the bottle may evaporate into the room air. For the same reason, store vaporizer-filling devices in a sealed plastic bag between uses.

## REVIEW QUESTIONS

1. Waste anesthetic gases are a potential hazard to personnel, but problems that arise are only of long-term nature.
   True          False

2. Long-term toxicity of inhalation anesthetics is thought to be caused by the release of toxic metabolites during the breakdown of these drugs within the body.
   True          False

3. The anesthetic most clearly associated with neurologic and adverse reproductive effects is:
   a. Isoflurane
   b. Halothane
   c. Methoxyflurane
   d. Nitrous oxide

4. In the United States, the National Institute for Occupational Safety and Health (NIOSH) recommends that the levels of waste anesthetic gases for anesthetics such as isoflurane, halothane, or methoxyflurane should not exceed ___ ppm.
   a. 0.2
   b. 2
   c. 20
   d. 200

5. The odor of halothane may be detected by a person when the levels reach a minimum of ___ ppm.
   a. 5
   b. 33
   c. 200
   d. 5000

6. Rooms in which animals are recovering from anesthesia may be highly contaminated with waste gas.
   True            False

7. Which of the following can be used to effectively monitor waste anesthetic gas levels?
   a. Odor of waste gas
   b. Passive dosimeter badge
   c. Radiation monitor
   d. Regular preventive maintenance by qualified personnel

8. How often should a test for low-pressure leaks be conducted?
   a. Each day that the machine is used
   b. At least once per week
   c. At least once per month
   d. When the anesthetist smells anesthetic gases

9. The safest way to transport a large high-pressure tank, such as an oxygen tank, is by:
   a. Carrying it
   b. Rolling it along the floor
   c. Using a handcart
   d. Dragging it by the neck

10. How many air changes per hour should be available in a room in which waste anesthetic gases are present?
    a. 5
    b. 10
    c. 15
    d. 30

For the following questions, more than one answer may be correct.

11. A technician may reduce the amount of waste gases by:
    a. Using cuffed endotracheal tubes
    b. Ensuring that the anesthetic machine has been tested for leaks
    c. Using an injectable agent rather than a mask or chamber
    d. Using high fresh gas flows

12. To conduct a low-pressure test on an anesthetic machine (circle system), you must:
    a. Close the pop-off valve and occlude the end of the circuit
    b. Turn off the oxygen tank
    c. Compress the reservoir bag
    d. Pressurize the circuit with a volume of gas

## SELECTED READINGS

Ad Hoc Committee on the effect of trace anesthetic gases on health of operating room personnel, American Society of Anesthesiologists: Occupational disease among operating room personnel: national study, *Anesthesiology* (41): 321-40.

American College of Veterinary Anesthesiologists: Commentary and recommendations on control of waste anesthetic gases in the workplace, *J Am Vet Med Assoc* 209(1):75-77, 1996.

American Society of Anesthesiologists Task Force on Trace Anesthetic Gases: www.asahq. org/ProfInfo/wasteanesgases.html.

Boivin J: Risk of spontaneous abortion in women occupationally exposed to anaesthetic gases: a meta-analysis, *J Environ Med* 54: 541-548, 1997.

Burkhart JE, Stobbe TJ: Real-time measurement and control of waste anesthetic gases during veterinary surgeries, *Am Ind Hyg Assoc J* 51(12):640-645, 1990.

Gross ME, Branson KR: Reducing exposure to waste anesthetic gas, *Vet Tech* 14(3):175-177, 1993.

Hoerauf K, Lierz M, Wiesner G, et al: Genetic damage in operating room personnel exposed to isoflurane and nitrous oxide, *Occup Environ Med* 56(7):433-437, 1999.

Johnson JA, Buchan RM, Reif JS: Effect of waste anesthetic gas and vapor exposure on reproductive outcomes in veterinary personnel, *Am Ind Hyg Assoc J* 48:62-66, 1987.

Lietzemayer DW: Current methods for removal of anesthetic gas, *Vet Tech* 11(4):213-220, 1990.

McKelvey D: *Safety handbook for veterinary hospital staff*, Lakewood, Colo, 1999, American Animal Hospital Association Press.

Meyer RE: Anesthesia hazards to animal workers. In Lanley RL, editor: *Occupational medicine state of the art reviews*, Philadelphia, 1999, Hanley and Belfus.

OSHA Office of Science and Technology Assessment: Anesthetic agents-workplace exposures, *OSHA Instruction TED* 1.15(H-2), 1996.

Schenker MB, Samuels SJ, Green RS, Wiggins P: Adverse reproductive outcomes among female veterinarians, *Epidemiol* 132:96-106, 1990.

Shirangi A, Fritschi L, Holman CD: Maternal occupational exposures and risk of spontaneous abortion in veterinary practice, *Occup Environ Med*, April 2008.

Short CE, Harvey RC: Anesthetic waste gases in veterinary medicine, *Cornell Vet* 73(4):363-374, 1983.

Shuhaiber S, Einarson A, Raddle IC, Sarkar M, Koren G: A prospective-controlled study of pregnant veterinary staff exposed to inhaled anesthetics and x-rays, *Ont Vet Med Assoc*, 1999.

Spence AA, Cohen EN, Brown BW, et al: Occupational hazards for operating physicians, *JAMA* 238:955-959, 1977.

Ward GS, Byland RR: Concentration of halothane in veterinary operating and treatment rooms, *J Am Vet Med Assoc* 180:174-177, 1982.

# ANSWER KEY

## ANSWERS FOR CHAPTER 1

1. d
2. a
3. c
4. b
5. a, b, d
6. a, d

## ANSWERS FOR CHAPTER 2

1. c
2. b
3. d
4. c
5. b
6. b
7. c
8. c
9. a
10. a
11. d
12. d
13. a
14. c
15. b
16. d
17. d
18. b
19. b
20. d

## ANSWERS FOR CHAPTER 3

1. c
2. False
3. True
4. a
5. True
6. d
7. b
8. c
9. a
10. c
11. True
12. a

13. c
14. d
15. c
16. d
17. a
18. a, b, c, d
19. a, b, c, d
20. c
21. a, b, c, d
22. a, b
23. b, d
24. a, c, d
25. b, d

## ANSWERS FOR CHAPTER 4

1. a
2. c
3. b
4. c
5. e
6. b
7. a
8. b
9. d
10. True
11. a
12. d
13. c
14. b
15. c
16. a, b, c
17. b, c, d
18. a, b
19. a, b, c, d
20. a, b, d

## ANSWERS FOR CHAPTER 5

1. True
2. b
3. b
4. c
5. a
6. False
7. b
8. b

9. c
10. False
11. c
12. d
13. a
14. b
15. c
16. c
17. a, b, c
18. a, b, c, d
19. a, b, c
20. b, c

## ANSWERS FOR CHAPTER 6

1. b
2. b
3. b
4. a
5. a
6. d
7. b
8. c
9. True
10. d
11. c
12. b
13. c
14. c
15. b
16. a
17. False
18. a
19. c
20. False
21. a, c, d
22. b, c, d
23. a, b, d
24. a, b, c, d
25. a, b, c

## ANSWERS FOR CHAPTER 7

1. b
2. c
3. c
4. c

5. b
6. b
7. a
8. d
9. c
10. False
11. d
12. c
13. c
14. d
15. True

## ANSWERS FOR CHAPTER 8

1. c
2. a
3. d
4. b
5. c
6. a
7. b
8. d
9. c
10. b
11. d
12. d
13. a
14. c
15. a, b, c, d
16. b, c, d
17. a, c, d
18. a, b, c, d
19. c
20. a, c, d

## ANSWERS FOR CHAPTER 9

1. c
2. a
3. b
4. a
5. c
6. a
7. d
8. c
9. True
10. b

## ANSWERS
## FOR CHAPTER 10

1. a
2. False
3. b
4. c
5. True
6. c
7. a
8. c
9. d
10. a

## ANSWERS
## FOR CHAPTER 11

1. b
2. a
3. b
4. d
5. b
6. c
7. b
8. b
9. c
10. a

## ANSWERS
## FOR CHAPTER 12

1. d
2. d
3. b
4. a
5. c
6. c
7. d
8. b
9. d
10. a
11. False
12. a, b, c, d
13. a, b
14. a, c
15. b, c, d
16. a, b, c, d
17. a, b, c, d
18. a, c
19. b
20. a, b, c
21. b, d
22. b
23. False
24. False
25. c

## ANSWERS
## FOR CHAPTER 13

1. False
2. True
3. d
4. b
5. b
6. True
7. b
8. a
9. c
10. c
11. a, b, c
12. a, c, d

# Appendix A

# American College of Veterinary Anesthesiologists Monitoring Guidelines Update, 2009

This document may be accessed on line at http://acva.org/under "ACVA Position Statements."

## Recommendations for Monitoring Anesthetized Veterinary Patients

### Position Statement

The American College of Veterinary Anesthesiologists (ACVA) has revised the set of guidelines for anesthetic monitoring that were originally developed in 1994 and published in 1995.* Since then many factors have caused a shift in the benchmark used to measure a successful anesthetic outcome, moving from the lack of anesthetic mortality toward decreased anesthetic morbidity.

This shift toward minimizing anesthetic morbidity has been facilitated by more objective definition and earlier detection of pathophysiologic conditions such as hypotension, hypoxemia, and severe hypercapnia. This has resulted from the incorporation of newer monitoring modalities by skilled attentive personnel during anesthesia.

The ACVA recognizes that it is possible to adequately monitor and manage anesthetized patients without specialized equipment and that some of these modalities may be impractical in certain clinical settings. Furthermore, the ACVA does not suggest that using any or all the modalities will ensure any specific patient outcome, or that failure to use them will result in poor outcome.

However, as the standard of veterinary care advances and client expectations expand, revised guidelines are necessary to reflect the importance of vigilant monitoring. The goal of the ACVA guidelines is to improve the level of anesthesia care for veterinary patients. Frequent and continuous monitoring and recording of vital signs in the perianesthetic period by trained personnel and the intelligent use of various monitors are requirements for advancing the quality of anesthesia care of veterinary patients.

*JAVMA 206:936-937, 1995.

### Circulation

#### Objective

To ensure adequate circulatory function

#### Methods

1. Palpation of peripheral pulse to determine rate, rhythm, and quality and evaluation of mucous membrane (MM) color and capillary refill time (CRT).
2. Auscultation of heartbeat (stethoscope; esophageal stethoscope or other audible heart monitor). Continuous (audible heart or pulse monitor) or intermittent monitoring of the heart rate and rhythm.
3. Pulse oximetry to determine the % hemoglobin saturation.
4. Electrocardiogram (ECG) continuous display for detection of arrhythmias.
5. Blood pressure:
   a. Noninvasive (indirect): oscillometric method—Doppler ultrasonic flow detector
   b. Invasive (direct): arterial catheter connected to an aneroid manometer or to a transducer and oscilloscope

#### Recommendations

Continuous awareness of heart rate and rhythm during anesthesia, along with gross assessment of peripheral perfusion (pulse quality, MM color, and CRT) are mandatory. Arterial blood pressure and ECG should also be monitored. There may be some situations where these may be temporarily impractical—for example, movement of an anesthetized patient to a different area of the hospital.

### Oxygenation

#### Objective

To ensure adequate oxygenation of the patient's arterial blood

#### Methods

1. Pulse oximetry (noninvasive estimation of hemoglobin saturation)
2. Arterial blood gas analysis for oxygen partial pressure ($Pao_2$)

### Recommendations

Assessment of oxygenation should be done whenever possible by pulse oximetry, with blood gas analysis being employed when necessary for more critically ill patients.

## Ventilation
### Objective

To ensure that the patient's ventilation is adequately maintained

### Methods

1. Observation of thoracic wall movement or observation of breathing bag movement when thoracic wall movement cannot be assessed
2. Auscultation of breath sounds with an external stethoscope, an esophageal stethoscope, or an audible respiratory monitor
3. Capnography (end-expired $CO_2$ measurement)
4. Arterial blood gas analysis for carbon dioxide partial pressure ($Pa_{CO_2}$)
5. Respirometry (tidal volume measurement)

### Recommendations

Qualitative assessment of ventilation is essential as outlined in either 1 or 2 above, and capnography is recommended, with blood gas analysis as necessary.

## Temperature
### Objective

To ensure that patients do not encounter serious deviations from normal body temperature

### Methods

1. Rectal thermometer for intermittent measurement
2. Rectal or esophageal temperature probe for continuous measurement

### Recommendations

Temperature should be measured periodically during anesthesia and recovery and if possible checked within a few hours after return to the wards.

## Neuromuscular Blockade
### Objective

To assess the intensity of and recovery from neuromuscular blockade

### Methods

1. Hand-held peripheral nerve stimulator
2. Spirometer

### Recommendations

For any patient in which neuromuscular blockade is used, it is essential to control ventilation, monitor closely for signs of awareness, and be certain of recovery of blockade before anesthesia recovery. Recovery of neuromuscular function may be assumed if the evoked response (twitch and/or tetanic fade) to a nerve stimulus, and respiratory tidal volume as measured with a spirometer, return to at least 70% of preblockade status. End tidal $CO_2$ may also be used as an indication of adequate ventilation in spontaneously ventilating patients.

## Record-Keeping
### Objectives

1. To maintain a legal record of significant events related to the anesthetic period
2. To enhance recognition of significant trends or unusual values for physiologic parameters and allow assessment of the response to intervention

### Recommendations

1. Record all drugs administered to each patient in the perianesthetic period and in early recovery, noting the dose, time, and route of administration, as well as any adverse reaction to a drug or drug combination.
2. Record monitored variables on a regular basis (minimum every 5 to 10 minutes) during anesthesia. The minimum variables that should be recorded are heart rate and respiratory rate, as well as oxygenation status and blood pressure if these were monitored.
3. Record heart rate, respiratory rate, and temperature in the early recovery phase.
4. Any untoward events or unusual circumstances should be recorded for legal reasons, and for reference should the patient require anesthesia in the future.

## Recovery Period
### Objective

To ensure a safe and comfortable recovery from anesthesia

### Methods

1. Observation of respiratory pattern
2. Observation of MM color and CRT
3. Palpation of pulse rate and quality
4. Measurement of body temperature, with appropriate warming or cooling methods applied if indicated
5. Observation of any behavior that indicates pain, with appropriate pharmaceutical intervention as necessary.
6. Other measurements as indicated by patient's medical status—for example, blood glucose, pulse oximetry, PCV, TP, blood gases, and so on.

## Recommendations

Monitoring in recovery should include *at the minimum* evaluation of pulse rate and quality, MM color, respiratory pattern, signs of pain, and temperature.

## Personnel
### Objective

To ensure that a responsible individual is aware of the patient's status at all times during anesthesia and recovery and is prepared either to intervene when indicated or to alert the veterinarian in charge about changes in the patient's condition

## Recommendations

1. Ideally, a veterinarian, technician, or other responsible person should remain with the patient continuously and be dedicated to that patient only.
2. If this is not possible, a reliable and knowledgeable person should check the patient's status on a regular basis (at least every 5 minutes) during anesthesia and recovery.
3. A responsible person may be present in the same room, although not necessarily solely occupied with the anesthetized patient (for instance, the surgeon may also be responsible for overseeing anesthesia).
4. In either 2 or 3 above, audible heart and respiratory monitors must be available.
5. A responsible person, solely dedicated to managing and caring for the anesthetized patient during anesthesia, remains with the patient continuously until the end of the anesthetic period.
   a. Recommended for all patients assessed as ASA status III, IV, or V
   b. Recommended for horses anesthetized with inhalation anesthetics and/or horses anesthetized for longer than 45 minutes

## Sedation without General Anesthesia

Sedation is a state characterized by central depression accompanied by drowsiness during which the patient is generally unaware of its surroundings but responsive to noxious manipulation.[†]

If a sedated patient is sufficiently obtunded to lose control of protective airway reflexes, it should be monitored as under general anesthesia.

## Objective

To ensure adequate oxygenation and hemodynamic stability in the obtunded patient

## Methods

1. Palpation of pulse rate, rhythm, and quality
2. Observation of MM color and CRT
3. Observation of respiratory rate and pattern
4. Auscultation
5. Pulse oximetry
6. Oxygen supplementation

## Recommendations

Intermittent monitoring of basic respiratory and cardiovascular parameters in the heavily sedated animal should be routine. Supplemental oxygen, an endotracheal tube, and materials for IV catheterization should always be readily available. Particular attention should be paid to brachycephalic breeds that are particularly at risk for airway obstruction under heavy sedation.

---

[†] Thurmon JC, Short CE: History and overview of veterinary anesthesia. In Tranquilli WJ, Thurmon JC, Grimm KA, eds: *Lumb and Jones' veterinary anesthesia and analgesia*, ed 4, Ames, Iowa, 2007, Blackwell, p. 5.

# Appendix B

## Nitrous Oxide

Nitrous oxide ($N_2O$) is a colorless, nonflammable gas with a pleasant odor that has been used in human patients since the mid 1800s to provide anesthesia and analgesia. It is not sufficiently potent to induce general anesthesia when used alone, but when used in combination with halogenated inhalant anesthetics, speeds induction and recovery, provides additional analgesia, and decreases the necessary dose and adverse effects of concurrently used agents.

### PHYSICAL PROPERTIES OF NITROUS OXIDE

Because $N_2O$ is a gas at room temperature, it is stored in blue compressed gas cylinders and does not require a vaporizer for delivery. It is delivered via a gas specific flow meter, mixed with $O_2$ in the anesthetic machine and then delivered to the patient as a part of the carrier gas flow.

The property that limits the use of $N_2O$ in veterinary anesthesia is its lack of potency (that is, a high minimum alveolar concentration [MAC]) in domestic animal species. The MAC of $N_2O$ in humans is approximately 100%, whereas the MAC in dogs and horses is close to 200% and in the cat is approximately 250%. Consequently, it is impossible to achieve surgical anesthesia in a healthy domestic animal using $N_2O$ alone.

Other properties of $N_2O$ can be summarized as follows:
- $N_2O$ reduces the MAC (and therefore the vaporizer setting) of other anesthetics by 20% to 30%. This reduces adverse effects and results in faster recoveries. $N_2O$ also has been shown to speed the uptake of other anesthetic gases into the bloodstream by the **second gas effect** when used at high concentrations (50% to 70% of the total gas flow). The second gas effect is an increase in the concentration of a gas in the alveoli resulting from the absorption of a second gas into the bloodstream. The absorption of $N_2O$ causes the concentration of the inhalant anesthetic gas in the alveoli to increase more rapidly than it would otherwise. This effect results in more rapid inductions.
- $N_2O$ has an extremely low solubility coefficient and by itself is associated with rapid induction and

recovery rates. It is therefore a helpful addition to slow-acting agents such as methoxyflurane. It does little to enhance induction with rapid-acting agents such as isoflurane and sevoflurane, however.

### EFFECTS OF NITROUS OXIDE ON MAJOR ORGAN SYSTEMS

#### Central Nervous System

$N_2O$ has a mild anesthetic effect, insufficient to produce general anesthesia when used alone, but does provide good analgesia.

#### Cardiovascular System

$N_2O$ usually has little effect on heart rate (HR), cardiac output (CO), and arterial blood pressure (BP), although there is a potential for tachycardia. It is considered to have a wide margin of safety.

#### Respiratory System

$N_2O$ causes minimal respiratory depression, although it will displace oxygen in the breathing circuit and the patient's lungs, leading to hypoxemia when used in concentrations of over 70% of total carrier gas flow. It is non-irritating to the respiratory system.

### OTHER EFFECTS

- $N_2O$ may accumulate within the gastrointestinal tract, causing distension and ileus.
- $N_2O$ crosses the placental barrier and may cause neonatal hypoxemia.
- $N_2O$ is not a muscle relaxant.

Despite the relative safety and advantages of $N_2O$, over the past several decades, its popularity has gradually decreased to the point that it is seldom used in general practices in North America. One reason is the increased cost of $N_2O$ anesthesia, compared with anesthesia with an inhalation agent alone. Another reason is the increased use of isoflurane and sevoflurane, which provide rapid inductions and recoveries even without the concurrent use of $N_2O$. Finally, the availability of good injectable analgesics has made the analgesic properties of $N_2O$ less advantageous.

## NITROUS OXIDE RISKS

The use of $N_2O$ is associated with several potential problems, including those described in the following paragraphs.

### Fire Hazard

$N_2O$ is not flammable, but like $O_2$ it supports combustion.

### Risk of Hypoxemia

The use of $N_2O$ in an anesthetic machine limits the amount of $O_2$ that is delivered to the patient to the extent that $N_2O$ replaces $O_2$ in the circuit. Because the minimal amount of $N_2O$ necessary to achieve analgesic effects is 50% (and values of 60% to 67% are recommended), the use of this agent decreases the amount of $O_2$ delivered to the patient by the same amount (50% to 67%). Therefore the patient breathing $N_2O$ should be monitored closely for adequate oxygenation with a pulse oximeter or blood gas analysis. Patients should also be monitored closely for cyanosis and cardiac arrhythmias. Because of the risk of hypoxemia, animals with preexisting lung disease are poor candidates for $N_2O$ anesthesia. For all patients, care should also be taken when adjusting the flow meter of the anesthetic machine to avoid confusing $O_2$ controls with those for $N_2O$.

### Diffusion into Air Pockets

Because of its low solubility coefficient, $N_2O$ is able to diffuse into trapped air pockets within the body. This diffusion may result in an increase in the amount of gas within an organ and consequent distension of the organ containing trapped gas. For this reason, the use of $N_2O$ is contraindicated in animals with intestinal obstruction, gastric torsion, pneumothorax, or diaphragmatic hernia. As there is normally a large amount of gas in the equine gut, $N_2O$ may cause undesirable dilation of the intestines in this species.

### Use in Closed (Total) Rebreathing Systems

$N_2O$ should never be used in a closed rebreathing system (that is, one with low $O_2$ flow rates) unless the anesthetist uses a monitor to determine $O_2$ levels in the inspired gas. Because $O_2$ is removed from a closed system by the animal's metabolism, the level of $N_2O$ in the circuit may increase to dangerous levels, resulting in hypoxemia.

### Diffusion Hypoxia

During recovery from anesthesia, $N_2O$ will readily exit from the body via the respiratory system. Because of the rapid outpouring of $N_2O$ into the lungs, a state of diffusion hypoxia may occur. In this condition, $O_2$ molecules normally found in the alveoli are displaced by the large numbers of $N_2O$ molecules exiting the blood. Diffusion hypoxia can be prevented by keeping the animal on high $O_2$ flow rates for at least 5 minutes after the $N_2O$ has been turned off and ensuring that the animal is frequently bagged with pure $O_2$.

### Waste Anesthetic Gas Hazards

Exposure of operating room personnel to waste $N_2O$ has been linked to several health disorders (see Chapter 13).

### Nitrous Oxide Storage

Some anesthetic machines are designed to deliver $N_2O$ gas in addition to $O_2$. $N_2O$ is contained in a compressed gas cylinder that is blue in color. As with $O_2$, this may be a large freestanding tank or a smaller tank attached to the machine. The pressure in a full $N_2O$ tank (745 psi or about 5140 kPa) is considerably less than the pressure in a full $O_2$ tank. This is because, unlike $O_2$, $N_2O$ is present in both the liquid and gas states within the pressurized tank.

The tank pressure gauge indicates the pressure of the gas within the tank but not that of the liquid and therefore does not indicate how full the tank is. As the gas leaves the tank, more liquid evaporates and enters the gas state. As a result, the pressure of the gas within the tank will not change until all of the liquid has evaporated, at which point the tank is nearly empty (5 to 10 minutes left, depending on the flow rate). The anesthetist therefore should not expect the $N_2O$ tank gauge reading to change, even after several hours of anesthesia, unless the tank is close to empty.

The amount of $N_2O$ in the tank can be determined only by weighing the tank before use. The full and empty weights are normally stamped on the outside of each cylinder. An E cylinder of $N_2O$ weighs approximately 8 kg (18 lb) when full and about 6.4 kg (14 lb) when empty. Because weighing the cylinder is not always an option, especially during a procedure, the anesthetist should change the tank as soon as the tank pressure gauge starts to drop below 745 psi.

## NITROUS OXIDE DELIVERY

As with $O_2$, $N_2O$ is delivered to the patient by a flow meter. So when this gas is used on a machine, there will be a flow meter for each gas (see Figure 4-25). These flow meters allow the anesthetist to accurately control the relative amounts of $O_2$ and $N_2O$ delivered. If the $N_2O$ flow meter is set to deliver 2 L/min and the $O_2$ flow meter is adjusted to deliver 1 L/min, the resulting mixture will be a 2:1 ratio of $N_2O$ to $O_2$. (This represents approximately 67% $N_2O$ and 33% $O_2$.)

Some machines automatically set the $O_2$ and $N_2O$ proportions, and an adjustment of the flow rate of one gas will automatically change the flow rate of the other. Some also have a device that discontinues $N_2O$ administration to the patient if the $O_2$ flow is cut off. This mechanism prevents inadvertent asphyxiation of the patient, which could occur if the patient breathed $N_2O$ in the absence of $O_2$.

## NITROUS OXIDE USE

When using $N_2O$, the anesthetist should ensure that the $N_2O/O_2$ ratio never exceeds 2:1, or the patient will receive insufficient $O_2$ and asphyxiation may result. It is also imperative to deliver a minimum $O_2$ flow of 10 to 15 mL/kg/min for large animal patients and 30 mL/kg/min for small animal patients receiving a mixture of $N_2O$ and $O_2$. Total flow rates less than 500 mL/min should be avoided.

For example, if a total carrier gas flow of 1 L/min is required, the 1 L may consist of pure $O_2$ or some combination of $N_2O$ and $O_2$. For example, 600 mL of $N_2O$ per minute and 400 mL of $O_2$ per minute (a ratio of 1.5:1) would be appropriate.

## Oxygen Depletion and Nitrous Oxide Accumulation

During any procedure, $O_2$ is gradually depleted as the patient breathes the circulating gas. This is normally compensated for by fresh $O_2$ entering the circuit. In a closed rebreathing system, the $O_2$ flow rate is low and the amount of fresh $O_2$ added to the circuit may not entirely compensate for this loss. This is particularly serious if $N_2O$ is used in addition to $O_2$, because the relative amount of $N_2O$ in the circuit may increase as the amount of $O_2$ decreases. As a result, the patient may breathe dangerously high levels of $N_2O$ gas. This effect is less likely to occur in a semiclosed rebreathing system, in which $N_2O$ escapes through the pop-off valve and $O_2$ flow rates are higher. The use of an $O_2$ flow above the minimum levels mentioned prevents $N_2O$ buildup, but this flow rate is not possible in a closed rebreathing system. Closed rebreathing systems therefore are not recommended if $N_2O$ is part of the anesthetic protocol, unless a monitor is used to measure inspired $O_2$.

# Use of Nonprecision Vaporizers

## DESCRIPTION AND FUNCTION OF NONPRECISION VAPORIZERS

Nonprecision vaporizers were originally designed for and used extensively for administration of low–vapor pressure liquid inhalant anesthetics, such as methoxyflurane, that are no longer available. These vaporizers are classified as variable-bypass, flow-over and non–temperature compensated. Because of their low resistance to gas flow, these vaporizers are located in the breathing circuit (vaporizer-in-circuit [VIC]).

Two examples of nonprecision vaporizers are the Ohio No. 8 vaporizer (Figure 4-26) and the Stephens vaporizer, both of which consist of a glass jar containing a wick and a control dial. The wick absorbs anesthetic contained in the jar and increases the surface area available for vaporization, thus increasing saturation of the carrier gas with anesthetic.

The imprecise control of anesthetic output characteristic of these vaporizers is adequate for methoxyflurane, which has a low vapor pressure and will achieve a maximum of only 4% concentration even if the vaporizer is fully open. This control is inadequate for more volatile anesthetics such as isoflurane, sevoflurane, or halothane, however, which can achieve very high concentrations and produce a dangerously excessive anesthetic depth.

Nonprecision vaporizers are sometimes used to deliver halothane or isoflurane. Ohio No. 8 vaporizers (nonprecision) can be used with halothane or isoflurane, but the wick should be removed and no more than 100 mL of anesthetic should be put into the vaporizer. For the first 2 minutes, a setting of 6 to "fully open" should be used, and thereafter a setting of 2 to 6 is usually adequate. If a Stephens vaporizer (nonprecision) is used to deliver halothane or isoflurane at low oxygen flow rates, the metal sleeve should be fully retracted and the anesthetic should be filled only to the anesthetic level line. A vaporizer setting of 4 is used for the first 2 minutes, and for the maintenance period a setting between "off" and 4 is usually adequate.

This practice of using nonprecision vaporizers to deliver isoflurane or halothane has become very uncommon in recent years, however, and will not be commonly encountered by the veterinary anesthetist.

## USE OF NONPRECISION VAPORIZERS

In a nonprecision vaporizer, the concentration of the anesthetic delivered to the patient is unknown because the vaporizer control dial settings ("0" through "10" for the Ohio, and "Off" to "On" with the distance between divided into eighths for the Stevens) are unrelated to specific anesthetic percentages. The anesthetist varies the relative amount of anesthetic delivered to the patient by turning the control dial, based on the patient's depth of anesthesia. When these vaporizers are used, the exact output at any given setting varies, is not known, and is influenced by a number of factors discussed in the next section.

## SAFETY

Nonprecision vaporizers are located in the breathing circuit (VIC) and do not compensate for changes in temperature, carrier gas flow rates, or back pressure. These factors have several serious implications that must be understood by the anesthetist using this type of vaporizer, so that appropriate adjustments can be made in the control dial position to compensate.

### Lack of Temperature Compensation

At any given setting the vaporizer will deliver a greater concentration of anesthetic if located in a warm room than if located in a cold room. In contrast, vaporizer output will decrease in response to the drop in temperature that occurs at high carrier gas flow rates. Therefore any change in temperature of the liquid anesthetic will change vaporizer output and consequently patient anesthetic depth.

### Lack of Flow Compensation

The amount of anesthetic delivered to the patient will increase if the patient's ventilation or carrier gas flow rate is increased because either of these situations will increase the flow of gas through the anesthetic chamber, which in turn will increase vaporization.

## Lack of Back-Pressure Compensation

Any buildup of pressure within the breathing circuit (as may occur when the patient is bagged, the $O_2$ flush valve is activated, or a ventilator is used) may result in increased concentration of anesthetic being delivered to the patient and may result in excessive anesthetic depth. Manual or mechanical ventilation is therefore more challenging when used with nonprecision vaporizers. The anesthetist must ensure that the vaporizer setting is greatly reduced (or in some cases turned off) when bagging the animal or when using a ventilator. In contrast, when using a precision out-of-circuit vaporizer [VOC], it is not normally necessary to turn the vaporizer off when bagging the patient because of the back-pressure compensation.

## Need for Vigilant Monitoring

The use of a nonprecision vaporizer to deliver a high–vapor pressure anesthetic such as isoflurane results in less precise control over anesthetic depth than does use of a standard precision vaporizer. Close monitoring of the patient is essential, particularly during the first 5 minutes of anesthesia, when patient depth increases rapidly.

## Inability to Use Non-Rebreathing Systems

Non-rebreathing systems are difficult to adapt to machines with nonprecision vaporizers because they require the use of a VOC.

# Procedure for Operation of a Closed Rebreathing System

A closed rebreathing system (also called a *total rebreathing system*) is one in which the pop-off valve can be kept nearly or completely closed and the flow of oxygen is relatively low, providing only the volume necessary to meet the patient's metabolic needs. If a closed (total) rebreathing system is used, the anesthetist should take the following steps to ensure patient safety:

- In a closed rebreathing system the oxygen flow rate is low, so any loss of oxygen or its dilution by room air may be detrimental. The pop-off valve is therefore nearly or completely closed, to prevent oxygen escape.
- Check the machine for leaks before use. If leaks are present, oxygen may escape from the circuit and room air may leak into and dilute the oxygen in the circuit.
- Induction is the most challenging period of anesthesia when low oxygen flows are used. The reservoir bag should be emptied and filled with oxygen 2 to 3 times during the first 15 minutes of anesthesia and every 30 minutes thereafter to help prevent patient hypoxemia and to eliminate nitrogen ($N_2$) that is being exhaled by the patient (a process known as *denitrogenization*). Alternatively, the anesthetist may provide 5 to 10 minutes of high oxygen flow (200 mL/kg/min) at the start of anesthesia, until the patient reaches a surgical plane. The pop-off valve should be open when high flow rates are used. This flushes room air out of the system and replaces it with oxygen. Thereafter, much lower flow rates (5 to 10 mL/kg/min for small animals and 3-5 mL/kg/min for large animals) can be used, and the pop-off valve should be nearly or completely closed. This amount of oxygen will meet the metabolic oxygen requirements of the anesthetized patient.
- Closely monitor the reservoir bag. If there is a leak in the system, if the pop-off valve is too far open, or if the flow rate of oxygen is inadequate, the bag will not remain inflated. On the other hand, if the fresh gas flow exceeds the patient's demand for oxygen and anesthetic (which can occur if the patient is too deeply anesthetized, the patient is too cold, or any other factor reduces patient demand for oxygen), the bag will become distended. In this case, after the patient has been checked and it is apparent that no other problems

exist, either the oxygen flow rate should be reduced or the pop-off valve should be opened. In any case, it is wise to leave the pop-off valve slightly open during low-flow anesthesia, in case pressure in the circuit rises and excess gas must be vented.
- It may be difficult to change the patient's anesthetic depth quickly. If a rapid change in anesthetic depth is required, the vaporizer setting should be changed and the breathing system converted to a semiclosed (partial) rebreathing system by increasing the oxygen flow rate and opening the pop-off valve. If low oxygen flow rates are maintained, changes in the vaporizer setting may not affect the concentration of anesthetic in the circuit for many minutes.
- If a precision out-of-circuit vaporizer is used for low-flow, closed-circuit anesthesia, the setting required during the maintenance period will often be well above the setting normally used to maintain surgical anesthesia with a semiclosed rebreathing system, at least until a state of equilibrium is reached (in which the concentration of anesthetic in the brain and blood is equal to the concentration of anesthetic in the circuit). In a closed system this may take a considerable period of time to occur, owing to the low gas flow rate (see Box 4-2).
- In contrast, if an in-circuit nonprecision vaporizer is used for low-flow, closed-circuit anesthesia, the required vaporizer setting will usually be lower than that used for a semiclosed rebreathing system. This is because the fresh gas flow is not adequate to dilute the anesthetic in the circuit.
- The low oxygen flow rates used in a closed rebreathing system may be inadequate for accurate delivery of anesthetic by some vaporizers. Consult the vaporizer manual for minimum recommended flow rates, and be aware that the anesthetic concentration indicated by the dial may be incorrect at lower flows. Closed rebreathing systems should not be used at all with certain vaporizers, including the Fluothane Tek-2, Copper Kettle, and Vernitrol.
- The low oxygen flow rates in a closed system are unsuitable for use with a Bain coaxial circuit or other non-rebreathing system.

# Appendix E

## Standard Volumes, Weights, Measures, and Equivalents

---

## METRIC SYSTEM

### Prefixes

| | | |
|---|---|---|
| "kilo" | *means* | One thousand |
| "milli" | *means* | One thousandth |
| "micro" | *means* | One thousandth of one thousandth, or one millionth |

### Weight to Volume Equivalents

1 gram (g) = the weight of 1 cc (cubic centimeter) of water at 4 degrees centigrade

### Volume Equivalents

| | | |
|---|---|---|
| 1 cc | = | 1 milliliter (mL) |
| 1000 mL *or* cc | = | 1 liter (L) |
| 1 mL *or* cc | = | 0.001 L |
| 1 deciliter (dL) | = | 100 mL |

### Weight Equivalents

| | | |
|---|---|---|
| 1000 microgram (mcg) | = | 1 milligram (mg) |
| 1 mcg | = | 0.001 mg |
| 1000 mg | = | 1 gram (g) |
| 1 mg | = | 0.001 g |
| 1 million mcg | = | 1 g |
| 1000 g | = | 1 kilogram (kg) |
| 1 g | = | 0.001 kg |

### Solution Equivalents

| | | |
|---|---|---|
| 1 part in 10 (1:10) | = | 10% (1 mL contains 100 mg) |
| 1 part in 100 (1:100) | = | 1% (1 mL contains 10 mg) |
| 1 part in 500 (1:500) | = | 0.20% (1 mL contains 2 mg) |
| 1 part in 1000 (1:1000) | = | 0.10% (1 mL contains 1 mg) |
| 1 part in 5000 (1:5000) | = | 0.02% (1 mL contains 0.2 mg) |
| 1 part in 10,000 (1:10,000) | = | 0.01% (1 mL contains 0.1 mg) |

The number of milligrams in 1 mL of any solution of known percentage strength is obtained by moving the decimal one place to the right. For example, a 1% solution contains 10 mg/mL. By definition, a percent solution contains the specified weight (in grams) of the solute in 100 mL of total solution. For example, a 5% dextrose and water solution contains 5 g of dextrose dissolved in each 100 mL of water.

### Metric to Household Equivalents

#### Weight

| | | | | | | | |
|---|---|---|---|---|---|---|---|
| 1 kg | = | 2.2 avoirdupois or imperial pounds | | | | | |
| 1 oz | = | 0.0625 lb | = | 28.4 (~30) g | = | ~0.03 kg | |
| 1 lb | = | 16 oz | = | 453.6 g | = | 0.454 kg | |

#### Volume

| | | | | |
|---|---|---|---|---|
| 1 liter | = | 1.06 U.S. quarts | = | 33.8 fluid ounces |
| 1 U.S. pint | = | 473.2 mL | | |
| 1 quart | = | 946.4 mL | | |

#### Length

| | | | | |
|---|---|---|---|---|
| 1 meter (m) | = | 39.37 inches (in) | | |
| 1 in | = | $\frac{1}{12}$ ft | = | 2.54 centimeters (cm) |

### Pressure Equivalents

#### Pressure

| | | | | |
|---|---|---|---|---|
| 1 lb/in$^2$ (psi) | = | 51.7 mm of mercury (Hg) | = | 70.3 cm of water (H$_2$O) |
| 1 mm Hg | = | 1.36 cm H$_2$O | | |
| 1 cm H$_2$O | = | 0.736 mm Hg | | |
| 1 atmosphere | = | 760 mm Hg = 14.7 psi = 100 kilopascals (kPa) | | |

---

## CONVERSION TABLES

Note: The conversions in each table are calculated using the rounded conversion factors noted and are therefore approximate. All conversions except for gas pressures in kPa and body weights over 100 kg are rounded to one decimal place.

## Conversion Table for a Pressure Manometer (cm H₂O to mm Hg)

Pressure (mm Hg) = Pressure (cm $H_2O$)/1.36

| cm $H_2O$ | mm Hg | cm $H_2O$ | mm Hg |
|---|---|---|---|
| 1 | 0.7 | 25 | 18.4 |
| 2 | 1.5 | 30 | 22.1 |
| 3 | 2.2 | 35 | 25.7 |
| 4 | 2.9 | 40 | 29.4 |
| 5 | 3.7 | 45 | 33.1 |
| 6 | 4.4 | 50 | 36.8 |
| 7 | 5.1 | 55 | 40.4 |
| 8 | 5.9 | 60 | 44.1 |
| 9 | 6.6 | 70 | 51.5 |
| 10 | 7.4 | 80 | 58.8 |
| 15 | 11.0 | 90 | 66.2 |
| 20 | 14.7 | 100 | 73.5 |

## Conversion Table for Gas Pressure in a Compressed Gas Cylinder (psi to kPa)

Pressure (kPa) = Pressure (psi) × 6.895

| psi | kPa | psi | kPa |
|---|---|---|---|
| 1 | 7 | 500 | 3448 |
| 5 | 34 | 600 | 4137 |
| 10 | 69 | 700 | 4827 |
| 15 | 103 | 800 | 5516 |
| 20 | 138 | 900 | 6206 |
| 30 | 207 | 1000 | 6895 |
| 40 | 276 | 1100 | 7585 |
| 50 | 345 | 1500 | 10343 |
| 100 | 690 | 2000 | 13790 |
| 200 | 1379 | 2200 | 15169 |
| 300 | 2069 | 2500 | 17238 |
| 400 | 2758 | 3000 | 20685 |

## Conversion Table for Endotracheal Tube and Catheter Internal Diameter (French to mm)

Internal diameter (French) = Internal diameter (mm) × 3

| French | mm | French | mm | French | mm |
|---|---|---|---|---|---|
| 1 | 0.3 | 9 | 3.0 | 40 | 13.3 |
| 1.5 | 0.5 | 10 | 3.3 | 45 | 15.0 |
| 2 | 0.7 | 12 | 4.0 | 50 | 16.7 |
| 2.5 | 0.8 | 14 | 4.7 | 55 | 18.3 |
| 3 | 1.0 | 16 | 5.3 | 60 | 20.0 |
| 3.5 | 1.2 | 18 | 6.0 | 65 | 21.7 |
| 4 | 1.3 | 20 | 6.7 | 70 | 23.3 |
| 4.5 | 1.5 | 22 | 7.3 | 75 | 25.0 |
| 5 | 1.7 | 24 | 8.0 | 80 | 26.7 |
| 5.5 | 1.8 | 26 | 8.7 | 85 | 28.3 |
| 6 | 2.0 | 28 | 9.3 | 90 | 30.0 |
| 7 | 2.3 | 30 | 10.0 | 95 | 31.7 |
| 8 | 2.7 | 35 | 11.7 | 100 | 33.3 |

## Conversion Table for Body Temperature (°F to °C)

Fahrenheit to Centigrade: °C = (°F − 32) × 5/9
Centigrade to Fahrenheit: °F = (°C × 9/5) + 32

| °F | °C | °F | °C | °F | °C |
|---|---|---|---|---|---|
| 32 | 0.0 | 92 | 33.3 | 102 | 38.9 |
| 68 | 20.0 | 93 | 33.9 | 103 | 39.4 |
| 84 | 28.9 | 94 | 34.4 | 104 | 40.0 |
| 85 | 29.4 | 95 | 35.0 | 105 | 40.6 |
| 86 | 30.0 | 96 | 35.6 | 106 | 41.1 |
| 87 | 30.6 | 97 | 36.1 | 107 | 41.7 |
| 88 | 31.1 | 98 | 36.7 | 108 | 42.2 |
| 89 | 31.7 | 99 | 37.2 | 109 | 42.8 |
| 90 | 32.2 | 100 | 37.8 | 110 | 43.3 |
| 91 | 32.8 | 101 | 38.3 | 212 | 100.0 |

## Conversion Table for Body Weight (lb to kg)

Body weight (kg) = Body weight (lb)/2.2

| lb | kg | lb | kg | lb | kg | lb | kg | lb | kg | lb | kg |
|----|----|----|----|----|----|----|----|----|----|----|----|
| 1 | 0.5 | 11 | 5.0 | 22 | 10.0 | 42 | 19.1 | 80 | 36.4 | 400 | 182 |
| 2 | 0.9 | 12 | 5.5 | 24 | 10.9 | 44 | 20.0 | 85 | 38.6 | 450 | 205 |
| 3 | 1.4 | 13 | 5.9 | 26 | 11.8 | 46 | 20.9 | 90 | 40.9 | 500 | 227 |
| 4 | 1.8 | 14 | 6.4 | 28 | 12.7 | 48 | 21.8 | 95 | 43.2 | 600 | 273 |
| 5 | 2.3 | 15 | 6.8 | 30 | 13.6 | 50 | 22.7 | 100 | 45.5 | 700 | 318 |
| 6 | 2.7 | 16 | 7.3 | 32 | 14.5 | 55 | 25.0 | 150 | 68.2 | 800 | 364 |
| 7 | 3.2 | 17 | 7.7 | 34 | 15.5 | 60 | 27.3 | 200 | 90.9 | 900 | 409 |
| 8 | 3.6 | 18 | 8.2 | 36 | 16.4 | 65 | 29.5 | 250 | 114 | 1000 | 455 |
| 9 | 4.1 | 19 | 8.6 | 38 | 17.3 | 70 | 31.8 | 300 | 136 | 1500 | 682 |
| 10 | 4.5 | 20 | 9.1 | 40 | 18.2 | 75 | 34.1 | 350 | 159 | 2000 | 909 |

# Appendix F

## Equipment and Drugs for Use in an Emergency Crash Kit

The following list of equipment and supplies may be altered depending on the veterinarian's preference. Some supplies (e.g., laryngoscope, Ambu bag, sterile fluids) that are easily accessible within the clinical setting may be omitted from the kit.

### IV Access and Injections
Needles: 18 to 25 gauge
Syringes: 1 to 60 mL
Over-the-needle catheters 24 to 18 gauge
IV catheter plugs
Bone marrow biopsy needle for IO access
Spinal needle
Surgical gloves sizes 6½-8 (2 of each size)

### Miscellaneous Supplies
Sterile water soluble lubricant
Sterile swabs (1 package)
Sterile 3×3 gauge sponges (2 packs of 20)
Tongue depressors (quantity 5)
Trocar catheter chest tube
18 Fr red rubber catheter (for chest tube)
12 Fr red rubber catheter
Umbilical tape
Penrose drain

### Bandaging Materials
1" and ½" porous tape (1 of each)
2" elastic gauge (quantity 3)
2" cohesive bandage (quantity 3)

### Airway Supplies
3 ×3 gauge sponges (quantity—at least 20)
Sponge forceps or Allis tissue forceps
Endotracheal tubes (ID 3-11 mm; whole sizes only)
Stylette for ET tubes
Laryngoscope with charged batteries
Laryngoscope blades (small, medium, and large)
2" length of IV tubing (to tie in ET tubes)
Cuffing syringe
Mouth gags (1 small and 1 large)
Tracheal cannula (made of macrodrip set)
Anesthetic masks (small, medium, and large)
Ambu bag
3.5, 5, 8, and 10 Fr polypropylene urinary catheters

### Oxygen Source
E-tank with at least 500 psi
Pressure-reducing valve and flow control for
oxygen tank

*Note:* A list of emergency drug doses should be posted or included in the kit.

# GLOSSARY

**Activated charcoal cartridge:** A type of passive scavenging system, consisting of a canister containing activated charcoal, designed to remove halogenated anesthetic agents from gases exiting from the pop-off or pressure-limiting valve of a breathing circuit.

**Adjunct:** A drug that is not a true anesthetic but that is used during anesthesia to produce other desired effects such as sedation, muscle relaxation, analgesia, reversal, neuromuscular blockade, or parasympathetic blockade.

**Agonal:** An abnormal breathing pattern seen during cardiopulmonary arrest, characterized by gasping and labored breathing.

**Agonist:** A drug that binds to and stimulates tissue receptors.

**Agonist-antagonist:** A drug that binds to more than one receptor type, simultaneously stimulating at least one and blocking at least one.

**Algesia:** Sensitivity to pain.

**Ambu bag:** A brand name of a self-inflating reservoir bag used to provide manual ventilation when an anesthetic machine is not available.

**Analeptic agent:** A drug that causes general central nervous system stimulation.

**Analgesia:** Absence of pain.

**Anatomic dead space:** *See Dead space*

**Anesthesia:** A loss of sensation.

**Anesthetic agent:** Any drug used to induce a loss of sensation with or without unconsciousness.

**Anesthetic chamber:** A clear, aquarium-like box used to induce general anesthesia in small patients that are feral, vicious, or intractable or that cannot be handled without undue stress.

**Anesthetic induction:** The process by which an animal loses consciousness and enters general anesthesia.

**Anesthetic maintenance:** The process of keeping a patient in a state of general anesthesia. The period between induction and recovery.

**Anesthetic mask:** A cone-shaped device, ideally made of transparent material, used to administer oxygen and anesthetic gases to nonintubated patients via the nose and mouth. Also used to administer pure oxygen to dyspneic, hypoxic, or other critically ill patients requiring supplemental oxygen.

**Anesthetic protocol:** A list of the anesthetic agents and adjuncts prescribed for a particular patient including doses, routes and order of administration.

**Anesthetic recovery:** The period between the time the anesthetic is discontinued and the time the animal is able to stand and walk without assistance.

**Anesthetic vaporizer:** The anesthetic machine system that vaporizes liquid inhalant anesthetic and mixes it with the carrier gases. Vaporizers are classified as precision or nonprecision and vaporizer-out-of-circuit (VOC) or vaporizer-in-circuit (VIC).

**Antagonist:** A drug that binds to but does not stimulate receptors.

**Anticholinergic:** An adjunct that lessens parasympathetic effects by blocking muscarinic receptors of the parasympathetic nervous system. Also known as a *parasympatholytic.*

**Apnea:** A temporary absence of spontaneous breathing.

**Apnea monitor:** A monitor used to alert the anesthetist when the patient has not taken a breath within a set period of time (e.g., 10, 20, or 30 seconds). Detects a change in the temperature of the air moving between the endotracheal tube and the breathing circuit as the patient breathes.

**Apneustic respiration:** A breathing pattern, most often seen during dissociative anesthesia, in which there is a pause for several seconds at the end of the inspiratory phase, followed by a short, quick expiratory phase.

**Asphyxiation:** The act of cutting off the supply of oxygen; suffocation.

**Assisted ventilation:** A type of ventilation in which the anesthetist ensures that an adequate volume of air is delivered to the patient, although the patient initiates each inspiration.

**Ataxia:** Inability to coordinate movement.

**Atelectasis:** Collapse of a portion or all of one or both lungs.

**Auscultate:** To listen to sounds made by internal organs with a stethoscope, especially the heart and lungs.

**Ayre's T-piece:** A non-rebreathing circuit with a fresh gas inlet entering at the patient end of the breathing tube at a 90-degree angle (like the base of the letter T) and without a reservoir bag at the opposite end of the breathing tube; Mapleson E circuit.

**Bagging:** Inflating the patient's lungs by squeezing the reservoir bag. Manual, positive-pressure ventilation.

**Bain coaxial circuit (Bain circuit):** A non-rebreathing circuit with a "tube within a tube" configuration that discharges fresh gas at the patient end of the breathing tube. Both the overflow valve and the reservoir bag are located away from the patient at the opposite end of the breathing tube; modified Mapleson D circuit.

**Balanced anesthesia:** Administration of multiple drugs concurrently in smaller quantities than would be required if each were given alone, to produce sedation, tranquilization, muscle relaxation, analgesia, or a variety of other effects needed for a particular patient.

**Blood gas analysis:** Measurement of the pH, bicarbonate level, and partial pressure of oxygen and carbon dioxide in the blood (most often arterial blood obtained via an intraarterial catheter).

**Blood pressure:** BP; The force exerted by flowing blood on vessel walls.

**Body condition score:** A numeric assessment of the patient's body weight compared with the ideal body weight.

**Bolus:** A pharmaceutical in the form of a large solid tablet or mass for oral administration; a relatively large volume of a liquid pharmaceutical for intravenous administration all at once; or a large mass of food ready to be swallowed.

**Borborygmus:** Intestinal noises audible with or without a stethoscope, caused by gas moving through the intestinal tract.

**Breathing circuit:** The anesthetic machine system that conveys the carrier gases and inhalant anesthetic to the patient and removes exhaled carbon dioxide. Breathing circuits are classified as rebreathing circuits or non-rebreathing circuits.

**Breathing tubes:** Corrugated tubes that complete a rebreathing circuit by carrying the anesthetic gases to and from the patient. Each tube is connected to a unidirectional valve at one end and to the Y-piece at the other end.

**Cachexia:** Weight loss, loss of muscle mass, and general debilitation that may accompany chronic diseases.

**Calculated oxygen content:** The total volume of oxygen in the blood including both dissolved and bound forms (expressed in milliliters per deciliter). $CaO_2$ = Calculated oxygen content in arterial blood. Arterial oxygen content is calculated using the following formula: $CaO_2 =$ (Hb $\times$ 1.39 $\times$ $SaO_2/100$) + ($PaO_2 \times$ 0.003), where Hb = hemoglobin in grams per deciliter, $SaO_2$ = oxygen saturation, and $PaO_2$ = partial pressure of oxygen.

**Capnogram:** The graphic representation of $CO_2$ levels generated by a capnograph.

**Capnograph:** Also known as an *end-tidal $CO_2$ monitor.* A monitoring device that measures the amount of $CO_2$ in the air that is breathed in and out by the patient, by sampling air passing between the endotracheal tube connector and the breathing circuit.

**Carbon dioxide absorber canister:** The part of a rebreathing circuit that holds the carbon dioxide absorbent granules. These granules, primarily made of calcium hydroxide, remove expired $CO_2$.

**Cardiac arrhythmia:** Any pattern of cardiac electrical activity that differs from that of the healthy awake animal.

**Cardiac output:** CO; Total blood flow from the heart per unit time.

**Catabolic state:** A metabolic state in which the rate of catabolism (the breakdown of body tissues and substances into simple molecules) exceeds the rate of anabolism (the synthesis of body tissues and substances from simple molecules).

**Cataleptoid state:** A state produced by dissociative agents, in which a patient does not respond to external stimuli and has a variable degree of muscle rigidity.

**Cauda equina:** A group of nerves located at the caudal termination of the spinal cord in the spinal canal. So called because they visually resemble a horse's tail.

**Central nervous system hypersensitivity:** A state, caused by constant nociceptive input from the periphery, in which neurons in the spinal cord become hyperexcitable and sensitive to low-intensity stimuli that would not normally elicit a pain response. Also referred to as *windup.*

**Central nervous system vital centers:** Areas of the brain that control cardiovascular function, respiratory function, and thermoregulation.

**Central venous pressure:** CVP; The blood pressure in a large central vein such as the anterior vena cava. Used to assess blood return to the heart and heart function.

**Closed rebreathing system:** A rebreathing system in which the pop-off valve is kept nearly or completely closed and the flow of oxygen is relatively low, providing only the volume necessary to meet the patient's metabolic needs.

**Colic:** Severe abdominal pain of sudden onset caused by a variety of conditions including obstruction, twisting, or spasm of the intestinal tract.

**Colloids:** Large–molecular-weight plasma proteins that provide oncotic pressure.

**Comatose:** In a sleeplike state. Unresponsive to all stimuli including pain.

**Common gas outlet:** The point where the oxygen, inhalant anesthetic, and $N_2O$, if used, exit the anesthetic machine on the way to the breathing circuit.

**Compressed gas cylinder:** A container that holds a large volume of highly pressurized gas. Oxygen, nitrous oxide, medical air, and carbon dioxide are stored in compressed gas cylinders.

**Compressed gas supply:** The anesthetic machine system that supplies carrier gases (oxygen and sometimes nitrous oxide).

**Consent form:** A form signed by the client confirming that he or she has been told about and understands the nature of the procedure to be performed, including the risks involved. Commonly includes a statement releasing the VIC, the hospital, and other health care providers from responsibility for uncontrollable outcomes.

**Constant rate infusion:** CRI; Slow continuous administration of a drug at a rate sufficient to achieve the desired effect.

**Controlled ventilation:** A type of ventilation in which the anesthetist controls the respiratory rate, the tidal volume, and the peak inspiratory pressure. In this type of ventilation, the patient does not make spontaneous respiratory efforts.

**Cortisol:** A natural steroid hormone, secreted by the adrenal cortex, which plays a role in protein, carbohydrate, and fat metabolism.

**Crystalloids:** Fluids that contain water and small–molecular-weight solutes (such as NaCl) and that pass freely through vascular endothelium.

**Cyanosis:** Blue discoloration of the mucous membranes.

**Dead space:** The breathing passages and tubes that convey fresh oxygen from the source (the atmosphere or the breathing circuit) to the alveoli, but in which no gas exchange can occur. *Anatomic dead space* includes the bronchi, trachea, larynx, pharynx, and nasal cavity. *Mechanical dead space* includes the Y-piece of the breathing circuit, where there is bidirectional flow of gases, and the portion of the endotracheal tube extending beyond the nose or the Y-piece and face mask.

**Debilitated:** Lacking strength; weak.

**Demand valve:** A valve attached to the endotracheal tube during anesthetic recovery that is used to deliver oxygen to the patient at a high flow rate.

**Diastolic blood pressure:** Arterial blood pressure when the heart is in its resting phase between contractions. (Compare with *Systolic blood pressure.*)

**Diffusion hypoxia:** A decrease in the concentration of oxygen in the alveoli after discontinuation of nitrous oxide administration. Caused by the sudden diffusion of nitrous oxide into the alveoli from the blood.

**Distress:** An extreme form of stress that leads to anxiety and suffering.

**Doppler blood flow detector:** A monitoring device that uses ultrasound frequency to convert the motion of red blood cells in small arteries into an audible "whooshing" sound. Used to monitor pulse rate and, if used in conjunction with a sphygmomanometer, systolic blood pressure.

**Dysphoria:** Anxiety, uneasiness, and restlessness most often produced by opioids; the opposite of euphoria.

**Dyspnea:** Difficult or labored breathing.

**Ecchymoses:** Large bruises. Discolorations of the skin or mucous membranes caused by leakage of blood into the tissues.

**Emergence delirium:** Disorientation that occurs during anesthetic recovery as consciousness returns. May be characterized by vocalization, aggression, thrashing, and locomotor activity.

**Enantiomer:** A mixture of two molecules that are mirror images of one another. The dextrorotatory enantiomer is a molecule that rotates the plane of polarized light to the right, and the levorotatory molecule rotates it to the left.

**Endotracheal tube:** ET tube; A flexible tube placed inside the trachea of an anesthetized patient and used to transfer anesthetic gases directly from the breathing circuit into the patient's trachea, bypassing the oral and nasal cavities, pharynx, and larynx.

**End-tidal CO$_2$ monitor:** *See Capnograph.*

**Epidural anesthesia:** Regional anesthesia produced by injection of a local anesthetic or analgesic into the epidural space surrounding the spinal cord.

**Epistaxis:** Nosebleed.

**Eructate:** Eject gas from the stomach; burp. Used most commonly in reference to ruminants.

**Esophageal stethoscope:** A monitoring device used to detect and amplify heart sounds via a catheter placed in the esophagus.

**Eutectic mixture:** A mixture of two substances with a melting point that is lower than the individual melting points. In the case of lidocaine and prilocaine, which are both solids at room temperature, mixture of the two drugs results in an oil that has a melting point of 16° C.

**Extra-label drug use:** The use of an approved drug in a manner that is not in accordance with the approved label directions.

**Fasciculation:** Involuntary muscle twitching.

**Field anesthesia:** General anesthesia performed away from the veterinary hospital at a farm or stable. Used most commonly for short procedures (20 to 45 minutes) in large animal patients.

**Flaccid:** Lacking any muscle tone.

**Flow meter:** A glass cylinder of graduated diameter that indicates carrier gas flow expressed in liters of gas per minute (L/min). Reduces the pressure of the gas in the intermediate-pressure line from about 50 psi (about 345 kPa) to 15 psi (about 100 kPa).

**Fresh gas inlet:** The point at which the carrier and anesthetic gases enter the breathing circuit.

**Functional residual volume:** The amount of air left in the lungs after expiration.

**Gastric dilatation–volvulus:** A dangerous gastrointestinal condition, occurring primarily in deep-chested large breed dogs, in which the stomach swells with air and twists on its long axis, leading to shock, loss of blood supply, and other serious consequences.

**General anesthesia:** A reversible state of unconsciousness, immobility, muscle relaxation, and loss of sensation throughout the entire body produced by administration of one or more anesthetic agents.

**Homeostasis:** A constant state within the body created and maintained by normal physiologic processes.

**Hypercarbia:** Elevated carbon dioxide levels in the blood.

**Hypnosis:** A sleeplike state from which the patient can be aroused with sufficient stimulation.

**Hypostatic congestion:** Pooling of blood in the dependent lung and tissues (those nearest the floor or table).

**Hypotension:** Low blood pressure; the opposite of hypertension.

**Hypothermia:** Low body temperature; the opposite of hyperthermia.

**Hypoventilation:** Slow and/or shallow ventilation, resulting in decreased minute volume; the opposite of hyperventilation.

**Hypoxemia:** Low blood oxygen level.

**Hypoxia:** Low tissue oxygen level.

**Icterus:** Yellow discoloration of the skin and mucous membranes.

**Idiopathic pain:** Pain of unknown or unidentifiable cause.

**Ileus:** Intestinal obstruction caused by inhibition of bowel motility; also referred to as *gastrointestinal stasis.*

**Infiltration:** Injection of local anesthetic into tissues, often in proximity to a nerve.

**Inotropy:** Force of heart muscle contraction.

**Insufflation:** Provision of oxygen by placement of an oxygen supply tube inside an endotracheal tube, nasopharyngeal tube, or nostril.

**Intact:** Possessing gonads. Not spayed or castrated.

**Intermittent mandatory ventilation:** Positive pressure ventilation throughout the entire anesthetic period as the sole source of the patient's ventilatory needs.

**Jackson-Rees circuit:** A non-rebreathing circuit with a fresh gas inlet at the patient end of the breathing tube and a reservoir bag at the opposite end. The fresh gas inlet enters the breathing tube at a 45- to 90-degree angle; Mapleson F circuit.

**Laryngoscope:** A device consisting of a handle, a blade, and a light source; used to increase visibility of the larynx during placement of an endotracheal tube.

**Laryngospasm:** A reflexive closure of the glottis in response to contact with any object or substance.

**Lethargic:** Depressed but able to be aroused with minimal difficulty.

**Level of consciousness:** The patient's responsiveness to stimuli. How easily the patient can be aroused. Often used to assess brain function.

**Line block:** Injection of a continuous line of local anesthetic in the subcutaneous or subcuticular tissues immediately proximal to the target area.

**Line pressure gauge:** A gauge that indicates the pressure in the intermediate-pressure gas line between the pressure-reducing valve and the flow meters.

**Local anesthesia:** A loss of sensation in a small area of the body produced by administration of a local anesthetic agent in proximity to the area of interest.

**Locomotor:** Relating to movement from place to place.

**Magill circuit:** A non-rebreathing circuit with an overflow valve at the patient end of the breathing tube. Both the fresh gas inlet and the reservoir bag are located away from the patient at the opposite end of the breathing tube; Mapleson A circuit.

**Manual ventilation:** Forced delivery of oxygen and anesthetic gases by squeezing of the reservoir bag of the anesthetic machine. May be used to provide periodic or intermittent mandatory ventilation.

**Mapleson circuit:** Any one of a number of non-rebreathing circuits as classified by WW Mapleson, in which the position of the fresh gas inlet, the reservoir bag, and the pressure-limiting valve varies.

**Mapleson classification system:** A system developed by W.W. Mapleson that is used to classify non-rebreathing circuits based on the position of the fresh gas inlet, the reservoir bag and the pressure-limiting valve.

**Mean arterial pressure:** MAP; The average arterial blood pressure. It may be calculated using the following equation: MAP = Diastolic pressure + ⅓ (Systolic pressure − Diastolic pressure).

**Mechanical dead space:** *See Dead space*

**Mechanical ventilation:** Forced delivery of oxygen and anesthetic gases by use of a mechanical ventilator. Usually used to provide intermittent mandatory ventilation.

**Mediators:** Chemical substances released from damaged cells or inflammatory cells that cause a response (such as increasing the sensitivity of peripheral pain receptors).

**Minimum patient database:** A compilation of pertinent information from the patient history, physical examination, and diagnostic tests. Used to diagnose and manage a case.

**Miosis:** Constriction of the pupil of the eye; opposite of mydriasis.

**Modulation:** The third step in nociception, in which sensory nerve impulses are amplified or suppressed by other neurons.

**Morbidity:** The incidence of disease.

**Moribund:** Near death.

**Mortality:** The death rate.

**Motor neuron:** A neuron that conveys impulses from the brain to muscle fibers and is responsible for initiating and controlling voluntary movements.

**Multimodal therapy:** Treatment of pain with analgesics that target two or more types of pain receptors.

**Mydriasis:** Dilatation of the pupil of the eye; opposite of miosis.

**Myopathy:** Muscle disease. In the context of anesthesia, this term refers to muscle damage caused by excessive pressure on dependent muscle tissue or insufficient blood flow to muscle tissue during the intraoperative period in large animals, particularly horses. Manifests during recovery as muscle hardness, pain, and weakness. Also known by the lay term "tying up."

**Narcosis:** A drug-induced sleep from which the patient is not easily aroused and that is most often associated with the administration of narcotics.

**Nerve block:** Loss of sensation in a particular anatomic site, produced by injection of local anesthetic in proximity to a nerve.

**Neuromuscular blocker:** An adjunct used to relax or paralyze skeletal muscles as a part of balanced anesthesia.

**Neuropathic pain:** Pain resulting from injury of a nerve.

**Neuropathy:** Disease or injury of a peripheral nerve.

**NIOSH:** National Institute for Occupational Safety and Health. The U.S. federal agency responsible for conducting research and making recommendations for the prevention of work-related injury and illness.

**Nociception:** Detection by the nervous system of the potential for or actual tissue injury.

**Non-rebreathing system:** An anesthetic machine fitted with a non-rebreathing circuit. In this system little or no exhaled gases are returned to the patient but are instead removed from the circuit by use of appropriately high flow rates of carrier gas and evacuated by a scavenger connected to a pressure-limiting valve or other exit port. Used most commonly for patients under 2.5 to 3 kg in body weight.

**Norman mask elbow:** A non-rebreathing circuit with a fresh gas inlet at the patient end of the breathing tube and a reservoir bag at the opposite end. The fresh gas inlet enters the breathing tube at a 45- to 90-degree angle, and the endotracheal tube connector is at right angles to the breathing tube; Mapleson F circuit.

**Noxious:** Painful or physically harmful.

**Nystagmus:** A rhythmic, involuntary oscillation of both eyes.

**Obtunded:** Depressed and unable to be fully aroused.

**Oncotic pressure:** Osmotic pressure provided by large–molecular-weight colloids such as albumin.

**Opisthotonus:** A severe spasm in which the back arches and the feet and head flex dorsally. Has several causes including drug reactions and brain lesions.

**Oscillometer:** A monitoring device used to measure systolic, mean, and diastolic blood pressure by detecting and analyzing pulsations of blood in the arteries of an extremity.

**OSHA:** Occupational Safety and Health Administration. U.S. federal agency responsible for ensuring a safe and healthful working environment for working men and women.

**Osmolarity:** A measurement of the number of dissolved solute particles per unit water in body fluids. Usually expressed as osmoles or milliosmoles per liter (mOsm/L) of water.

**Osmotic pressure:** The pressure required to prevent water flow through a semipermeable membrane from a region of lower solute concentration to a region of higher solute concentration.

**Oxygen flush valve:** A button or lever that rapidly delivers a large volume of pure oxygen (at a flow rate of 35 to 75 L/min) directly to the common gas outlet or breathing circuit of a rebreathing system, bypassing the anesthetic vaporizer and oxygen flow meters.

**Pain:** An aversive sensory and emotional experience that elicits protective motor actions, results in learned avoidance, and may modify species-specific behavior.

**Pain scale:** Any assessment tool used to rate the intensity of pain.

**Paralysis:** Inability to move a particular muscle group or body part such as a limb because of loss of nerve function. May also involve a loss of sensation in the affected part.

**Parasympatholytic:** *See Anticholinergic.*

**Paresis:** Weakness of a body part caused by loss of nerve function. Partial paralysis.

**Partial agonist:** A drug that binds to and partially stimulates tissue receptors.

**Partial pressure of oxygen:** $Po_2$; A measurement of the unbound $O_2$ molecules dissolved in the plasma expressed in millimeters of mercury (mm Hg). $Pao_2 = Po_2$ in arterial blood; $Pvo_2 = Po_2$ in venous blood.

**Pathologic pain:** Pain that occurs after tissue injury.

**Percent oxygen saturation:** $So_2$; A measurement of the percentage of the total hemoglobin binding sites occupied by oxygen molecules. $Sao_2 = So_2$ in arterial blood; $Svo_2 = So_2$ in venous blood; $Spo_2 = So_2$ as measured by a pulse oximeter; $Sto_2 = So_2$ in the tissues.

**Perception:** The final step of nociception, in which sensory impulses are transmitted to the brain, where they are processed and recognized.

**Perioperative analgesia:** Pain control before and/or after surgery.

**Petechiae:** Small or pinpoint purple discolorations of the skin or mucous membrane resulting from hemorrhage. Smaller than purpura.

**Pharmacodynamics:** The effect that a drug has on the body. Drug action.

**Pharmacokinetics:** The effect that the body has on a drug, including movement of a drug in the body.

**Physical status classification:** A graded assessment of a patient's physical condition. Used to plan patient management prior to administering anesthetics and to gauge patient risk.

**Physiologic anemia:** A relative decrease in red blood cell (RBC) mass caused by an increase in plasma volume without a corresponding increase in the number of RBCs. Seen in pregnant patients.

**Physiologic pain:** The protective sensation of pain that occurs when there is no or minimal tissue injury.

**Pleural effusion:** Abnormal accumulation of fluid in the space between the lungs and the chest wall (pleural space).

**Pneumomediastinum:** The presence of air in the space between the lungs that contains the heart and great vessels.

**Pneumothorax:** The presence of air in the space between the lungs and the chest wall (pleural space) associated with collapse of the lungs.

**Pop-off valve:** Also known as the *pressure relief valve, exhaust valve, adjustable pressure limiting (APL) valve,* or *overflow valve;* this valve is the point of exit of anesthetic gases from the breathing circuit.

**Porcine stress syndrome:** Also known as *malignant hyperthermia.* A hereditary, metabolic condition of swine caused by a mutation in one of the genes that controls calcium metabolism in muscle fibers. Occurs in affected swine in response to some anesthetic agents including inhalant agents. Signs include muscle rigidity, rapid rise in temperature, hypercapnia, hyperkalemia, and death.

**Positive inotrope:** A drug that increases inotropy (the force of heart muscle contractions).

**Positive pressure ventilation:** PPV; Any procedure by which the anesthetist assists or controls the delivery of oxygen and anesthetic gas to the patient's lungs. Includes both manual and mechanical ventilation.

**Preanesthetic medication:** An anesthetic agent or adjunct administered during the preanesthetic period to provide one or more of a variety of desired effects, including analgesia, sedation, and muscle relaxation.

**Preemptive analgesia:** Provision of analgesia before tissue injury, including surgery.

**Pressure manometer:** A gauge that indicates the pressure of the gases within the breathing circuit, and by extension the pressure in the animal's airways and lungs. Expressed in centimeters of water (cm $H_2O$), millimeters of mercury (mm Hg), or kilopascals (kPa).

**Pressure-reducing valve:** A valve that reduces the pressure of a compressed gas to a constant safe operating pressure of 40 to 50 psi (275 to 345 kPa) regardless of pressure changes within the tank.

**Pressure transducer:** An instrument designed to measure fluid pressure that converts the pressure wave form into an electrical signal.

**Primary hyperalgesia:** A state of increased sensitivity near a site of tissue injury, in which stimulation with a normally non-noxious stimulus is painful (compare with *Secondary hyperalgesia*).

**Pulmonary contusion:** Bruising of lung tissue caused by blunt trauma.

**Pulmonary thromboembolism:** The presence of one or more blood clot in the lungs.

**Pulse oximeter:** A monitoring device used to estimate (1) the percent oxygen saturation of hemoglobin ($Spo_2$) by measuring subtle differences in light absorption, and (2) the pulse rate by detecting blood pulsations in the small arterioles.

**Purpura:** Purple discolorations of the skin or mucous membrane caused by hemorrhage. Larger than petechiae.

**Rebreathing system (Circle system):** An anesthetic machine fitted with a rebreathing circuit. In this system exhaled gases minus carbon dioxide are recirculated and rebreathed by the patient, along with variable amounts of fresh oxygen and anesthetic. Appropriate for most patients over 2.5 to 3 kg in body weight.

**Regional anesthesia:** A loss of sensation in a limited area of the body produced by administration of a local anesthetic or other agent in proximity to sensory nerves.

**Regurgitation:** Flow of stomach contents into the esophagus and mouth unaccompanied by retching; as distinguished from vomiting, which is a forceful expulsion of stomach contents into the esophagus and mouth preceded by retching.

**Regurgitus:** Regurgitated ruminal contents consisting of saliva and ingesta.

**Reproductive status:** Whether or not the patient has been spayed or castrated. If intact, whether or not the patient is being used for breeding. In the case of female patients, whether pregnant or not.

**Reservoir bag:** Also called a *rebreathing bag.* A rubber or plastic bag that serves as a flexible storage reservoir for expired and inspired gases. It also allows the anesthetist to observe respirations, confirm proper endotracheal tube placement, and ventilate for the patient.

**Respiration:** The processes by which oxygen is supplied to and used by the tissues, and carbon dioxide is eliminated from the tissues.

**Respiratory minute volume:** RMV; The amount of air that moves into and out of the lungs in a minute. The tidal volume multiplied by the respiratory rate.

**Respirometer:** A monitoring device used to measure the tidal volume and respiratory minute volume.

**Reversal agent:** A drug used to lessen or abolish the effects of anesthetic agents or adjuncts, and which is therefore used to "wake" the patient after sedation or anesthesia.

**Ring block:** A type of line block that completely encircles an anatomic part, such as a digit or teat.

**Scavenging system:** The anesthetic machine system that disposes of excess and waste anesthetic gases outside of the building, so that inhalation by occupationally exposed individuals is minimized.

**Scoliosis:** Lateral curvature of the spine. Seen in cattle that have had a paravertebral block.

**Second gas effect:** An increase in the concentration of a gas in the alveoli resulting from the absorption of a second gas into the bloodstream.

**Secondary hyperalgesia:** A state of increased sensitivity distant from a site of tissue injury, in which stimulation with a normally non-noxious stimulus is painful (compare with *Primary hyperalgesia*).

**Sedation:** A drug-induced central nervous system depression and drowsiness.

**Semiclosed rebreathing system:** A rebreathing system in which the pop-off valve is positioned partially open, and the flow of oxygen is relatively high, providing more volume than is necessary to meet the patient's metabolic needs.

**Sensory neuron:** A neuron that conveys sensations (i.e., pain, heat, cold, and pressure) from the skin, muscles, and other peripheral tissues to the brain.

**Sequestration:** Loss of blood or plasma into tissues or spaces within the body, resulting in a decreased circulating blood volume.

**Signalment:** The species, breed, age, sex, and reproductive status of a patient.

**Sloughing:** Separation of dead tissue from surrounding live tissue in a wound. Often used in reference to tissue death and loss secondary to drug-induced damage.

**Solute:** An atom or molecule dissolved in body water.

**Somatic analgesia:** Absence of pain of the skin, muscle, bone, and connective tissue.

**Somatic pain:** Pain originating from the musculoskeletal or integumentary system. Subclassified as superficial (i.e., skin) and deep (i.e., joints, muscles, bones).

**Sphygmomanometer:** A monitoring device consisting of a pressure gauge and cuff used to measure arterial blood pressure.

**Splash block:** Local anesthesia produced by direct application of local anesthetic to a wound or open surgical site. Most often applied as a spray or with a soaked gauze sponge.

**Standing chemical restraint:** A type of chemical restraint used in horses in which the patient is heavily sedated but remains standing throughout the procedure.

**Status epilepticus:** Continuous seizures, or a series of seizures in rapid succession.

**Stertor:** A heavy snoring sound during inspiration; often caused by partial upper airway obstruction. Seen in patients with laryngospasm, laryngeal edema, and in brachycephalic dogs.

**Stridor:** Noisy breathing caused by turbulent air flow in the upper airways.

**Stuporous:** In a sleeplike state. Can be aroused only with a painful stimulus.

**Surgical anesthesia:** A specific stage of general anesthesia in which there is a sufficient degree of analgesia and muscle relaxation to allow surgery to be performed without pain or movement.

**Sympathetic blockade:** Loss of function of sympathetic nerves supplying the heart and blood vessels resulting from diffusion of local anesthetic into the thoracic spinal cord. Signs include bradycardia, decreased cardiac output, and hypotension. Blockade of the caudal sympathetic nerves results in less severe hypotension and tachycardia.

**Syncope:** Fainting episodes caused by brain hypoxia.

**Systolic blood pressure:** Arterial blood pressure during contraction of the ventricles. (Compare with *Diastolic blood pressure.*)

**Tachyarrhythmia:** Any arrhythmia in which the heart rate is abnormally increased.

**Tachycardia:** Rapid heart rate; the opposite of bradycardia.

**Tachypnea:** Rapid respiratory rate.

**Tank pressure gauge:** A device attached to the yoke of an anesthetic machine or the pressure regulator of an H tank. Indicates the pressure of gas remaining in a compressed gas cylinder measured in pounds per square inch (psi) or kilopascals (kPa).

**Therapeutic index:** TI; A ratio of the toxic to the therapeutic dose of a drug, used to measure relative safety. A drug with a wide therapeutic index (much more of the drug is required to intoxicate a patient than is required to treat it) is relatively safer than a drug with a narrow therapeutic index (one for which the toxic and therapeutic doses are similar).

**Thoracocentesis:** Surgical puncture of the pleural space with a needle or tube for the purpose of removing fluid or air.

**Thrombocytopenia:** Low platelet count.

**Tidal Volume ($V_T$):** The volume of a normal breath (approximately 10 to 15 mL/kg body weight).

**Tilt table:** A specialized table used to restrain cattle, and occasionally horses, undergoing anesthetic procedures, by securing the patient to the table with ropes and straps and tilting the table to the desired angle.

**Titration:** Administration of an anesthetic agent in small increments until the desired depth of anesthesia is reached, as opposed to administration of the entire calculated dose.

**TKX:** A combination of Telazol, ketamine, and xylazine, widely used to produce heavy sedation to total intravenous anesthesia in pigs.

**Topical anesthesia:** A loss of sensation of a localized area produced by administration of a local anesthetic directly to a body surface or to a surgical or traumatic wound.

**Total injectable anesthesia:** Induction and maintenance of anesthesia by intramuscular injection of an anesthetic agent or combination of agents with no concurrent use of inhalant agents. A technique commonly employed in swine.

**Total intravenous anesthesia:** Induction and maintenance of anesthesia by intravenous injection of ultra–short-acting anesthetics with no concurrent use of inhalant agents. Accomplished using repeat bolus injections or a constant rate infusion.

**Tranquilization:** A drug-induced state of calm in which the patient is reluctant to move and is aware of but unconcerned about its surroundings.

**Transduction:** The first step in nociception, in which noxious thermal, chemical, or mechanical stimuli are transformed into electrical signals called *action potentials.*

**Transmission:** The second step in nociception, in which sensory impulses are conducted to the spinal cord.

**Unidirectional valve:** The inspiratory valve or expiratory valve of a rebreathing circuit. Controls the direction of gas flow through a rebreathing circuit as the patient breathes.

**Vaporizer-in-circuit:** VIC; A vaporizer that is located in the breathing circuit. Nonprecision vaporizers are often positioned this way.

**Vaporizer-out-of-circuit:** VOC; A vaporizer in which carrier gas from the flow meters flows into the vaporizer before entering the breathing circuit. Precision vaporizers are positioned this way.

**Vasodilation:** (Also *vasodilatation.*) Dilation of the blood vessels; the opposite of vasoconstriction.

**Ventilation:** The movement of gases into and out of the alveoli.

**Ventilation-perfusion mismatch:** A lack of equality in the quantity of oxygen that reaches the alveoli per minute and the volume of blood that perfuses the alveoli per minute. Results in alveoli that are oxygenated but are not perfused and/or alveoli that are perfused but are atelectatic and not oxygenated.

**Vesicants:** Drugs that damage tissues if injected perivascularly.

**Veterinarian-in-charge:** The veterinarian responsible for the management and welfare of a particular patient.

**Visceral analgesia:** Absence of pain in the internal organs.

**Visceral pain:** Pain originating from the internal organs.

**Waste anesthetic gas:** Any inhalation anesthetic (including isoflurane, other halogenated compounds, and nitrous oxide) that is breathed out by the patient or that escapes from the anesthetic machine.

**Wasting:** A decrease in body mass, energy, or vigor often caused by disease.

**Windup:** *See Central nervous system hypersensitivity.*

# Index

## A

Abdominal organ abnormality, anesthetic response to, 13
Abdominal pain, in small mammals, 313-314
Abdominal palpation/auscultation, 22
Absolute leukocyte count, 23
Acepromazine, 3
  adverse effects of, 60
  as antiemetic, 26, 60
  as antihistamine, 60
  boxer/giant breed sensitivity to, 10
  cardiovascular effects of, 53t
  cardiovascular system, effect on, 59-60
  CNS, effect on, 52t, 59-60
  contraindications for, 10
  decrease in PCV, 60
  dog reaction to, 11
  dosage of, 60-61, 60b
  effects of, 55t-56t, 226
  mode of action/pharmacology of, 59
  opioids combining with, 68
  penile prolapse and, 60
  respiratory/gastrointestinal effects of, 54t
  respiratory system, effect on, 60
  in ruminants, 285b
  in small mammals, 304, 305t
  toxicity of, 60
  use of, 59-61, 226
Acepromazine-butorphanol, 305t
Acetaminophen
  codeine and, 226
  species/route/dosage of, 215t-217t
Acetate, 30-32
Acetylcholine, PNS receptors for, 57
Acidotic, 169
Action potential, transformation into, 207-208
Activated charcoal cartridge, 358, 358b
Active scavenging system, 356, 357f
Activity level/temperament, 18
Acupuncture, for pain control, 228
Addiction
  morphine and, 218
  opioid causing, 68
Adjunct
  adverse effects of, 55
  as agonist, 51
  analgesic effect of, 51-52
  cardiovascular effects of, 53t
  classification of
    by administration, 51

Adjunct (Continued)
    by chemistry, 51
    by effect of, 51
    by time period for, 51
  CNS, effect on, 51, 52t
  combination of, 52-53
  definition of, 50
  nonpharmacologic therapies as, 228
  respiratory/gastrointestinal effects of, 54t
  solubility of, 53, 53b
Adjusting pressure limit (APL), 117
Age
  anesthetic response by, 10, 10b
  hydration assessment, 17
  water concentration and, 28-29
Agonal phenomenon, 335
Agonist, role of, 51
Agonist-antagonist
  effects of, 56t
  use of, 51, 68-69
Air embolism, 28
Air intake valve
  description/function of, 121
  negative pressure and, 121
Airway blockage
  anticholinergic and, 57
  cause of, 9
  stridor indicating, 19
Albumin
  colloid/blood plasma, administration of, 30
  diffusion, 30
  movement within body, 29
Allergy, patient history and, 11
Alpha$_2$-adrenergic, 51
Alpha$_2$-adrenoceptor agonist
  adverse effects of, 64b
  anticholinergic and, 64b
  effects of, 63b
  epidural use of, 225
  mode of action/pharmacology of, 62-63
  for pain control, 225
  in small mammals, 305
  type/route/dosage of, 215t-217t
  use/risks of, 59
  See also Alpha$_2$-agonist
Alpha$_2$-agonist
  adverse effects of, 55, 63-64
  cardiovascular system, effect on, 53t, 63-64
  CNS, effect on, 52t, 63
  drug combining with, 64

Alpha$_2$-agonist (Continued)
  effects of, 55t-56t, 63b
  gastrointestinal system, effect on, 54t, 64
  in horses, 275
  hyperglycemia and, 63
  hypothermia and, 63
  metabolization of, 63
  mode of action/pharmacology of, 62-63
  as muscle relaxant, 63
  respiratory depression and, 92
  respiratory system, effect on, 54t, 63-64
  risks with use of, 59
  use of, 62-65
  vagus nerve, stimulation of, 57
  See also Alpha$_2$-adrenoceptor agonist
Alpha$_2$-antagonist
  adverse effects of, 65-66, 65b
  dosage of, 66
  effects of, 65
  mode of action/pharmacology of, 65
  use of, 65-66
Alpha-adrenergic receptor, blockage of, 59
Alphaxalone, 308
Amantadine, 215t-217t
Ambu bag
  example of, 338f
  indications for, 337
American College of Veterinary Anesthesiologists (ACVA), guidelines by
  anesthetic monitoring, 139, 367-369
  body temperature, 368
  circulation monitoring, 143
  neuromuscular blockade, 368
  oxygenation, 157, 367-368
  personnel, 369
  record-keeping, 176, 368
  recovery period, 255b, 368-369
  sedation without general anesthesia, 234b, 369
  ventilation, 163, 368
American Society of Anesthesiologists (ASA)
  physical status classification system, 24, 25t
  tiletamine-zolazepam, recommendations for, 82
  waste anesthetic gas, risks from, 354
Amethocaine, 186
Amitraz, 11
Amitriptyline
  effects of, 11
  species/route/dosage of, 215t-217t
Amnesia, dissociative agent and, 80

Page numbers followed by b indicate boxes; t, tables; f, figures.

Analgesia
  adjunct for, 50
  anesthetic agent/adjunct producing,
    51-52
  definition of, 2
  dissociative agent and, 79
  general anesthesia and, 52
  at home, 227
  opioid as, 67
  preanesthetic agent providing, 56t
  technician role in, 206
Analgesic
  constant rate infusion for, 27
  multimodal therapy with, 208b
  selection of, 212
  in small mammals, 314-315, 314t
    administration of, 315-316
  type/route/dosage of, 215t-217t
Anal sac impaction, 13
Anaphylaxis
  local anesthetic causing, 190
  patient history and, 11
Anatomic dead space, 245
Anemia
  anesthetic protocol for, 25
  anesthetic response to, 13
  blood products for, 32
  cause of, 18
  mucous membrane color and, 21b
  PCV/RBC decrease and, 23
  in trauma patient, 328
Anesthesia
  adjunct and, 50
  body characteristics during, 140
  body temperature, effect on, 169b
  in canines/felines, 233
  consent form for, 11-12, 12f
  definition of, 1
  delaying in trauma patients, 330
  in equines, 265
    extending duration of, 275
    preparation for, 279b
  fluid needs during, 30
  history and terminology of, 1-3
  horse recovery from, 9
  hypothermia and, 169
  in large animals, 9, 283
  maintenance of, 251-252
  newborn nursing after, 327-328
  in obese patient, 16-17
  optimum depth of, 142-143
  preparing dog/cat for, 258b
  prolonged, intravenous catheterization
    for, 27
  recording information during, 176-177
    form for, 178f-179f
  regurgitation during/after, 341-342
  respiratory depression and, 92
  of rodents/rabbits, 298
  in rodents/rabbits, 303
  in ruminants, 283-289
    preparation for, 295b

Anesthesia (Continued)
  tissue perfusion during, 152
  use of, 2b
  veterinary technician, role of, 3
  vital signs during, 144t
  waste anesthetic gas and, 355
  See also Monitoring; Recovery period;
    Ruminant anesthesia
Anesthetic agent
  adverse effects of, 55
    as anesthetic emergency/problem, 323
    minimizing, 235
  as agonist, 51
  analgesic effect of, 51-52
  carbon dioxide absorbents and, 120-121
  cardiovascular effects of, 53t
  checking levels of, 125
  classification of
    by administration, 51
    by chemistry, 51
    by effect of, 51
    by time period for, 51
  CNS, effect on, 51, 52t
  combination of, 52-53
  constant rate infusion for, 27
  definition of, 50
  dosage/calculation of, 3
  drugs influencing, 10
  effect of, 3
  MAC of, 88
  mal-effects of, 3
  metabolizing/excretion problems, 13
  oral administration in feral cats, 244
  pain control by, 52
  premedication with, 240
  respiratory disease causing, 332
  respiratory/gastrointestinal effects of,
    54t
  response to
    by age, 10, 10b
    by breed, 10
    by species, 9-10
  in small mammals, 306t
  solubility of, 53, 53b
  species response to, 9-10
  sympathomimetic and, 10
  therapeutic index and, 3, 14
  unfamiliarity with, as anesthetic emer-
    gency/problem cause, 320
Anesthetic chamber
  advantage/disadvantage of, 99
  complications with, 244
  example of, 100f
  materials for, 99
  parts of, 244
  for small mammals, 308f
  use of, 99
  waste anesthetic gas and, 355
Anesthetic depth, 139
  adjustments for, 239
  antagonist decreasing, 236
  assessment of, case study for, 177b

Anesthetic depth (Continued)
  eye positioning and, 174, 174b
  flow rate and, 128
  heart/respiratory rate and, 176
  as inadequate, 335
  indicators by stages/planes, 141t
  indicators of, 171t
    muscle tone as, 173-174
    reflexes as, 170-176
    spontaneous movement as, 173
  inhalation induction and, 308-309
  intramuscular agent and, 236
  jaw tone and, 173b, 174
  monitoring for, 139
  monitoring of, 309-310
  muscle-paralyzing agent and, 195
  muscle relaxation and, 174
  nonprecision vaporizer and, 374
  pupil size and, 174-175
  salivary/lacrimal secretions and, 175
  too deep, 335-336
  treating excessive, 345b
Anesthetic drug
  CNS depression and, 2f
  decreasing heart rate, 330-331
  effect of, 2-3
Anesthetic emergency/problem, 319
  anesthetic agent/adverse effects on, 323
  anesthetic machine misassembly as
    cause of, 322
  approach to, 334
  brachycephalic dog as, 325-326
  carbon dioxide absorber exhaustion as,
    321
  cardiac arrest as, 337-341
  cardiovascular disease causing, 330-331
  cause of, 320
  cesarean patient as, 326-328
  for dogs/cats
    for CPR, 340t
    for treatment of, 340t
  dyspnea/cyanosis as, 336
  empty oxygen tank as, 321-322
  endotracheal tube problems as cause
    of, 322
  equipment failure as, 321-323
  geriatric patient as, 323-325
  hepatic disease causing, 333
  human error causing, 320-321, 320b
    anesthetic agent/machine, unfamiliar-
      ity with, 320
    drug administration, incorrect,
      320-321
    fatigued personnel, 321
    history/examination, not obtaining,
      320
    inattentiveness, 321
    preoccupied/hurried personnel, 321
  hypotension as, 336
  mortality rate from, 319-320
  obese animals as, 326
  pale mucous membranes as, 336

Anesthetic emergency/problem *(Continued)*
  patient factors as, 323-334, 324t
  pediatric patient as, 325
  pop-off valve as cause of, 322-323
  prolonged capillary refill time as, 336
  renal disease and, 333-334, 334b
  respiratory arrest as, 337
  respiratory depression and, 312
  respiratory disease causing, 331-333
  responding to, 345b
  response to, 334-343
    veterinary technician, role of, 334
  sighthound as, 326
  tachypnea as, 336
  trauma patient as, 328-330
  types of, 334-341
    inadequate depth, 335
    too deeply anesthetized, 335-336
  vaporizer problems as cause of, 322
Anesthetic emergency. *See* Anesthetic
    emergency/problem
Anesthetic equipment, 96
  care/maintenance of, 132b
    compressed gas cylinder, 132
    E tank, removal/replacement of, 132
    H tank, detachment/reattachment
      of, 132
    ongoing, 131-132
  chemical solution, exposure to, 134
  development of, 97
  disinfection of, 133-134
  failure of, as anesthetic emergency/
    problem cause, 321-323
  leak testing, 355, 358-359, 358b
  malfunctioning, effects of, 167
  preparation of, 239-240, 267-268
  setup checklist for, 135b
Anesthetic induction
  in horses, 269-272
    patient positioning/safety/comfort
      during, 275
    protocol for, 279b
  with intramuscular agent/combination,
    236, 236f
  intubation and, 241-242, 241b
  with IV of ultra-short-acting agent, 237
  process of, 240
  in ruminants, 285
    patient positioning/safety/comfort
      and, 288
  in swine, 290
  *See also* Induction
Anesthetic machine
  air intake valve for
    description/function of, 121
    negative pressure and, 121
  assembly of, 125
  checking before use, case study for, 127b
  components of, 100-101
  example of, 102f
  flow meter for
    description/function of, 109

Anesthetic machine *(Continued)*
  example of, 109f
  use of, 109
  function/cost of, 100
  gas leak from, 358-359, 358b
  for large animals, 267-268, 267f,
    283-284
    example of, 284f
  for large versus small animals, 100f
  misassembly of, as anesthetic emergency/
    problem cause, 322
  operation of, daily setup of, 125
  oxygen and, 101
  parts of, 101b
  preparation of, 239-240
  schematic of
    with common gas outlet, 102f
    without common gas outlet, 101f
  selection of, 125
  setup checklist for, 135b
  unfamiliarity with, as anesthetic emer-
    gency/problem cause, 320
  waste anesthetic gas from, 355
Anesthetic maintenance, 251
  constant rate infusion with, 259b-260b
  with CRI of propofol, 262b
  in dogs/cats, 262b
  in horses, 273-275
    with inhalation agent, 273-275, 281b
    with injectable/inhalation agents, 275
    patient positioning/safety/comfort,
      275
  with IM injection, 254b, 262b
  with inhalation agent, 258b, 262b
  with injectable/inhalation agents,
    260b-261b
  intubation and, 309-311
  in PSC P1/P2 cats/dogs, 251b
  in PSC P1/P2 horses, 274b
  in PSC P1/P2 ruminants, 287b
  with repeat bolus of propofol/ultra-
    short-acting agent, 256b, 262b
  in ruminants, 287-288
    with inhalation agent, 287-288, 294b
    with IV agent, 288
    patient positioning/safety/comfort
      and, 288
  in swine, 290-292
    monitoring during, 292
Anesthetic mask
  advantages/disadvantages of, 99
  example of, 99f
  fitting for, 243
  materials for, 99
  use of, 99
Anesthetic overdose, 142
Anesthetic protocol
  disease and, 24-25
  factors influencing, 25-26
    cost, 26
    facilities and equipment, 25
    familiarity with agent, 25

Anesthetic protocol *(Continued)*
    procedure, nature/circumstances of, 25
    urgency, degree of, 26
  illness and, 24-25
  selection of, 24, 235-236
Anesthetic recovery period. *See* Recovery
    period
Anesthetic risk. *See* Anesthetic emergency/
    problem
Anesthetic spill, waste anesthetic gas and,
    355-356
Anesthetic stages/planes, 140-142, 140f,
    141b
  anesthetic overdose, stage of, 142
  depth indicators of, 141t
  involuntary movement, period of,
    141-142
  voluntary movement, period of, 141
Anesthetic vapor, 351
Anesthetic vaporizer, 100, 102f
  description/function of, 110
  indicator window of, 115f
  parts of, 101b
  types of, 110-111
Anesthetist
  minimum patient database,
    development of, 5-6
  personal responsibility of, 3, 3b
  preinduction care by, 5-6
  role of, 3
Anion, 29
Anorexia, 11
Antagonist
  anesthetic depth and, 236
  role of, 51
Antibiotic
  anesthetic agent and, 10
  as preanesthetic care, 39
Anticholinergic
  acetylcholine and, 57
  adverse effects of, 55, 58, 58b
  alpha$_2$-adrenoceptor agonist and, 64b
  bradycardia and, 330-331
  bronchodilatation, 57
  cardiovascular system, effect on, 53t, 57
  CNS, effect on, 52t
  effects of, 55t-56t, 58b
  intestinal peristalsis, inhibition of, 58
  lacrimal secretions, effect on, 57
  mode of action/pharmacology of, 57
  pupillary light reflex and, 19, 57
  respiratory/gastrointestinal effects of, 54t
  respiratory system, effect on, 58
  in ruminants, 285, 285b
  ruminants and, 9
  in small mammals, 304
  tricyclic antidepressants and, 11
  use of, 51, 56, 58
Anticonvulsant
  benzodiazepine as, 61
  cardiac arrhythmia and, 10
  as preanesthetic care, 39

Antiemetic, 26
  acepromazine as, 60
  as preanesthetic care, 39
  propofol as, 76
Antihistamine
  acepromazine as, 60
  effects of, 11
Antiinflammatory drug, 39
Anxiety
  opioid causing, 67
  preanesthetic agent for, 55
Anxiousness, 18
Apnea
  barbiturates and, 72-73
  capnogram and, 167
  propofol effect on, 76
Apnea monitor, 164, 164f
Appetite stimulant
  diazepam/midazolam as, 61
  propofol as, 76
Arousal
  extubation and, 255-256
  in horse after sedation, 269b
Arrhythmia. *See* Cardiac arrhythmia
Arterial blood pressure, in small animals,
  310
Arterial oxygen saturation, 159
Asphyxiation, 98
Aspiration, 9
Aspiration pneumonia, 341-342
Aspirin, 215t-217t
Assisted ventilation, 190-194
Asystole, 341
Ataxia, 59
Atelectasis, 118-119
  alveoli and, 191
  in horse, 266
  predisposing factors for, 191
  reversal of, 163-164, 164b
Atipamezole
  administration/dosage of, 66
  for anesthetic emergency in dogs/cats,
    340t
  in small mammals, 305, 306t
  use of, 65
Atom, 29
Atracurium besylate, 195
Atrial fibrillation, 150f, 176
Atrioventricular heart block
  treatment of, 331
  types of, 147
Atropine
  bradycardia from, 58
  for cardiac arrest, 341
  cardiovascular system, effect on, 57-58
  CNS, effect on, 57
  in dogs/cats
    for anesthetic emergency, 340t
    for CPR, 340t
  mode of action of, 57
  respiratory system, effect on, 58
  in small mammals, 304, 304b, 305t

Atropine *(Continued)*
  strengths of, 58, 58b
  use/administration of, 56, 58
Auscultation, 19-20
Autoclaving, 134
Autonomic nervous system, 185
AV heart block, 147
AVPU scale, 17
Ayres T-piece, 123
Ayres T-piece (Mapleson E system), 124,
  124f
  oxygen flow rate for, 131

B
Back pressure, 113
Bacteria, anesthetic equipment harboring,
  133-134
Bagging. *See* Reservoir bag
BAG protocol, 58
Bain coaxial circuit, 123
Bain coaxial circuit (modified Mapleson D
  system), 123-124, 124f
  oxygen flow rate for, 128b, 130t, 131
Balanced analgesia, 226
Balanced anesthesia
  effect of, 3b
  technique for, 3
Balanced fluid, 31
  isotonic, polyionic replacement solution
    as, 31-32
Barbiturate
  action/pharmacodynamics of, 70-71
  adverse effects of, 73-74, 74b
  cardiac arrhythmia and, 10
  cardiovascular system, effect on, 53t, 72
  chloramphenicol and, 11
  classes of, 70
  classification of, 70
  CNS, effect on, 52t, 70-72
  as controlled substance, 53-54
  critically ill and, 74
  development of, 70
  effects of, 55t, 73, 73b
  excitement from, 74
  geriatric animals and, 324
  ionization of, 71
  lipid solubility of, 71
  muscle relaxants and, 74
  potency of, 73
  redistribution of, 71
  respiratory/gastrointestinal effects of,
    54t
  respiratory system, effect on, 72-73
  sighthounds and, 8, 74
  in small mammals, 307
  tissue irritation and sloughing, 74
  types of
    methohexital as, 75
    pentobarbital as, 75
    thiopental as, 74-75
  use of, 70b, 72

Barium hydroxide lime, 120-121
Basophil count, normal values for, 23t
Behavior
  by anesthetic depth, 141t
  changes in, 11
  pain-associated, 209, 211f
Behavior-modifying drug, cardiac
  arrhythmia and, 10
Benzodiazepine
  administration of, 61-62
  adverse effects of, 61-62, 62b
  cardiovascular/respiratory system, effect
    on, 61
  cardiovascular system, effect on, 53t
  classification of, 62
  CNS, effect on, 52t, 61
  as controlled substance, 53-54
  effects of, 55t-56t, 61b
  mode of action/pharmacology of, 61
  preanesthetic agent for, 56
  respiratory/gastrointestinal effects of, 54t
  risks with use of, 59
  in rodents/rabbits, 304
  as skeletal muscle relaxant, 61
  use of, 62
Bicarbonate ($HCO_3^-$), 29
Bier block, 189
  in dog, procedure for, 203b
Bifid, 146
Bilateral stifle arthroscopy, multimodal
  therapy for horse, 228b
Bile acid, monitoring levels of, 224-225
Bird, anesthesia in, 10
Bleeding
  cause of, 11
  from clotting disorder, 13
  IV infusion rates for, 33
Blink reflex. *See* Palpebral reflex
Bloat, in ruminants, 9
  eructate and, 284
Blood-brain barrier, 57
Blood carbon dioxide level, factors
  determining, 165, 165b
Blood chemistry test, 24
Blood coagulation screen, 24
Blood flow, body weight and, 72f
Blood gas analysis, 157
  of oxygenation, 163
  sample collection for, 167
Blood gas machine, 333f
Blood-gas partition coefficient
  of desflurane, 90b
  importance of, 87
  inhalation agent and, 87
  of isoflurane, 88
  of methoxyflurane, 91
  of sevoflurane, 89
  significance of, 87b
  solubility and, 87
Blood loss
  sequestration and, 328
  in small mammals, 310, 312

Blood oxygen
    measurement of, 158
    saturation levels, 159
Blood plasma, administration of, 30
Blood pressure
    anesthetic agent/adjunct effect on, 53t
    capnogram and, 167
    cuff placement for, 155
    determination of, 152-157
    isoflurane effect on, 60
    measurement, with Doppler probe, 180b
    monitoring, 139
        in horses, 274, 274f
        instruments used for, 152, 154-157
    pulse and, 21, 153-154
    of swine, 293f
    systolic versus diastolic, 152
    tissue perfusion and, 152-153, 152b
    in trauma patient, 328-329
Blood pressure cuff, 155b, 157f
Blood product
    administration of, 30
    composition/uses for, 32
Blood volume
    increasing/decreasing of, 30
    total body weight and, 29
Body condition score
    five-level versus nine-level system, 15-16
    importance of, 16
Body condition system, 15f-16f
Body fat, water and, 28-29
Body fluid
    composition of, 28-29
    water as, 28-29
Body fluid compartment
    total body weight and, 29f
    water and, 28-29
Body openings, examination of, 19
Body temperature
    ACVA guidelines for, 368
    anesthesia and, 169b
    anesthetic agent/adjunct effect on, 52t
    conversion table for, 377t
    determination of, 18
    indicators of, 169-170
    monitoring in small mammals, 311b
    opioid effect on, 67
    regulation of, 169
    by species, 18t
    See also Temperature
Body weight. See Weight
Bolus, 285-286
Boxer, acepromazine and, 10
Brachycephalic animal, intubation of, 10
Brachycephalic dog, as increased anesthetic
        risk, 324t, 325-326
Bradycardia
    during anesthesia, 144
    anticholinergic and, 56-57
    atropine and, 57-58
    cause of, 55, 330
    definition/cause of, 337

Bradycardia (Continued)
    endotracheal intubation and, 176
    opioid causing, 67
    preanesthetic agent minimizing, 56t
    treatment of, 330-331, 337
Breathing circuit, 100, 102f, 116
    breathing tube for, 121-122
    leaks, checking for, 126
    parts of, 101b
    pop-off valve, 117
    pressure manometer for
        description/function of, 121
        safe readings for, 121b
        use of, 121
    selection of, 125
Breathing tube
    care/maintenance of, 133
    description/function of, 121-122
    selection/use of, 122
    sizes of, 122b
    Universal F-circuit as, 121-122
Breed, anesthetic response by, 10
British Government Health Advisory
        Committee, waste gas and, 354
Bronchodilatation, anticholinergic and, 57
Bruising
    anesthetic response to, 13
    cause of, 11
Buccal bleeding time, 42b-43b
Bupivacaine
    administration of, 186
    cardiotoxicity from, 189b
    onset of action/administration of, 184
    pharmacology of, 185t
    for skin infiltration, 184
    in stifle joint, 188
Buprenorphine
    classification of, 220
    mode of action of, 66-67
    neuroleptanalgesia and, 68
    piroxicam and, 226
    respiratory depression from, 220
    as reversal agent, 220
    route of administration of, 220
    in small mammals, 314t
        duration of action, 314b
        effects of, 314-315
    species/route/dosage of, 215t-217t
Burette, 35, 36f
Butorphanol
    classification of, 220
    duration of effect, 219
    effectiveness of, 219
    epidural use of, 221
    for home analgesia, 227
    intravenous infusion of, 221
    neuroleptanalgesia and, 68
    route/forms of administration of, 219
    in ruminants, 285b
    in small mammals, 314t
    species/route/dosage of, 215t-217t
    use of, 69, 219-220

C
Cachexia, body condition score and,
        15-16
Calcium ($Ca^{2+}$), 29
    plasma concentration in, 30, 30b
Calculated oxygen content, 158
Calf
    endotracheal intubation in, 286, 287f
    oxygen flow rate for, 128b
Capillary refill time
    assessment of, 21
    procedure for, 151-152, 151f
    prolonged, 152, 319, 336
    in rodents/rabbits, 310
Capnogram
    appearance of
        abnormal, 167
        normal vital signs of, 165-167
    changes/cause of, 168t
    generation of, 165
    interpretation of, 167, 167b
    normal
        appearance of, 165-167
        example of, 166f
Capnograph, 143
    carbon dioxide measurement by,
        164
    End-tidal $CO_2$ measurement by, 165f
    parts of, 164-165
    for small mammals, 311
Carbocaine, 185t
Carbon dioxide
    accumulation of, 131
    capnograph measuring, 164
    transportation of, 167-168
Carbon dioxide absorbent (granule)
    characteristics of, 120
    exhaust, signs of, 120b
    safety with use of, 120-121
Carbon dioxide absorber canister, 116
    care/maintenance of, 133
    description/function of, 119-120
    example of, 117f, 120f
    use of, 120
Carbon dioxide absorber exhaustion, as
        anesthetic emergency/problem cause,
        321
Carbon monoxide
    isoflurane and, 89
Cardiac arrest
    airway and breathing, 339
    atropine for, 341
    capnogram and, 167
    CPCR for, 338
    dopamine/dobutamine for, 341
    drugs for, 339-341
    effects of, 341
    epinephrine for, 341
    from general anesthesia, 319-320
    as increased anesthetic risk, 337-341
    in small mammals, 313t
    vasopressin for, 341

Cardiac arrhythmia
   during anesthesia, 144-145
   anesthetic agent/adjunct effect on, 53t
   anticholinergic effect on, 58
   cause of, 10, 331, 337
   definition of, 145, 337
   detection of, 331
   halothane causing, 90
   nitrous oxide and, 371
   in trauma patient, 330-331
   treatment of, 346b
Cardiac compression
   external versus internal, 339
   initiation of, 338
   for large dog/foal/ruminant, 338
   location for, 338f
   for medium dog, 338
   procedure for, 339
   rate of, 339
   for small dog/cat, 338
Cardiac conduction system, 146f
Cardiac disease
   capnogram and, 167
   ECG for, 24
   signs of, 11
Cardiac dysrhythmia, 145, 145b
Cardiac failure
   in small mammals, 312
Cardiac output, 28
   acepromazine effect on, 59
   anesthetic agent/adjunct effect on, 53t
   isoflurane and, 88-89
Cardiac rhythm. See Heart rhythm
Cardiopulmonary-cerebrovascular
     resuscitation (CPCR)
   atropine and, 57
   cardiac arrest, repeat of, 341
   cardiac arrest reversal using, 338
   compressions, correct location for, 338f
   consent form for, 13
   steps for, 338
Cardiopulmonary function
   anesthetic agent affecting, 28
Cardiopulmonary resuscitation (CPR)
   for dogs/cats, drugs for, 340t
Cardiotoxicity, from bupivacaine, 189b
Cardiovascular collapse, 141t
Cardiovascular depression
   alpha$_2$-agonist effect on, 63-64
Cardiovascular disease
   anesthetic response to, 13
   cause of, 18
   as increased anesthetic risk, 324t,
     330-331
Cardiovascular function
   by anesthetic depth, 141t
   by anesthetic stage/plane, 141
Cardiovascular system
   acepromazine effect on, 59-60
   alpha$_2$-agonist effect on, 63-64
   anesthetic agent/adjunct effect on, 53t
   anticholinergic effect on, 57

Cardiovascular system (Continued)
   barbiturate effect on, 72
   benzodiazepine as, 61
   dissociative agent effect on, 80
   etomidate effect on, 83
   function of, 28
   halogenated organic compound effect
     on, 85
   halothane effects on, 90
   nitrous oxide effect on, 370
   opioid effect on, 67
   pain-related changes in, 209b
   propofol effect on, 76
   xylazine effect on, 225-226
Cardiovascular system examination
   heart rate/rhythm determination, 19-21
   mucous membrane color/capillary refill
     time, 21
   for murmur, 21
   pulse palpation, 21
Carprofen
   for home analgesia, 227
   liver disease and, 224-225
   in small mammals, 314t
   species/route/dosage of, 215t-217t
Carrier gas flow rate, 111-113
   determination of, 126-127
   with Mapleson A system, 131
   waste anesthetic gas and, 355
Castration
   multimodal therapy
     for cat, 227b
     for dog, 227b
   undescended testicle and, 14
Cat
   airway blockage in, 9
   analgesics for, 215t-217t
   anesthetic emergency, drugs for, 340t
   anesthetic maintenance in, 262b
   anesthetic preparation for, 258b
   body fluids and weight of, 29
   cardiac compression for, 338
   chamber induction in, 260b
   CPR, drugs for, 340t
   dissociative agent and, 9
   dissociative anesthesia in, 79f
   dyspnea in, 343
   fasting recommendations for, 26t
   general anesthesia in, 234
     mortality rate of, 319-320
     recovery from, 262b
   heart rhythm in, 20
   hypoxemia/hypercarbia in, 9
   IM anesthetic protocol for, 252b
   inhalation induction in, 243b
   intravenous induction for, 242b
   intubation in, 260b-261b
   intubation of, anatomy showing, 245f
   IV induction in, 259b
   ketamine and, 81b
   MAC of, 86t
   mask induction in, 259b-260b

Cat (Continued)
   multimodal therapy for
     onychectomy, 227b
     ovariohysterectomy/castration, 227b
   neuroleptanalgesics in, 68-69
   normal hematologic value for, 23t
   normal vital signs of, 144t
   opioid and, 9-10
   opioid effect on, 67
   pain in, 211f
   patient positioning/safety/comfort and,
     254b
   preanesthetic diagnostic testing for, 22t
   premedication/sedation of, 241b
   propofol effect on, 77
   reversal agents for, 254b
   ventricular bigeminy in, 73f
   vital signs for, 18t
Catabolic state, untreated pain producing,
   208
Catalepsy, 79
Catheter
   placement/maintenance of, 28
   types of, 27
   See also Intravenous catheterization
Catheter internal diameter, conversion
    table for endotracheal tube, 377t
Catheterization. See Intravenous catheterization
Cation
   function and types of, 29
Cattle. See Cow
Cauda equina, 189-190
Ceiling effect, 220
Cell membrane
   water and, 28-29
Central nervous system (CNS)
   acepromazine effect on, 59-60
   alpha$_2$-agonist effect on, 63
   anesthetic agent/adjunct effect on, 51, 52t
   anticholinergic effect on, 57
   barbiturate effect on, 72
   benzodiazepine effect on, 61
   dissociative agent effect on, 79-80
   dissociative effect on, 2f
   etomidate effect on, 82-83
   halogenated organic compound effect
     on, 85
   nitrous oxide effect on, 370
   nociception and, 207
   opioid effect on, 67
   propofol effect on, 76
   untreated pain and, 208
Central nervous system (CNS) depression
   anesthesia and, 2f
   antihistamines and, 11
   barbiturate causing, 70-72
   benzodiazepine causing, 61
   sedation and tranquilization, 2
   tricyclic antidepressants and, 11
Central nervous system (CNS) disease,
   signs of, 11

Central nervous system (CNS) vital center, 235
Central nervous system hypersensitivity, 208
Central venous pressure (CVP), 143
 importance of, 157
 procedure for, 157
Cerebral edema, 341
Cesarean patient
 anesthetic concerns for, 327b
 anesthetic techniques for, 326
 hypotension in, 327
 as increased anesthetic risk, 324t, 326-328
 physiologic anemia in, 327
 respiratory/circulatory depression in, 327
Chamber induction
 in dog/cat, 260b
 flow rate during, 127-128
 monitoring during, 243b
 in rabbits, 308b
 use of, 243
Chamber. See Anesthetic chamber
Chemical solution, anesthetic equipment exposure to, 134
Chemistry testing, for hydration status, 17
Chest tap, in trauma patient, 329-330
Chest trauma, ECG for, 24
Chloramphenicol, effects of, 11
Chlorhexidine gluconate, 134
Chloride (Cl⁻), 29
Chlorpromazine, 59
Cholinergic effects, 57
Chronic pain, in small mammals, 315
Circle system, 116
Circulation, 143
 cardiac compression and, 338-339
 indicators of, 143-157
Circulatory depression, 327
Circulatory failure, 312-313
Cisatracurium, 195
Client communication, 6-7, 6b
Clomipramine, 11
Closed rebreathing system
 advantages/disadvantages of, 125
 cost of, 125-126
 flow rate for, 126-127
 flow rate with, 130-131
 nitrous oxide and, 371
 operation of, 375
 oxygen flow rate for, 128b, 130t
 safety concerns with, 131
 semiclosed system versus, 116
 waste gas from, 126
 See also Non-rebreathing system; Rebreathing system
Clotting disorder, bruising and, 13
Coagulation disorder, 11
 blood products for, 32
Coagulation test, 23b
Coat condition, 19
Codeine, 226
Cold application, for pain control, 228

Colic
 alpha₂-adrenoceptor agonist and, 225-226
 cause of, 58
Colloid, 29
 administration of, 30, 328-329
 administration/side effects of, 35
 classification of, 31
 composition/uses for, 32-33
 diffusion of, 30
 indications for, 328
 intravenous solution as, 30
 types of, 328
Colloid solution, administration of, 30
Comatose patient, 17
Combination therapy, 226
Common gas outlet
 care/maintenance of, 133
 description/function of, 115
 safety with use of, 115-116
 use of, 115
Communication
 omissions in, example of, 7b
 with patient, 6-7, 6b
 procedure confirmation and, 9
Complete blood cell count, 22-23
Compressed gas, handling of, 359
Compressed gas cylinder
 care/maintenance of, 132
 cautions for, 105b
 characteristics/capacity/pressure of, 105t
 conversion table for gas pressure in, 377t
 description/function of, 103-104
 label for, 108f
 outlet port for, 104
 oxygen flush valve for, 109-110
  description/function of, 109-110
  safety with, 110
  use of, 110
 oxygen volume in, 108
 parts of, 105f-106f
 pressure-reducing valve
  description/function of, 108
  use of, 108
 risks from, 105
 setup checklist for, 135b
 size E
  attachment for, 103-104
  in cart, 103f
  removal/replacement of, 132
 size H, 103-104, 103f-104f
  detachment/reattachment of, 132
 size of, 103-104
 tank pressure gauge
  description/function of, 107
  use of, 107-108
 turning on/off, 106f
 use of, 104f
 use/storage of, 359-360
 valve for, 104
 vaporizer inlet port
  description/function of, 114
  use of, 115

Compressed gas supply, 100, 101b, 102f
 parts of, 101b
Congestive heart failure, 29-30
Consciousness
 AVPU scale measuring, 17
 definition of, 17
 See also Loss of consciousness (LOC)
Consensual reflex, 19
Consent form
 for CPCR, 13
 example of, 12f
 for surgery/anesthesia, 11-12
Constant rate infusion (CRI)
 anesthetic maintenance with, 259b-260b, 262b
 intravenous catheterization for, 27
 tachyarrhythmia and, 331
 total intravenous anesthesia by, 237, 238f
Controlled substance
 benzodiazepine as, 62
 drug schedules for, 53-54
 regulatory considerations for, 53-54
 storage of, 54
 types of, 53-54
Controlled ventilation, 190-194
 risks of, 194
 types of, 192-194
Conversion table, 376
 body temperature for, 377t
 for body weight, 378t
 for endotracheal tube/catheter internal diameter, 377t
 for gas pressure in compressed gas cylinder, 377t
 for pressure manometer, 377t
Corneal drying, 57
Corneal reflex, 173
 assessment of, 173f
 presence of, 173b
Corrugated breathing tube, 121-122
 example of, 122f
Corticosteroid, 226
Cortisol, 83
Coughing, 11
Cough reflex, 171
Cow
 alpha₂-agonist effect on, 63-64
 analgesics for, 215t-217t
 endotracheal intubation in, 286-287
 fasting recommendations for, 26t
 induction in, 285-286
 intravenous induction in, 295b
 intubation of, 295b-296b
 locomotor pain in, 211f
 normal hematologic value for, 23t
 opioid effect on, 67
 oxygen flow rate for, 128b
 pain tolerance of, 209
 paravertebral anesthesia, procedure for, 197b-198b
 vital signs for, 144t
 vital signs of, 18t

COX-1 selective NSAID, 223
  type/route/dosage of, 215t-217t
COX-2 selective NSAID, 223
  type/route/dosage of, 215t-217t
Crash kit, emergency, equipment and
  drugs for, 380
Cross placental barrier, anesthetic agent/
  adjunct effect on, 55t
Crystalloid
  classification of, 31
  composition of, 31-32
  intravenous solution as, 30
  solute composition of, 31t
  use of, 31
Cyanosis, 22, 22b
  cause of, 158
  as increased anesthetic risk, 332, 336
  indications by, 158, 158b
  nitrous oxide and, 371
  vomiting causing, 341-342
Cyclohexamine
  cardiac arrhythmia and, 10
  in small mammals, 307
Cyclooxygenase (COX), NSAIDs and, 223

D

Database, minimum patient, 5-6
Dazzle reflex, 173
Dead space
  anatomic, 245
  increase in, 57
  mechanical, effect of, 9
Debilitated patient, intravenous
  catheterization for, 27
Deep surgical anesthesia, 142, 142b
Defibrillation, 347b
Dehydration
  anesthetic protocol for, 25
  anesthetic response to, 13
  fluid loss and, 30
  hyperproteinemia and, 23
  intravenous catheterization for, 27
  osmolarity and, 29-30
  PCV/RBC elevation and, 23
  signs of, 17t
  in small mammals, 303b, 304
  *See also* Hydration
Delivery rate, 36b
Delta (δ), 66
Demand valve, oxygen support using, 276,
  277f
Dental cleaning, 19, 19b
Dental disease, 13
Dental tartar, 19
Dependent atelectasis, 9
Dependent lung, 163-164
Depolarizing agent, 195
Deracoxib, 215t-217t
Descriptive scale, simple, 210, 211f
Desflurane, 84
  anesthetic maintenance with, 251b
  blood-gas partition coefficient of, 90b

Desflurane (Continued)
  effects/adverse effects of, 90
  MAC of, 90
  metabolization of, 90
  properties of, 86t, 90
  use of, 90
  vapor pressure of, 86, 90
Detomidine
  in ruminants, 285b
  species/route/dosage of, 215t-217t
  use of, 65
Dexamethasone, 340t
Dexmedetomidine
  dosage of, 65
  drug combining with, 65
  effects of, 140
  epidural use of, 225
  opioids combining with, 68
  for pain control, 225
  pharmacology of, 64
  in small mammals, 305
  species/route/dosage of, 215t-217t
  use of, 64
Dextran, 32
Dextromethorphan, 215t-217t
Dextrose solution
  composition/uses for, 32
  IV fluids as, 30
Diagnostic testing, 303
Diameter-index safety system (DISS), 104f,
  106-107
Diaphragmatic hernia, 332-333
Diarrhea, 11
  osmolarity and, 29-30
Diastolic blood pressure, 152
Diazepam, 3
  administration/use of, 61
  adverse effects of, 61
  for anesthetic emergency in dogs/cats, 340t
  as appetite stimulant, 61
  drug combining with, 62, 62b
  effects of, 226
  intravenous catheterization of, 27
  midazolam versus, 62
  mode of action/pharmacology of, 61
  opioids combining with, 68
  preanesthetic agent for, 56
  in rodents/rabbits, 304
  route of administration, 61
  in small mammals, 305t
  solubility of, 53, 53b
  storage of, 62, 62b
  use of, 62, 226
Diethyl ether
  pain-relieving properties of, 1
  use/contraindications for, 84
Differential white blood cell count, 23
Diffusion
  of albumin, 30
  of ion, 30
Dilation, of pupil, 175f
Direct BP monitoring, 154

Direct patient preparation, 6b
Disease
  fluid loss and, 30
  moderate/severe pain from, 209, 209b
  signs of, 11
Disorientation, opioid and, 67
Dissociative agent
  administration/use of, 81
  adverse effects of, 80-81, 80b
  amnesia from, 80
  cardiovascular system, effect on, 53t, 80
  cats/dogs and, 9
  characteristics of, 79-80
  CNS, effect on, 52t, 79-80
  as controlled substance, 53-54
  drug combining with, 79
  effects of, 2f, 55t, 79-80, 79b
  as injectable anesthetic, 70
  mode of action/pharmacology of, 78-79
  respiratory/gastrointestinal effects of, 54t
  respiratory system, effect on, 80
  use of, 78-82
Distended uterus, in cesarean patient, 327
Distress, stress response and, 208
Dobutamine
  for anesthetic emergency in dogs/cats,
    340t
  blood pressure and, 274-275
  for cardiac arrest, 341
  use in horses, 275b
    preparation/administration of, 281b
Dog
  acepromazine and, 10
  alpha$_2$-agonist effect on, 64
  analgesics for, 215t-217t
  anesthetic emergency, drugs for, 340t
  anesthetic maintenance in, 262b
  anesthetic preparation for, 258b
  barbiturates and, 8
  body fluids and weight of, 29
  cardiac compression for, 338
  chamber induction in, 260b
  CPR, drugs for, 340t
  dissociative agent and, 9
  fasting recommendations for, 26t
  general anesthesia in, 234
    mortality rate of, 319-320
  heart rhythm in, 20
  hypoxemia/hypercarbia in, 9
  inhalation induction in, 243b
  intravenous induction for, 242b
  intubation in, 260b-261b
  IV induction in, 259b
  MAC of, 86t
  mask induction in, 259b-260b
  multimodal therapy
    for fractured humerus, 228b
    for ovariohysterectomy/castration,
      227b
  normal hematologic value for, 23t
  normal vital signs of, 144t
  opioid effect on, 67

Dog (Continued)
   patient positioning/safety/comfort and, 254b
   preanesthetic diagnostic testing for, 22t
   premedication/sedation of, 241b
   propofol effect on, 76
   recovery period for, 262b
   reversal agents for, 254b
   sinus arrhythmia in younger, 21b
   vital signs for, 18t
Dopamine
   for anesthetic emergency in dogs/cats, 340t
   for cardiac arrest, 341
Dopamine receptor, blockage of, 59
Doppler blood flow detector, 143-144, 154
   monitor base unit for, 155f
   parts/method of, 154-156
   probe placement for, 155f
   problems with, 156
   use/operation of, 154-155
Doppler probe
   blood pressure, measuring, 180b
   swine and, 293f
Dorsal pedal artery, pulse strength at, 153f
Double drip
   as bolus, 285-286
   example of, 286f
   in ruminants, 285b
Down lung, 163-164
Doxapram
   administration of, 92
   adverse effects of, 92
   dosage of, 92, 92b
   effects of, 92
   indications for, 92
   mode of action/pharmacology of, 92
   in small mammals, 306t
      dosage for, 313t
Draft horse, sedatives in, 10
Drip rate
   calculation of, 38b-39b
   definition of, 36b, 37
Droperidol, 305
Drug administration
   for anesthetic emergency in dogs/cats, 340t
   incorrect, as anesthetic emergency/ problem cause, 320-321
   intravenous catheterization for, 28
Drug Enforcement Administration (DEA), 53-54
Drug-induced CNS depression, 2
Drug reaction
   intravenous catheterization and, 27
   patient history and, 11
Dysphoria, 61
   opioid effect on, 67
Dyspnea, 22, 22b
   cause of
      in cats, 343
      in dogs, 343

Dyspnea (Continued)
   as increased anesthetic risk, 332-333, 336
   prevention of, 343
   during recovery period, 343
   signs of, 22
   vomiting causing, 341-342
Dysuria, 11

E

Ear, examination of, 19
Ear mite, 13
Electrocardiogram (ECG)
   cardiac rhythm and, 341
   indications for, 24
   pulseless electrical activity pattern, 342f
Electrocardiography, 145
   electrode placement for, 147b
Electrolyte
   composition of, 29
   concentration in ICF/ECF, 30f
   constant rate infusion for, 27
   IV fluids as, 30
Electrolyte disturbance
   anesthetic protocol for, 25
   cause of, 18
   ECG for, 24
   intravenous catheterization for, 27
Electromechanical dissociation, 341
Electroneutrality, 29
Emergence delirium, 210
Emergency crash kit, equipment and drugs for, 380
Emergency. See Anesthetic emergency/ problem
Endocrine disease, 11
Endogenous opioid peptide, 66
Endotracheal intubation
   advantages of, 245
   adverse effects of, 57
   bradycardia from, 176
   of calf, 286, 287f
   complications of, 250-251, 250b
   cuff inflation after, 248-249, 249b
   equipment for, 245-246, 245f
   in horses
      complications of, 273
      equipment for, 270b, 272
      procedure for, 272-273, 273f, 280b
   during laryngospasm, 249
   laryngospasm from, 172
   patient positioning/safety/comfort after, 252
   placement of, 245, 247b
   procedure for, 247-248
   in rabbits, 316b-317b
   readiness for, 247b
   in ruminants, 286-287
      equipment for, 286
      procedure for, 286-287
      tube selection for, 286
   in small mammals, 309

Endotracheal intubation (Continued)
   tube selection for, 246, 246t, 246b
   ventilation with, 245
   See also Intubation
Endotracheal tube (ET tube)
   airway
      blocked, 253f
      maintaining, 252
   catheter internal diameter, conversion table for, 377t
   cuff of
      cautions for, 98
      importance of, 98
      use of, 98
   for dogs/cats
      preparation of, 247
      selection of, 246t, 246b
   example of, 249f
   for horses
      preparation of, 272-273
      selection of, 272
   lengths of, 97, 99b
   materials for, 97
   parts of, 98-99, 98f
   placement/management of, 98, 246f
   problems with, 322
   in ruminants
      preparation of, 286
      selection of, 286
   securing, 248
   selection of, 246
   sizes of, 97-98
   for small mammals, 309
   types of, 97, 98f
   use of, 97
End-tidal $CO_2$, 165, 165f
End-tidal $CO_2$ monitor
   carbon dioxide measurement by, 164-167
   example of, 165f
Enflurane, 84
   adverse effects of, 91
Eosinophil count, normal values for, 23t
Epidural analgesia
   alpha$_2$-adrenoceptor agonist and, 225
   opioid and, 221-222
Epidural anesthesia
   anatomic considerations for, 189
   in dog, procedure for, 200b-202b
   drug selection for, 189
   spinal anesthesia versus, 189
   use of, 3, 188-189
Epidural block, 185
Epinephrine
   for cardiac arrest, 341
   cardiac arrhythmia and, 10
   in dogs/cats
      for anesthetic emergency, 340t
      for CPR, 340t
   intravenous catheterization for, 27
   lidocaine and, 187
   in small mammals, 313t
   ventricular arrhythmia from, 187

Equilibrium, 86
Equine anesthesia, 265
    preparation for, 267
    protocol for, 267
Equine anesthetic induction gate, 269-270, 270f
Equine. *See* Horse
Equipment preparation, 6b
Eructate, 284
Erythrocyte count, 22-23
Esophageal reflux
    during anesthesia, 26
    fasting and, 26
Esophageal stethoscope, 143
    example of, 145f
    maintenance of, 145
    parts of, 145
    use of, 145
Estimate of charges, 11-12, 12b
Estrous cycle status, 10
Ether. *See* Diethyl ether
Ethyl chloride, 186
Ethylene oxide gas, 134
Etodolac
    for home analgesia, 227
    species/route/dosage of, 215t-217t
Etomidate
    adverse effects of, 83, 83b
    cardiovascular system, effect on, 53t, 83
    characteristics of, 82-83
    CNS, effect on, 52t, 82-83
    effects of, 55t, 82-83, 82b
    mode of action/pharmacology of, 82
    muscle relaxation and, 83
    respiratory/gastrointestinal effects of, 54t
    respiratory system, effect on, 83
    to effect, 259b
    use/administration of, 83
    use/indications for, 82
Eutectic mixture, 186
Examination. *See* Cardiovascular system examination; Physical examination; Respiratory system examination
Excitement, 18
    acepromazine effect on, 60
    from barbiturates, 74
    opioid effect on, 67
    during postanesthetic period, 342-343
    preanesthetic agent for, 55
    pupillary light reflex and, 19
    *See also* Involuntary excitement
Excitement stage, 141
Exercise, osmolarity and, 29-30
Exercise intolerance, 11
    cause of, 18
Exhalation, 21
Exhaust valve, 117
Exotic animal
    anesthesia for, 10
        sensitivity to, 10
    heart rhythm in, 20

Expiration, 164
Expiratory breathing tube, 121-122
Extracellular fluid
    concentration of, 29
    total body weight and, 29, 29f
Extracellular fluid compartment
    electrolyte concentration in, 30f
    fluid loss in, 30
    water and, 28-29
Extra-label drug use, 13
Extubation
    arousal/swallowing reflex and, 255-256
    delaying, 256
    of horse, 277
    preparation for, 255
    respiratory distress after, 256
    of ruminant, 289
    of swine, 292
Eye
    anesthetic agent/adjunct effect on, 55t
    dilation of, 175f
    examination of, 19
    nystagmus of, 175
    vagus nerve and iris of, 57
    *See also* Pupil size
Eye position, 140
    anesthetic depth and, 174, 174b
    by anesthetic stage/plane, 141
    central and ventromedial, 174f

F
Facial expression/appearance/attitude, pain and, 210
Fainting, 11
Fasciculation, 61
Fasting
    before anesthesia, 26-27, 26t
        in ruminants, 284
    in pediatric patients, 26t, 325
    time period for, 26t, 27
    vomiting despite, 26
Fatigue, as anesthetic emergency/problem cause, 321
Fat solubility, 86t
Fecal analysis history, 11
Feline immunodeficiency virus, 11
Feline leukemia, 11
Femoral artery, pulse strength at, 153f
Fentanyl
    administration/dosage of, 219
    classification of, 219
    effects/adverse effects of, 219
    intravenous infusion of, 221
    species/route/dosage of, 215t-217t
Fentanyl-droperidol (Innovar Vet), 305
    in small mammals, 305t
Fentanyl-fluanisone (Hypnorm), 305
    in small mammals, 305t
Fentanyl-fluanisone (Hypnorm) and diazepam, 306t
Fentanyl-fluanisone (Hypnorm) and midazolam, 306t

Fentanyl patch
    absorption of
        breakthrough pain, 222
        death and, 222
        delay in, 222
        high concentrations of, 222
    adverse effects of, 222
    application of, 230b
    for home analgesia, 227
    mechanism of action, 222
    meloxicam and, 226
Feral cat, anesthetic agent, oral administration of, 244
Ferret, heart rhythm in, 20
Fibrillation, 176
    atrial fibrillation, 176
    ventricular fibrillation, 176
Field anesthesia, 266
    horses and
        recovery period for, 275-278
        using TIVA, 275, 275b
Firocoxib, 215t-217t
First-degree atrioventricular (AV) heart block, 20, 147
    example of, 148f
Five freedoms, 208, 209b
Five-level body score system, 15-16
Flaccid, 141
Flea infestation, 13
Flow-by oxygen, 329
Flow meter, 109f
    accuracy assessment of, 132
    description/function of, 109
    example of, 109f
    leaks, checking for, 126
    use of, 109
Flow rate
    for breathing systems, 126-127, 127b
    calculation of, 126, 129b
    with closed rebreathing system, 130-131
    conditions of, 126-127
    maintenance level and, 129
    during mask/chamber induction, 127-128
    for non-rebreathing system, 131
    for oxygen, 126, 128b
    during recovery, 129
    for semiclosed rebreathing system
        anesthetic depth changes, 128
        induction with injectable agent, 128
    *See also* Oxygen flow rate
Fluid administration, 28-39
    purpose of, 27
Fluid administration set chamber
    types of, 37, 37f
Fluid homeostasis
    during anesthesia, 30
    maintenance of, 29
Fluid overload
    pulmonary edema and, 328f
    signs of, 328

Fluid rate calculation, flow chart for, 40f-41f
Fluid therapy
administration of
calculating rates for, 35-39, 38b-39b
flow chart for, 40f-41f
rate of, 34t-35t
adverse effects of, 35
choices/administration rates for, 33
hypertonic saline solution as, 33-35
isotonic crystalloid as, 33, 33b
in small mammals, 304t
solutes in, 29
volume/administration rates, 304
Flumazenil, 62
Flunixin meglumine
in small mammals, 314t
species/route/dosage of, 215t-217t
Foal
cardiac compression for, 338
inhalation induction in, 272, 272b
via nasotracheal intubation, 280b
oxygen flow rate for, 128b
Food and Drug Administration (FDA), 13
Fresh gas, 110
Fresh gas inlet, 110
care/maintenance of, 133
description/function of, 116
leaks, checking for, 126
use of, 116
Fresh gas outlet
description/function of, 115
safety with use of, 115-116
use of, 115
Functional residual volume, 327

G
Gabapentin, 215t-217t
Gait, 18
in small mammals postoperatively, 313-314
Gallamine, 195
Gas line, 103-104
Gastric dilatation-volvulus, 24
Gastrointestinal (GI) tract, 57
Gastrointestinal secretion
anesthetic agent/adjunct effect on, 54t
anticholinergic and, 57
Gastrointestinal system
alpha$_2$-agonist effect on, 64
anesthetic agent/adjunct effect on, 54t
NSAIDs effect on, 224
opioid effect on, 68
xylazine effect on, 225-226
Gelatin product, 32
General anesthesia
definition of, 2
in dogs/cats, 234
mortality rate of, 319-320
recovery from, 262b
in horses, 266
agents for, 270

General anesthesia (Continued)
duration of, 270
recovery from, 281b
indications for, 234
induction techniques/agents, 306-309
by intravenous induction, 242
with IV agent induction, 258b
local anesthesia and, 184, 184b
maintenance of, 239
with inhalation agent, 251-252
in PSC P1/P2 cats/dogs, 251b
optimum depth of, 142-143
pain control by, 52
renal disease and, 333
risks of, 319
in ruminants
equipment for, 284-285
recovery from, 296b
sedation and, 234, 234b
sedation without, ACVA guidelines for, 369
sedatives for, 55
stages/planes of, 140
vagus nerve, stimulation of, 57
See also Anesthetic stages/planes; Monitoring
General anesthetic procedure, dynamics of, 236
General condition, 18-19
Gerbil
analgesic agents in, 314t
anesthetic/related drugs for, 306t
biologic data for, 299t
fluid administration in, 304t
handling/restraint of, 301
preanesthetic agent for, 305t
Geriatric patient
anesthesia in, 10
characteristics of, 323
hypotension/kidney function of, 324-325
hypothermia in, 324
as increased anesthetic risk, 324, 324t
Giant breed dog
acepromazine and, 10
sedatives and, 10
Gingiva, mucous membrane color and, 157-158
Gluconate, 30-32
Glucose, 29
IV fluids as, 30
Glutaraldehyde solution, 134
Glycopyrrolate
cardiovascular system, effect on, 57-58
CNS, effect on, 57
mode of action of, 57
respiratory system, effect on, 58
in small mammals, 304, 304b, 305t
strengths of, 58
use/administration of, 56, 58
Goat. See Ruminant
Greyhound, barbiturates and, 8

Guaifenesin
administration for use of, 84
adverse effects of, 83
cardiovascular system, effect on, 53t
CNS, effect on, 52t
effects of, 55t, 83
in horses, 275
mode of action/pharmacology of, 83
for rapid infusion, 270f
respiratory/gastrointestinal effects of, 54t
use of, 83
Guedel, Arthur, MD, 140
Guedel's stages/planes of anesthesia, 140, 140f
Guinea pig
analgesic agents in, 314t
anesthetic/related drugs for, 306t
biologic data for, 299t
fluid administration in, 304t
handling/restraint of, 301, 302f
preanesthetic agent for, 305t
Gut motility, alpha$_2$-adrenoceptor agonist causing, 225-226
Gut stasis, 58

H
Halogenated inhalant
cardiovascular system, effect on, 53t
CNS, effect on, 52t
effects of, 55t
respiratory/gastrointestinal effects of, 54t
Halogenated organic compound
cardiovascular system, effect on, 85
CNS, effect on, 85
effects/adverse effects of, 85b
mode of action/pharmacology of, 84-85
respiratory system, effect on, 85-86
supply/storage of, 84-85
use of, 88-91
Halothane, 84
cardiac arrhythmia and, 10
concentration of, 355t
effects/adverse effects of, 90-91
MAC of, 88, 90
metabolization of, 91
partition coefficient of, 90
properties of, 86t, 90
respiratory system, effect on, 91
rubber solubility of, 90
stability of, 90
vapor pressure of, 86, 90
Hamster
analgesic agents in, 314t
anesthetic/related drugs for, 306t
biologic data for, 299t
fluid administration in, 304t
handling/restraint of, 300-301, 301f
injection in, 301f
life span of, 299
preanesthetic agent for, 305t

Heart, vagus nerve and, 57
Heart block, 55
Heart disease. *See* Cardiac disease
Heart rate
    acepromazine effect on, 59
    during anesthesia, 140, 144t
    anesthetic agent/adjunct effect on, 53t
    anesthetic depth and, 141t, 176
    anesthetic drug decreasing, 330-331
    by anesthetic stage/plane, 141
    anticholinergic increasing, 57
    assessment of, 143-144
    body size and, 20
    determination of, 19-20
        in small animals, 20b
    as increased anesthetic risk, 336-337
    instruments used for, 145-151
    pulse and, 21
    in rodents/rabbits, 310
Heart rhythm
    during anesthesia, 144t
    assessment of, 144-151
    determination of, 19-20
    ECG for, 24
    electrocardiogram for, 341
    first-degree atrioventricular (AV) heart
        block, 20
    as increased anesthetic risk, 336-337
    instruments used for, 145-151
    normal sinus rhythm
        definition of, 20
        by species, 20
    in rodents/rabbits, 310
    second-degree atrioventricular (AV)
        heart block, 20-21
    sinus arrhythmia
        definition of, 20
        by species, 20
    by species, 20
    types of, 341
Heartworm disease, 11
Heartworm test, 24
Heat application, for pain control, 228
Heat stroke, 29-30
Hematocrit, for hydration status, 17
Hematologic effect, of waste gas, 353
Hematology testing
    for hydration status, 17
    normal values for, 23t
Hemodilution, 35
Hemoglobin, normal values for, 23t
Hemoglobin-based oxygen carrier, 32-33
Hemoglobin saturation
    measurement of, 159
    pulse oximeter measuring, 159-160
Hemorrhage
    capnogram and, 167
    fluid loss and, 30
Hepatic disease, 333
    as increased anesthetic risk, 324t
Hepatocellular toxicosis, from carprofen,
    224-225

Herbal remedy, for pain control, 228
Hetastarch, 32
High-pressure system test, 361b
Histamine receptor, blockage of, 59
History, of anesthesia, 1-3
Hoisting, of horse to surgery table, 270,
    271f
Holmes, Oliver Wendell, 1
Home analgesia, 227
Homeopathic remedy, for pain control,
    228
Homeostasis
    definition of, 29-30
    *See also* Fluid homeostasis
Horse
    acepromazine effect on, 60
    alpha$_2$-agonist effect on, 63-64
    analgesics for, 215t-217t
    anesthesia preparation in, 279b
    anesthetic induction gate for, 269-270,
        270f
    anesthetic induction in, 269-272
        protocol for, 279b
    anesthetic machine for, 267-268, 267f
    anesthetic maintenance in, 273-275
        with inhalation agent, 281b
        with IV agent (TIVA), 275
    anesthetic recovery in, 9
    atelectasis in, 266
    blood pressure monitoring in, 274, 274f
    body weight, formula for, 14
    colic pain in, 211f
    dobutamine in, 275b
        blood pressure and, 274-275
        preparation/administration of, 281b
    endotracheal intubation in
        equipment for, 272
        procedure for, 280b
    endotracheal tube for
        preparation of, 272-273
        selection of, 272
    fasting recommendations for, 26t
    general anesthesia in, 266
        agents for, 270
        recovery from, 281b
    heart rhythm in, 20
    hypotension in, 274-275
    hypoventilation in, 274
    hypoxemia in, 275
    inhalation anesthetics and, 9
    IV drug, dosage calculations for, 267b
    IV induction in, 269-270, 270b
    MAC of, 86t
    multimodal therapy, for bilateral stifle
        arthroscopy, 228b
    myopathy prevention in, 270, 270b
    normal hematologic value for, 23t
    opioid effect on, 9-10, 67
    orotracheal intubation in, 273b
    oxygen flow rate for, 128b
    patient positioning/safety/comfort and,
        275

Horse (*Continued*)
    preanesthetic diagnostic testing for,
        22t
    premedication/sedation of, 268-269,
        268b
    recovery period for
        extubation and, 277
        monitoring during, 276
        nasopharyngeal tube for, 276f
        preparation for, 276
        restraining during, 276f
        rope placement for, 276f, 277-278
        signs of, 277
        standing after, 275, 277-278
    sedatives and, 10
    surgery table for
        hoisting to, 270, 271f
        padding for, 271f
    vital signs for, 18t, 144t
    *See also* Field anesthesia
Human error
    as anesthetic emergency/problem,
        320-321, 320b
        anesthetic agent/machine, unfamiliar-
            ity with, 320
        drug administration, incorrect,
            320-321
        fatigued personnel, 321
        history/examination, not obtaining,
            320
        inattentiveness, 321
        preoccupied/hurried personnel, 321
Humerus fracture, multimodal therapy for
    dog, 228b
Hydration
    assessment of, 17
    chemistry/hematology test for, 17
    *See also* Dehydration
Hydromorphone
    classification of, 219
    intravenous catheterization of, 27
    intravenous infusion of, 221
    neuroleptanalgesia and, 68
    pharmacology of, 218
    species/route/dosage of, 215t-217t
Hypercarbia, 191
    cause of, 9
    predisposing factors for, 191
    respiratory rate and, 176
Hyperglycemia, 63
Hyperkalemia, 27
Hyperproteinemia, 23
Hypertension, 152
Hyperthermia
    capnogram and, 167
    cause of, 170
    halothane causing, 91
    nursing care for, 257
Hypertonic fluid, 31
Hypertonic saline solution, 32
    administration of, 30
    side effects of, 33-35

Hyperventilation
    capnogram and, 167
    doxapram causing, 92
Hypnorm (fentanyl-fluanisone), 305, 305t
Hypnosis
    definition of, 2
    etomidate causing, 82-83
Hypoglycemia
    in rodents/rabbits, 303
    signs of, 11
Hypoproteinemia
    blood products for, 32
    cause of, 23
Hypotension
    acepromazine effect on, 59-60
    in anesthetized horses, 274-275
    blood pressure and, 152
    capnogram and, 167
    cause of, 28, 152b
    in cesarean patient, 327
    dehydration causing, 13
    in geriatric patients, 324-325
    as increased anesthetic risk, 336
    intravenous catheterization and, 27
    IV infusion rates for, 33
    opioid causing, 68
    prevention of, 153b
    propofol effect on, 76
    signs of, 21b
    in trauma patient, 328
Hypothermia
    acepromazine effect on, 59
    from alpha₂-agonist, 63
    anesthesia and, 169
    capnogram and, 167
    in geriatric patients, 324
    minimizing, techniques for, 170
    in pediatric patients, 10, 325
    rewarming techniques for, 170
    in small mammals, avoiding, 311
Hypotonic fluid, 31
Hypoventilation, 85
    in anesthetized horses, 274
    capnogram and, 167
Hypoxemia, 191
    anemia causing, 13
    in anesthetized horses, 275
    anticholinergic and, 57
    cause of, 9, 169
    nitrous oxide and, 371
    predisposing factors for, 191
    respiratory rate and, 176
    signs of, 11
Hypoxia
    nitrous oxide and, 371
    in pediatric patients, 10

I

Icterus, 162
Identification collar, 14b
Identification of patient, 14
Ileus, 26

Illness
    history of, 11
    moderate/severe pain from, 209, 209b
    patient stabilization from, 27
    signs of, inquiring about, 8
Inattentiveness, as anesthetic emergency/
        problem cause, 321
In-circle vaporizer, 194
Incompatible drug, intravenous catheteri-
        zation and, 27
Indirect BP monitoring
    photoplethysmograph for, 154
    types of, 154, 154b
Induction
    in brachycephalic dogs, 325-326
    in cattle, 285-286
    with IM injection, 262b
    with inhalation agent, 237-239, 239f
    with IV agent, 258b
    respiratory depression and, 332-333
    See also Anesthetic induction
Induction agent, 51
Induction period
    flow rate during, 127-128
        semiclosed rebreathing system,
            128-129
    involuntary excitement during, 55
    preanesthetic agent for, 56t
Infection, WBC count indicating, 23
Infectious agent, anesthetic equipment
        transferring, 133-134
Infiltration, 184
    procedure for, 186
    techniques for, 187
    use of, 186
Inflammatory bowel disease, 11
Informed consent, 11-12
Infusion pump, 35, 36f
Infusion rate
    calculation of, 37-39, 38b-39b, 40f-41f
    definition of, 36b, 37
Infusion time, 36b
Infusion volume, 36b
Inhalation, 21
Inhalation agent
    administration of, 51, 242
    anesthetic maintenance with, 262b
    blood-gas partition coefficient and, 87
    development of, 84
    diethyl ether as, 1
    horse and, 9
    induction/maintenance with, 237-239,
        239f
    intravenous induction/maintenance
        with, 239, 240f
    maintenance with, 260b-261b
        in dogs/cats, 251-252, 258b
        in horses, 273-275, 281b
    partition coefficient of, 87
    for pediatric patients, 325
    percent concentration levels of, 113
    physical/chemical properties of, 86-88

Inhalation agent (Continued)
    properties of, 86t
    solubility of, 87
    types of, 84
    via face mask in swine, 291f
Inhalation induction
    anesthetic depth and, 308-309
    in foals, 272, 272b
        via nasotracheal intubation, 280b
    for PSC P1/P2 cats/dogs, 243b
    in small mammals, 308, 308b
    via nasotracheal tube, 272
Injectable agent
    administration of, 51
    dosage calculations for, 235b
    maintenance with
        in dogs/cats, 260b-261b
        in horses, 275
injectable anesthetic
    accidental exposure to, 360
    administration of, 70
    characterization of, 70
    flow rate after induction with, 128
    oral routes of, 244
    types of, 70
Injection rate, case study for
    too fast, 77b
    too slowly, 78b
Innovar Vet (fentanyl-droperidol), 305
    in small mammals, 305t
Inotropy, 28
Insensibility to pain, state of, 1
Inspiration, time period for, 164
Inspiratory breathing tube, 121-122
Inspired air, oxygen level in, 101
Insufflation, 276
Insulin
    constant rate infusion for, 27
    as preanesthetic care, 39
Intact, reproductive status and, 10
Intact female patient, 10
Intermediate-acting barbiturate, 70
Intermittent mandatory ventilation, 192
    technical consideration for
        in-circle versus out-of-circle
            vaporizer, 194
        rebreathing system versus non-
            rebreathing, 194
Interstitial fluid, 29, 29f
Interstitial fluid compartment, 30
Intestinal peristalsis, 58
Intraarticular use, of opioids, 221
Intracardiac injection, 341
Intracellular fluid
    concentration of, 29
    total body weight and, 29, 29f
Intracellular fluid compartment
    electrolyte concentration in, 30f
    water and, 28-29
Intracranial pressure
    anesthetic agent/adjunct effect on, 52t
    dissociative agent and, 81

Intracranial pressure *(Continued)*
  halothane causing, 91
  opioid causing, 68
  propofol effect on, 76
Intramuscular anesthetic agent
  induction/maintenance with, 262b
  induction with, 236, 236f
  maintenance with, 254b
  for PSC P1/P2 cats, 252b
Intramuscular induction
  agents for, 244
  IV induction versus, 244
  in rabbit, 306
Intramuscular injection
  in mouse, 300f
  in rabbit, 302
  in rat, 301f
Intramuscular route
  preanesthesia administration by, 56
  sedative administered by, 56b
  swine sedation by, 289-290
Intraocular pressure
  dissociative agent and, 81
  opioid causing, 68
  propofol effect on, 76
Intraoperative analgesia, multimodal
      therapy
  for bilateral stifle arthroscopy, 228b
  for fractured humerus, 228b
Intraosseous route, 304
Intraperitoneal fluid administration, 304t
Intraperitoneal injection
  in mouse, 299, 300f
  in rat, 300f
  in small mammals, 306
Intravascular fluid, 29, 29f
Intravascular fluid compartment, 30
Intravascular volume, 28
Intravenous administration set port, IV
      injection through, 46b-47b
Intravenous agent, 288
Intravenous catheterization
  for drug administration, 28
  indications for, 27
  necessity of, 27
  in pediatric patients, 325
  placement/maintenance of, 28
  in small animals, 44b-46b
  of swine, 291f
  types of, 27
Intravenous fluid
  administration of
    adverse effects of, 35
    calculating rates for, 34t-35t, 35-39,
        38b-39b
    flow chart for, 40f-41f
  choices/administration rates for, 33
  classification of, 30-33
  hypertonic saline solution as, 33-35
  isotonic crystalloid as, 33, 33b
  morphine/lidocaine/ketamine, adding,
      231b

Intravenous fluid *(Continued)*
  renal disease and, 333
  as replacement/maintenance, 31
Intravenous induction
  by bolus injection, 242
  in cattle, 295b
  in dog/cat, 259b
  of general anesthesia, 258b
  in horses, 269-270, 270b
  IM induction versus, 244
  with inhalation agent, 239, 240f
  loss of consciousness from, 241-242
  for PSC P1/P2 cats/dogs, 242b
  in ruminants, 285-286
  to effect, 259b
  types of, 242
Intravenous infusion, of opioids, 221
Intravenous injection, 302
Intravenous injection, through IV admin-
      istration set port, 46b-47b
Intravenous method, 56
Intravenous propofol, 251b
Intravenous regional anesthesia (Bier
      block), 189
Intubation
  anesthetic induction and, 241-242,
      241b
  of brachiocephalic animal, 10
  of cow, 295b-296b
  in dog/cat, 260b-261b
  in pediatric patients, 10, 325
  of swine, 290, 292f
  *See also* Endotracheal intubation
Involuntary excitement, 55
Involuntary movement, stage II, 141-142
Ion, 29
  diffusion of, 30
Ionization, of barbiturates, 71
Iris, 57
Isoflurane, 3, 84
  anesthetic maintenance with
    in dogs/cats, 251b
    in PSC P1/P2 horses, 274b
  blood-gas partition coefficient of, 88
  blood pressure, effect on, 60
  carbon monoxide and, 89
  effects/adverse effects of, 88-89
  elimination of, 89
  MAC of, 88
  as muscle relaxant, 89
  nonprecision vaporizer delivering, 110
  properties of, 86t, 88-91
  rubber solubility of, 88
  use of, 88-91
  vapor pressure of, 86, 88
Isolyte S (IS), 31-32, 31t
Isotonic, polyionic maintenance solution,
      32
Isotonic, polyionic replacement solution,
      31-32
Isotonic crystalloid, 33, 33b
Isotonic fluid, 31

J
Jackson-Rees circuit, 123
Jackson-Rees circuit (Mapleson F system),
      124-125
Jaw tone
  anesthetic depth and, 174
  assessment of, 173b, 174f

K
Kappa (χ), 66
Ketamine, 3, 78
  action/administration of, 81
  adverse effects of, 55, 57, 226
  in cats, 81b
  chloramphenicol and, 11
  drug combining with, 53, 81
  in horses, 275
  midazolam and, 62
  mode of action of, 79
  *N*-methyl-D-asparte (NMDA) receptor
      and, 208
  pharmacology of, 226
  recovery from, 81
  respiratory pattern from, 164
  route of administration, 56
  in small mammals, 307
  species/route/dosage of, 215t-217t
  supply of, 81
  tissue irritation from, 80
  use of, 81
Ketamine-acepromazine, in rabbits, 307
Ketamine-diazepam combination
  administration of, 82
  advantages of, 81-82
  in horses, 279b
  pharmacology of, 81
  in rabbits, 307
  in ruminants, 285b
  to effect, 259b
Ketamine-medetomidine, 306t
Ketamine-midazolam
  in horses, 279b
  in rabbits, 307
Ketamine-xylazine, 306t
Ketoprofen
  in small mammals, 314t
  species/route/dosage of, 215t-217t
Ketorolac, 215t-217t
Kidney, 353
Kidney damage, 13
Kidney function, importance of, 23, 333

L
Lack circuit, 123
Lack circuit (modified Mapleson A
      system), 123, 124f
  oxygen flow rate for, 128b, 130t
Lacrimal secretion
  anesthetic depth and, 175
  reduction of, 57
Lactate, 30-32
Lactated Ringer's (LR) solution, 31-32, 31t

Large animal
    anesthetic machine for, 283-284
        example of, 284f
    oxygen flow rate for, 128b
Large animal anesthesia, 283
Laryngeal mask, 309
Laryngeal reflex, 172
Laryngoscope
    handles/blades for, 99, 99f
    use of, 99
Laryngospasm
    barbiturate induction causing, 73
    definition of, 343
    endotracheal intubation and, 172, 249
    lidocaine preventing, 186, 246
    prevention of, 249
Laser therapy, for pain control, 228
L-block, 188
Leading question, 8
Length, in metric system, 376
Lethargy, 17
Leukemia, 23
Leukocyte count, normal values for, 23t
Lidocaine, 3
    administration of, 184
    in dogs/cats
        for anesthetic emergency, 340t
        for CPR, 340t
    dosing requirements for, 9
    epinephrine and, 187
    laryngospasm and, 186, 246
    pharmacology of, 185t
    skin application of, 186
    for skin infiltration, 184
    in small mammals, 313t
    use of, 186
Lidocaine patch, 186
Ligamentum interarcuatum, 189
Light surgical anesthesia, 142, 142b
Line block, 187
    locations for, 188f
    positioning for, 187-188
    use of, 188
Line pressure, 105
Line pressure gauge
    description/function of, 108
    example of, 107f
    use of, 108-109
Lipid solubility, 71
    of inhalation anesthetics, 86t
    of methoxyflurane, 91
    of phenobarbital, 71
Liver
    NSAIDs effect on, 224-225
    waste gas effect on, 353
Liver enlargement, anesthetic response
    to, 13
Local analgesia, 183
Local anesthesia
    advantages of, 184
    definition of, 2-3, 183
    general anesthesia and, 184, 184b

Local anesthetic
    administration, routes of, 185-189
    administration of, 189
    adverse effects of, 189-190
    anaphylaxis from, 190
    characteristics of, 184
    duration of effect, 187
    infiltration of, 186-188
    intraarticular administration of, 188
    mechanism of action, 184-185
    mucous membranes and, 186
    neurons and, 184-185
    pharmacology of, 185t
    in small mammals postoperatively,
        315
    spinal cord trauma from, 190
    surgery and, 225
    testing effectiveness of, 186
    tissue irritation from, 189-190
    topical use of, 186
    toxicity of, 190
    types of, 184
Locomotor activity, 210
    morphine and, 214-217
Long-acting barbiturate, 70
Lorazepam
    route of administration, 61
    use/administration of, 61
Loss of consciousness (LOC)
    assessment of, 18t
    indication/cause of, 17
    intravenous induction producing,
        241-242
    lethargy and, 17, 141
    See also Anesthetic stage/plane
Low blood pressure, signs of, 11
Low dead space T-piece system, 309, 310f
Low-pressure system, 126, 361
Lung
    auscultation of, 22
    vagus nerve and, 57
Lymph node, 19
Lymphocyte count, normal values for, 23t

M
Macrodrip set chamber
    administration rates for, 37
    example of, 37f
    use of, 37
Magill circuit (Mapleson A system),
        123, 124f
    carrier gas flow with, 131
    oxygen flow rate for, 128b, 130t
Magnesium ($Mg^{2+}$), 29, 31-32
Magnetic therapy, for pain control, 228
Mainstream capnograph, 164-165
Mainstream sampler, 165
Maintenance
    flow rate during, 129
    with inhalation agent, 237-239, 240f
Maintenance agent, 51
Maintenance fluid, 31, 31b

Malignant hyperthermia (MH), 170
    in swine, 292
Mammary gland(s), 19
Manual ventilation, 113, 192
    endotracheal intubation and, 245
    example of, 120f
    performance of, 192
    respiratory depression and, 192
    ventilation rate for, 192-193
    weaning from, 193
    See also Reservoir bag
Mapleson A system, 123, 124f
    carrier gas flow with, 131
    oxygen flow rate for, 128b, 130t
Mapleson classification system, 123
    non-rebreathing system flow rates using,
        131
Mapleson D system, 124f
Mapleson E system, 124, 124f
    oxygen flow rate for, 131
Mapleson F system, 124-125, 124f
    oxygen flow rate for, 131
Marcaine, 185t
Mask induction
    anesthetic stages and, 243
    cautions with use of, 243
    challenges with, 243
    in dog/cat, 259b-260b
    flow rate during, 127-128
    inhalation agent for, 243
    monitoring during, 243
    waste anesthetic gas and, 355
Mask. See Anesthetic mask
Massage therapy, for pain control,
        228
Mean arterial pressure (MAP), 152b
    calculation of, 152
    tissue perfusion and, 152, 152b
Mechanical dead space
    effect of, 9
    endotracheal tube causing, 246
Mechanical ventilation, 192-193
    endotracheal intubation and, 245
    gas delivery with, 193
    respiratory rate with, 193-194
    ventilators for, 193
Medetomidine, 305, 305t
Mediator, 208
Medical problem, history of, 11
Medium surgical anesthesia, 142, 142b
Meloxicam
    fentanyl patch and, 226
    for home analgesia, 227
    in small mammals, 314t
    species/route/dosage of, 215t-217t
Meperidine
    adverse effects of, 68
    classification of, 219
    pharmacology of, 219
    in rodents, 314-315
    in small mammals, 314t
    species/route/dosage of, 215t-217t

Mepivacaine
　pharmacology of, 185t
　for skin infiltration, 184
Metabolic alkalosis, 169
Metabolic disorder, signs of, 11
Metabolism
　capnogram and, 167
　of inhalation anesthetics, 86t
Methadone
　intravenous infusion of, 221
　for moderate/severe pain, 219
　species/route/dosage of, 215t-217t
Methohexital
　effects/pharmacology of, 75
　redistribution of, 71
　use of, 72
Methoxyflurane, 84
　blood-gas partition coefficient of, 91
　lipid solubility of, 91
　MAC of, 91
　metabolization of, 91
　properties of, 86t
　rubber solubility of, 91
　use of, 91
　vapor pressure of, 86-87, 91
Metric system
　conversion tables, 376
　metric to household equivalents
　　length, 376
　　volume, 376
　　weight, 376
　prefixes in, 376
　pressure equivalents, 376
　weight to volume equivalents in, 376
　　solution equivalents in, 376
　　volume equivalents in, 376
　　weight system in, 376
Microdrip set chamber
　administration rates for, 37
　example of, 37f
　use of, 37
Midazolam
　as appetite stimulant, 61
　diazepam versus, 62
　drug combining with, 62
　ketamine and, 62
　mode of action/pharmacology of, 61
　opioids combining with, 68
　in rodents/rabbits, 304
　in ruminants, 285b
　in small mammals, 305t
　storage of, 62
　use/administration of, 61
Minimum alveolar concentration (MAC), 88, 88b
　of desflurane, 90
　of halothane, 90
　of inhalation anesthetics, 86t
　of isoflurane, 88
　of methoxyflurane, 91
　of sevoflurane, 89

Minimum patient database
　appointment for, 8b
　development of, 5-6
　information in, 8
　purpose of, 7
　See also Patient history
Minor tranquilizer, 61
Miosis, 19
　opioid causing, 67
Modified Mapleson A system, 123, 124f
　oxygen flow rate for, 128b, 130t
Modified Mapleson D system, 123-124, 124f
　oxygen flow rate for, 128b, 130t, 131
Modulation
　drug effectiveness in, 208b
　nociception pathway, step of, 207-208, 207f
Molecule, 29
Monitoring
　anesthetic depth and, 309-310
　of blood oxygen levels, 158
　definition of, 139
　guidelines for, 139
　importance of, case study for, 166b
　necessity of, 139, 139b
　nonprecision vaporizer, use of, 374
　parameters for, 139
　principle of, 140, 140b
　during recovery period, 255
　　horses and, 276
　　ruminants and, 288
　of swine, 292
　time period for, 139
Monoamine oxidase inhibitor, 11
Monocyte count, normal values for, 23t
Morbidity, stress response and, 208
Morphine, 3, 214-217
　adverse effects of, 68
　classification of, 218
　epidural use of, 221
　intraarticular administration of, 221
　intravenous infusion of, 221
　locomotor activity from, 214-217
　mode of action of, 66-67
　monoamine oxidase inhibitor and, 11
　neuroleptanalgesia and, 68
　NSAIDs and, 226
　route of administration of, 217-218
　in small mammals, 314t
　　duration of action, 314-315, 314b
　species/route/dosage of, 215t-217t
　use/adverse effects of, 214-218
Morphine/lidocaine/ketamine (MLK)
　as combination therapy, 226-227
　for interoperative analgesia, 226
　IV fluid, adding to, 231b
Mortality
　fentanyl patch and, 222
　from general anesthesia, 319-320
　stress response and, 208
Morton, Dr. William T. G., 1

Motor neuron, 185
　local anesthetic affecting, 189
Mouse
　analgesic agents in, 314t
　anesthetic/related drugs for, 306t
　biologic data for, 299t
　fluid administration in, 304t
　handling/restraint of, 299-302, 299f
　IM injection in, 300f
　intraperitoneal injection in, 299, 300f
　preanesthetic agent for, 305t
Mu (μ), 66
Mucosal bleeding time, 42b-43b
Mucous membrane color, 157-158
　assessment of, 21
　paleness
　　cause of, 336
　　treatment of, 345b
Multimodal therapy, 207-208, 208b
　for cat
　　onychectomy, 227b
　　ovariohysterectomy/castration, 227b
　for dog
　　for fractured humerus, 228b
　　ovariohysterectomy/castration, 227b
　for horse, for bilateral stifle arthroscopy, 228b
　for pain control, 226
　for perioperative analgesia, 211-212
Murmur, 21
Murphy eye, 98
Muscarinic receptor, 57f
　acetylcholine binding to, 57
　anticholinergic and, 57
　location of, 57
Muscle fasciculation, 61
Muscle-paralyzing agent, 194
　anesthetic depth and, 195
　dosage/duration of action of, 195
Muscle relaxation
　adjunct for, 50
　alpha$_2$-agonist effect on, 63
　anesthetic depth and, 174
　benzodiazepine for, 61
　effect of, 51
　etomidate causing, 83
　isoflurane and, 89
　preanesthetic agent for, 56, 56t
　sevoflurane and, 68
　surgical anesthesia and, 2
Muscle tone
　during anesthesia, 140
　anesthetic agent/adjunct effect on, 55t
　anesthetic depth and, 173-174
　by anesthetic stage/plane, 141
　as flaccid, 141
　during recovery period, 254
Mydriasis, 57, 209b
Myopathy, prevention in horses, 270, 270b

N

Nalbuphine, 220

Naloxone hydrochloride
    for anesthetic emergency in dogs/cats,
        340t
    effects of, 69
    use/administration of, 69
Narcosis
    definition of, 2
    opioid causing, 67
Narcotic, 2
Nasal catheter, 329
    example of, 329f
Nasal congestion, nasopharyngeal tube
        for, 276b
Nasopharyngeal tube, equine recovery
        period, 276f
    nasal congestion and, 276b
Nasotracheal tube, inhalation induction
        via, 272, 280b
National Institute for Occupational Safety
        and Health (NIOSH), waste gas and,
        352, 354b
Necrosis, pressure, 9
Negative pressure, 121
Negative pressure relief valve. *See* Air
        intake valve
Neonate
    anesthesia in, 10
    barbiturate effect in, 73
    benzodiazepine effect on, 61
    fasting recommendations for, 26t
Nerve block, 184, 187
    procedure for, 187-188
Neuroleptanalgesia
    administration of, 69, 69b
    contraindications for, 68-69
    opioids and, 68-69
    procedures performed under, 234b
    to effect, 259b
    use of, 68, 234
Neuroleptanalgesic, 307
Neurologic effect, of waste gas, 353
Neuromuscular blockade
    ACVA guidelines for, 368
    adjunct for, 50
    barbiturates and, 74
    use of, 51
Neuromuscular blocking agent
    administration of, 195
    use of, 194-195
Neuron
    local anesthetic targeting, 184-185
    untreated pain and, 208
Neuropathic pain, 207
Neutrophil count, normal values for, 23t
Nicotinic receptor, 57f
    location of, 57
Nightshade plant, 56
Nine-level body score system, 15-16
Nitrous oxide, 84
    accumulation of, oxygen depletion and,
        372
    advantages of, 91, 91b

Nitrous oxide (Continued)
    characteristics of, 92, 370
    compressed gas cylinder risks and, 105
    delivery of, 371-372
    effects of, 370-371
        on cardiovascular system, 370
        on central nervous system, 370
        on respiratory system, 370
    flow rate determination of, 126
    induction/recovery from, 91
    physical properties of, 370
    properties of, 86t
    risks of, 371
        closed rebreathing system, use in, 371
        diffusion hypoxia, 371
        diffusion into air pockets, 371
        as fire hazard, 371
        hypoxemia, 371
        storage of, 371
        waste anesthetic gas and, 371
    use of, 91, 370-372
*N*-methyl-D-asparte (NMDA) receptor,
        208
Nociception, 207
Nociception pain pathway
    drug effectiveness in, 208b
    steps of, 207-208, 207f
Noise sensitivity, 67
Non-breathing circuit
    parts of, 123
    patient weight and, 239-240
Nondepolarizing neuromuscular blocking
        agent
    atropine/glycopyrrolate as, 58
    reversal of, 195
    types/adverse effects of, 195
Nonpharmacologic therapy, for pain,
        207-208
Nonprecision vaporizer, 86, 110, 110f
    back-pressure compensation, lack of,
        374
    checking before use, 113, 113b
    description/function of, 373
    flow compensation, lack of, 373
    monitoring during use of, 374
    non-rebreathing system and, 374
    respiratory rate/depth of, 113
    safety with use of, 373-374
    temperature compensation, lack of, 373
    use of, 373
Non-rebreathing circuit, 101f-102f, 116
    configuration of, 122-123
    Mapleson classification system for, 123
    parts of, 103f
Non-rebreathing system
    advantages/disadvantages of, 125
    flow rate for, 126-127, 131
    indications for, 122
    intermittent mandatory ventilation
        using, 194
    nonprecision vaporizer and, 374
    oxygen flow rate for, 128b, 130t

Non-rebreathing system (Continued)
    during maintenance, 129
    pop-off valve and, 135b
    rebreathing system versus, 123t,
        125-126
    *See also* Closed rebreathing system
Nonsteroidal antiinflammatory drug
        (NSAID)
    absorption of, 223
    advantages of, 223
    adverse effects of, 223-225
    elimination of, 223
    for home analgesia, 227
    mechanism of action, 223
    morphine and, 226
    opioids and, 226
    preoperative administration of, 212
    in small mammals
        opioid and, 314-315
        pain management in, 315
    species/route/dosage of, 215t-217t
    types of, 222
    ulcerogenic activity of, 224
Non-water-soluble drug, combining,
        53
Normal saline solution, 32
Normal sinus rhythm (NSR), 146-150
    definition of, 20
    example of, 148f
    by species, 20
Norman mask elbow, 123
Norman mask elbow (Mapleson F system),
        124-125, 124f
    oxygen flow rate for, 131
Normosol-R (NR), 31-32, 31t
Nose, examination of, 19
Novocaine, 185t
Noxious stimulation, 2
NSAID. *See* Nonsteroidal antiinflamma-
        tory drug (NSAID)
Numeric rating scale, 210, 212f
Nursing care, 227-228
Nystagmus, 76, 175

**O**

Obesity
    anesthesia and, 16-17
    body score system and, 15-16
    heart assessment and, 19-20
    as increased anesthetic risk, 324t,
        326-328
Obtundity, 17
Occupational Safety and Health Adminis-
        tration (OSHA), waste gas and, 352
Ocular. *See* Eye
Oculovagal reflex, 57
Oncogenic effect, of waste gas, 353
Oncotic pressure, 30
Onychectomy, 227b
Open-ended questions, patient history
        and, 8, 8b
Open rebreathing system, 97, 97f, 122

Opioid
    addiction from, 68
    adverse effects of, 67-68, 68b
    analgesic effect of, 67, 214
    as antagonist, 51
    body temperature, effect on, 67
    cardiovascular system, effect on, 53t, 67
    classification of, 66
    CNS, effect on, 52t, 67
    as controlled substance, 53-54
    disadvantages of, 220
    drug interaction with, 68
    effects of, 55t-56t, 67b
    for epidural anesthesia, 189
    excitement/dysphoria from, 342
    gastrointestinal system, effect on, 68
    horse sweating and, 67
    mode of action/pharmacology of, 66-67
    for moderate/severe pain, 214-220
    monoamine oxidase inhibitor and, 11
    mydriasis and, 67
    neuroleptanalgesia and, 68-69
    noise sensitivity and, 67
    NSAIDs and, 226
    pain control by, 52
    as partial agonist/agonist-antagonist, 51
    pupillary light reflex and, 19
    respiratory depression and, 92
    respiratory/gastrointestinal effects of,
        54t
    respiratory system, effect on, 67-68
    route of administration, 220-221
        epidural use, 221-222
        intraarticular use, 221
        intravenous infusion, 221
    in small mammals, 304-306
        NSAIDs and, 314-315
    species response to, 9-10
    species/route/dosage of, 215t-217t
    tranquilizers and, 68
    types/administration of, 66
    urine production and, 67
    use of, 68, 214
    vagus nerve, stimulation of, 57
Opioid antagonist
    advantages of, 69
    duration of action, 70
    effects/adverse effects of, 69-70
    mode of action/pharmacology of, 69
    use/administration of, 69b, 70
Opioid receptor
    stimulation of, 66
    types of, 66
Opisthotonus, 342
Optimum depth, 142-143
Oral agent, 51
Oral cavity, examination of, 19
Organ dysfunction, 11
    anesthetic response to, 13
    intravenous catheterization for, 27
Orotracheal intubation, 273b
Oscillometer, 143, 154b

Oscillometric blood pressure monitor,
    156f
    advantages of, 156
    parts/method of, 156-157
    problems with, 157
    use/operation of, 156-157
Osmolarity, 29-30
Osmotic pressure, 30
Otitis externa, 13
Outlet port, 104, 106f-107f
    care/maintenance of, 133
    for H tank, 106-107
    oxygen flow from, 104
Outlet valve, 106f
Out-of-circle vaporizer, 194
    for small mammals, 309
Ovariohysterectomy/castration,
        multimodal therapy
    for cat, 227b
    for dog, 227b
Overflow valve, 117
    setting of, 135b
Overgrown nail(s), 13
Overhydration, 33
    avoidance of, 35
    signs of, 35b
Over-the-needle catheter
    placement/maintenance of, 28
    use of, 27
Oxybarbiturate, 70
Oxygen
    checking levels of, 125
    compressed gas cylinder for
        outlet port, 104
        size E, 103f
        size H, 103f
        sizes of, 103-104
        volume in, 108
    compressed gas cylinder risks and,
        105
    during equine recovery period, 276
    function of, 103
    methods of, 329
    need for, 28
    partial pressure of, 158
    percentage in body, 101
    for rat, 309f
    during recovery period, 255, 255b
    for respiratory dysfunction, 333
Oxygenation, 143
    ACVA guidelines for, 367-368
    blood gas analysis of, 163
    indicators of, 157-163
Oxygen collar, 329
    example of, 329f
Oxygen delivery, 329f
Oxygen demand valve, 276, 277f
Oxygen dissociation curve, 160b-161b
Oxygen flow meter. See Flow meter
Oxygen flow rate, 128b
    determination of, 126
    maintenance level and, 129

Oxygen flow rate (Continued)
    with Mapleson system, 131
    for non-rebreathing system, 130t
    for rebreathing system, 130t
    during recovery, 129
    See also Flow rate
Oxygen flush valve, 108-109
    description/function of, 109-110
    safety with, 110
    use of, 110
Oxygen saturation, 161b
    partial pressure and, 159
Oxygen tank
    bulk, 107, 107f
    empty, as anesthetic emergency/problem
        cause of, 321-322
Oxygen transport, 158-159
Oxymorphone
    classification of, 218
    effects/adverse effects of, 218
    epidural use of, 221
    intravenous infusion of, 221
    route of administration of, 218
    in small mammals, 314t
    species/route/dosage of, 215t-217t

P
Packed cell volume (PCV), 22-23
    decrease in, 23, 23b
        acepromazine effect on, 60
    elevation in, 23
    normal values for, 23t
Packed red blood cell, 32
Pain
    adverse effects of, 207
    assessment of, 17, 207b
    behavioral responses to, 209, 211f
    chronic, in small mammals, 315
    definition of, 207
    disease/surgery causing, 209, 209b
    facial expression/appearance attitude
        and, 210
    mechanism of, 207
    neuroendocrine changes from, 208
    nonpharmacologic therapies for,
        207-208
    opioid effect on, 52, 68, 214-220
    pathway/receptors of, 207f
    physical changes relating to, 210
    physiologic changes from, 208, 209b
    physiology of, 207-208
    postoperative assessment of, 210-211
    preanesthetic agent for, 56
    quality of life with, 208
    severity, classification of, 207
    signs of, 208-210
    technician role in, 206
    untreated, consequences of, 208
    vocalization and, 210
Pain assessment
    form for, 213f
    in small mammals, 313-314

Pain assessment tool
  limitations of, 210
  requirements for, 210
  types of, 210
Pain management
  perioperatively, 211-212
  in small mammals
    analgesic, administration of,
      315-316
    NSAIDs and, 315
  in surgical patient, 212
Pain scale, 210
Pain score, 17
Pale mucous membrane
  cause of, 336
  treatment of, 345b
Palpebral reflex
  absence of, 172b
  assessment of, 172f
Pancuronium, 195
Panting
  heart assessment and, 19-20
  hydration assessment and, 17
  stopping of, 20
Paralysis, local anesthetic causing, 185
Parasitism, 23
Parasympathetic blockade, 50
Parasympathetic innervation, 57
Parasympathetic nervous system (PNS)
  acetylcholine, receptors for, 57
  anticholinergic and, 51
  parts/role of, 57f
Parasympatholytic, 57
  See also Anticholinergic
Paravertebral anesthesia, 188
  in cow, procedure for, 197b-198b
Paresis, local anesthetic causing, 185
Paresthesia, local anesthetic causing, 190
Partial agonist
  effects of, 56t
  opioid receptor, stimulation of, 66
  use of, 51, 68
Partial pressure of carbon dioxide
    ($Paco_2$)
  low/high levels of, 168, 168b
  measurement of, 168
Partial pressure of oxygen ($Po_2$)
  blood oxygen and, 158
  oxygen saturation and, 159
Partial rebreathing system. See Semiclosed
    rebreathing system
Partition coefficient, 71, 87b
  of halothane, 90
Parvovirus, 11
Passive diffusion, 29
Passive scavenging system, 356, 357f
Pathologic pain, 207
  classification of, 207
  untreated, consequences of, 208
Patient
  anesthetic risks to, 3
  client bond with, 6

Patient (Continued)
  minimum patient database, develop-
    ment of, 5-6
  preparation of, 5, 6b
  stabilization of, 27
  status as anesthetic emergency/problem,
    323-334
Patient history, 6b, 8
  allergy/drug reactions, 11
  illness, signs of, 8
  information for, 10b
  in minimum patient database, 8-13
  open-ended questions and, 8b
  signalment and, 9
    by age, 10
    by breed, 10
    sex/reproductive status, 10
    by species, 9-10
Patient identification
  collar for, 14b
  importance of, 14
Patient positioning
  for dogs/cats, 254b
  for horses, 275
  for ruminants, 288
Patient preparation, 234-235
Patient safety
  assessment of, 143-170
  for dogs/cats, 254b
  for horses, 275
  for ruminants, 288
Pedal reflex
  assessment of, 172f
  presence of, 172b
  in rodents, 309
Pediatric patient
  anesthesia in, 10
  drug dosages for, 325
  fasting recommendations for, 26t, 325
  hypothermia in, 325
  as increased anesthetic risk, 324t, 325
  inhalation agent for, 325
  IV catheterization/intubation in, 325
Pediatric scale, 14, 14b
Penile prolapse, 60
Penlon Sigma Delta vaporizer, 114f
Pentastarch, 32
Pentazocine, 215t-217t
Pentobarbital
  action/pharmacodynamics of, 75
  lipid solubility of, 71
  respiratory system, effect on, 73
Pentobarbitone, 306t
Percent concentration, of inhalation agent,
    113
Percent oxygen saturation ($So_2$), 159
Perception
  drug effectiveness in, 208b
  nociception pathway, step of, 207-208,
    207f
Perfusion, capnogram, 167
Perioperative analgesia, 211-212

Perioperative hemorrhage, 30
Perioperative pain management, 211-212
Peripheral vasodilatation
  acepromazine effect on, 59
  local anesthetic and, 185
Personnel, ACVA guidelines for, 369
pH, 30
Pharmacodynamics, 51
Pharmacokinetics, 51
Pharmacologic analgesia, nonpharmaco-
    logic therapies and, 228
Pharmacologic analgesic therapy,
    212-227
Pharynx, anatomy of, 247f
Phencyclidine, 78
Phenobarbital, 71
Phenothiazine tranquilizer, 59-61
  as antiemetic, 56
  CNS, effect on, 61
  effects of, 60b
  in small mammals, 304
  temperament/activity level affecting, 18
  use/risks of, 59
Phenylbutazone, 215t-217t
Phosphate ($HPO_4^{2-}$, $H_2PO_4^{-}$), 29
Photoplethysmograph, 154
Physical assessment
  anesthetic management and, 13
  hydration and, 17
  law regulations for, 14
  level of consciousness, 17
  pain score and, 17
  physical examination versus, 13
  before procedure, 13
  technique for, 14
Physical examination, 6b
  anesthetic management and, 13
  of body openings, 19
  of EENT, 19
  of exterior surfaces
    coat condition, 19
    lymph nodes/mammary glands, 19
    skin, 19
  physical assessment versus, 13
  of pupillary light reflex, 19
  of small mammals, 302-303
  of swine, 289
  technique for, 13-14
Physical status classification
  anesthetic protocol and, 24b
  by ASA, 24, 25t
  determination of, 24
Physiologic anemia, 326
  in cesarean patient, 327
Physiologic pain, 207
Physiologic saline, 32
Physiotherapy, for pain control, 228
Pig. See Swine
Piroxicam
  buprenorphine and, 226
  species/route/dosage of, 215t-217t
Plasma, 32

Plasma-Lyte A and R (PA and PR), 31-32, 31t
Plasma protein
  decrease in, 23b
  elevation in, 23
  normal values for, 23t
test, for hydration status, 17
Platelet aggregation, NSAIDs and, 224
Platelet count
  decrease in, 23b
  importance of, 23
  normal values for, 23t
Platelet function, testing, 42b-43b
Pleural effusion, thoracentesis for, 329-330
Pneumothorax
  stabilization of, 27
  thoracocentesis for, 329
Polydipsia, 11
Polyuria, 11
Pontocaine, 185t
Poor tissue fusion, 13
Pop-off valve, 116-118
  adjustment of, 126
  checking before use, 118, 133
  closing of, 118f
  description/function of, 117
  example of, 117f
  problems with, 322-323
  for semiclosed rebreathing system, 118
  setting of, 135b
Porcine stress syndrome, 292
Positive pressure ventilation (PPV), 191
Postanesthetic period
  in dogs/cats, 256-257
  in horses, 277-278
  in ruminants, 289
  seizure/excitement during, 342-343
  See also Recovery period
Postganglionic neuron, 57f
Postoperative analgesia
  multimodal therapy
    for bilateral stifle arthroscopy, 228b
    for fractured humerus, 228b
    for onychectomy, 227b
    for ovariohysterectomy/castration, 227b
  in small mammals, 313-316
Postoperative care, 312
Postoperative pain
  NSAIDs effect on, 225
  opioid injection for, 220-221
Potassium (K+)
  as cation, 29
  movement within body, 29
  plasma concentration in, 30, 30b
Preanesthetic agent, 51
  benzodiazepine as, 61
  hepatic disease and, 333
  purpose of, 54
  route of administration, 56
  selection of, 56, 240
  in small mammals, 304-306

Preanesthetic diagnostic workup
  complete blood cell count, 22-23
  test recommendations
    considerations for, 22
    by species, 22t
    types of, 22
Precision vaporizer, 86
  carrier gas flow rate in, 112-113
  checking before use, 113, 113b
  example of, 111f
  use of, 110, 113-114
Prednisone sodium succinate, for dogs/cats
  for anesthetic emergency, 340t
  for CPR, 340t
Preemptive analgesia, 39
  multimodal therapy
    for bilateral stifle arthroscopy, 228b
    for fractured humerus, 228b
    for onychectomy, 227b
    for ovariohysterectomy/castration, 227b
  for perioperative analgesia, 211-212
  before surgery, 209b
  tissue injury and, 209
Prefix, in metric system, 376
Preganglionic neuron, 57f
Pregnancy status, 10
Preinduction patient care, 5-6
  fasting, 26-27
Preload, 330-331
Premature complex, 148
Premature contraction, 148
Premedication
  definition of, 240
  for PSC P1/P2 cats, 241b
  for PSC P1/P2 dogs, 241b
  for PSC P1/P2 horses, 268-269, 268b
  for PSC P1/P2 ruminants, 285b
  for PSC P1/P2 swine, 290b
  of ruminants, 285
Preoxygenation, 331
Prescribed rate, 36b
Pressure manometer
  description/function of, 121
  safe readings for, 121b
  use of, 121
Pressure manometer, conversion table for, 377t
Pressure necrosis, 9
Pressure-reducing valve (pressure regulator)
  care/maintenance of, 132
  description/function of, 108
  example of, 107f
  use of, 108
Pressure relief valve, 117
Pressure transducer, 154
Preventive care, 11
Primary hyperalgesia, 208
PR interval, 146, 146f
Problem. See Anesthetic emergency/problem

Procaine
  pharmacology of, 185t
  for skin infiltration, 184
Procedure confirmation, 9
Prolonged anesthesia, intravenous catheterization for, 27
Proparacaine, 186
Propofol
  adverse effects of, 76-77, 77b, 163
  anesthetic maintenance with, 256b, 262b
    in dogs/cats, 251b
  cardiovascular system, effect on, 53t, 76
  chloramphenicol and, 11
  CNS, effect on, 52t, 76
  cost of, 78
  dog reaction to, 76
  effects of, 55t, 76, 76b
  handling/storage of, 77-78, 78b
  mode of action/pharmacology of, 76
  respiratory/gastrointestinal effects of, 54t
  respiratory system, effect on, 76
  in ruminants, 285b
  in small mammals, 307-308
  status epilepticus and, 75
  to effect, 259b
  use/administration of, 76-78
Prostacyclin, NSAIDs and, 224
Prostaglandin, role of, 223
Prostaglandin synthesis, NSAIDs and, 223
Protein
  as anion, 29
  in urine, 23
Pulmonary aspiration, 26
Pulmonary disease, 167
Pulmonary edema, 328f
Pulse, palpation of, 21
Pulseless electrical activity
  definition of, 151
  electrocardiogram and, 341
  example of, 342f
Pulse oximeter, 143
  hemoglobin saturation levels and, 159-160
  maintenance of, 162
  probe types/placement of, 162f
  for rabbits, 311, 311f
  signal loss troubleshooting, 162, 162b
  for small mammals, 311
  for swine, 293f
  with transmission lingual probe, 161f
  use/operation of, 161-163
Pulse strength, 153-154
  assessment of, 153f
Pupillary light reflex (PLR), 173
  anticholinergic and, 57
  assessment of, 19, 20f
Pupil size, 175f
  anesthetic depth and, 174-175
Purkinje fiber, 146, 146f
Purring
  heart assessment and, 19-20
  stopping of, 20
P wave, 146, 146f

## Q

QRS complex, 146, 146f
Quality of life
  five freedoms and, 208
  pain and, 208
Question
  leading, 8
  open-ended, 8, 8b
  in patient history, 9-13
Quick-release connector, 103-104
  DISS and, 106-107

## R

Rabbit
  alphaxalone in, 308
  analgesic agents in, 314t
  anesthesia in, 298
    withholding food in, 303
  anesthetic/related drugs for, 306t
  benzodiazepine in, 304
  biologic data for, 299t
  capillary refill time in, 310
  chamber induction in, 308b
  endotracheal intubation in,
    316b-317b
  fluid administration in, 304t
  heart rate/rhythm monitoring in,
    310
  heart rhythm in, 20
  hypoglycemia in, 303
  IM injection in, 302
  induction techniques/agents for,
    306
  IV injection in, 302
  lifting/support of, 302f
  pain assessment postoperatively in,
    314
  patient evaluation of, 298-303
  preanesthetic agent for, 305t
  pulse oximeter for, 311, 311f
  restraint of, 302, 302f
  sedative/tranquilizer in, 304
  transportation of, 299
  weight of/kick from, 301-302
Radiography
  indications for, 24
  use of, 332
Rare breed animal, anesthesia sensitivity
  in, 10
Rat
  analgesic agents in, 314t
  anesthetic/related drugs for, 306t
  biologic data for, 299t
  fluid administration in, 304t
  handling/restraint of, 300, 300f
  IM injection in, 301f
  intraperitoneal injection in,
    300f
  oxygen delivery for, 309f
  preanesthetic agent for, 305t
  ventilation in, 312f
Rebreathing bag. See Reservoir bag

Rebreathing circuit, 101f-102f
  parts of, 116-122, 117f
  unidirectional valves and
    description/function of, 117
    use of, 117
Rebreathing system
  advantages/disadvantages of, 125
  closed versus semiclosed systems, 116
  intermittent mandatory ventilation
    using, 194
  non-rebreathing system versus, 123t,
    125-126
  oxygen flow rate for, 128b, 130t
    during maintenance, 129
  safety with use of, 125
  use of, 116
  See also Closed rebreathing system
Receptor, untreated pain and, 208
Record-keeping, ACVA guidelines for,
  368
Recovery, signs of, 254-255
Recovery period
  ACVA guidelines for, 368-369
  anesthetist role in, 253-254
  definition of, 253
  dyspnea during, 343
  expediting, 347b
  heating sources during, 257b
  horses and, 275-278
    extubation of, 277
    monitoring during, 276
    nasopharyngeal tube for, 276f
    oxygen support during, 276
    preparation for, 276
    restraining during, 276f
    rope placement for, 276-278, 276f
    signs of, 277
    standing after, 275
  hypostatic congestion and, 256
  with intramuscular agent/combination,
    236f
  involuntary excitement during, 55
  length of, factors influencing, 253
  minimizing discomfort during, 256
  monitoring during, 255
  oxygen flow rate during, 129
  oxygen therapy during, 255, 255b
  preanesthetic agent for, 56t
  prolonged, 343
  regurgitation during, 341-342
  as rough/stormy, 254-255
  ruminants and, 288
    extubation of, 289
    from general anesthesia, 296b
    monitoring during, 288
    preparation for, 288
    signs of, 288
    sternal recumbency for, 289b
  seizure/excitement during, 342
  shivering to, 255
  stimulation hastening, 256
  swine and, 292

Red blood cell count, 22-23
  decrease in, 23
  elevation in, 23
  normal values for, 23t
Redistribution, 71
Reflective probe, 162
Reflex
  anesthetic depth and, 170-176
  dissociative agent effect on, 79
  monitoring, 139
  as protective, 171-173
  during recovery period, 254
  tiletamine-zolazepam effect on, 82
  types of, 171-172
Regional anesthesia
  definition of, 3
  technique for, 188-189
Regurgitation, anesthesia and, 9, 26
  during and after, 341-342
  in ruminants, 284
Regurgitus, 284
Renal disease, 324t, 333-334, 334b
Renal function test, 333
Renal toxicity, NSAIDs and, 224
Renarcotization, 70
Replacement fluid, 31, 31b
Reproduction, waste gas effect on, 352-
  353
Reproductive status, 10
Reptile, anesthesia in, 10
Reservoir bag
  benefits of, 118
  care/maintenance of, 133
  description/function of, 118-119
  guidelines for selecting, 119b
  inflation of, 119, 119b
  safety with use of, 119
  sizes of, 119, 119f
  use of, 119
Respiration, 163
  ketamine and, 164
  in obese anesthetized animals, 326
Respiratory acidosis, 169
Respiratory arrest
  as increased anesthetic risk, 337
  treatment of, 347b
Respiratory character, 21, 164
Respiratory depression
  anesthesia and, 92
  antihistamines and, 11
  from buprenorphine, 220
  in cesarean patient, 327
  halothane causing, 91
  after induction, 332-333
  isoflurane and, 89
  in large animals, 9
  manual ventilation and, 192
  opioid causing, 67-68
  sevoflurane and, 68
  in small mammals, 312
Respiratory depth, in VIC nonprecision
  vaporizer, 113

Respiratory disease
    anesthetic response to, 13
    as increased anesthetic risk, 324t,
        331-333
Respiratory distress, after extubation, 256
Respiratory drive, 125
Respiratory dysfunction
    cause of, 332
    oxygen for, 333
    treatment of, 346b
Respiratory infection, upper, 11
Respiratory minute volume (RMV), 113b
    definition of, 191
Respiratory rate, 21-22
    during anesthesia, 140, 144t
    anesthetic agent/adjunct effect on, 54t
    anesthetic depth and, 141t, 176
    by anesthetic stage/plane, 141
    assessment of, 163
    hypercarbia/hypoxia increasing, 176
    with mechanical ventilation, 193-194
    in small mammals, 310-311
    tachypnea and, 163
    in VIC nonprecision vaporizer, 113
Respiratory secretion
    anesthetic agent/adjunct effect on, 54t
    anticholinergic and, 56-57
Respiratory system
    acepromazine effect on, 60
    alpha$_2$-agonist effect on, 63-64
    anesthetic agent/adjunct effect on, 54t
    anticholinergic effect on, 58
    barbiturate effect on, 72-73
    benzodiazepine as, 61
    compromised, in trauma patient, 329
    dissociative agent effect on, 80
    etomidate effect on, 83
    function of, 28
    halogenated organic compound effect
        on, 85-86
    nitrous oxide effect on, 370
    opioid effect on, 67-68
    pain-related changes in, 209b
    propofol effect on, 76
Respiratory system examination
    abdominal palpation/auscultation, 22
    lung auscultation, 22
    respiratory rate/character, determina-
        tion of, 21-22
Respirometer, 164
Restraining
    of gerbil, 301
    of guinea pig, 301, 302f
    of hamster, 300-301, 301f
    of horse during recovery, 276f
    of mouse, 299-302, 299f
    of rabbit, 302f
    in rabbit, 302
    of rat, 300, 300f
    of small animals, 299b
Reticular activating center of brain,
        depression, 59

Return of spontaneous circulation
        (ROSC), 338
    aftercare for, 341
    agents for, 341
    cardiac compressions for, 339
Reversal agent
    adjunct as, 50
    adverse effects of, 195
    antagonist as, 51
    atropine/glycopyrrolate as, 58
    for cats, 254b
    for dogs, 254b
    role of, 66
    types of, 195
    use of, 51
Ring block, 187
    use of, 188
Risk. See Anesthetic emergency/problem
Rodent
    anesthesia in, 298
        withholding food in, 303
    benzodiazepine in, 304
    capillary refill time in, 310
    heart rate/rhythm monitoring in, 310
    heart rhythm in, 20
    hypoglycemia in, 303
    patient evaluation of, 298-303
    pulse oximeter for, 311
    tiletamine-zolazepam in, 307
Romifidine
    species/route/dosage of, 215t-217t
    use of, 65
Room air, oxygen in, 101
Room ventilation, waste anesthetic gas
        and, 355, 355b
Rope placement, during equine recovery
        period, 276-278, 276f
Rubber solubility
    of halothane, 90
    of inhalation anesthetics, 86t
    of isoflurane, 88
    of methoxyflurane, 91
Ruminant
    airway blockage in, 9
    anesthesia, preparation for, 295b
    anesthetic induction in, 285
        with IV agent, 294b
    anesthetic maintenance in, 287-288, 287b
        with inhalation agent, 287-288, 294b
        with IV agent, 288
    anticholinergic and, 9, 285, 285b
    bloat in, 9
    cardiac compression for, 338
    double drip in, 285b, 286f
    endotracheal intubation in, 286-287
    epidural anesthesia in, 188
    fasting recommendations for, 26t
    general anesthesia recovery in, 296b
    heart rhythm in, 20
    intravenous induction in, 285-286
    ketamine-diazepam combination in,
        285b

Ruminant (Continued)
    opioid effect on, 67
    oxygen flow rate for, 128b
    paravertebral anesthesia in, 188
    patient positioning/safety/comfort and,
        288
    postanesthetic period in, 289
    preanesthetic diagnostic testing for, 22t
    premedication/sedation of, 285, 285b
    regurgitation in, 284
    vital signs of, 18t
    xylazine and, 9, 285b
Ruminant anesthesia, 283-289
    equipment for, 284-285
    preparation for, 284
    protocol for, 284
    recovery period for, 288
        extubation of, 289
        monitoring during, 288
        preparation for, 288
        signs of, 288
        sternal recumbency for, 289b

S
Safety. See Patient safety; Workplace safety
0.9% saline solution, 32
Salivary secretion
    anesthetic depth and, 175
    anticholinergic and, 57
Salivation
    anesthetic agent/adjunct effect on, 54t
    anticholinergic and, 56
    preanesthetic agent minimizing, 56t
Saluki, barbiturates and, 8
Scavenging system, 100, 102f
    active versus passive, 356, 357f
    parts of, 101b
    use of, 356-358, 356b
    waste anesthetic gas and, 354-355
Scoliosis, 188
Secondary hyperalgesia, 208
Second-degree atrioventricular (AV) heart
        block, 20-21, 147-148
    example of, 149f
Second gas effect, 370
Secretory gland, vagus nerve and, 57
Sedation
    arousal after in horse, 269b
    CNS depression and, 2
    premedication and, 240
    procedures performed under, 234b,
        266b
    for PSC P1/P2 cats, 241b
    for PSC P1/P2 dogs, 241b
    for PSC P1/P2 horses, 268-269, 268b
    for PSC P1/P2 swine, 290b
    of ruminants, 285
    of swine, 289-290
        protocol for, 290b
    use of, 234
    without general anesthesia, 234, 234b
        ACVA guidelines for, 369

Sedative
    adjunct as, 50
    classes of, 59
    draft horse/giant breed sensitivity to, 10
    effect of, 51
    general anesthesia and, 55
    preanesthetic agent as, 55
    in rabbits, 304
    route of administration, 56b
Seizure, 11
    acepromazine effect on, 60
    characteristics of, 342
    during postanesthetic period, 342-343
Selegiline, 11
Semiclosed rebreathing system, 116
    closed system versus, 116
    cost of, 125
    flow rate for, 126-127, 127b
        anesthetic depth changes, 128
        induction with injectable agent, 128
    oxygen flow rate for, 128b, 130t
    pop-off valve and, 118, 135b
Semiopen rebreathing system, 122
Sensation, loss of, anesthesia and, 1
Sensory neuron, 185
Sensory stimulation, 80
Sequestration, 328
Sevoflurane, 84
    administration of, 89b
    anesthetic maintenance with
        in dogs/cats, 251b
        in PSC P1/P2 horses, 274b
    blood-gas partition coefficient of, 89
    effects/adverse effects of, 89
    elimination of, 68
    MAC of, 89
    muscle relaxation and, 68
    nonprecision vaporizer delivering, 110
    properties of, 86t, 89
    vapor pressure of, 86, 89
Sex, confirmation of, 10
Sheep, vital signs in, 18t
Shivering, during recovery period, 255
Shock
    capnogram and, 167
    intravenous catheterization and, 27
    IV infusion rates for, 33
    signs of, 21b
    in trauma patient, 330
    treatment of, 346b
Short-acting barbiturate, 70
Sidestream capnograph, 165f
Sidestream sampler, 165
Sighing
    atelectasis and, 163-164
    manual ventilation and, 192
Sighthound
    barbiturate effect on, 8, 74
    as increased anesthetic risk, 324t, 326
    propofol effect on, 77
Sigma Delta vaporizer, 114f

Signalment
    by age, 10
    by breed, 10
    importance of, 9
    sex/reproductive status, 10
    by species, 9-10
Simple descriptive scale, 210, 211f
Sinoatrial node, 146, 146f
Sinus arrhythmia (SA), 146
    definition of, 20
    example of, 148f
    by species, 20
    in young dogs, 21b
Sinus bradycardia, 146
Sinus tachycardia, 58, 147
Skeletal muscle relaxant, 61
Skin, examination of, 19
Sleep, drug-induced, 2
Sloughing
    barbiturates and, 74
    cause of, 27
Small animal
    anesthetic techniques in, 234
    oxygen flow rate for, 128b
    restraining of, 299b
Small mammal
    abdominal pain in, 313-314
    alpha$_2$-adrenoceptor agonist in, 305
    analgesic, administration of, 315-316
    analgesic agents in, 314t
    anesthetic chamber for, 308f
    anesthetic/related drugs for, 306t
    anticholinergic in, 304
    arterial blood pressure in, 310
    atropine/glycopyrrolate in, 304, 304b
    barbiturates in, 307
    biologic data for, 299t
    blood loss in, 310, 312
    body temperature, monitoring, 311b
    capnograph for, 311
    cardiac failure in, 312
    circulatory failure in, 312-313
    cyclohexamine in, 307
    dehydration in, 303b, 304
    diagnostic tests in, 303
    emergency drugs in, 313t
    endotracheal intubation in, 309
    endotracheal tube for, 309
    fluid administration in, 304t
    gait postoperatively for, 313-314
    hypothermia, avoiding, 311
    inhalation induction in, 308, 308b
    intraperitoneal injection in, 306
    local anesthetic, postoperatively, 315
    neuroleptanalgesic in, 307
    opioids and, 304-306
    pain assessment postoperatively, 313-314
    phenothiazine in, 304
    physical examination of, 302-303
    postoperative analgesia in, 313-316
    postoperative care in, 312

Small mammal (Continued)
    preanesthetic agent for, 304-306
    propofol effect on, 307-308
    pulse oximeter for, 311
    respiratory depression in, 312
    respiratory rate/depth in, 310-311
    thermoregulation in, 311
Sneezing, 11
    barbiturate induction causing, 73
Sodium (Na$^+$)
    as cation, 29
    movement within body, 29
Sodium bicarbonate
    in dogs/cats
        for anesthetic emergency, 340t
        for CPR, 340t
    in small mammals, 313t
Sodium channel, local anesthetic effect on, 184-185
Sodium chloride (NaCl), 29
Sodium chloride (NaCl) 0.9%, 32
Solubility, 87b
Solute
    balance of, 29
    composition/importance of, 29
    composition of, 31t
    concentration of, 29
    movement within body, 29
    osmotic pressure by, 30
    plasma concentration in, 30, 30b
    purpose of, 29
    as replacement/maintenance fluid, 31
Solution equivalents, in metric system, 376
Somatic pain, 207
Species
    anesthetic response by, 9-10
    heart rhythm by, 20
    vital signs by, 18t
Sphygmomanometer, 155
Spinal anesthesia, 189
Spinal cord, 57f
    local anesthetic affecting, 190
Splash block, 186
Splenic disease, ECG for, 24
Spontaneous movement, 173
Standing, horse need after anesthesia, 275, 277-278
Standing chemical restraint, 266
    dynamics of, 268-269
    procedures performed under, 266b
    sedation, signs of, 269
Standing general anesthesia, 268-269
Status epilepticus
    pentobarbital for, 75
    propofol for, 75
Sternal recumbency, for ruminant anesthetic recovery, 289b
Stevens vaporizer, 86, 111
Stifle joint, bupivacaine for, 188
Stomach ulcer, NSAIDs and, 224
Stool, blood in, 11
Stress response, 208

Stridor, 19
Stuporous patient, 17
Subcutaneous fluid administration, 304t
Subcutaneous induction, 306
Subcutaneous route
    preanesthesia administration by, 56
    sedative administered by, 56b
Sublingual artery, pulse strength at, 153f
Succinylcholine, 195
Sucralfate suspension, 224
SuperBAG protocol, 58
Supraventricular premature complex
    (SPC), 148-149
    example of, 149f
Supraventricular tachycardia, 149
    example of, 149f
Surgery
    comfort, signs of, 214f
    consent form for, 11-12, 12f
    diethyl ether for, 1
    history of, 11
    local anesthetic and, 225
    moderate/severe pain from, 209, 209b
    pain assessment postoperatively,
        210-211
    pain management in, 212
    preemptive analgesia before, 209b
    stabilization before, 27
    vagus nerve, stimulation of, 57
Surgery table, for horse
    hoisting to, 270, 271f
    padding for, 271f
Surgical anesthesia, 2
    anesthetic depth in, 251
    objectives of, 143, 143b
    period of
        characteristics of, 142
        plane I, 142
        plane II, 142
        plane III, 142
        plane IV, 142
Surgical stimulation, 176
Swallowing reflex, 26, 171-172, 172b
    extubation and, 255-256
Sweating, opioids causing, 67
Swine
    anesthetic induction in, 290
    anesthetic maintenance in, 290-292
    blood pressure of, 293f
    catheterization of, 291f
    inhalation anesthetics in, 291f
    intubation of, 292f
    physical examination of, 289
    porcine stress syndrome in, 292
    premedication/sedation of, 290b
    pulse oximetry, 293f
    recovery period for, 292
        extubation of, 292
    sedation of, 289-290
        protocol for, 290b
        with TKX, 290
Sympathetic blockade, 185

Sympathetic nervous system (SNS)
    local anesthetic affecting, 185, 190
    receptors for, 62-63
Sympathetic storm, 90
Sympathomimetic, 10
Syncope, 11
Synthetic colloid solution, 32
    administration rates for, 35, 35b
Syringe pump, example of, 78f
Systemic administration, of local
    anesthetic, 189
Systemic disease, 25
Systemic toxicity, local anesthetic causing, 190
Systolic blood pressure, 152
    determination of, 155-156

T
Tachyarrhythmia, 331
Tachycardia, 58
    cause of, 336
Tachypnea, 163
    as increased anesthetic risk, 336
    treatment of, 346b
Tail pinch, 309
Tank pressure gauge, 107f
    description/function of, 107
    example of, 107f
    use of, 107-108
Tape scale, 35, 36f
Tec 3 vaporizer, 114f
Telazol, 62
    administration of, 78
    in ruminants, 285b
Telazol-ketamine-xylazine (TKX)
    preparation/administration of, 296b
    swine sedation by, 289b, 290
Telephone number, importance of, 13
Temperament/activity level, 18
Temperature
    during anesthesia, 144t
    indicators of, 169-170
    vaporizer output affecting, 111
    See also Body temperature
Tenesmus, 11
Tepoxalin, 215t-217t
Terminology, of anesthesia, 1-3
Tetanus antitoxoid history, 11
Tetracaine
    pharmacology of, 185t
    use of, 186
Therapeutic index, 3, 14
Thermoregulation, 169
    in small mammals, 311
Thiobarbiturate, 70
    adverse effects of, 57
Thiopental, 27
Thiopental sodium
    adverse effects of, 163
    dosage of, 74-75
    IV induction with, 75
    metabolization of, 71
    pharmacology of, 74

Thiopental sodium (Continued)
    redistribution of, 71
    supply of, 75b
    to effect, 259b
    use of, 72
Third-degree atrioventricular (AV) heart
    block, 148
    example of, 149f
Third eyelid prolapse, 59, 59f
Thoracocentesis
    in trauma patient, 329-330
    use of, 332
Three-point nerve block, 199b
Throat, examination of, 19
Thrombocytopenia, 23
    blood products for, 32
Through-the-needle catheter
    placement/maintenance of, 28
    use of, 27
Tidal volume ($V_T$), 101
    anesthetic agent/adjunct effect on, 54t
    assessment of, 163-164
    definition of, 191
    respirometer measuring, 164
Tiletamine
    administration of, 78
    effects of, 82
    tissue irritation from, 80
    zolazepam and, 62
    See also Tiletamine-zolazepam
Tiletamine-zolazepam
    advantages of, 82
    contraindications for, 82
    disadvantages of, 82
    drugs combining with, 82
    in rodents, 307
    in small mammals, 306t
Tilt table
    bull restrained on, 288f
    for large animals, 283
Time constant, 113b
Time management, for veterinary
    technician, 234
Tissue fusion, poor, dehydration causing, 13
Tissue injury
    preemptive analgesia and, 209
    stress response and, 208
Tissue irritation, 152b
    cause of, 27
    from dissociative agent, 80
    local anesthetic and, 189-190
Tissue perfusion, 152-153
Titration, 242
Toe amputation, bier block for, 203b
To effect
    definition of, 242
    IV anesthetic to, 259b
Tolazoline
    dosage of, 66
    use of, 65
Topical agent, 51
Topical anesthesia, 2-3

Total blood volume, 22-23
Total injectable anesthesia, 290
Total intravenous anesthesia (TIVA)
    by constant rate infusion, 237, 238f
    field anesthesia using, 275b
    in horses, 267, 275
    by IV bolus of ultra-short-acting agent, 237, 238f
Total leukocyte, 23, 23t
Total rebreathing system. *See* Closed rebreathing system
Total white blood cell count, 23, 23t
Toxicity
    from acepromazine, 60
    from bupivacaine, 189b
    local anesthetic causing, 190
Toxin ingestion, signs of, 11
Tramadol
    for home analgesia, 227
    mechanism/pharmacology of, 226
    species/route/dosage of, 215t-217t
Tranquilization
    CNS depression and, 2
    preanesthetic agent for, 56, 56t
Tranquilizer
    classes of, 59
    effects of, 51, 226
    opioids and, 68
    in rabbits, 304
Transdermal patch, 222
Transduction
    drug effectiveness in, 208b
    nociception pathway, step of, 207-208, 207f
Transformation, of action potentials, 207-208
Transient excitement, 2f
Transmission
    drug effectiveness in, 208b
    nociception pathway, step of, 207-208, 207f
Transmission probe, 161-162
Trauma patient
    anemia in, 328
    arrhythmia in, 331
    blood pressure, changes in, 328-329
    delaying anesthesia in, 330
    hypotension in, 328
    as increased anesthetic risk, 324t, 328-330
    respiratory problems in, 329-330
    thoracocentesis in, 329-330
Tricyclic antidepressant, 11
Triflupromazine, 59
Triple drip, preparation/administration of, 281b
T wave, 146, 146f

U
Ultra–short-acting agent
    anesthetic maintenance with, 256b, 262b
    induction with IV injection of, 237
    TIVA by IV bolus of, 237, 238f
Ultra–short-acting barbiturate, 70
Unbalanced fluid, 31

Unconsciousness. *See* Loss of consciousness
Undescended testicle, castration and, 14
Unidirectional valve
    breathing tube and, 121-122
    care/maintenance of, 133
    description/function of, 117
    example of, 117f
    use of, 117
Universal F-circuit, 122
Upper respiratory infection, 11
Urinalysis, 23
    abnormalities of, 23
Urinary blockage, 11
Urinary obstruction, 324t
Urine
    blood in, 11
    opioid effect on production of, 67
    protein in, 23
Urine specific gravity, 23
Urogenital system, 55t

V
Vaccine history, 11
Vagus nerve, 57
Vaporizer
    care/maintenance of, 132-133
    checking before use, 113, 113b
    indicator window of, 115f
    leaks, checking for, 126
    liquid anesthetic levels in, 115f
    problems with, 322
    safety with use of, 114, 114b
    setting adjustments for, 239
    setup checklist for, 135b
Vaporizer-in-circuit (VIC), 100
    respiratory rate/depth and, 113
    vaporizer-out-of-circuit versus, 111
        schematic of, 112f
    *See also* Nonprecision vaporizer
Vaporizer inlet port
    care/maintenance of, 133
    description/function of, 114
    use of, 115
Vaporizer outlet port
    description/function of, 115
    safety with use of, 115-116
    use of, 115
Vaporizer-out-of-circuit (VOC), 100, 101f-102f
    vaporizer-in-circuit versus, 111
        schematic of, 112f
Vaporizer output, factors affecting, 111-113
    temperature, 111
Vapor pressure, 86-87, 86b
    of desflurane, 90
    of halothane, 90
    of inhalation anesthetics, 86t
    of isoflurane, 88
    of methoxyflurane, 91
    of sevoflurane, 89
Vapor. *See* Anesthetic vapor

Variable-bypass, flow-over vaporizer, 110
Vasoconstriction
    signs of, 21b
    sympathetic stimulation causing, 208
Vasodilation, 28, 33
    local anesthetic and, 185
Vasopressin
    for cardiac arrest, 341
    in dogs/cats
        for anesthetic emergency, 340t
        for CPR, 340t
Venipuncture, prolonged bleeding after, 11
Venous oxygen saturation, 159
Ventilation, 143
    ACVA guidelines for, 368
    in anesthetized animal, 191-192
    assisted and controlled, 190-194
    in awake animal, 191
    capnogram and, 167
    definition of, 163
    indicators of, 163-169
    in rat, 312f
    waste anesthetic gas and, 355
Ventilator, 192
    example of, 193f
    types of, 193
Ventilatory support, 9
Ventricular arrhythmia, 58
    epinephrine causing, 187
Ventricular bigeminy, 73f
Ventricular fibrillation, 151f, 176
    electrocardiogram and, 341
Ventricular premature complex (VPC), 149-150, 150f
Ventricular tachycardia, 150f, 175
Verbal rating scale, 210
Vesicant, 27
Vessel-rich group, 71
Veterinarian-in-charge (VIC)
    anesthetic protocol selection by, 235
    minimum patient database, development of, 5-6
Veterinary practice, anesthesia and, 1
Veterinary technician
    analgesia/pain management, role in, 206
    patient history and, 8-13
    role of
Veterinary technician *(Continued)*
        in anesthesia, 3
        in emergency care, 334
    time management for, 234
Virus, anesthetic equipment harboring, 133-134
Visceral pain, 207
Viscerovagal reflex, 57
Visual analogue scale, 210, 212f
Vital signs
    during anesthesia, 144t
    assessment of, 143
    monitoring, 139
        tools for, 143
    by species, 18t

Vocalization, pain and, 210
Volume equivalents, in metric system, 376
Voluntary movement, stage I, 141
Vomiting, 11
    alpha₂-agonist causing, 63
    anesthesia and, 26
        during and after, 341-342
    endotracheal intubation for, 342
    fasting and, 26
    osmolarity and, 29-30

W

Waste anesthetic gas
    anesthesia duration and, 355
    anesthetic machine maintenance and, 355
    anesthetic spills and, 355-356
    anesthetic technique and, 355, 359
    carrier gas flow rate and, 355
    concentration of, 351, 352b, 355t
    contamination, sources of, 355t
    exposure to, reducing, 356-359, 356b
    hazards of, 351-359
    hematologic effects from, 353
    kidney, effect on, 353
    levels, measurement of, 354-356, 359
    liver, effects on, 353
    long-term effects of, 352-353, 352b
    minimizing, procedure for, 362b-363b
    neurologic effects from, 353
    nitrous oxide and, 371
    oncogenic effects of, 353
    reproduction, effects on, 352-353
    risk from, 353-356

Waste anesthetic gas (Continued)
    room ventilation and, 355, 355b
    scavenging system and, 355
    short-term effects of, 352
Wasting, untreated pain and, 208
Water
    balance of, 29
    body weight and, 28-29
    movement within body, 29
Water-soluble drug, combining, 53, 53b
Waveform. See Capnogram
Weakness, 11
    cause of, 18
Weaning, from manual ventilation, 193
Weight
    anesthetic response by, 10b
    blood flow and, 72f
    conversion table for, 378t
    in horse, formula for, 14
    hydration assessment and, 17, 17b
    non-rebreathing circuit and, 239-240
    technique for, 14
    water and, 28-29
Weight equivalents, in metric system, 376
Weight to volume equivalents, in metric system, 376
Whole blood, 32
Windup, 208
Workplace safety, 351

X

Xylazine
    adverse effects of, 64, 225-226
    analgesic effect of, 225

Xylazine (Continued)
    cardiac arrhythmia and, 10
    contraindications for, 10
    drug combining with, 64
    in horses, 275
    opioids combining with, 68
    for pain control, 225
    in ruminants, 9, 285b
    in small mammals, 305, 305t
    species/route/dosage of, 216t
    supply of, 64
    use of, 225-226
    vomiting and, 26
Xylocaine, 185t

Y

Yohimbine
    for anesthetic emergency in dogs/cats, 340t
    dosage of, 66
    in small mammals, 305
    use of, 65
Yoke, 106f
    of E tank, 106-107
Y-piece
    breathing tube and, 121-122
    care/maintenance of, 133
    sizes of, 121-122

Z

Zolazepam
    drug combining with, 62
    mode of action/pharmacology of, 61
    use/administration of, 61